CW01116765

Small and Large Intestine

Requisites in Gastroenterology
Anil K. Rustgi (ed.)

Books in the series:

Volume 1: Esophagus and Stomach, David A. Katzka, David C. Metz (eds)
Volume 2: Small and Large Intestine, Gary R. Lichtenstein, Gary D. Wu (eds)
Volume 3: Hepatobiliary Tract and Pancreas, K. Rajender Reddy,
    William B. Long (eds)
Volume 4: Endoscopy and Gastrointestinal Radiology, Gregory G. Ginsberg, Michael L.
    Kochman (eds)

Commissioning Editor: *Rolla Couchman*
Project Development Manager: *Hilary Hewitt*
Project Manager: *Alan Nicholson*
Illustration Manager: *Mick Ruddy*
Designer: *Andy Chapman*

The Requisites in Gastroenterology

Anil K. Rustgi MD (ed.)
T. Grier Miller Professor of Medicine and Genetics
Chief, Division of Gastroenterology
University of Pennsylvania School of Medicine
Philadelphia, PA
USA

Volume 2: Small and Large Intestine

Edited by

Gary R. Lichtenstein, MD
Professor of Medicine
Director, Center for Inflammatory Bowel Diseases
Division of Gastroenterology
University of Pennsylvania School of Medicine
Philadelphia, PA
USA

Gary D. Wu, MD
Associate Professor of Medicine
Associate Director,
NIH Center for Molecular Studies in Digestive and
  Liver Diseases
Division of Gastroenterology
University of Pennsylvania School of Medicine
Philadelphia, PA
USA

Mosby
An Affiliate of Elsevier Inc.
Edinburgh • London • New York • Philadelphia • St Louis • Sydney • Toronto 2004

Mosby
An Affiliate of Elsevier Inc.

© 2004, Elsevier Inc. All rights reserved.

The right of Anil K. Rustgi, Gary R. Lichtenstein and Gary D. Wu to be identified as editors of this work has been asserted by them in accordance with the Copyright, Designs and Patents Act 1988

No part of this publication may be reproduced, stored in a retrieval system, or transmitted in any form or by any means, electronic, mechanical, photocopying, recording or otherwise, without either the prior permission of the publishers (Permissions Manager, Permissions Office, Elsevier, Inc. The Curtis Center, 625 Walnut Street, 3rd Floor, Philadelphia, PA 19106, USA), or a licence permitting restricted copying in the United Kingdom issued by the Copyright Licensing Agency, 90 Tottenham Court Road, London W1T 4LP.

First published 2004

ISBN 0-3230-1895-5

British Library Cataloguing in Publication Data
A catalogue record for this book is available from the British Library

Library of Congress Cataloging in Publication Data
A catalog record for this book is available from the Library of Congress

Note
Medical knowledge is constantly changing. As new information becomes available, changes in treatment, procedures, equipment and the use of drugs become necessary. The editors/contributors and the publishers have taken care to ensure that the information given in this text is accurate and up to date. However, readers are strongly advised to confirm that the information, especially with regard to drug usage, complies with the latest legislation and standards of practice.

Printed in the UK

The publisher's policy is to use **paper manufactured from sustainable forests**

Contents

Series Foreword vii
Preface ix
Contributors xi
Dedication xiii

1 Abnormalities of Gastrointestinal Organogenesis 1
Jonathan P. Katz, Gary D. Wu

2 Evaluation of Acute Diarrhea 21
Faten N. Aberra, Stephen J. Gluckman

3 Evaluation of Chronic Diarrhea 31
Lawrence R. Schiller

4 Ulcerative Colitis 53
Jeffry A. Katz, Thomas A. Judge

5 Crohn's Disease 77
Chinyu Su, Gary R. Lichtenstein

6 Evaluation of Malabsorption and
Maldigestion 111
Melissa Teitelman, Julius J. Deren

7 Diverticular Disease 127
James D. Lewis, Howard M. Ross

8 Intestinal Polyposis Syndromes and
Hereditary Colorectal Cancer 135
Jonathan P. Terdiman

9 Colorectal Neoplasia 159
Elizabeth E. Half, Robert S. Bresalier

10 Motility Disorders of the Small Bowel
and Colon 195
Henry P. Parkman

11 Mesenteric Ischemia and Intestinal
Vascular Disorders .217
Ross Milner, Omaida C. Velazquez

12 Irritable Bowel Syndrome 243
Kevin W. Olden

13 Anorectal Diseases 257
Samantha K. Hendren, John L. Rombeau

Index 285

… quickly!

The Requisites in Gastroenterology

Series editor **Anil K. Rustgi**

The information you need to know...
...quickly!

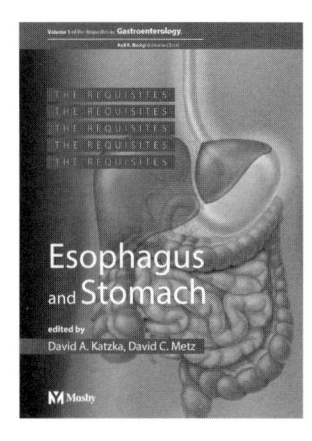

Volume 1:
Esophagus and Stomach

David A. Katzka, MD
David C. Metz, MD

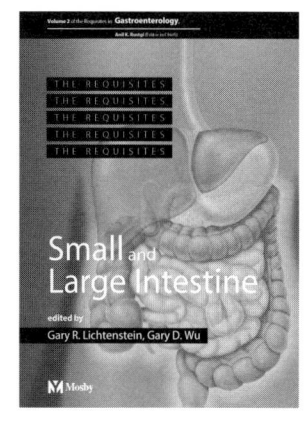

Volume 2:
Small and Large Intestine

Gary R. Lichtenstein, MD
Gary D. Wu, MD

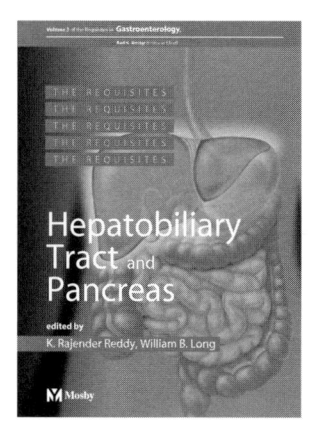

Volume 3:
Hepatobiliary Tract and Pancreas

K. Rajender Reddy, MD
William B. Long, MD

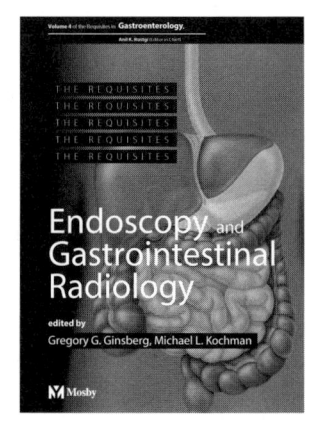

Volume 4:
Endoscopy and Gastrointestinal Radiology

Gregory G. Ginsberg, MD
Michael L. Kochman, MD

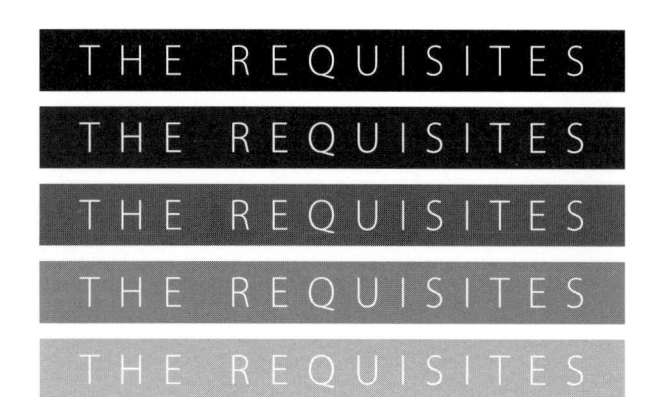

Each volume in the series offers concise, practice-proven information from internationally recognized authorities. They cover all the information that you must know for exams and for clinical practice in an easily digestible format. Packed with illustrations, boxes, and tables, there is no quicker way to gain the knowledge that you need.

To order these or any other Elsevier titles please visit www.elsevierhealth.com today!

Series Foreword

This exciting and innovative *Requisites in Gastroenterology* series takes a broad-based and fundamental approach to the pathophysiology, diagnosis and management of gastrointestinal, hepatic and pancreatic diseases and disorders. The series is divided into 4 interrelated volumes, each of which in turn is edited by nationally and internationally renowned editors who are supported by excellent contributors. The contributors represent a breadth of disciplines and expertise, and are drawn from a number of different institutions and academic medical centers. At the same time, the University of Pennsylvania provides a 'home' base for the series, and indeed, its gastroenterology, surgery, radiology and pathology departments have been a foundation for clinical care, teaching and investigation for several generations.

Volume 1 deals with diseases and disorders of the esophagus and stomach, edited by Drs David Katzka and David Metz. Volume 2 covers small and large intestinal diseases and disorders, edited by Drs Gary Lichtenstein and Gary Wu. Volume 3 delineates hepatobiliary and pancreatic diseases and disorders, edited by Drs Rajender Reddy and William Long. Finally, Volume 4, edited by Drs Gregory Ginsberg and Michael Kochman, brings together the important diagnostic and therapeutic modalities of endoscopy, interventional endoscopy and radiological imaging that are of direct relevance to topics covered in Volumes 1, 2 and 3. While each volume is self-sufficient, all volumes provide the reader with a focused, cohesive and integrated view of the principles and practice of gastroenterology, hepatology and pancreatology. Each volume is well illustrated and contains tables and figures that highlight salient features of different topics. Of note, boxes are provided that encapsulate key information covered in each chapter. These collective features are meant to assist the reader. The references are pivotal ones from the literature, and are not meant to be exhaustive.

In the evolution of this series, our collective thinking was to target the audience of medical students, residents, gastrointestinal fellows, allied health professionals (nurses, nurse practitioners, physician assistants), and those physicians (gastroenterologists, hepatologists, oncologists, surgeons, pathologists, radiologists) who require overviews for certifying examinations. The series is unique in the library of books that span the discipline of gastroenterology. The reader will find the volumes 'user-friendly' and will be imparted with expert knowledge and insights, making this an engaging overview and refresher course. We hope and trust that we will succeed in this mission.

The volumes that form the kernel of this series were profoundly influenced on the one hand by students, residents and fellows, and on the other hand, by the pioneering advances of T. Grier Miller, Thomas Machella, Frank Brooks, Sidney Cohen, Richard McDermott, Peter Traber and Ed Raffensperger. It is to these past and future leaders to whom I wish to give my special gratitude.

Anil K. Rustgi, MD
Editor-in-Chief

Preface

The small and large intestine are multifunctional organs responsible solely for nutrient, water, and electrolyte absorption. Examples of the remarkable efficiency by which the intestinal tract accomplishes these tasks include the ability to absorb 98% of the fluid (approximately nine liters per day), as well as 93% of the fat introduced to the intestinal tract each day. The small intestinal folds, as well as the villi and microvilli of the intestinal epithelium provide the large surface area required for these and other functions. In turn, the delicately balanced activity of the mucosal immune system protects us from the toxic, antigenic, and bacteria-laden environment of the intestinal lumen to which this large mucosal surface is exposed. Movement of the luminal contents through the intestinal tract requires the coordinated function of the enteric nervous system and the intestinal musculature.

It is no surprise, therefore, that alterations of any of the anatomical and physiological components of the intestinal tract results in pathologic disease states, many of which are major causes of morbidity and mortality. For example, anatomic abnormalities, whether developmental or acquired, can result in disorders such as congenital intestinal anomalies (Chapter 1) or diverticulosis (Chapter 7), respectively. Alteration of the intestinal epithelium can result in acute or chronic diarrhea (Chapters 2 and 3), malabsorption (Chapter 6), or intestinal polyposis and/or neoplasia (Chapters 8 and 9). Perturbation of the delicately balanced mucosal immune system can result in unrestrained intestinal inflammation characteristic of inflammatory bowel diseases (Chapters 4 and 5) whereas abnormalities of the enteric nervous system may result in intestinal dysmotility (Chapter 10) that may be associated with symptoms of irritable bowel syndrome (Chapter 12).

In this volume of *The Requisites in Gastroenterology* series, we provide reviews of the most common disease entities associated with the small and large intestine. We have focused each chapter to include not only essential clinically relevant information on the diagnosis and treatment of each disorder but also pertinent information dealing with pathophysiology and epidemiology. As the reader will observe, information regarding the pathogenesis, diagnosis, and treatment of each intestinal disease process is a combination of long-established information as well as more recent innovative approaches. Advances in molecular technology have provided new insights into the pathogenesis of intestinal disease processes that, in turn, have led to new diagnostic tests. For example, using the power of genetics, it is now possible to identify family members who are at risk for developing intestinal neoplasia associated with familial adenomatous polyposis (FAP) as well as hereditary nonpolyposis colorectal cancer syndrome (HNPCC) (Chapter 8). In turn, using molecular technology, newer 'designer' drugs have been developed to target specific cellular signaling pathways to achieve a clinical outcome. Examples of such approaches include the newer 'biologic' agents now available to treat inflammatory bowel diseases (Chapter 5).

Now that sequencing of the human genome has been completed, interactions between basic scientists as well as experienced clinicians are providing invaluable information correlating disease phenotypes with specific genotypes. This information will ultimately lead to new discoveries regarding disease pathophysiology and treatment of patients suffering from disorders of the small and large intestine.

**Gary R. Lichtenstein
and Gary D. Wu**

Contributors

Faten N. Aberra MD
Division of Gastroenterology
University of Pennsylvania School of Medicine
Philadelphia, PA
USA

Robert S. Bresalier MD
Professor of Medicine and Chairman
Department of Gastrointestinal Medicine and
  Nutrition
The University of Texas MD Anderson Cancer Center
Houston, TX
USA

Julius J. Deren MD
Professor of Medicine
Division of Gastroenterology
University of Pennsylvania School of Medicine
Philadelphia, PA
USA

Stephen J. Gluckman MD, FACP
Professor of Medicine
University of Pennsylvania School of Medicine
Chief, Infectious Diseases Clinical Services
Hospital of the University of Pennsylvania
Philadelphia, PA
USA

Elizabeth E. Half MD
Instructor
Department of Gastrointestinal Medicine and
  Nutrition
University of Texas MD Anderson Cancer Center
Houston, TX
USA

Thomas A. Judge MD
Assistant Professor of Medicine
Division of Gastroenterology
University of Pennsylvania School of Medicine
Philadelphia, PA
USA

Samantha K. Hendren MD
Mount Sinai Hospital
Department of Surgery
University of Toronto
Toronto, Ontario
Canada

Jonathan P. Katz MD
Assistant Professor of Medicine
Division of Gastroenterology
University of Pennsylvania School of Medicine
Philadelphia, PA
USA

Jeffry A. Katz MD
Assistant Professor of Medicine
Case Western Reserve University
University Hospitals of Cleveland
Cleveland, OH
USA

James D. Lewis MD, MSCE
Assistant Professor of Medicine and Epidemiology
University of Pennsylvania, Center for Clinical
  Epidemiology and Biostastistics
Philadelphia, PA
USA

Gary R. Lichtenstein MD
Professor of Medicine
Director, Center for Inflammatory Bowel Diseases
University of Pennsylvania School of Medicine
Philadelphia, PA
USA

Ross Milner MD
Assistant Professor of Surgery
Division of Vascular Surgery
Emory University School of Medicine
Atlanta, GA
USA

Kevin W. Olden MD, FACG, FAPA
Associate Professor of Medicine and Psychiatry
Mayo Clinic Scottsdale
Scottsdale, AZ
USA

Contributors

Henry P. Parkman MD
Associate Professor of Medicine and Physiology
Gastroenterology Section
Department of Medicine
Temple University Hospital
Philadelphia, PA
USA

Howard M. Ross MD
Clinical Assistant Professor of Surgery
Department of Surgery
University of Pennsylvania School of Medicine
Philadelphia, PA
USA

John L. Rombeau MD
Professor of Surgery
Department of Surgery
Division of Colon and Rectal Surgery
University of Pennsylvania School of Medicine
Philadelphia, PA
USA

Lawrence R. Schiller MD
Program Director
Gastroenterology Division
Baylor University Medical Center
Clinical Professor of Internal Medicine
University of Texas Southwestern Medical Center
Dallas, TX
USA

Chinyu Su MD
Assistant Professor of Medicine
Division of Gastroenterology
University of Pennsylvania School of Medicine
Philadelphia, PA
USA

Jonathan P. Terdiman MD
Associate Professor of Clinical Medicine
University of California
San Francisco, CA
USA

Melissa Teitelman MD
Division of Gastroenterology
University of Pennsylvania School of Medicine
Philadelphia, PA
USA

Gary D. Wu MD
Associate Professor of Medicine
Division of Gastroenterology
Department of Medicine
University of Pennsylvania School of Medicine
Philadelphia, PA
USA

Omaida C. Velazquez MD
Department of Surgery
University of Pennsylvania School of Medicine
Philadelphia, PA
USA

Dedication

We would like to acknowledge and thank our wives Nancy and Betty for their support and love, and our children – Julie and Danielle, and Steven and Katie for their understanding.

Chapter 1

Abnormalities of Gastrointestinal Organogenesis

Jonathan P. Katz and Gary D. Wu

CHAPTER OUTLINE

INTRODUCTION

FOREGUT DEVELOPMENT AND ANOMALIES

Normal esophageal development

Esophageal anomalies

Normal gastric development

Gastric anomalies

Normal duodenal development

Duodenal anomalies

Normal pancreatic development

Pancreatic anomalies

Normal development of the liver and biliary tree

Anomalies of the liver and biliary tree

MIDGUT DEVELOPMENT AND ANOMALIES

Normal midgut development

Midgut anomalies

HINDGUT DEVELOPMENT AND ANOMALIES

Normal hindgut development

Hindgut anomalies

CONCLUSIONS

FURTHER READING

Introduction

The origins of the organs of the gastrointestinal tract can be traced to the period of gastrulation in the third week of embryonic life. Gastrulation is the process by which the three germ layers – ectoderm, endoderm, and mesoderm – emerge within the embryonic disc. In the fourth week, the embryo begins to fold in both the median and horizontal planes, converting the flat embryonic disc into a cylinder. The endoderm is incorporated into the embryo as it folds, giving rise to the primordial gut.

Human development can be divided into three related phases: growth, morphogenesis, and differentiation. The cells of each germ layer divide, migrate, gather, and differentiate in precise and consistent patterns to form the tissues and organs of the developing fetus. From the ectoderm come the central and peripheral nervous systems, epidermis, mammary glands, subcutaneous glands, pituitary gland, and sensory epithelia of the eye, ear, and nose. The mesoderm produces the connective tissue, cartilage, bone, striated and smooth muscle, blood and lymphatic vessels, heart, kidneys, ovaries and testes, genital ducts, spleen, adrenal cortex, and serous membranes lining the body cavities. The endoderm gives rise to the liver, pancreas, thyroid and parathyroid glands, epithelia of the auditory tube and gastrointestinal, respiratory, and urinary tracts, and parenchyma of the tonsils. Note that while the epithelia of the gastrointestinal tract are derived from the endoderm, the musculature and connective tissue arise from the mesoderm. Complex interactions define the morphogenesis and the differentiation of the organs of the gastrointestinal tract. In the normal human, these organs must be able to perform highly specialized functions.

Foregut development and anomalies

The primitive gut can be recognized in the developing human fetus by 4 weeks of age. The gut can be divided anatomically into three segments – the foregut, the midgut, and the hindgut. The foregut contributes the luminal organs of the gastrointestinal tract, i.e. the esophagus, stomach, and duodenum (proximal to the ligament of Treitz), and the glandular organs, i.e. the liver and the pancreas. In addition, the foregut contributes the lower respiratory system including the trachea, the pharynx, and the oral cavity. The organs of the foregut, with the exception of the respiratory tract, pharynx, oral cavity, and most of the esophagus, are supplied by the celiac axis.

Normal esophageal development

The esophagus develops from the foregut immediately caudal to the primordial pharynx (Figure 1.1). At 22 to 23 days of gestation, a median ventral diverticulum, the laryngotracheal diverticulum, can be observed in the posterior region of the developing foregut (Figure 1.1A). This diverticulum will become the cranial portion of the trachea and esophagus (Figure 1.1B and C). As the laryngotracheal diverticulum elongates, it forms a groove and the proliferation of endodermal cells leads to ridges or folds along the lateral aspects (Figure 1.1D). By 34 to 36 days of gestation, a division is created between the trachea and the esophagus (Figure 1.1E and F). As the folds progress, a dilation forms along the caudal aspect of the foregut. This dilation will become the stomach. All tissues between the laryngotrachealtracheal diverticulum and this dilation comprise the developing esophagus. Initially, the esophagus is relatively short, but it elongates rapidly because of the growth and descent of the heart and lungs. By the seventh week of gestation, the esophagus has reached its final relative length.

The esophageal lumen is initially lined by columnar epithelial cells which eventually become ciliated. Proliferation of the esophageal epithelium partly or completely obliterates the lumen by 7 to 8 weeks gestation. By week 10, vacuoles appear and subsequently coalesce. Recanalization is complete by the end of the fetal period. Starting at approximately 4 months of age, the columnar epithelium lining the esophagus is replaced by a stratified squamous epithelium. This process is completed by birth. The upper third of the esophagus contains

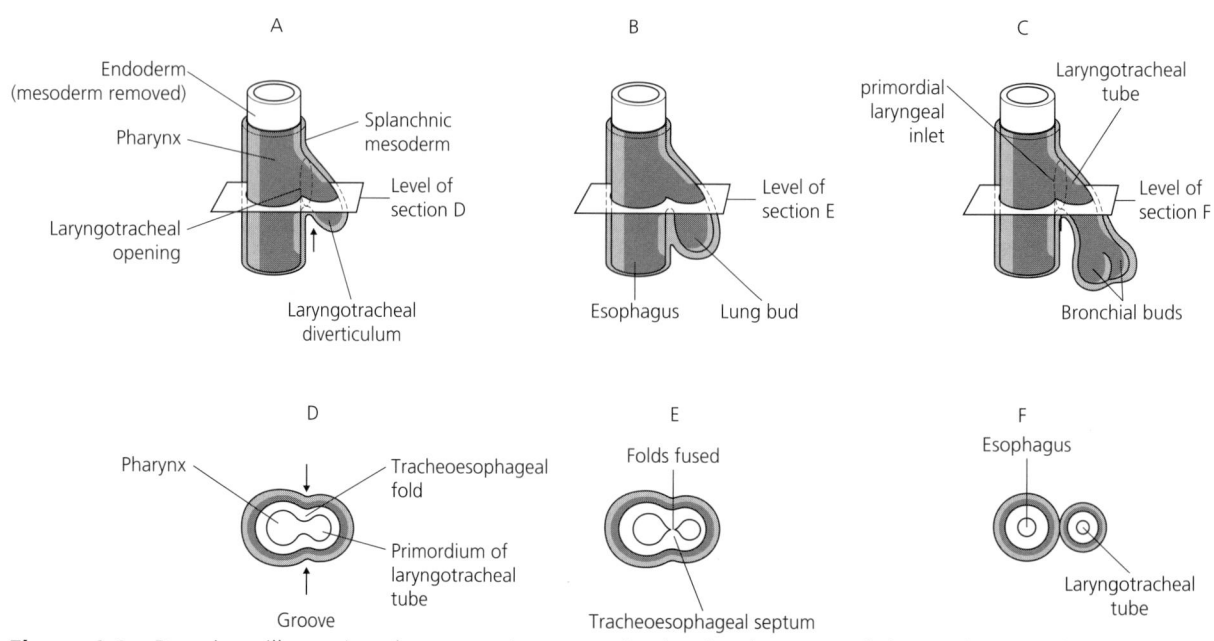

Figure 1.1 Drawings illustrating the successive stages in the development of the tracheoesophageal septum during the fourth and fifth weeks. (A, B and C) Lateral views of the caudal part of the primordial pharynx showing the laryngotracheal diverticulum and partitioning of the foregut into the esophagus and laryngotracheal tube. (D, E and F) Transverse sections illustrating the formation of the tracheoesophageal septum and showing how it separates the foregut into the laryngotracheal tube and esophagus (reproduced with permission from Moore KL, Persaud TVN. *The Developing Human: Clinically Oriented Embryology* 6th edn. Philadelphia PA, Saunders, 1998: Fig. 11.2).

Foregut development and anomalies

striated muscle derived from the mesenchyme of the caudal pharyngeal arches. Smooth muscle from the splanchnic mesenchyme comprises the lower two thirds. Both types of muscle are innervated by branches of the vagus nerve.

Esophageal anomalies

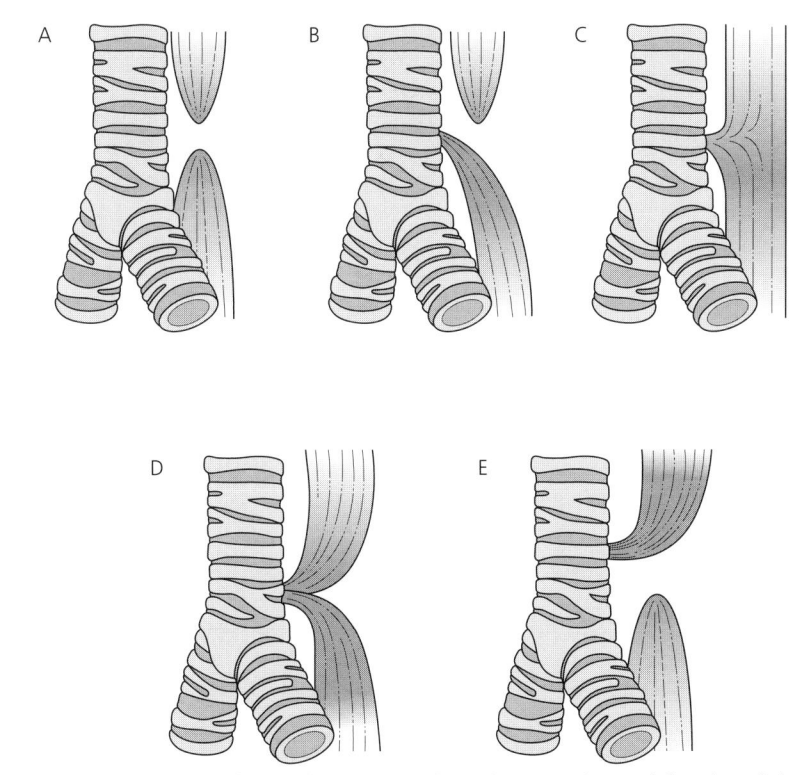

Esophageal atresia and tracheoesophageal fistula

Esophageal atresia and tracheoesophageal fistulas occur in 1 in 3000 to 1 in 4500 live births. These anomalies are found concurrently in approximately 85% of all cases, and the esophagus is the most common site of atresia (complete luminal occlusion) in the alimentary tract. Approximately one third of cases arise in infants born prematurely. Tracheoesophageal fistula and esophageal atresia result from incomplete division of the proximal foregut into the respiratory and esophageal components. The tracheoesophageal folds fail to fuse completely (Figure 1.1E), leading to an abnormal communication between the trachea and esophagus.

At least five different configurations of tracheoesophageal fistula and esophageal atresia may be seen (Figure 1.2). The most common form, representing 85% of all cases, is a blind proximal esophageal pouch associated with a distal tracheoesophageal fistula. Approximately 50% of neonates with tracheoesophageal fistula and esophageal atresia have other anomalies as well. Several syndromes have been recognized including VATER (vertebral defects, imperforate anus, tracheoesophageal fistula with esophageal atresia, radial and renal dysplasia), VACTERL (VATER plus cardiac and limb), and CHARGE (coloboma, heart disease, choanal atresia, retarded growth and development, genital hypoplasia, ear anomalies and deafness). Half of all mothers of a fetus with esophageal atresia

Figure 1.2 Esophageal atresia and tracheoesophageal fistulas. (A) Esophageal atresia and (B, C, D, and E) tracheoesophageal fistulas are the most common developmental anomalies of the esophagus. The most common tracheoesophageal fistula is that in which the trachea communicates with the distal segment of the atretic esophagus (B). The next most common is the H-type tracheoesophageal fistula, in which the trachea communicates with an otherwise normal esophagus (C). The tracheoesophageal fistulas in which the trachea communicates with both uper and lower segments of an atretic esophagus (D) or only the upper segment of an atretic esophagus (E) are rare (reproduced with permission from Sleisenger MH, Fordtran JS, Feldman M, Scharschmidt B. *Sleisenger & Fordtran's Gastrointestinal and Liver Disease: Pathophysiology, Diagnosis, Management* 6th edn. Philadelphia PA, Saunders, 1998: Fig. 31.7).

have polyhydramnios, increasing the likelihood of a prenatal diagnosis. Normally, the fetus swallows amniotic fluid, passing the fluid to the intestine for transfer through the placenta into the maternal blood. In esophageal atresia, the fetus is unable to swallow the fluid and polyhydramnios results. Surgical management of tracheoesophageal fistula and esophageal atresia leads to survival rates greater than 85%.

Congenital esophageal stenosis

Congenital esophageal stenosis occurs less commonly than esophageal atresia. Most cases of esophageal stenosis in children and adults are the result of an acquired anomaly. Congenital esophageal stenosis usually results from incomplete recanalization of the esophageal lumen, but it may occur from a failure of blood-vessel development in the affected area, leading to atrophy of a segment of the esophageal wall. Congenital esophageal stenosis most commonly occurs in the distal third of the esophagus, either as a web or as a long segment of narrowed esophagus, but may occur anywhere along the length of the esophagus. In rare cases, abnormal tissue, usually respiratory, may form within the esophageal wall, leading to a ring-like narrowing of the distal esophagus. Symptoms of congenital esophageal stenosis vary from feeding difficulties, with vomiting and choking in infants, to no symptoms. While an ectopic respiratory focus is best treated surgically, stenoses of other etiologies may be amenable to endoscopic management.

Congenital short esophagus

When the esophagus fails to elongate sufficiently as the other organs of the neck and thorax form, congenital short esophagus develops. The lengthening of the esophagus creates the descent of the stomach. If the elongation terminates prematurely, a portion of the stomach may be displaced through the esophageal hiatus and into the thorax. Supradiaphragmatic displacement of part of the stomach due to congenital short esophagus is distinct from hiatal hernia. Hiatal hernia develops from weakening and widening of the esophageal hiatus, usually in people of middle age.

Other esophageal anomalies

Several other common esophageal anomalies are rarely symptomatic. As many as 70% of normal individuals have heterotopic mucosa within the esophagus. During differentiation of the esophageal mucosa, if glandular columnar epithelium develops instead of stratified squamous epithelium, gastric-type epithelium can occur within the esophagus. In rare instances, other ectopic tissues, such as thyroid, may be seen. The Schatzki ring, located at the distal margin of the esophagus, is seen in 10% to 15% of subjects having a routine upper gastrointestinal series. The ring is lined by a squamous epithelium on the upper surface and a columnar epithelium on the lower surface, thus demarcating the squamocolumnar junction. Schatzki ring is likely to be congenital, although a relationship to gastroesophageal reflux disease has been proposed. While most patients are asymptomatic, Schatzki ring can cause dysphagia to solids and solid-food impaction.

Normal gastric development

The stomach develops as a slight dilation of the distal foregut around the fourth week of gestation (Figure 1.3). While the stomach begins its development at the C3 to C5 level, it eventually "descends" to its final location between T10 and L3 because of the marked cephalic growth of the foregut. Initially, the primitive stomach is oriented in the median plane (Figure 1.3B). As the stomach develops, the dorsal border grows more rapidly than the ventral border so that a 90-degree clockwise rotation occurs on its longitudinal axis (Figure 1.3C). Eventually, the dorsal border rotates to the left and becomes the greater curvature, the ventral border rotates to the right and becomes the lesser curvature, the original left side is anterior, and the original right side is posterior (Figure 1.3D and E). Consequently, the left vagus nerve innervates the ventral wall of the adult stomach and right vagus nerve supplies the dorsal wall. The rotation of the stomach is completed by approximately 8 weeks of gestation, and the final position of the longitudinal axis of the stomach is nearly perpendicular to the long axis of the body. The columnar epithelium lining the stomach is first noted at 6 to 9 weeks, and, unlike the esophagus and duodenum, the stomach does not undergo a phase of epithelial occlusion of the lumen during development.

The stomach is suspended from the dorsal and ventral walls of the abdominal cavity by two mesenteries, the dorsal mesogastrium and the ventral mesogastrium. These mesenteries originally lie in the median plane but are carried with the rotating stomach to the left and the right respectively. Individual cavities develop in the dorsal mesogas-

Foregut development and anomalies

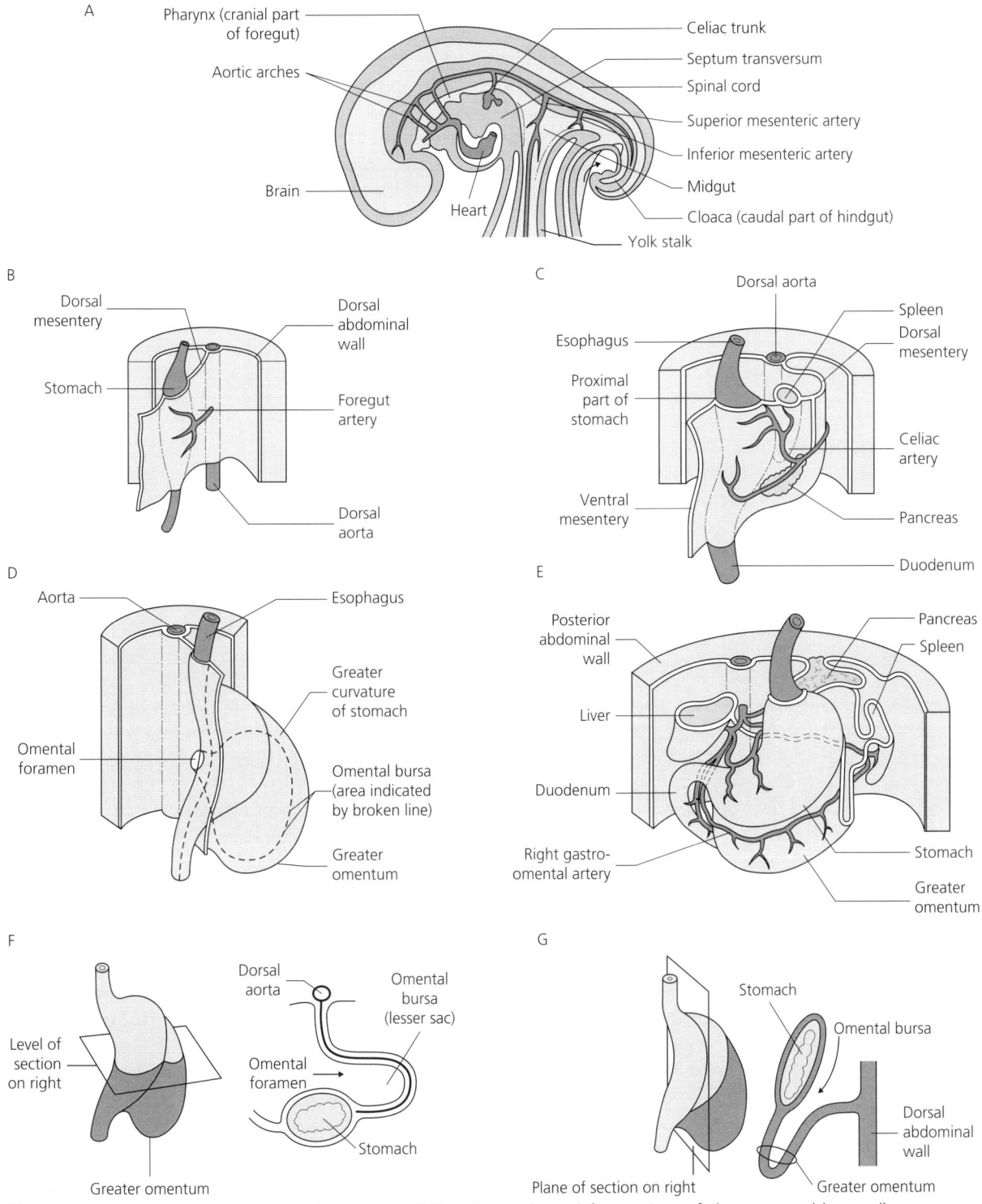

Figure 1.3 The development and rotation of the stomach and formation of the omental bursa (lesser sac and greater omentum. (A) Median section of a 128-day-old embryo. (B) Anterolateral view of a 28-day-old embryo. (C) Embryo about 35 days. (D) Embryo about 40 days. (E) Embryo about 48 days. (F) Lateral view of the stomach and greater omentum of an embryo at about 52 days. The transverse section shows the omental foramen and omental bursa. (G) Sagittal section showing the omental bursa and greater omentum (reproduced with permission from Moore KL, Persaud TVN. *The Developing Human: Clinically Oriented Embryology* 6th edn. Philadelphia PA, Saunders, 1998: Fig. 12.2).

trium and coalesce to form the omental bursa or lesser sac of the peritoneum (Figure 1.3F). The omental bursa grows as the stomach rotates and is eventually located between the stomach and the posterior abdominal wall. At the inferior portion of the omental bursa, a recess develops between layers of the dorsal mesogastrum. These layers fuse, forming the greater omentum, which overlies the developing intestines (Figure 1.3G).

Gastric anomalies

Gastric agenesis and atresia

While total agenesis of the stomach is not encountered in otherwise viable infants, microgastria may occur. This anomaly is nearly always associated with megaesophagus and incomplete gastric rotation, although isolated microgastria may be seen. Other associations include situs inversus, and asplenia. Microgastria is believed to result from the incomplete development of the caudal foregut. The stomach is small and tubular, but the mucosa of the gastric wall is otherwise normal.

Gastric atresia, which is almost always partial, is usually the result of membranous diaphragms in the antral or pyloric regions. Complete, solid atresia of a portion of the stomach is uncommon. Unlike atresia of the esophagus and duodenum, gastric atresia is not the result of failure of canalization. It is likely that discontinuity of the endodermal tube and areas of endodermal redundancy lead, respectively, to segmental defects and membranous webs. Congenital gastric-outlet obstruction from either solid atresia or webs is extremely rare and usually presents in the newborn. The diagnosis is suggested by a large, dilated stomach with a single gas bubble with no gas in the distal bowel, although gastric hypotonia may have similar findings. An upper gastrointestinal series typically reveals absence of the beak sign (seen with pyloric stenosis or duplication) and presence of the pyloric dimple sign (due to a shallow pyloric cavity at the proximal point of the atresia). Treatment is initially supportive followed by operative repair.

Pyloric stenosis

Pyloric stenosis was first recognized in 1788 and accurately described by Hirschsprung in 1888. Initially, surgical intervention resulted in mortality greater than that of conservative management, but in 1912, splitting of the pyloric muscle alone was shown to be curative, resulting in decreased operative mortality. The incidence of pyloric stenosis is increased in the children of affected parents and in first-born children. Males are affected four to six times more frequently than females. While the cause of pyloric stenosis is unknown, the pathology is hypertrophy of the muscle of the pyloric channel, especially the circular muscle. In most cases, children present in the second or third week after birth with non-bilious vomiting, but the onset of symptoms may occur as early as at birth or as late as 5 months of age. Vomiting may or may not be projectile but is usually progressive, and dehydration, malnutrition, electrolyte abnormalities, and failure to thrive may result. On physical examination a small, movable mass similar in size and shape to an olive may be palpated in the midepigastrum in 80% of cases and is pathognomonic. Sonography is the procedure of choice to confirm the diagnosis; upper gastrointestinal series should be reserved only for cases where neither physical examination nor sonography provides the diagnosis. Surgical treatment with pyloromyotomy produces excellent results with minimal complications, and a mortality less than 0.5%.

Gastric duplications

Gastric duplications are spherical structures which develop along the greater curvature or on the anteroposterior walls of the stomach. They may be tubular, communicating with the stomach, or cystic, lacking such communication, and most are lined by gastric mucosa. Abnormal adhesions between the endoderm and the notochord, a cellular rod which defines the primordial axis of the embryo, presumably lead to the formation of a traction diverticulum, disorganizing the endoderm as the embryo grows. Most cases of gastric duplication present in the first year of life with symptoms that include gastric-outlet obstruction, palpable abdominal mass, abdominal pain, weight loss, and failure to thrive. Treatment is surgical, by excision of the cyst if possible or by marsupialization with internal drainage if resection is not technically possible.

Gastric volvulus

Gastric volvulus is rare in infants, being encountered much more frequently in adults. Volvulus in children is usually the result of errors in gastric rotation, resulting in laxity or lack of the normal attachments of the stomach to the body. These attachments include the gastrophrenic ligaments, gastrocolic ligament, short gastric vessels, and fixation of the duodenum. Diaphramatic abnormalities such as eventration, herniation, and elevation of the left hemidiaphragm are often associated. Rotation of the stomach may occur along the longitudinal axis (organoaxial volvulus) or along the transverse axis (mesenteroaxial volvulus). Approximately two thirds of the cases of gastric volvulus in children are of the organoaxial type. Complete obstruction is rare, and patients usually present with intermittent vomiting. Acute gastric volvulus in children is a surgical emergency as strangulation may occur. Chronic gastric volvulus often presents with postprandial pain, belching, vomiting, and early satiety. In select cases, chronic volvulus can be managed by endoscopic correction.

Heterotopic mucosal tissue

Heterotopic mucosal tissue can be found anywhere in the gastrointestinal tract but is most common in the stomach. Pancreatic tissue (pancreatic rest) is the most common tissue found, appearing as a submucosal 1.2 cm mass in the gastric antrum. Both translocation of embryonic pancreatic cells and metaplasia *in situ* have been proposed as etiologies. Heterotopic intestinal epithelium is seen in the stomach on rare occasions. Intestinal epithelial cells are found in abundance within the pylorus and cardia of newborns, suggesting that hetertopic intestinal mucosa results from the persistence of a primitive form of gut epithelium rather than *in situ* metaplasia. Treatment of heterotopic mucosal tissue is usually not necessary.

Normal duodenal development

The duodenum begins to develop early in the fourth week of embryonic life from the caudal portion of the foregut and the cranial portion of the midgut. As a watershed between the foregut and the midgut, the duodenum is supplied by branches of both the celiac and superior mesenteric arteries. The duodenum grows rapidly, forming a C-shaped loop which is originally oriented in an anterior position. As gastric rotation occurs, the duodenal loop moves to the right, settling in the right upper quadrant with the loop convex to the right. The duodenum and adjacent pancreas are pressed against the posterior abdominal wall, and fusion of these structures with the wall causes them to become retroperitoneal. The duodenum is thus fixed.

Duodenal atresia and stenosis arise from the same embryologic defect, the failure of the lumen to recanalize during the solid stage of duodenal development. During the fourth week of gestation, the duodenal mucosa begins to proliferate, and extensive proliferation occurs through the tenth week of gestation. The cellular proliferation is so marked that, during the fifth and sixth weeks of gestation, the lumen is completely occluded by proliferating epithelial cells. As these cells degenerate, vacuoles form and eventually coalesce. By the end of the embryonic period, the duodenum is normally recanalized.

Duodenal anomalies

Duodenal atresia and obstruction

Duodenal atresia, complete luminal occlusion, is uncommon, but the consequences are usually severe. Polyhydramnios often occurs because of obstruction of the normal intestinal absorption of amniotic fluid, and bilious vomiting is usually seen within 12 hours after birth. The occlusion is typically located in the second or third portion of the duodenum, just distal to the opening of the bile duct. Classically, the stomach and duodenal bulb are distended by air, producing the "double bubble sign" seen on plain films of the abdomen. This finding may also be seen in complete duodenal obstruction of other etiologies. Between 20% and 30% of infants with duodenal atresia have Down's syndrome, and another 20% are premature. Most cases of duodenal stenosis, a luminal narrowing, result from mucosal webs, also the result of defective vacuolization. The stenosis is typically located in the third or fourth portion of the duodenum. In very rare cases, complete obstruction may result from the mucosal webs. Management of duodenal atresia and stenosis is surgical.

Duodenal obstruction may also occur from a number of other developmental anomalies. If the midgut fails to rotate normally, the cecum may persist above the second portion of the duodenum. Overlying attachments of the cecum to the lateral body wall (Ladd bands) may obstruct the duodenum. Duodenal obstruction may also result from annular pancreas or from a preduodenal portal vein. A preduodenal portal vein results from the abnormal development of the anastomoses of the vitelline vein, which returns poorly oxygenated blood from the yolk sac, and is frequently associated with other serious malformations, often of a rotational variety.

Normal pancreatic development

The organogenesis of the pancreas is very closely related to that of the duodenum. During the fifth

Abnormalities of Gastrointestinal Organogenesis

week of development, dorsal and ventral buds of endodermal cells appear in the caudal portion of the foregut, the region which is developing into the proximal duodenum (Figure 1.4 A and B). These buds, also called the dorsal and ventral pancreatic anlagen, eventually fuse to create the pancreas (Figure 1.4C and D). The dorsal pancreatic bud develops first, just cranial to the ventral bud, and grows between the layers of dorsal mesentery. The ventral pancreatic bud develops at the site of the entry of the bile duct into the duodenum and grows between the layers of the ventral mesentery. As the duodenum rotates to the right, the ventral pancreatic bud is carried dorsally along with the bile duct, eventually lying caudal to the dorsal bud. By the seventh week of gestation, both buds are normally fused. The course of the ventral pancreatic bud may be quite variable, and errors in rotation commonly lead to pancreatic anomalies. Complete agenesis of the pancreas is incompatible with postnatal life. Partial agenesis, the result of agenesis of the dorsal or ventral segment, is exceedingly rare.

Most of the pancreas is derived from the dorsal bud. The ventral pancreatic bud forms only the uncinate process in the inferior portion of the head of the pancreas. The pancreatic ducts normally anastomose as the pancreatic buds fuse (Figure 1.4D). The main pancreatic duct (duct of Wirsung) forms from the duct of the ventral bud and the distal part of the duct of the distal bud. The proximal part of the duct of the dorsal bud persists as an accessory pancreatic duct (duct of Santorini) in about 70% of people. In about 5% to 10% of people, the pancreatic duct systems fail to fuse (pancreas divisum). In such cases the main pancreatic duct drains into the minor papilla and has no connection with the common bile duct. Although pancreatic divisum is often listed as an etiologic factor in the pathogenesis of acute pancreatitis, its role in this disorder remains controversial. The parenchyma of the pancreas is derived from the endoderm of the pancreatic buds. Islets and acini develop from cell clusters around the end of the primordial pancreatic ducts. Like the duodenum, the

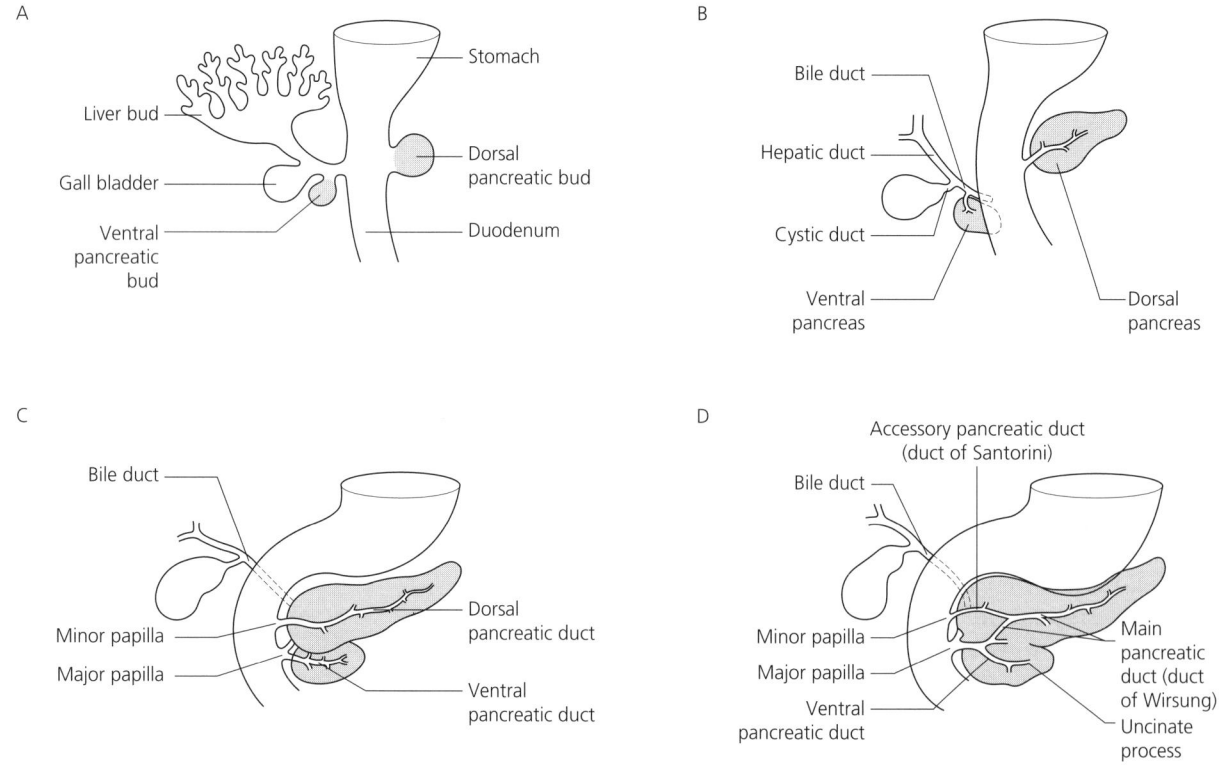

Figure 1.4 Anatomic maturation of the pancreas and its ductal system. (A) The pancreas at 4 weeks' gestation. (B) At 5 weeks, the dorsal bud grows rapidly and elongates. (C) During the 6th week of gestation, the ventral pancreatic bud migrates to join the inferior portion of the dorsal bud. (D) As the buds merge, the main pancreatic duct joins the bile duct to enter the duodenum at the major papilla. The accessory pancreatic duct enters the duodenum at the minor papilla. (Adapted from Sadler TW, ed. *Langman's medical embryology*. Baltimore. Williams and Wilkins. 1985)

pancreas comes to lie retroperitoneal as a result of normal rotation.

Pancreatic anomalies

Annular pancreas

Annular pancreas, while uncommon, is a well-known cause of duodenal obstruction. The ring-like or annular part of the pancreas is a thin flat band of pancreatic tissue surrounding the second portion of the duodenum. The tissue is histologically normal and continuous with the head of the pancreas. Annular pancreas probably results from the growth of a bifid ventral pancreatic bud around the duodenum or an aberration in the rotation of the ventral bud. The ventral bud then fuses with the dorsal bud to produce a ring of pancreatic tissue. Duodenal obstruction from annular pancreas may be partial or complete and may present just after birth or much later. Pancreatitis and peptic ulcer disease are seen with increased frequency. Treatment of obstruction due to annular pancreas is usually by surgical bypass.

Normal development of the liver and biliary tree

The liver, gallbladder, and biliary duct system develop as a ventral outgrowth of foregut in the fourth week of gestation. The liver forms from two primordia, the hepatic diverticulum or liver bud and the septum transversum. The hepatic diverticulum develops from the proliferation of endodermal cells at the caudal end of the foregut. As it grows, the diverticulum expands into the septum transversum, a mass of mesodermal tissue located between the developing heart and midgut. The rapid growth of the hepatic diverticulum leads to the development of a solid cranial portion and a hollow caudal portion. The larger cranial portion becomes the liver primordium, differentiating into proliferating cords of hepatocytes and the intrahepatic bile ducts. The smaller caudal portion forms the gallbladder, common duct, and cystic duct. The central tendon of the diaphragm, the fibrous and hematopoetic tissue of the liver, and the Küppfer cells all arise from the mesenchymal cells of the septum transversum.

The liver grows rapidly from the fifth to tenth weeks of gestation, and by the tenth week it constitutes 10% of the body weight (compared to 2% in the adult). The large size of the fetal liver is primarily because of hepatic hematopoesis, which begins during the sixth week. The right and left lobes of the liver are initially the same size, but the right lobe eventually becomes larger. The quantity of oxygenated blood flow from the umbilical vein determines the relative sizes of the hepatic lobes. Minor variations of liver lobulation are common.

The intrahepatic bile ducts form from primitive hepatocytes in close proximity to branches of the portal vein. In the later stages of fetal development extensive biliary remodeling and reabsorption occurs to form the normal portal tracts, but, even at 40 weeks, the process may not be complete. Also, in some cases, small branches of the portal vein may not be associated with individual bile ducts or the bile ducts and bile cannaliculi may be discontinuous. Such anomalies are referred to as "ductal plate malformations". Segmental dilation of some intrahepatic bile ducts may result.

Much of the extrahepatic biliary system arises from the caudal portion of the hepatic diverticulum. Initially, the gallbladder and the extrahepatic bile ducts are occluded by solid cords of proliferating epithelial cells. Around 5 weeks gestation, many of these cells degenerate, vacuolization occurs and the bile ducts are canalized. By the third month of gestation, the gallbladder is patent. The common bile duct initially attaches to the ventral aspect of the duodenum. As the duodenum rotates, the attachment of the common duct moves to the dorsal aspect of the duodenum. In the adult, the common bile duct passes posterior to the duodenum and head of the pancreas. Bile secretion begins by the fourth month of gestation, and bile draining into the duodenum imparts a dark green color to the intestinal contents (meconium).

Anomalies of the liver and biliary tree

Congenital abnormalities of the liver parenchyma

Congenital abnormalities of the liver parenchyma are rare. The liver may be located higher than normal in a patient with diaphragmatic hernia or on the left side in a patient with situs inversus. Accessory lobes may be seen, but absent right or left hepatic lobes are rare. Hepatic cysts are usually asymptomatic, and up to half of all cases of multiple hepatic cysts are due to adult polycystic kidney disease. Clinically, the most important abnormality of hepatic parenchyma is congenital hepatic fibrosis, an autosomal recessive disease which may present with signs of portal hypertension. The ductal plate malformation may be seen with dilated segments of intrahepatic biliary ducts.

Biliary atresia

Biliary atresia is an idiopathic disorder of the newborn resulting in complete obstruction of the biliary tract. Both the intrahepatic and extrahepatic biliary ducts are affected by an ongoing inflammatory process. Bilary obstruction leads to cholestasis, progressive fibrosis, and ultimately cirrhosis. Biliary atresia is seen in approximately 1 in 15 000 live births and is the leading indication for liver transplantation in children. The disease is slightly more common in females than males and is not felt to be inherited. Possible causes for biliary atresia include failure of the ducts to canalize during the solid stage of bile-duct formation and infection of the liver during the late stages of fetal development.

Two forms of biliary atresia have been recognized, embryonic and perinatal. The embryonic or fetal type occurs in 10% to 35% of cases. Neonatal cholestasis occurs early and there is no interval between physiologic jaundice of the newborn and cholestasis. At surgical exploration, bile-duct remnants are rarely seen. Other congenital malformations including the laterality sequence (polysplenia, cardiovascular defects, asplenia, abdominal situs inversus, intestinal malrotation, and vascular malformations of the portal vein and hepatic artery) and isolated anomalies of the gastrointestinal, urinary, and cardiac systems, are seen in 10% to 20% of patients with the embryonic type of biliary atresia. Perinatal biliary atresia occurs in 65% to 90% of cases. Patients present at 4 to 8 weeks of life with persistent cholestasis and jaundice. The prior history is usually unremarkable, with patients born at full term and normal birth weight. Jaundice typically disappears after the initial physiologic period but returns progressively. Bile-duct remnants may be found at surgery.

The first step in the diagnosis of biliary atresia is to fractionate the serum bilirubin. Conjugated hyperbilirubinemia in a newborn is always pathologic. Typical findings on liver biopsy include bile-duct proliferation, canalicular and hepatocyte bile stasis, periportal edema, and fibrosis. If performed early, a Kasai portoenterostomy (excision of the extrahepatic biliary tree, identification of a ductal remnant, and anastomosis of this remnant to the bowel) can re-establish bile flow in up to 80% of patients. Approximately one third of these patients will still require liver transplantation within 1 year.

Alagille's syndrome

Alagille's syndrome is a multisystemic disorder which includes arteriohepatic dysplasia, intrahepatic biliary hypoplasia, and syndromic paucity of interlobular bile ducts. The disease is inherited in an autosomal dominant fashion with variable penetrance and has been linked to deletion of the Jagged1 gene on human chromosome 20. Spontaneous cases may also occur. The classic syndrome includes five characteristics

- chronic cholestasis with pruritis, hypercholesterolemia, and a paucity of interlobular bile ducts
- congenital heart disease
- bone defects including butterfly vertebrae and hemivertebrae
- eye findings, especially posterior embryotoxon
- typical facies including a broad forehead, deep, wide-set eyes, and a small and pointed mandible, imparting a triangular appearance to the face.

Short stature is frequently seen. Not all patients have all of the classic findings.

The timing of presentation and severity of the liver disease is variable. Patients may develop jaundice as early as the first 6 weeks of life, although symptoms may improve. Severely affected individuals may develop intractable pruritis and xanthomas, and a small number will progress to end-stage liver disease. Treatment, including supplementation of fat-soluble vitamins, is aimed mainly at the complications of cholestasis. Bilary diversion is not effective, and liver transplantation is indicated for severe complications including bone fractures, refractory pruritis, portal hypertension, growth failure, and end-stage liver disease.

Choledochal cysts

Choledochal cysts occur in approximately 1 in 13 000 live births in western countries. About half of the cases are diagnosed in infancy, and the occurrence of cysts is more common in females and in Asians. The etiology remains unclear but may be related to congenital weakness of the bile-duct wall, congenital obstruction, reflux of pancreatic secretions, or an abnormality of biliary proliferation, remodeling, and reabsorption during development. Choledochal cysts can be broadly classified into five categories (Figure 1.5).

1. Type I cysts, which account for 80% to 90% of cases, exhibit segmental or diffuse dilation of the common bile duct.

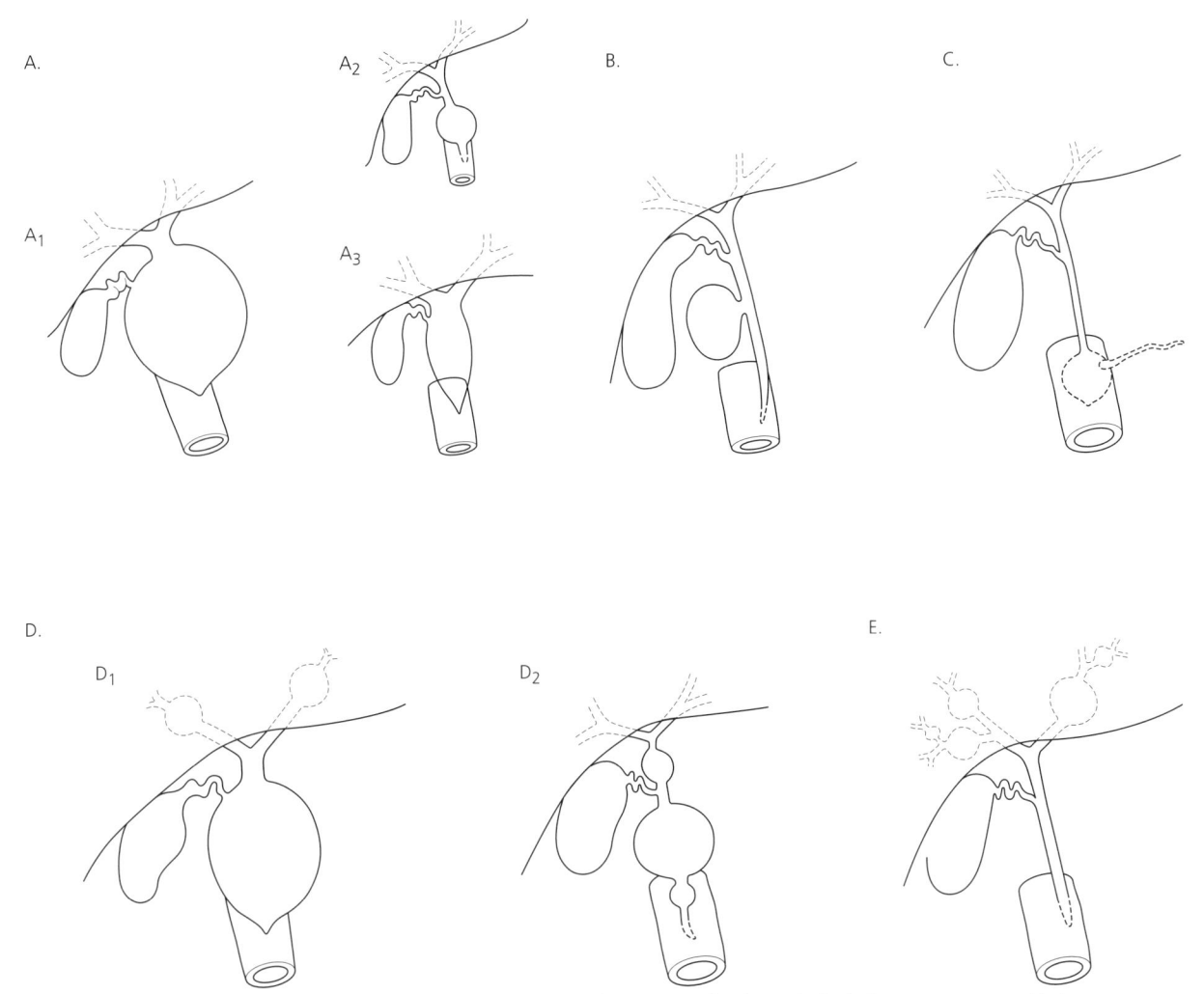

Figure 1.5 Classification of choledochal cysts according to Todani et al. (A₁) Common type. (A₂) Segmental dilatation. (A₃) Diffuse dilatation. (B) Diverticulum. (C) Choledochocoele. (D₁) Multiple cysts (intra- and extrahepatic). (D₂) Multiple cysts (extrahepatic). (E) Single or multiple dilatations of the intrahepatic ducts (reproduced with permission from Sleisenger MH, Fordtran JS, Feldman M, Scharschmidt B. *Sleisenger & Fordtran's Gastrointestinal and Liver Disease: Pathophysiology, Diagnosis, Management* 6th edn. Philadelphia PA, Saunders, 1998: Fig. 52.8).

2. Type II cysts have a true diverticulum of the common bile duct.
3. "Choledochocele," a dilation of the intraduodenal portion of the common bile duct, is the hallmark of type III cysts.
4. Type IV cysts consist of multiple extrahepatic cysts with or without intrahepatic cysts.
5. In Caroli's disease, type V, there are single or multiple non-obstructive dilations of the intrahepatic ductal system, with stone formation and recurrent cholangitis frequently noted. Many consider Caroli's disease to be a ductal-plate malformation and not a true choledochal cyst.

Classically, choledochal cysts present with pain, jaundice, and a palpable abdominal mass, although this triad is seen in less than 20% of patients. In neonates, choledochal-cyst disease must be distinguished from other hepatobiliary disease, particularly biliary atresia. Up to 80% of patients present with cholestatic jaundice and acholic stools within the first months of life. Approximately 50% of patients have a palpable abdominal mass. Vomiting, irritability, and failure to thrive are occasionally seen and hepatomegaly is usually present. In older patients, epigastric pain, possibly due to pancreatitis, is the most common symptom. Patients may experience recurrent bouts of cholangitis, with intermittent jaundice and fever.

Treatment for choledochal cyst types I to IV is surgical excision. Since the epithelial lining of the cysts has a high risk of malignant transformation, biliary drainage alone is reserved for patients with complicated anatomy. Patients who previously underwent drainage procedures without excision of the cyst should have complete excision of the cyst if possible. Patients with type V choledochal cysts have an especially poor prognosis, and complications include sepsis, hepatic abscesses, and cholangiocarcinoma. Ursodeoxycholic acid may be helpful in the management of intrahepatic stones, and hepatic resection is indicated for disease confined to a single lobe. For more extensive Caroli's disease, liver transplantation may be required.

Midgut development and anomalies

Normal midgut development

The midgut consists of the small bowel beginning with the duodenum distal to the ampulla of Vater and includes the cecum, appendix, ascending colon, and right one half to two thirds of the transverse colon. All of the organs of the midgut are supplied by branches of the superior mesenteric artery. The organogenesis of the midgut is one of the more fascinating stories of fetal development (Figure 1.6). By the beginning of the sixth week of gestation, the midgut elongates at a faster rate than the body. The rapid growth of the midgut results in the formation of a ventral U-shaped loop, the midgut loop (Figure 1.6A). This loop projects anteriorly into the remains of the extraembryonic coelom, a large fluid-filled cavity that surrounds the definitive yolk sac, in the proximal part of the umbilical cord. The movement of the intestine results in a physiologic umbilical herniation. During this herniation, the midgut loop rotates 90 degrees counterclockwise around the axis of the superior mesenteric artery (Figure 1.6B).

The midgut structures develop within the umbilical cord until about the tenth week of gestation, when the bowel begins its return to the abdomen (Figure 1.6C). The site of the connection between the yolk stalk and the apex of the midgut loop is the omphalomesenteric (or vitelline) duct. This point of attachment is directly in line with the axis of the superior mesenteric artery and defines the cranial and the caudal limbs of the midgut. The cranial limb grows rapidly and forms the small intestine. The caudal limb undergoes very little change except for the formation of the cecal diverticulum, the primodium of the cecum and appendix, at 6 to 7 weeks of gestation. Histogenesis in the midgut proceeds in a cranial-to-caudal direction and complete occlusion of the lumen does not seem to occur.

The return of the bowel to the abdomen occurs rapidly, possibly because of external pressure or a relative decrease in the size of the kidneys and liver. The small intestine returns first, passing posterior to the superior mesenteric artery and occupying the central part of the abdomen. As the cecum and large intestine return, they undergo an additional 180-degree counterclockwise rotation to lie in front of the superior mesenteric artery, on the right side of the abdomen (Figure 1.6D). At this point, the cecum and developing appendix lie below the liver, but the growth of the ascending colon forces these structures down into the right lower quadrant (Figure 1.6E). The appendix arises as a small diverticulum at the apex of the cecal pouch but increases rapidly in length before birth. Because of the rotation of the cecum, the position of the appendix may vary widely, passing posterior to the cecum (in about two thirds of people), posterior to the colon, or descending over the brim of the pelvis. The attachment of the appendix is generally located along the medial aspect of the cecum.

Formal fixation of the intestines begins in approximately the twelfth gestational week. By this point, the midgut has already returned to the abdomen. The force of the mesentery of the ascending colon against the posterior abdominal wall causes these surfaces to fuse, and the ascending colon becomes retroperitoneal. While the duodenum, except for the first few centimeters, has no mesentery (because of pressure against the posterior abdominal wall by the enlarged colon), the jejunum, ileum, and transverse colon retain their mesenteries. The remaining mesentery of the small bowel, as a result of the disappearance of the mesentery of ascending colon, becomes fan shaped, extending from the left upper quadrant to the right lower quadrant. This broad attachment normally prevents midgut volvulus from occurring around the axis of the superior mesenteric artery. If intestinal rotation is incomplete, the mesenteric attachment may be insufficient to prevent midgut volvulus.

Midgut anomalies

Abdominal wall defects

Omphalocele Failure of the midgut to return to the abdominal cavity is a frequently encountered

Midgut development and anomalies

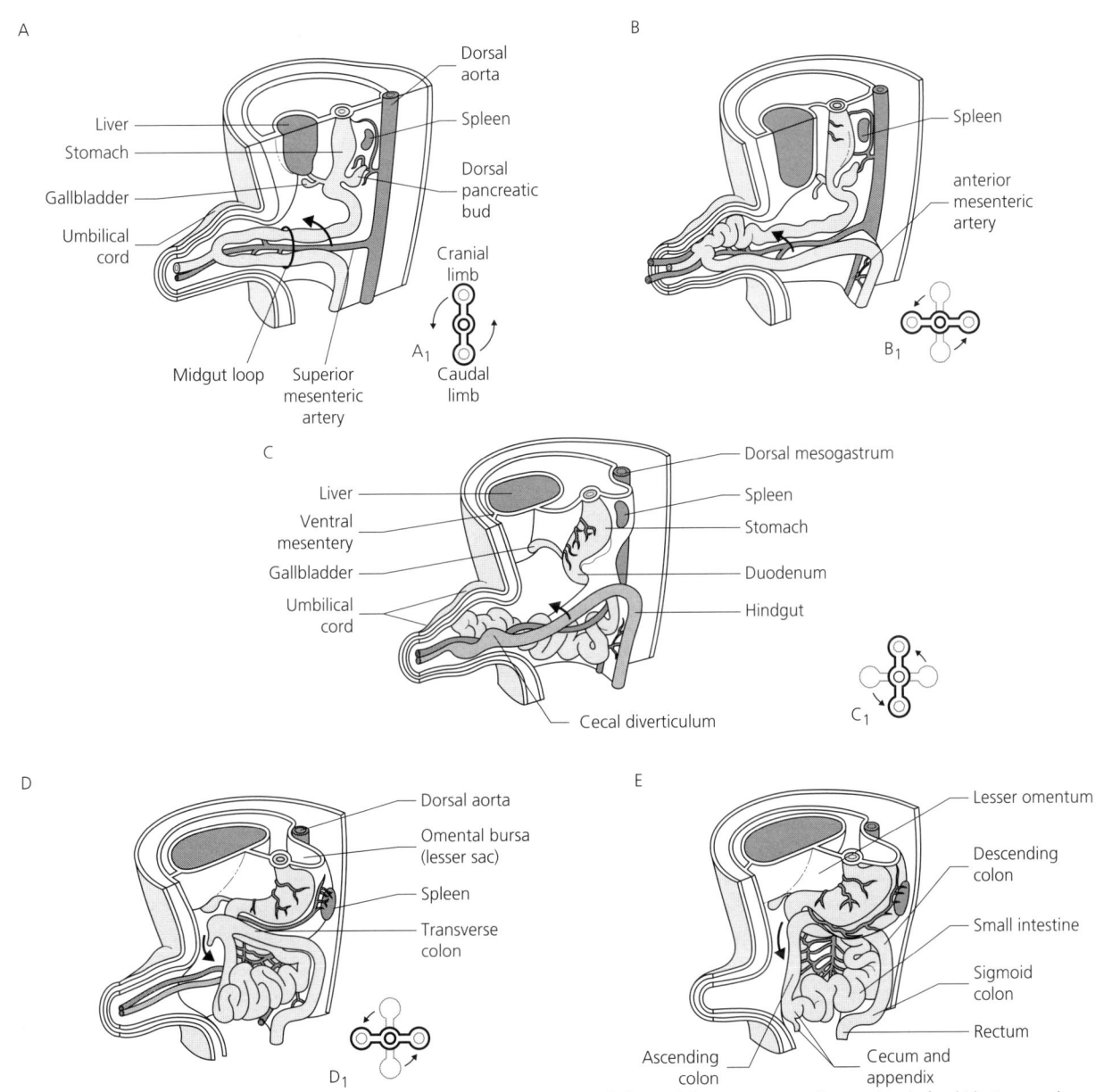

Figure 1.6 Schematic drawings illustrating the rotation of the midgut as seen from the left. (A) Around the beginning of the sixth week, showing the midgut loop in the proximal part of the umbilical cord. (A₁) Illustration of the transverse section through the midgut loop, illustrating the initial relationship of the limbs of the midgut loop to the artery. (B) Later stage showing the beginning of midgut rotation. (B₁) Illustration of the 90-degree counterclockwise rotation that carries the cranial limb of the midgut to the right. (C) About 10 weeks, showing the intestines returning to the abdomen. (C₁) Illustration of a further rotation of 90 degrees. (D) About 11 weeks after return of intestines to the abdomen. (D₁) Illustration of a further 90-degree rotation of the gut, for a total of 270 degrees. (E) Later fetal period, showing the cecum rotating to its normal position in the lower right quadrant of the abdomen (reproduced with permission from Moore KL, Persaud TVN. *The Developing Human: Clinically Oriented Embryology* 6th edn. Philadelphia PA, Saunders, 1998: Fig. 12.13).

congenital anomaly known as omphalocele. In about 1 in 5000 births, persistent herniation of the intestine into the umbilical cord is seen. Herniation of both the intestine and the liver is seen in 1 in 10 000 births. Unless ruptured, the omphalocele is covered by the epithelium of the umbilical cord, a derivative of the amnion. The abdominal cavity is proportionately small, but it is unclear whether this is the cause or effect of the failure of the abdominal contents to return. Normal midgut rotation does not occur, so intestinal rotation is incomplete. The presence of omphalocele necessitates surgical repair. Umbilical hernia, the herniation through an imperfectly closed umbilicus, is distinct from omphalocele, as the protruding mass is covered by a layer of subcutaneous tissue and skin. Surgery is not usually performed unless the hernia persists until age 3 to 5 years.

Gastroschisis Gastroschisis, the more common of the congenital abdominal wall defects, results from incomplete closure of the lateral folds during the fourth week of gestation. The term gastroschisis, which means "split stomach", is a misnomer as the defect is in the anterior abdominal wall. The linear defect, usually located on the right side near the median plane, permits extrusion of the abdominal viscera into the amniotic cavity. The umbilical cord is not involved and there is no membrane covering the extruded bowel. Females are more commonly affected than males and exposure to environmental drugs and chemicals may be involved in the etiology of gastroschisis. As in omphalocele, the intestinal rotation is incomplete and surgical repair is required.

Intestinal anomalies

Midgut malrotation The term malrotation is commonly used to describe a large spectrum of defects in midgut rotation. As a result of incomplete intestinal rotation, the normal wide-based mesenteric attachment of the midgut is lacking, allowing the bowel to twist along the axis of the superior mesenteric artery. Volvulus is a concern in all patients with malrotation, and midgut volvulus with evidence of peritonitis requires emergent surgical correction. Intestinal obstruction may also occur in the absence of volvulus. As a result of the failed midgut rotation, the ascending colon remains in the upper abdomen, and the peritoneal attachments of the ascending colon still exist. The peritoneal bands (Ladd bands) cross the second or third portion of the duodenum to attach to the lateral body wall, and duodenal obstruction may result.

It is likely that anomalies of intestinal rotation are quite common, although the true incidence is unknown as many remain asymptomatic. If the midgut loop fails to rotate as it re-enters the abdomen (non-rotation) the caudal limb or large intestine returns first. The small intestine lies on the right side of the abdomen with the entire large intestine on the left. Non-rotation of the midgut is usually asymptomatic. In very rare cases, the midgut loop rotates in a clockwise rather than a counterclockwise rotation. The duodenum thus lies anterior to the superior mesenteric artery and the transverse colon posterior to it. In these cases, the transverse colon may become obstructed by pressure from the superior mesenteric artery. Patients with anomalies of midgut rotation who are asymptomatic should still undergo surgical treatment, regardless of age or symptoms, as volvulus can develop without pre-existing symptoms.

Between 30% and 60% of patients with defects in intestinal rotation have other associated anomalies. Rotational defects occur in one third to one half of infants with duodenal atresia and one third of infants with jejunal atresia. Other gastrointestinal anomalies associated with midgut malrotation include esophageal atresia, biliary atresia, annular pancreas, meconium ileus, intestinal duplications, mesenteric cysts, Meckel's diverticulum, Hirschsprung's disease, and imperforate anus. Heterotaxia, an abnormal arrangement of body organs distinct from situs inversus, also coexists with abnormalities of intestinal rotation. Features of heterotaxia include midline liver, malpositioned stomach, non-retroperitoneal pancreas, major cardiac anomalies, and asplenia or polysplenia.

Intestinal atresia and stenosis Atresia and stenosis are the most common congenital anomalies of the midgut. Intestinal atresia is more common than stenosis and occurs in approximately 1 in 3000 live births. Atresia of the small intestine is significantly more common than colonic atresia. In contrast to duodenal atresia, atresia of the jejunal, ileal, or colonic region typically results from fetal vascular accidents leading to intestinal ischemia, necrosis, and subsequent development of a fibrous cord connecting the proximal and distal ends of normal intestine. Mechanisms for the ischemic event may include volvulus, internal hernia, obstruction with perforation, and constriction of the mesentery in an abdominal wall defect. Lack of intestinal fixation, which may occur as the intestines return to the abdomen during the tenth week of gestation, predisposes to such events. Most patients with atresia present within the first days of postnatal life, usually with bilious vomiting or abdominal distension. Surgical intervention is required.

Meckel's diverticulum The omphalomesenteric duct or vitelline duct is a vestige of the embryonic yolk stalk. Remnants of the omphalomesenteric duct are found in 1% to 4% of infants, making these the most common congenital gastrointestinal anomalies. The congenital ileal diverticulum, the most common remnant of the omphalomesenteric duct, was initially described more than four centuries ago. In the early 19th century Meckel's landmark paper resulted in the association of his name with this anomaly. Other omphalomesenteric duct remnants, including a patent duct, solid cord, cystic remant, or umbilical remnant, have been described, but Meckel's diverticulum represents more than 80% of cases and is the most significant clinically. In children, Meckel's diverticulum is the most common cause of lower gastrointestinal tract bleeding and is an occasional cause of hemorrhage in adults. In other cases, the diverticulum may become inflamed and mimic appendicitis or cause intussusception and intestinal obstruction. None the less, only a small percentage of Meckel's diverticula are symptomatic.

Meckel's diverticulum contains all three layers of the intestinal wall and is usually located 40 to 50 cm from the ileocecal junction. The diverticulum originates from the border of the bowel opposite the mesentery and is typically a finger-like pouch 3 to 6 cm long and slightly smaller in diameter than the lumen of the small intestine. In some cases, including up to 80% of symptomatic patients, the lining of the diverticulum may contain ectopic tissue, such as gastric, pancreatic, bile-duct, duodenal, or colonic tissues. Gastric mucosa, the most common ectopic tissue, typically secretes acid, producing ulceration and bleeding. The "Meckel's scan" takes advantage of this finding by using ^{99m}technetium pertechnetate, which binds to parietal cells in the ectopic gastric mucosa. This test has a sensitivity of 85% and specificity of 95% in children, but rates are lower in adults. Surgical resection is the treatment of choice in symptomatic patients.

Midgut duplications Duplications of the gastrointestinal tract are extremely rare occurrences and may be found anywhere from the mouth to the anus. The most common location of duplication is in the derivatives of the midgut. Duplications are more prevalent in the small intestine than the colon, and the most common small-intestinal site is the ileum. While the etiology of intestinal duplication is unknown, theories include errors in recanalization of epithelial plugs within the small intestine and diverticula which develop from adhesions between germ layers during embryogenesis. The result is the formation of a second intestinal lumen, with a seromuscular wall and mucosal lining which is usually similar to that of the neighboring bowel. The duplication nearly always arises on the mesenteric side of the bowel and receives branches from the same arteries which supply the adjacent intestine.

Intestinal duplications are broadly categorized as either cystic or tubular. Cystic duplications are much more common and usually do not communicate with the intestinal tract. Tubular duplications generally communicate with the intestinal lumen. About 25% of tubular duplications contain heterotopic gastric mucosa. Both types of duplication may present with obstruction, mass effect, and abdominal pain and are usually identified by early childhood. Treatment is surgical resection of the duplication along with the adjacent intestine.

Hindgut development and anomalies

Normal hindgut development

The hindgut consists of the left one half to one third of the transverse colon and the descending colon, sigmoid colon, rectum, and superior portion of the anal canal. The epithelium of the urinary bladder and most of the urethra are also derivatives of the hindgut. All of the organs of the hindgut are supplied by branches of the inferior mesenteric artery. The watershed area between the superior and inferior mesenteric arteries (located in the mid- to distal transverse colon) marks the border between the tissues of the midgut and hindgut. The growth of the hindgut and the caudal limb of the midgut lag behind the cranial limb. Thus, when the intestine returns to the abdomen in the tenth week of gestation, the caliber of the colon is much smaller than that of the small intestine. With rotation, the descending colon becomes retoperitoneal as its mesentery fuses with the peritoneum of the posterior abdominal wall and disappears. The mesentery of the sigmoid colon remains but is shorter than in the embryo. Transient occlusion of the colonic lumen by epithelial plugs is seen between the fifth and eight weeks of gestation, but colonic atresia and stenosis are exceedingly rare.

The most complex region of hindgut development is the terminal portion known as the cloaca (Figure 1.7). Beginning around the thirteenth day of gestation, a ventral diverticulum, the allantois, forms from the yolk sac and grows toward the hindgut (Figure 1.7A and B). The cloaca is an expanded cavity of the hindgut at the junction of the allantoic stalk. While the cloaca is endodermally lined, it abuts a depression of the surface ectoderm called the proctodeum or anal pit. The endoderm from the cloaca and the ectoderm from the proctodeum together form the cloacal membrane (Figure 1.7C and D). The margins of the

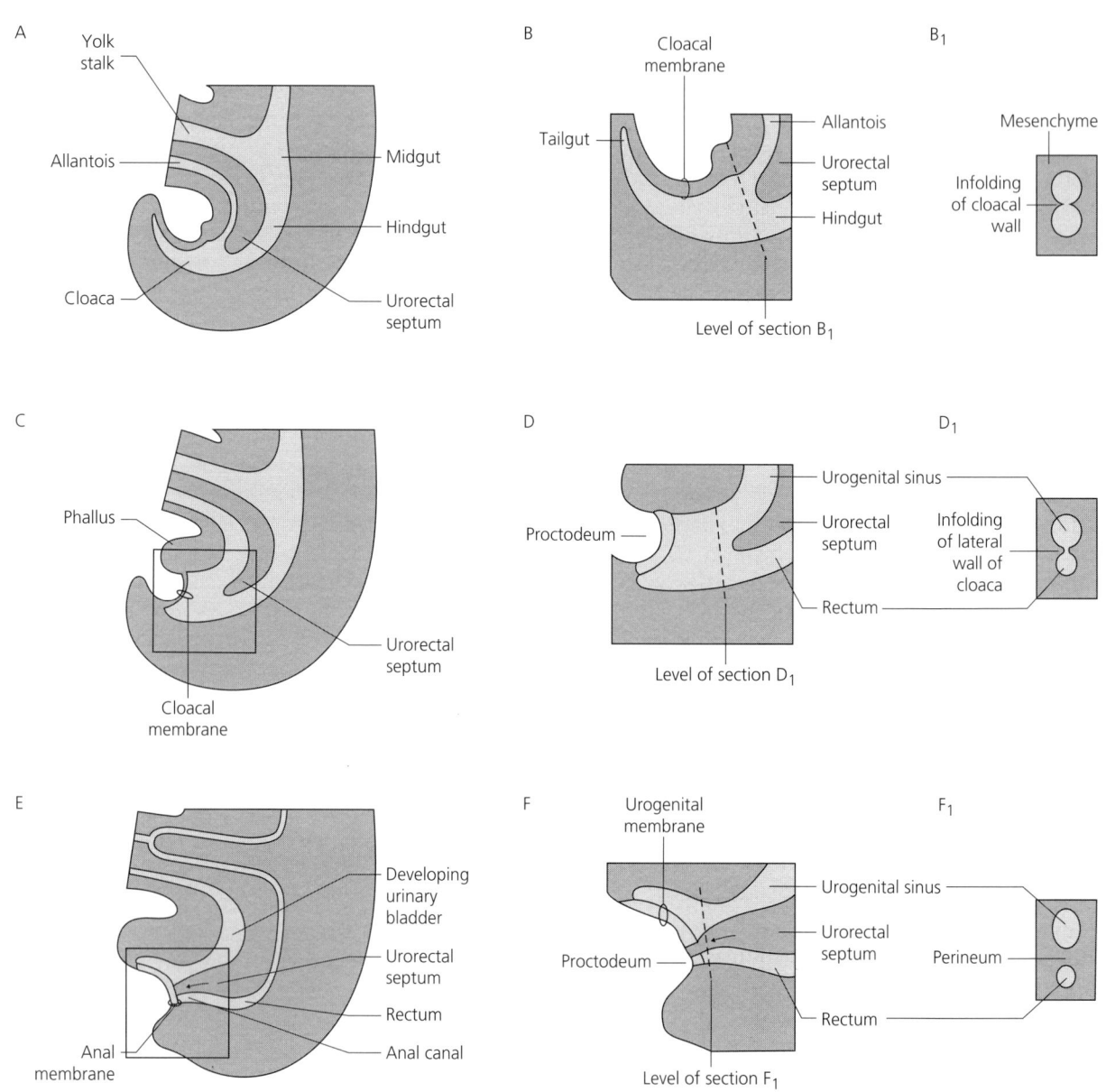

Abnormalities of Gastrointestinal Organogenesis

Figure 1.7 Drawings illustrating successive stages in the partitioning of the cloaca into the rectum and urogenital sinus by the urorectal septum. (A, C, and E) Views from the left side at 4, 6, and 7 weeks respectively. (B, D, and F) Enlargements of the cloacal region. (B₁, D₁, and F₁) Transverse sections of the cloaca at the levels shown in B, D, and F respectively. Note that the tailgut (shown in B) degenerates and disappears as the rectum forms from the dorsal part of the cloaca (shown in C) (reproduced with permission from Moore KL, Persaud TVN. *The Developing Human: Clinically Oriented Embryology* 6th edn. Philadelphia PA, Saunders, 1998: Fig. 12.25).

cloaca are thus the allantois ventrally and the cloacal membrane dorsally. A more posterior region of the hindgut, the tailgut, remains small and disappears by approximately 6 weeks gestation.

As organogenesis continues, the cloaca is partitioned into dorsal and ventral sections by a wedge of mesenchyme known as the urorectal septum. The urorectal septum develops in the angle between the allantois and the hindgut and grows caudally towards the cloacal membrane. As the septum grows, infoldings develop in the lateral walls of the cloaca. These folds grow towards one another and fuse, dividing the cloaca into two parts. The dorsal region forms the rectum and cranial part of the anal canal while the ventral portion becomes the urogenital sinus.

By the seventh week of gestation, the urorectal septum and cloacal membrane fuse (Figure 1.7E and F). The site of this fusion becomes the perineal body, the tendinous center of the perineum in the adult. The cloacal membrane is now divided into a dorsal anal membrane and a larger ventral urogenital membrane. The descent of the urorectal septum also defines the cloacal sphincter, which forms the external anal sphincter posteriorly and the superficial transverse perineal, bulbospongiosus, and ischiocavenosus muscles anteriorly. All of these muscles are supplied by the branches of the pudendal nerve.

At approximately 8 weeks gestation, the anal membrane ruptures. At this point, the anal canal is in direct communication with the amniotic cavity. The superior two thirds of the anal canal are derived from the hindgut while the inferior one third comes from the proctodeum. The junction of hindgut and proctodeum is roughly indicated in the adult by the irregular pectinate line, the approximate site of the anal membrane in the embryo. This region also represents a watershed between the superior rectal artery (from the inferior mesenteric artery), which supplies the upper portion of the anal canal, and the inferior rectal artery (from the internal pudendal artery), which supplies the lower portion. About 2 cm above the anus, the columnar epithelium of the upper anal canal transitions to a stratified squamous epithelium.

The venous and lymphatic drainage and the innervation of the anal canal make sense embryologically and are important clinically. The superior portion of the anal canal drains into the portal system via the superior rectal vein, a tributary of the inferior mesenteric vein. The inferior part of the anal canal drains through the inferior rectal vein, entering the systemic circulation via the internal iliac vein. The lymphatic drainage of the superior part of the anal canal goes to the inferior mesenteric lymph nodes and inferior part to the superficial inguinal lymph nodes. The autonomic nervous system innervates the anal canal derived from the hindgut while the lower part has its nerve supply from the inferior rectal nerve and thus is sensitive to pain, temperature, touch, and pressure. All of these factors contribute to the differences in sensation and to alterations in the spread of tumors from the upper and lower portions of the anal canal.

Hindgut anomalies

Anomalies of the anorectal region

Imperforate anus is a term used to describe a spectrum of anorectal anomalies from small defects to complex malformations (Figure 1.8). Because of the complex development of the cloacal region anorectal malformations are quite common and affect approximately 1 in 5000 newborns with a male predominance. Most anorectal anomalies result from abnormal partitioning of the cloaca by the urorectal septum. Lesions are commonly characterized as low or high, depending on whether the blind end of the rectum is above or below the level of the puborectalis muscle. The high type of lesion is more common and usually more complex. A slight dorsal deviation of the urorectal septum leads to anal stenosis (Figure 1.8B). If the anal membrane fails to perforate, membranous atresia results (Figure 1.8C). The anus is separated from the exterior by only a thin layer of tissue. In anal agenesis, another low anorectal malformation, the anal canal may end blindly or there may be an ectopic opening into the vagina in women, the urethra in men, or onto the perineum (Figure 1.8D and E). Anorectal agenesis, a high anorectal anomaly, accounts for about two thirds of all anorectal defects (Figure 1.8F and G). The rectum ends blindly, but a fistula is usually present to the urethra in males, the vagina in females, or the bladder. Rectal atresia has an etiology similar to atresia elsewhere in the midgut and hindgut but distinct from most of the other anorectal anomalies (Figure 1.8H and I). Both the anal canal and rectum are present and often separated by a fibrous cord.

Hirschsprung's disease

Hirschsprung's disease or congenital megacolon results from failure of the normal migration of autonomic ganglion cells in the submucosal (Auerbach) and myenteric (Meissner) plexuses. Neural crest cells, which normally migrate caudally along the vagus and enter the bowel wall, fail to complete their migration into the wall of the colon. The defect probably arises during the fifth to seventh weeks of gestation. As a result, the parasympathetic ganglion cells in the Auerbach and Meissner plexuses do not develop in the affected segment. The lack of parasympathetic stimulation leads to decreased intestinal relaxation, and the unopposed sympathetic activity results in increased tone. The colon is seen to be dilated, but the enlarged colonic segment is actually normal colon which dilates in response to failed peristalsis in the distal aganglionic segment. In most cases, only the rectosigmoid region of the colon is affected, but total colonic and even total intestinal aganglionosis have been reported.

Congenital megacolon is the most common cause of neonatal obstruction of the colon, occurring

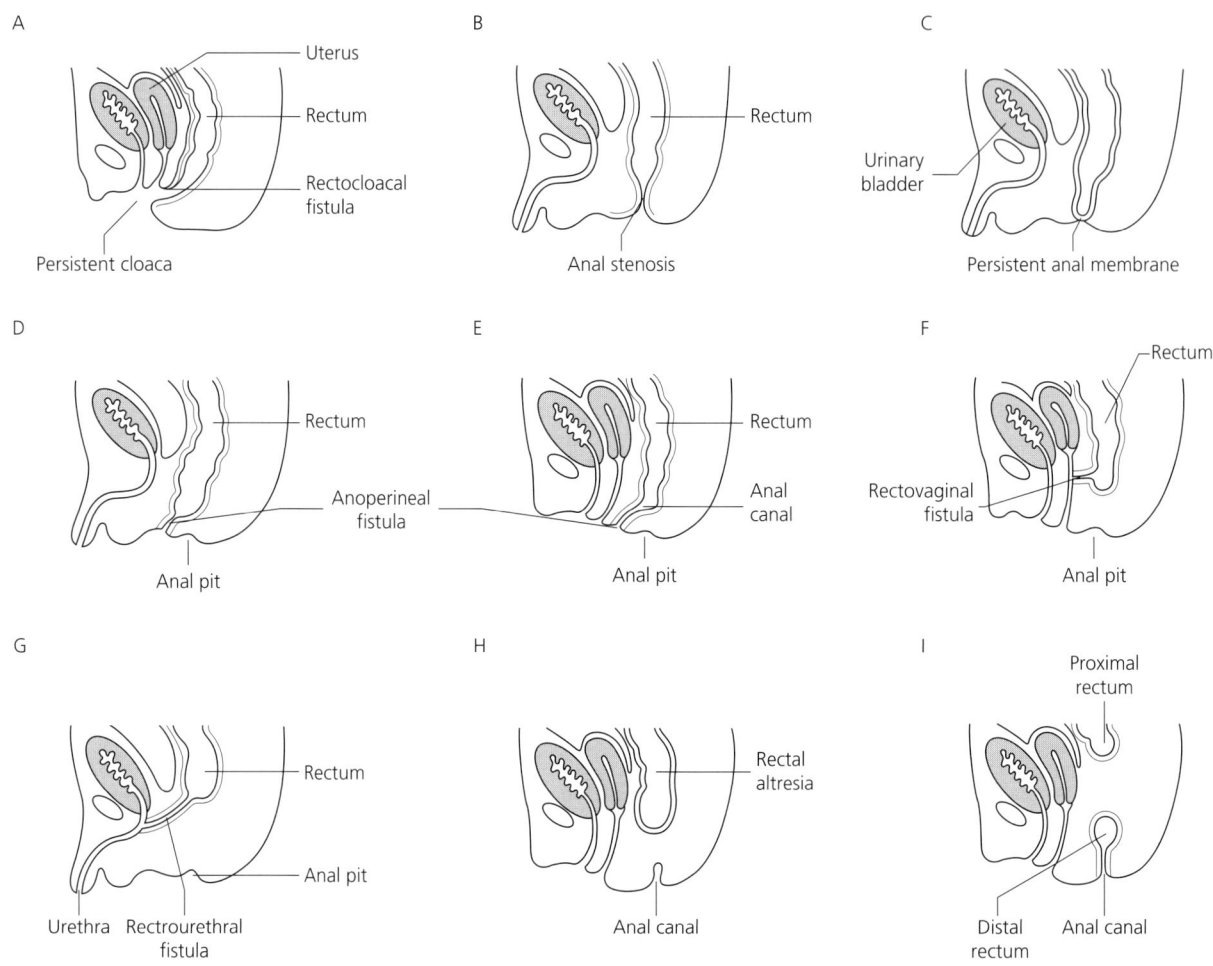

Figure 1.8 Drawings illustrating various types of anorectal anomaly. (A) Persistent cloaca. Note the common outlet for the intestinal, urinary, and reproductive tracts. (B) Anal stenosis. (C) Membranous anal atresia (covered anus). (D and E) Anal agenesis with a perineal fistula. (F) Anorectal agenesis with a rectovaginal fistula. (G) Anorectal agenesis with a rectourethral fistula. (H and I) Rectal atresia (reproduced with permission from Moore KL, Persaud TVN. *The Developing Human: Clinically Oriented Embryology* 6th edn. Philadelphia PA, Saunders, 1998: Fig. 12.29).

in approximately 1 in 5000 live births, and is seen in males four times more often than in females. Barium enema and manometry may be helpful in establishing the diagnosis, but the finding of aganglionosis on full-thickness rectal biopsy is the gold standard. Treatment of Hirschsprung's disease is surgical resection of the aganglionic bowel, but surgery is usually deferred until the child reaches 1 year of age. Enterocolitis is a major, life-threatening complication of Hirschsprung's disease. It may be seen preoperatively, but occurs more often within 6 to 12 months after surgical repair.

Genetic studies regarding the pathogenesis of this disease have identified several specific molecular mechanisms underlying the development of Hirschsprung's disease. Perhaps the most extensively studied mechanisms include mutations in the ret receptor tyrosine kinase gene and the endothelin-B receptor gene. The ret protooncogene has also been implicated in up to 90% of families with multiple endocrine neoplasia 2. The ret protooncogene is normally expressed early in fetal development in neurocrest cells and enteric glia. The ligand for this receptor is glial cell line derived neurotrophic factor (GDNF). Together with a second receptor, GDNFRα, ret and GDNF form a multiprotein-signaling complex. In support of this model, inactivation of ret in transgenic mice results in the loss of enteric neurons throughout the entire gastrointestinal tract, a phenotype nearly identical to that observed in mice with a targeted disruption of the GDNF gene. Additional studies are needed to determine the mechanism by which disruption of this complex prevents the development of the enteric nervous system.

Conclusions

The development of the human gastrointestinal tract is a complex process, yet multiple interactions define the gastrointestinal growth and development in a remarkably consistent manner. From gastrulation to the origins of the primordial gut, to the morphogenesis of the individual organs, the human gastrointestinal tract undergoes dynamic changes to attain functionality. Slight perturbations can lead to malformations which are incompatible with life or which necessitate early recognition for postnatal survival. An appreciation of all of the complex interactions of normal gastrointestinal development is invaluable. By understanding the origins of the gastrointestinal tract, we can not only learn to recognize abnormalities of gastrointestinal organogenesis but also to comprehend the causes and to predict the courses of many gastrointestinal disorders in the adult.

Further reading

Berrocal T, Lamas M, Gutieerrez J, Torres I, Prieto C, del Hoyo ML. Congenital anomalies of the small intestine, colon, and rectum. *Radiographics* 1999; 19(5): 1219–1236.

Berrocal T, Torres I, Gutierrez J, Prieto C, del Hoyo ML, Lamas M. Congenital anomalies of the upper gastrointestinal tract. *Radiographics* 1999; 19(4): 855–872.

Lebenthal E. *Human Gastrointestinal Development*. Raven Press, New York, 1989.

Montgomery RK, Mulberg AE, Grand RJ. Development of the human gastrointestinal tract: twenty years of progress. *Gastroenterology* 1999; 116(3): 702–731.

Moore KL, Persaud TVN. *The Developing Human: Clinically Oriented Embryology* 6th edn. Saunders, Philadelphia PA, 1998.

Ross III AJ. Organogenesis, innervation, and histologic development of the gastrointestinal tract. In: Polin RA, Fox WW (eds) *Fetal and Neonatal Physiology* 2nd edn. Saunders, Philadelphia PA, 1998: pp. 1342–1353.

Sleisenger MH, Fordtran JS, Feldman M, Scharschmidt B. *Sleisenger & Fordtran's Gastrointestinal and Liver Disease: Pathophysiology, Diagnosis, Management* 6th edn. Saunders, Philadelphia PA, 1998.

Wyllie R, Hyams JS. *Pediatric Gastrointestinal Disease: Pathophysiology, Diagnosis, Management* 2nd edn. Saunders, Philadelphia PA, 1999.

Chapter 2

Evaluation of Acute Diarrhea

Faten N. Aberra and Stephen J. Gluckman

CHAPTER OUTLINE

DEFINITION

TYPES OF DIARRHEA

EVALUATION
   History
   Physical examination
   Diagnostic tests

SPECIAL CONSIDERATIONS
   Acute diarrhea in the elderly
   Hospital-acquired diarrhea
   Traveler's diarrhea
   Enterohemorrhagic Escherichia coli
   Diarheogenic (non-hemorrhagic) Escherichia coli
   Outbreak diarrhea
   Immunocompromised patients

TREATMENT
   Volume expansion
   Antidiarrheal agents
   Antibiotics

FURTHER READING

Definition

Diarrhea is defined as stool weight greater than 200 g per day or the passage of three or more watery stools in a 24-hour period. When diarrhea is present for less than 2 to 4 weeks it is acute.

There are numerous etiologies for acute diarrhea with infection being the most common cause (Box 2.1).

Types of diarrhea

Most of the pathogens that cause acute infectious diarrhea are listed in Table 2.1. Special consideration should be taken in certain groups of patients to help identify the likely diagnoses and structure the management of the disease (Figure 2.1). These groups include people over 65 years old, travelers, immunocompromised individuals, and cases of antibiotic-associated enterocolitis, hemorrhagic colitis, and outbreak diarrhea. Immunodeficiency may occur because of human immunodeficiency virus (HIV), steroids, chemotherapy, or other immunosuppressive drugs. In addition, precautions should be taken with patients who have underlying diseases such as diabetes, hypertension, heart disease, chronic lung disease, chronic renal failure, and cirrhosis because the diarrhea may make the primary disease more difficult to manage.

There are four pathophysiological mechanisms that can cause diarrhea

- osmotic diarrhea
- exudative diarrhea
- secretory diarrhea
- altered intestinal transit.

Evaluation of Acute Diarrhea

> **Box 2.1** Causes of acute diarrhea
>
> Infectious agents
>   bacteria
>   viruses
>   parasites
> Medications
>   antacids
>   antiarrhythmics
>   antibiotics
>   antihypertensives
>   antineoplastics
>   cholinergics
>   laxatives
>   magnesium supplements
>   non-steroidal anti-inflammatory drugs
>   potassium supplements
>   prokinetics
>   prostaglandins
>   proton pump inhibitors
>   theophylline
> Dietary causes
>   foods containing
>   sorbitol
>   mannitol
>   xylitol
> Intestinal ischemia
> Fecal impaction
> Pelvic inflammation

Most cases of acute diarrhea result from more than one mechanism.

Osmotic diarrhea is the result of an osmotically active agent in the intestinal lumen that cannot be absorbed and which draws fluid into the lumen. This can be due to the presence of medications such as laxatives that contain magnesium hydroxide, phosphate or sulfate, or antacids that contain magnesium, colchicine, cholestyramine, neomycin, lactulose, and para-aminosalicylic acid. Diseases that result in malabsorption can also produce a large number of osmotically active particles in the gastrointestinal tract. These are varied and include such entities as disaccharidase deficiencies, fructose malabsorption, abetalipoproteinemia, congenital lymphangiectasia, cystic fibrosis, postenteritis disaccharidase deficiency, pancreatic exocrine insufficiency, bacterial overgrowth, celiac sprue, thyrotoxicosis, adrenal insufficiency, bile-salt diarrhea, and infections caused by rotavirus, *Giardia*, and *Coccidia*.

Exudative or inflammatory diarrhea is commonly the result of an infection. Other causes include graft-versus-host disease, food allergy, celiac sprue, eosinophilic gastroenteritis, Crohn's disease, ulcerative colitis, and lymphocytic and collagenous colitis.

Secretory diarrhea occurs as a result of mucosal stimulation of active chlorine ion secretion. The endogenous offenders include bacterial toxins such as those from *Escherichia coli* and *Vibrio cholerae*. Other offenders include hormone-producing tumors such as vipoma and gastrinoma, mastocy-

Table 2.1 Organisms that cause acute diarrhea.

Bacteria	Viruses	Parasites
Shigella dysenteriae	Rotavirus	*Giardia lamblia*
Salmonella	Norwalk-like viruses	*Entamoeba histolytica*
Campylobacter jejuni	Enteric adenoviruses	*Cryptosporidium*
Escherichia coli	Astroviruses	*Cyclospora*
Yersinia enterocolitica	Coronoviruses	*Isospora belli*[1]
Staphylococcus aureus	Herpes simplex	*Microsporida*[1]
Bacillus cereus	Cytomegalovirus[1]	*Stronglyoides*
Vibrio spp.	Small round viruses	*Trichinella spiralis*
Listeria monocytogenes	Human immunodeficiency virus	*Balantidium coli*
Treponema pallidum and other *Spirillum* spp.		Schistosomiasis (acute)
Neisseria gonorrhea		
Aeromonas hydrophila		
Plesiomonas shigelloides		
Clostridium difficile		
Clostridium perfringens		
Mycobacterium avium intracellulare[1]		
Chlamydia		
[1]organisms that cause diarrhea in immunocompromised patients.		

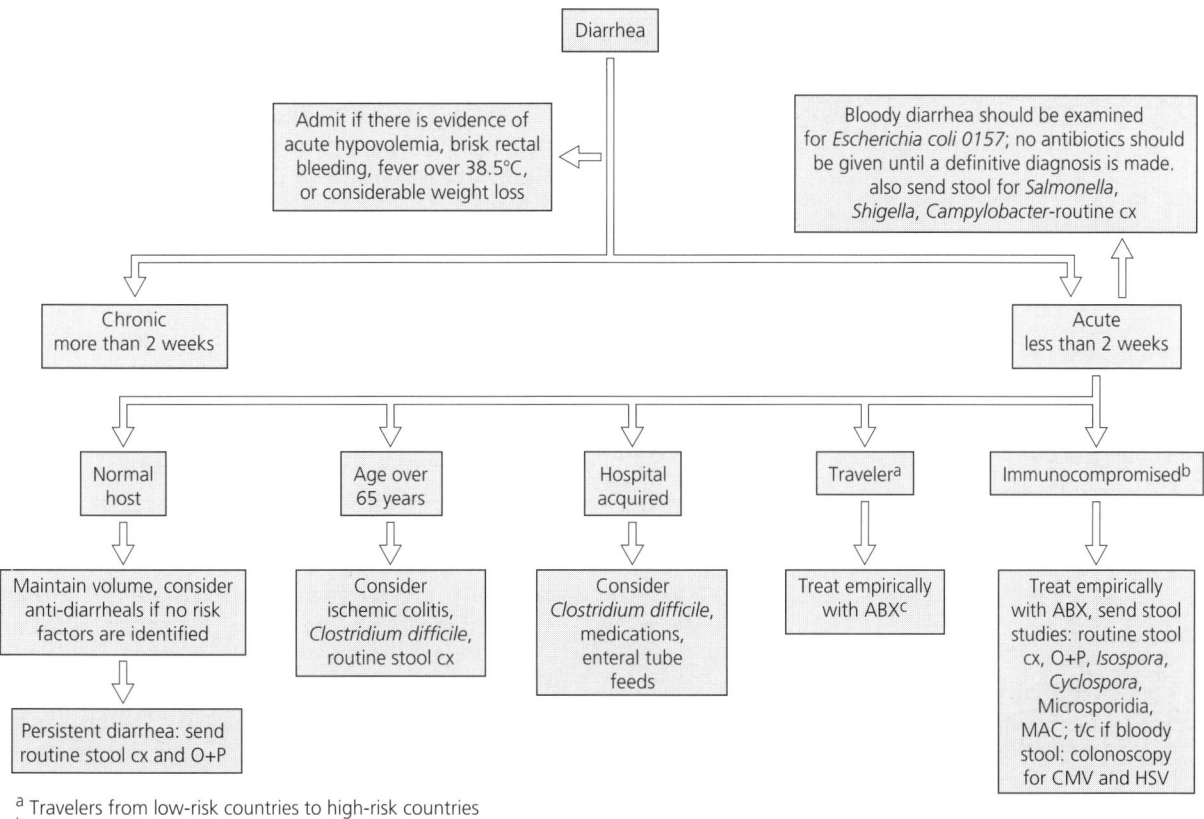

```
                          Diarrhea
                             │
    ┌────────────────────────┼────────────────────────┐
    │                        │                        │
Admit if there is evidence of                  Bloody diarrhea should be examined
acute hypovolemia, brisk rectal                for Escherichia coli O157; no antibiotics should
bleeding, fever over 38.5°C,                   be given until a definitive diagnosis is made.
or considerable weight loss                    also send stool for Salmonella,
                                               Shigella, Campylobacter-routine cx
```

```
        Chronic                                      Acute
    more than 2 weeks                            less than 2 weeks
            │                    ┌──────────┬──────────┬──────────┬──────────┐
            │                    │          │          │          │          │
        Normal              Age over     Hospital   Traveler[a]  Immunocompromised[b]
         host              65 years     acquired
            │                    │          │          │          │
   Maintain volume, consider  Consider   Consider   Treat empirically   Treat empirically
   anti-diarrheals if no risk ischemic colitis,  Clostridium difficile,  with ABX[c]  with ABX, send stool
   factors are identified     Clostridium difficile,  medications,                studies: routine stool
            │                 routine stool cx   enteral tube                     cx, O+P, Isospora,
   Persistent diarrhea: send                     feeds                             Cyclospora,
   routine stool cx and O+P                                                        Microsporidia,
                                                                                   MAC; t/c if bloody
                                                                                   stool: colonoscopy
                                                                                   for CMV and HSV
```

[a] Travelers from low-risk countries to high-risk countries
[b] HIV infection, autoimmune diseases, hematologic malignancy, acute graft-versus-host, corticosteroid use, immunosuppressive therapy, chemotherapy
[c] If febrile and/or severe diarrhea stool cx and O+P should be sent

Figure 2.1 Management algorithm.

tosis, and endogenous laxatives such as bile acids and long chain fatty acids.

Evaluation

History

Several elements in the patient's history can often help to suggest possible diagnoses from the long list of causes of diarrhea. Bloody or heme-occult positive stools may suggest inflammatory diarrhea and colonic location. Tenesmus is suggestive of an inflammatory cause with anorectal involvement. Voluminous and watery stools are suggestive of disorders of the small bowel. Secretory diarrhea persists despite fasting, and occurs night and day in contrast to osmotic diarrhea. Mucus in the stools may be suggestive of irritable bowel syndrome. If vomiting overshadows diarrheal symptoms then "food poisoning" by toxin-producing bacteria or viruses should be considered. Patients should be asked about their travel history, especially travel to developing countries, and their dietary history.

Detailed information about the use of medications must be taken. Common offenders are magnesium-containing antacids, antibiotics (over the previous 8 weeks), laxatives, digitalis, propranolol (Inderal®), colchicine, and cancer chemotherapeutic agents. If acute diarrhea occurs in a hospitalized or recently hospitalized person *Clostridium difficile* should be strongly considered. Social history should include occupation (working at a day-care center may increase the risk for rotavirus, farmers may at be at higher risk for *Salmonella* and *Campylobacter*) and a sexual history. Recipients of anal sex are at risk of proctitis, due to herpes simplex, *Chlamydia*, *Treponema pallidum*, and *Neisseria gonorrhoeae*. Table 2.2 provides information about the route of infection of many pathogens.

In addition to a history reviewing the duration, frequency, and characteristics of the stool, it is extremely important to determine the severity of illness. Markers of severe disease include profuse watery diarrhea with dehydration, passage of many small-volume stools containing blood and mucus, temperature 38.5°C or above, passage of more than six unformed stools per 24 hours or an illness that has lasted more than 48 hours, severe abdominal

Evaluation of Acute Diarrhea

Table 2.2 Route by which certain pathogens infect humans.

Vehicle	Pathogen
Water	*Vibrio cholerae*, Norwalk agent, *Giardia*, *Cryptosporidium*
Food	
poultry	*Salmonella, Campylobacter, Shigella*
beef, unpasteurized fruit juice	enterohemorrhagic *Escherichia coli*
seafood, shellfish, raw sushi	*Vibrio cholerae, Vibrio parahaemolyticus, Vibrio vulnificus, Salmonella* spp., hepatitis A and B
cheese, milk	*Listeria* spp.
eggs	*Salmonella* spp.
mayonnaise-containing food and cream pies	Staphylococcal and clostridial food poisonings
fried rice	*Bacillus cereus*
fresh raspberries	*Cyclospora*
canned vegetables or fruits	*Clostridium botulinum*
Animal-to-person (pets and livestock)	*Salmonella, Campylobacter, Brucella, Cryptosporidium, Giardia* spp.
Person-to-person (fecal–oral)	all enteric bacteria, viruses, and parasites
Day-care centers	Rotavirus, astrovirus, *Shigella, Salmonella, Campylobacter, Cryptosporidium, Giardia, Clostridium difficile*
Hospitals, antibiotics, or chemotherapy	*Clostridium difficile*
Chronic-care facilities	*Clostridium difficile*
Swimming pools	*Giardia* and *Cryptosporidium* spp.
Foreign travel	*Escherichia coli* spp., *Salmonella, Shigella, Campylobacter, Giardia, Cryptosporidium, Entamoeba histolytica, Cyclospora cayetanensis, Aeromonas* spp., rotavirus

pain in a patient over the age of 50 years, and diarrhea in elderly (over 70 years of age) or immunocompromised individuals. Patients with any of these symptoms require thorough evaluation. Indications for hospitalization include signs of acute volume loss (orthostatic hypotension, poor skin turgor, and increased urine and plasma specific gravity), brisk rectal bleeding, fever with a tender abdominal mass, and diarrhea with considerable weight loss.

Physical examination

A physical examination may provide important information about the severity of the diarrhea and occasionally provides information for diagnosis of diarrhea type. On skin examination rose spots may be seen suggesting *Salmonella typhi* (typhoid fever). A tender abdominal mass may be indicative of an abcess and a rectal fistula or peri-rectal abscess may suggest Crohn's disease.

Diagnostic tests

Most diarrheal illnesses are self-limited and of mild to moderate severity. They require minimal evaluation. However, patients with severe disease must have an evaluation to make a definitive diagnosis. Routine stool cultures should be sent and usually identify *Salmonella, Shigella, Campylobacter, Yersinia* and *Aeromonas* (Table 2.3). Some laboratories may need to be notified if *Yersinia* and *Aeromonas* are of interest. Stools should be checked for blood if there is no gross blood. In patients with bloody stools the clinician should consider sending the stool for *Escherichia Coli* O157 culture or the associated verotoxin. The yield from sending stools for ova and parasites is generally very small and such an evaluation should be initiated only in certain specific situations, for example in patients with a history of travel to a resource-poor country, camping, advanced immunosuppression, exposure to children at day-care centers, community waterborne outbreak, or with otherwise undiagnosed diarrhea. If *Entamoeba histolytica* is suspected and the stool specimen is negative, then serologic examination, an indirect hemagglutination test, for *E. histolytica* should be performed. However, the sensitivity of this test is variable and is more likely to be positive in amoebic colitis than is mere diarrhea. Patients that have taken antibiotics over the 8 weeks prior to diarrhea or have hospital-acquired diarrhea should have a sample sent for *Clostridium difficile* toxin A assay. A single test is about 85% sensitive so several may have to be sent on successive days. If the toxin A assay is repeatedly negative and *C. difficile* infection is still highly suspected

Table 2.3 Organisms classified by presentation of diarrhea: non-inflammatory versus inflammatory diarrhea.

Non-inflammatory (watery) diarrhea	Inflammatory (bloody) diarrhea
Viruses	**Viruses**
Rotavirus	Cytomeglovirus[1]
Caliciviruses	
Enteric adenovirus (types 40, 41)	**Bacteria**
Hepatitis A, hepatitis B	Shigella spp.[1]
	Enteroinvasive Escherichia coli[2]
	Enterohemorrhagic Escherichia coli
Bacteria	Plesiomonas shigelloides[1]
Clostidium perfingens	Clostridium difficile[1]
Bacillus cereus	Campylobacter jejuni[1,2]
Staphylococcus aureus	Vibrio parahaemolyticus
Aeromonas spp.	Salmonella typhi, non-typhi Salmonella
Enteropathogenic Escherichia coli	Yersinia enterolitica[1]
Enterotoxigenic Escherichia coli	Trichenella spiralis
Vibrio cholerae[3]	Spirillum spp.
Listeria monocytogenes	
Pleisiomona sp.	**Parasites**
	Balantidium coli
Parasites	Entamoeba histolytica[2]
Giardia	Schistosoma
Cryptosporidium	
Microsporidia	
Isospora belli	
Cyclospora	

[1] may cause watery or bloody diarrhea.
[2] usually causes bloody diarrhea which may initially present as watery.
[3] to be considered in developing countries.

then a stool specimen for toxin B should be sent. If the history suggests proctitis, rectal swabs for *Neisseria gonorrhoeae*, *Chlamydia trachomatis*, and herpes simplex, should be sent.

A method of differentiating between secretory and osmotic diarrhea is to obtain stool electrolytes and calculate the osmotic gap. The sum of stool sodium and potassium multiplied by two subtracted from 290 mOsm/kg (290 − 2(Na + K)) equals the stool osmotic gap. If the osmotic gap is greater than 125 mOsm/kg, then diarrhea is likely to be osmotic. If the osmotic gap is less than 50 mOsm/kg then the diarrhea is likely to be secretory. Another method to further characterize osmotic diarrhea is to perform a clinitest. A clinitest tablet is mixed in the stool that has been diluted with water and detects the presence of glucose. A positive test in combination with a fecal pH less than 5.5 suggests carbohydrate intolerance.

Sigmoidoscopy is beneficial when diarrhea is severe and persistent, and stool examinations for pathogens are non-diagnostic. In HIV-infected patients presenting with diarrhea and a low CD4+ cell count, endoscopy and colonoscopy are indicated if the initial stool examinations are negative. Colonoscopy or sigmoidoscopy may also be indicated if ischemic colitis is suspected. In such situations, the examination should be done without prior evacuation of the bowel. Yellow lenticular plaques in the colon are suggestive of pseudomembranous colitis. Colonic ulcerations are usually present in patients with Crohn's disease, radiation proctitis, shigellosis, or amebiasis. A fecal aspirate in the area of the ulceration may reveal mobile trophozoites of amebiasis. Anorectal fistulas, deep anal fissures, and peri-rectal abscesses are signs suggestive of Crohn's disease, tuberculosis, and sexually transmitted diseases. Biopsies should be obtained of any abnormal area and in HIV-infected patients random biopsies for CMV inclusions should be obtained even from normal appearing mucosa.

Additional laboratory testing that may be helpful include a complete blood count with differential looking for eosinophilia. Eosinophilia may be suggestive of eosinophilic gastroenteritis. Hypocalcemia or anemia may indicate malabsorption. Hypercalcemia associated with Zollinger–Ellison syndrome may suggest multiple endocrine neoplasia syndrome type 1.

Special considerations

Acute diarrhea in the elderly

There is a considerable impact caused by diarrheal illnesses in the elderly (those older than 65 years), with 51% of diarrheal deaths occurring in adults over the age of 75 years from 1979 to 1987. It is likely that concomitant diseases associated with the aging process, rather than age itself, increases the risk of diarrheal illness. Ischemic colitis should be considered in patients presenting in this age group, as well as neoplasia creating a partially obstructive lesion of the intestinal tract, dysmotility with impaction, malabsorption, uremia, and diabetes. If the patient resides in a nursing home or has a nosocomial diarrhea *Clostridium difficile* should be considered. Older patients are also more likely to be exposed to *Clostridium perfringens* and toxigenic *Escherichia coli*.

Hospital-acquired diarrhea

The most common cause of acute diarrhea in hospitalized patients is *Clostridium difficile* infection. Other infectious causes are uncommon, but those to be considered include ingestion of elixir containing sorbitol or mannitol (acetaminophen and theophylline may contain these products), a medication side effect, or enteral tube feedings.

Traveler's diarrhea

Individuals traveling from resource-rich to resource-poor countries are at risk of acquiring traveler's diarrhea. The risk of acquiring diarrhea is 40% when traveling from the US to most parts of Latin America, Haiti, Dominican Republic, Africa, and southern Asia. Intermediate risk areas with a 10% to 15% risk of acquiring diarrhea, include northern Mediterranean countries, the Middle East, China, and Russia. Low risk regions are the US, Canada, western Europe, Japan, South Africa, Australia, and New Zealand. Enterotoxigenic *Escherichia coli* is a leading cause of diarrhea worldwide and is the most common cause of traveler's diarrhea. This organism produces disease by adhering to the intestinal mucosa and generating toxins.

Other common pathogens are *Campylobacter* which is relatively common in north Africa and southeast Asia, enteraggregative *E. coli*, *Salmonella* spp., *Shigella* spp., rotavirus, Norwalk agent, *Giardia*, *Cryptosporidium*, and *Cyclospora*. Other parasites are uncommon causes of traveler's diarrhea. Of note during winter months in the US more than 75% of fresh produce is imported from developing countries and can be the source of outbreaks in this country.

To reduce the risk of infection, diet recommendations for travelers to developing countries are to consume steaming-hot cooked food, hot beverages, bottled carbonated drinks without ice, dry foods such as bread, acidic foods such as citrus fruits, and foods with a high-sugar content such as syrups and jellies. Antimicrobial prophylaxis should be given to patients with AIDS, prior gastric surgery and people taking a proton pump inhibitor. They are generally not indicated for other travelers. The suggested approach is for the traveler to carry an antibiotic treatment dose and to initiate treatment at the earliest onset of the illness. This strategy will be effective within 24 hours and will lessen excessive use of antibiotics with the associated risk of antibiotic resistance. Antimicrobials recommended for prophylaxis and treatment are mentioned in the section on treatment.

Enterohemorrhagic *Escherichia coli*

In patients presenting with bloody diarrhea, enterohemorrhagic *Escherichia coli* should be considered as a possible cause, especially in the setting of an outbreak. This is particularly important because of the association of enterohemorrhagic *E. coli* with hemolytic uremic syndrome, that mostly affects children between the ages of 5 and 10 years. The syndrome consists of renal failure, microangiopathic hemolytic anemia, and thrombocytopenia. Symptoms of hemolytic uremic syndrome occur in about 15% of cases following an infection with enterohemorrhagic *E. coli*, and typically begin 5 to 10 days after the onset of diarrhea.

Several studies suggest that antibiotic treatment of enterohemorrhagic *E. coli* increases the risk for the development of hemolytic uremic syndrome. Therefore, antibiotics should not be given if enterohemorrhagic *E. coli* is suspected. It has been noted that other gram negative rods can acquire the ability to make the verotoxin and produce an identical syndrome.

Diarheogenic (non-hemorrhagic) *Escherichia coli*

In addition to enterotoxigenic *Escherichia coli* and enterohemorrhagic *E. coli*, *E. coli* can cause gastrointestinal illness by a number of other mechanisms. None is identifiable using routine laboratory testing. If one of these types of *E. coli* is suspected, then consultation with an expert is recommended. There are five additional types of *E. coli* that produce a watery diarrhea

- enteropathogenic *E. coli*
- enteroinvasive *E. coli*
- enteroaggregative *E.coli*
- diarrhea-associated hemolytic *E. coli*
- cytolethal distending toxin *E. coli*.

Enteropathogenic *E. coli*, a major cause of infantile diarrhea, may cause diarrhea by adhering to intestinal mucosa and then causing localized destruction to the intestinal mucosa. Enteroaggregative *E. coli* is a significant cause of diarrhea in developing countries and in travelers to endemic countries. The name enteroaggregative *E. coli* is based on the bacteria forming a stacked brick-like appearance of adherence to the intestinal mucosa. The pathogenic properties of enteroaggregative *E. coli* are still not well understood. The pathological mechanism of diarrhea-associated *E. coli* is also poorly understood, but it is believed that bacterial toxins, α-hemolysin, and cytotoxic necrotizing factor 1, contribute to cause diarrhea. The final class of *E. coli* that may possibly cause diarrhea is cytolethal distending toxin *E. coli*. Cytolethal distending toxin causes distension and disintegration of cells.

Outbreak diarrhea

If acute diarrhea occurs in two or more individuals from the same exposure, then it is considered to be an outbreak. Acute diarrhea occurring in an outbreak situation should be reported to the area health officials. Identification of the outbreak pathogen is important for containing the spread and appropriate treatment.

Immunocompromised patients

A patient may be immunocompromised if they have any of the following conditions: HIV infection, autoimmune diseases, hematologic malignancy, acute graft-versus-host disease, or use corticosteroids or other immunosuppressive therapy. Since these patients are more prone to septicemia, antibiotics should be started early. In addition to the routine pathogens, *Crytosporidium*, *Isospora belli*, *Cyclospora*, Microsporum, *Mycobacterium avium-intracellulare*, Cytomegalovirus, adenovirus, and herpes simplex virus should be considered.

Treatment

Volume expansion

Volume expansion is the first step in managing patients with acute diarrhea. If a patient is not hypovolemic then they should be advised to continue drinking plenty of fluid. If signs of mild hypovolemia are present, then oral rehydration therapy should be used. There are several formulas of oral rehydration therapy which include the World Health Organization formula, Pedialyte, Rehydralyte, Rice-Lyte, and Resol. If ready made formulas are not available a home-made formula can be prepared. In one glass add 8 oz of juice of choice, 1/2 teaspoon of corn syrup or honey, and a pinch of salt. In another glass add 8oz of water bottle and 1/4 teaspoon of baking soda. Both glasses of fluid are to be ingested alternately until thirst abates. Another formulation is 1/2 cup of dry, precooked baby rice cereal combined with 2 cups of bottled water and 1/4 teaspoon salt. To maintain energy and water losses during an acute bout of diarrhea, a diet containing boiled starches such as potatoes, noodles, rice, wheat, and oats with additional salt may be helpful. Also helpful are crackers or toast, bananas, yogurt, soup, and boiled vegetables. Milk and other lactose-containing products should be eliminated from the diet since lactose intolerance may occur during infectious gastroenteritis which may aggravate diarrhea.

If a patient is severely hypovolemic or vomiting is a significant part of the clinical course and adequate hydration by mouth cannot be maintained, then intravenous fluids should be given.

Antidiarrheal agents

Most cases of acute infectious diarrhea resolve on their own and therapy is primarily supportive.

Therapy may help in reducing volume loss and the duration of clinical symptoms. There are several types of antidiarrheal agents including antimotility agents, anticholinergics, adsorbents, probiotics, and antisecretory drugs.

Commonly prescribed antimotility agents include loperamide (Imodium®) and diphenoxylate (Lomotil®). Other less commonly prescribed medications include codeine and tincture of opium. These agents should not be prescribed if a high fever and bloody diarrhea is present because they may enhance tissue invasion by the organism and slow intestinal motility.

Bismuth subsalicylate (Pepto-Bismol®), dioctahedral smectite, attapulgite (anhydrous aluminum silicate or Kaopectate®) are adsorbents. Bismuth subsalicylate is also an antisecretory agent. Adsorbents have the advantage of adsorbing toxins, improving stool consistency, and reducing the frequency of bowel movements. They should not be combined with antimicrobials since they may decrease efficacy by adsorbing antibiotics. Bismuth subsalicylate has been shown to be effective in preventing traveler's diarrhea if taken prophylactically. A common, but inconsequential, side effect of bismuth is blackened stool and sometimes tongue as well.

Probiotics such as *Lactobacillus acidophilus* and *Saccharomyces boulardii* may reduce the course of acute diarrhea by increasing the acidity of the stool and inhibiting growth of enteropathogens.

In refractory cases of diarrhea octreatide, an antisecretory agent, may be useful, though it is generally reserved for refractory *chronic* diarrhea. Anticholinergics such as atropine, hycoscyamine, and dicyclomine are generally not as helpful in reducing diarrhea, but may be helpful in reducing abdominal cramping. Diphenoxylate, an antimotility agent, is commonly prepared with atropine as Lomotil to reduce diarrhea and cramping.

Antibiotics

Most cases of acute infectious diarrhea are self-limiting and therapy is primarily supportive. In these situations antibiotics are of limited, if any, benefit and may result in complications. In Table 2.4, indications and preferred antibiotics are listed for common pathogens. Sensitivity to antimicrobials should be checked when an enteropathogen is identified to assure effective treatment and narrow spectrum therapy.

Travelers going to high-risk destinations should carry a treatment dose of an antibiotic to prevent gastroenteritis. Recommended antibiotics include ciprofloxacin 500 mg twice a day for 3 days, bismuth subsalicylate 524 mg with every meal and before bedtime for 5 days, or trimethoprim sulfamethoxazole, one double strength tablet twice a day for 3 days.

Table 2.4 Preferred antimicrobial treatment regimens for specific types of infectious diarrhea.

Pathogen/disease	Antibiotic of choice	Alternative agents
Traveler's diarrhea	Ciprofloxacin 500 mg p.o. b.i.d. × 3 days.	Other quinolones, trimethoprim sulfamethoxazole.
Amebiasis	Metronidazole 750 mg p.o. t.i.d. × 10 days, followed by iodoquinol 650 mg p.o. t.i.d. × 20 days or paromomycin 500 mg p.o. t.i.d. × 7 days.	Tetracycline 500 mg p.o. q.i.d. × 14 days and dehydroemetine 0.5–0.75 mg/kg i.m. q. 12 h × 5 days
Aeromonas	Ciprofloxacin 500 mg p.o. b.i.d. or other fluoroquinolone[1].	Trimethoprim sulfamethoxazole, third generation cephalosporin, chloramphenicol, tetracycline.
Campylobacter	Erythromycin 250–500mg p.o. q.i.d. × 7 days.	Quinolone × 5 days.
Clostridium difficile	Metronidazole 500 mg p.o. t.i.d.× 10–14 days	Vancomycin 125 mg p.o. q.i.d. × days
Cryptosporidia[2]	No proven effective treatment.	Paromomycin 500 mg t.i.d. has been used.
Cyclospora	Trimethoprim sulfamethoxazole 1 double strength tablet p.o. b.i.d. × 7 days.	
Escherichia coli enterotoxigenic enteropathogenic enteroinvasive	Ciprofloxacin 500 mg p.o. b.i.d. × 3 days or other fluoroquinolone.[3]	Trimethoprim sulfamethoxasole 160/800 mg p.o. b.i.d. × 3 days.
Escherichia coli enteraggregative	Ciprofloxacin 500 mg p.o. b.i.d. × 3 days or other fluoroquinolone.	
Escherichia coli enterohaemorrhagic	Antibiotics should not be given since they may predispose to hemolytic uremic syndrome.	

Table 2.4 Preferred antimicrobial treatment regimens for specific types of infectious diarrhea — Cont'd

Pathogen/disease	Antibiotic of choice	Alternative agents
Giardia	Metronidazole 250 mg p.o. t.i.d. × 5 days.	
Isospora	Trimethoprim sulfamethoxazole 1 double strenght tablet p.o. q.i.d. × 10 days, then b.i.d. for 3 weeks.	Pyrimethamine plus folinic acid.
Microsporum	Albendazole 200–400 mg p.o. b.i.d. × 3 months[4].	Fumagillin[5].
Plesiomonas	Ciprofloxacin 500 mg p.o. b.i.d. × 3 days[6].	Trimethoprim sulfamethoxazole 160–800 mg p.o. b.i.d. × 3 days[7].
Salmonella non-typhoid[8]	Ciprofloxacin 500 mg p.o. b.i.d. × 5–7 days or other fluoroquinolone[9].	Trimethoprim sulfamethoxazole 160–800 mg p.o. b.i.d. × 5–7 days.
typhoid	Ciprofloxacin 500 mg b.i.d. × 10 days or third generation cephalosporin.	Azithromycin 500 mg q.d. × 6 days.
Shigella	Ciprofloxacin 500 mg p.o. b.i.d. × 5 days or other fluoroquinilone.	Trimethoprim sulfamethoxazole or ampicillin Ceftriaxone 1 g i.v. b.i.d. × 5–7 days[10].
Vibrio spp. cholera O1 cholera O139[11]	Tetracycline 500 mg p.o. q.i.d. × 3 days.	Doxycycline 300 mg p.o. × 1 dose, trimethoprim sulfamethoxazole 160–800 mg b.i.d. × 3 days, or fluoroquinolone × 3 days.
Vibrio non-cholera, O139	Antibiotics are usually not required. Tetracycline 500 mg p.o. q.i.d. × 3 days.	Doxycycline 300 mg p.o. × 1 dose, fluoroquinolone × 3 days.
Yersinia	Antibiotics are not usually required. Ciprofloxacin 500 mg p.o. b.i.d. × 3 days or other fluoroquinolone.	Doxycycline and aminoglycoside or trimethoprim sulfamethoxazole

[1] antibiotics are usually not needed unless the patient is immunocompromised.
[2] infection may spontaneously resolve in immunocompetent patients and in HIV patients with a CD4 count over 150 cell/mm³.
[3] antibiotics are needed if the patient is severely ill, immunocompromised, septicemic prone, an uncontrolled diabetic, or in traveler's diarrhea.
[4] not effective for all species.
[5] fumagillin is not licensed in the US, but can be obtained through the Centers for Disease Control and Prevention.
[6] antibiotics are usually not needed unless the patient is immunocompromised or severely ill.
[7] bacterial antibiotic sensitivity should be checked.
[8] if the illness is mild, antimicrobial therapy is not indicated. If the patient is immunosuppressed or 50 years old antibiotics are indicated.
[9] antibiotics are usually not needed unless the patient is severely ill, under 6 months or over 65 years old, immunocompromised, an uncontrolled diabetic or septicemic prone conditions.
[10] used in septicemic cases.
[11] Vibrio cholera 0139 is not susceptible to trimethoprim-sulfamethoxazole.

Further reading

Aranda-Michel J, Giannella RA. Acute diarrhea: a practical review. *Am J Med* 1999; 106: 670–676.

Bennett RG, Greengough WB. Approah to acute diarrhea in the elderly. *Gastroenterol Clin North Am* 1993; 22: 517–533.

Bruckstein AH. Acute diarrhea. *Am Fam Physician* 1988; 38: 217–228.

Dupont HL. Guidelines on acute infectious diarrhea in adults. *Am J Gastroenterol* 1997; 92: 1962–1975.

Guerrant RL, Van Gilder T, Steiner TS. Practice guidelines for the management of infectious diarrhea. *Clin Infect Dis* 2001; 32: 331–351.

Ilnyckyj A. Clinical evaluation and management of acute infectious diarrhea in adults. *Gastroenterol Clin* 2001; 30: 599–609.

Kelsall BL, Guerrant RL. Evaluation of diarrhea in the returning traveler. *Infect Dis Clin North Am* 1992; 6: 413–425.

Kroser JA, Metz DC. Evaluation of the adult patient with diarrhea. *Gastroenterology* 1996; 23: 629–647.

Manatsathit S, Dupont HL, Farthing M. Guideline for the management of acute diarrhea in adults. *J Gastroenterol Hepatol* 2002; 17: S54–S71.

Mandell GL, Bennett JE, Dolin R. *Mandell, Douglas, and Bennett's Principles and Practice of Infectious Diseases* 5th edn. Churchill Livingstone, 2002: pp. 1098–1136.

Scheidler MD, Gianenella RA. Practical management of acute diarrhea. *Hosp Pract* 2001; 36: 49–56.

Yamada T, Alpers DH, Laine L et al. *Textbook of Gastroenterology* 3rd edn. Lippincott Williams and Wilkens, 1999: pp. 867–873.

Chapter 3

Evaluation of Chronic Diarrhea

Lawrence R. Schiller

CHAPTER OUTLINE

INTRODUCTION
   Clinical definition of chronic diarrhea
PATHOPHYSIOLOGY
   Gastrointestinal water transport
   Major mechanisms of chronic diarrhea
CLASSIFICATION OF CHRONIC DIARRHEA
   Osmotic versus secretory diarrhea
   Watery versus fatty versus inflammatory diarrhea
DIFFERENTIAL DIAGNOSIS OF CHRONIC DIARRHEA
   Watery diarrhea
   Fatty diarrhea
   Inflammatory diarrhea
INITIAL EVALUATION AND CLASSIFICATION OF PATIENTS WITH CHRONIC DIARRHEA
   History
   Physical examination
   Routine laboratory testing
   Stool analysis
   Classification of diarrhea
FURTHER EVALUATION OF CHRONIC SECRETORY DIARRHEA
   Exclude infection
   Exclude structural disease
FURTHER EVALUATION OF CHRONIC OSMOTIC DIARRHEA
FURTHER EVALUATION OF CHRONIC INFLAMMATORY DIARRHEA
FURTHER EVALUATION OF CHRONIC FATTY DIARRHEA
DIFFICULT-TO-DIAGNOSE DIARRHEAS
   Fecal incontinence
   Iatrogenic diarrhea
   Surreptitious laxative ingestion
   Microscopic colitis
   Bile-acid induced diarrhea
   Small-bowel bacterial overgrowth
   Pancreatic exocrine insufficiency
   Carbohydrate malabsorption
   Peptide-secreting tumors
   Chronic idiopathic secretory diarrhea
FUNCTIONAL DIARRHEA
FURTHER READING

Introduction

Chronic diarrhea is a common problem among Americans, with a prevalence of up to 5%. Gastroenterologists are often called upon to deal with these patients in a variety of settings. With a broad-ranging differential diagnosis of hundreds of conditions and dozens of diagnostic tests to choose among, every clinician feels some trepidation in evaluating these patients. Yet a thoughtful, systematic approach to evaluation is often rewarded by a correct diagnosis and effective treatment.

Clinical definition of chronic diarrhea

Diarrhea means different things to different people. For most patients, diarrhea is the production of loose or unformed stools usually with increased frequency. For physicians, diarrhea is the production of excessively voluminous stools (typically more than 200 grams per 24 hours). These two clinical definitions do not always coincide; patients may complain of diarrhea yet have normal stool output. This is particularly likely to occur if fecal incontinence is present. Patients have a very poor notion of stool volume and it is impossible to extrapolate stool frequency to stool volume, for example ten bowel movements a day may only produce a total of 200 grams of stool if each bowel movement averages 20 grams. Thus the only way to accurately assess stool output is to measure the output quantitatively.

The differentiation between acute and chronic diarrhea is arbitrary but useful. For most purposes, a duration of 4 weeks or more excludes acute infectious conditions which should have run their course during that time (see Chapter 2). Infections can still be responsible for chronic diarrhea, but the likely pathogens are quite different and attention can be directed to other conditions.

Pathophysiology

Gastrointestinal water transport

Loose, voluminous stools are the result of too much water being retained intraluminally. Thus, understanding gastrointestinal water transport is the key to understanding the pathophysiology of diarrhea.

Normal stool output averages 100 g/24 h (slightly less in women and slightly more in men) and stool water makes up about 70% of that amount (70 mL). Increasing stool water by as little as 10% can result in loosening of stool, depending on the water-binding characteristics of stool solids. Stool solids interact with stool water by solvation and other chemical reactions. Not all solids interact with water to a similar extent. For example, fat interacts very little with water and thus for any given percentage of water in stool, fatty stools will be looser than stools with less fat. The ability of fiber to bind water is the reason that adding fiber to the diet of a patient with diarrhea can improve stool consistency (although it may increase stool weight).

In health, the gastrointestinal tract transports large amounts of water into the lumen in the form of digestive secretions, and absorbs that large volume and almost all of the ingested fluid volume to produce stools containing very little water. Each day 1 to 2 liters of water is ingested as food and drink and is complemented by 7 to 8 liters of secretions from the salivary glands, stomach, pancreas, and biliary tract. Thus the volume of fluid flow past the ligament of Trietz is approximately 9 to 10 liters daily. Fluid is avidly absorbed by the jejunum and ileum and fluid flow at the ileocecal valve is reduced to only 1 to 1.5 liters per day. The colon removes 90% of this load, and so stool water represents only about 1% of the fluid entering the gut each day.

Diarrhea develops if the efficiency of water absorption declines by as little as 1%. Reduction of net water absorption may be due to a reduced rate of water absorption by the mucosa, stimulation of secretion, or speeding fluid through the intestines thereby reducing the time for absorption to take place. Relatively minor disturbances may produce sufficient water malabsorption to result in diarrhea.

Major mechanisms of chronic diarrhea

Several mechanisms can reduce net water absorption enough to cause chronic diarrhea. These include infection, inflammation, reduction of the mucosal surface area, ingestion of poorly absorbed, osmotically active substances, absence of an ion-transport mechanism, dysregulation, and circulating secretagogues.

Infection

Several microbes can be responsible for chronic diarrhea. Bacteria causing chronic diarrhea include *Plesiomonas*, *Aeromonas*, *Mycobacterium tuberculosis*, and *Yersinia* spp. These organisms produce diarrhea by releasing enterotoxins or by producing chronic inflammation. Normal gut bacteria may also produce diarrhea by overgrowth in the small intestine, thereby disrupting the absorptive process by deconjugating bile acids, and perhaps by toxin production. Viruses that may be responsible for chronic diarrhea include cytomegalovirus and herpes, especially in immunosuppressed patients. The role of HIV as a direct cause of enteropathy and diarrhea remains controversial. Protozoa that can cause chronic diarrhea include *Giardia, Entamoeba histolytica, Cryptosporidium,* and *Microsporidia*. The pathogenicity of *Blastocystis hominis* is less certain.

Inflammation

Many inflammatory conditions that involve the intestine are associated with diarrhea. While diarrhea may be the consequence of structural changes due to inflammation, such as fistula formation, diarrhea is usually due to the release of cytokines and other inflammatory mediators that have affect enterocytes and the enteric nervous system reducing the rate of absorption or speed of transit through the intestine.

Reduction of the mucosal surface area

Intestinal resection or mucosal disease causing extensive ulceration reduces the surface area available for absorption to take place. In many instances, more distal parts of the small intestine and colon can compensate for the loss of surface area. There are two situations in which this is not possible however. First, so much surface area may have been resected or may be diseased that there is not enough functional mucosa more distally to compensate. Second, the missing or dysfunctional area may have a specialized function that cannot be duplicated by more distal areas. For instance, loss of the terminal ileum compromises bile acid and vitamin B_{12} absorption and the colon cannot actively absorb these substances. Thus, loss of the terminal ileum produces bile acid and vitamin B_{12} malabsorption, even though the colon may be intact.

Ingestion of poorly absorbed, osmotically active substances

Unlike the renal tubule, the intestine cannot maintain an osmotic gradient between luminal contents and the plasma because of its high permeability to water. Thus intestinal contents come into osmotic equilibrium with plasma within the jejunum and remain isosmolar with body fluids (approximately 290 mOsm/kg) thereafter. If an osmotically active substance that cannot be absorbed is ingested, it will remain in the lumen and obligate retention of water to keep intraluminal contents isosmolar with plasma. Electrolyte absorption continues, reducing sodium and potassium concentrations to low levels and eventually luminal contents are close to being an isosmolar solution of the poorly absorbed substance. If a sufficient amount of the poorly absorbed substance is ingested and is not metabolized, enough water may be retained intraluminally to produce diarrhea. Common causes of osmotic diarrhea include ingestion of magnesium salts, lactose ingestion by lactase-deficient individuals, excessive fructose ingestion, and ingestion of mannitol or sorbitol.

Absence of an ion-transport mechanism

In rare individuals mutations impair the activity of specific transport proteins. For example, the apical chloride–bicarbonate exchanger of the ileum and colon is dysfunctional in congenital chloridorrhea. As a result of this mutation, chloride becomes poorly absorbed in the distal intestine and patients lose water osmotically into the stool. Congenital abnormalities of sodium transport have also been described.

Dysregulation

Absorption and secretion are carefully regulated by the enteric nervous system and by release of local mediators, such as 5-hydroxytryptamine (serotonin) and various peptides. Dysfunction of this regulatory system can lead to reduced absorption and consequent diarrhea. It is likely that many "functional" diarrheas, such as irritable bowel syndrome, are due to this mechanism. More concrete examples are those diarrheas occurring after vagotomy or sympathectomy in which regulatory nerves are destroyed surgically.

Circulating secretagogues

Tumors of the enteroendocrine cells in the gut wall or pancreas can result in the secretion of large amounts of peptide hormones that can cause diarrhea. These tumor syndromes are quite rare and usually present with a group of symptoms, such as flushing or hives, that are characteristic of the particular secretagogues that are released.

Classification of chronic diarrhea

The rationale for differentiating acute from chronic diarrhea has already been discussed. Other classification schemes can help to organize the physician's thinking about chronic diarrhea and direct the evaluation in productive ways.

Osmotic versus secretory diarrhea

Ingestion of poorly absorbed, osmotically active substances has already been discussed as a mechanism for the production of diarrhea. At best this mechanism accounts for only a small fraction of cases of diarrhea. Many more are due to "secretory" processes in which net intestinal electrolyte absorption is reduced because of diminished rates of electrolyte absorption or increased rates of intestinal secretion. This classification is of most use in the evaluation of chronic watery diarrhea in which osmotic diarrheas need to be identified early in the diagnostic process (see below).

Watery versus fatty versus inflammatory diarrhea

For clinical purposes the most useful classification of chronic diarrhea is based on the gross characteristics of stool and simple laboratory testing

- watery diarrhea is characterized by its fluidity and the absence of blood or pus
- fatty diarrhea is typified by greasy, often light-colored stools that have an excess of fat globules when examined under the microscope with Sudan or other lipophilic stains
- inflammatory diarrhea is epitomized by the presence of blood and pus.

Thus the patient's description of the stools, gross inspection of the stools, fecal occult blood testing, and microscopic inspection of the stool for excess fat globules and white blood cells can be used to identify the type of diarrhea and thereby limit the differential diagnosis.

Differential diagnosis of chronic diarrhea

Watery diarrhea

Most patients with substantial chronic diarrhea (more than 500 g/24 h) have watery diarrhea. Causes for chronic watery diarrhea are numerous (Box 3.1).

Osmotic diarrheas

Osmotic diarrheas are due to ingestion of poorly absorbed, osmotically active substances. These include poorly absorbed anions and cations, such as phosphate, sulfate, and magnesium. These substances may be ingested surreptitiously as a form of factitious diarrhea due to laxative ingestion, but more often are accidently ingested as components of mineral supplements or antacids. For example, many calcium supplements contain magnesium, both for its intrinsic benefits and to offset the constipating effect of calcium.

Another cause for osmotic diarrhea is ingestion of poorly absorbed carbohydrates and carbohydrate derivatives, such as the sugar alcohols, mannitol and sorbitol. Disaccharides, such as sucrose and lactose, must be cleaved into monosaccharides in order to be transported into enterocytes. Sucrase and lactase, the disaccharidases present in the highest amounts in the small intestine, may be congenitally absent or inactive because of mutations in their respective genes. Patients with these problems will have symptoms from infancy.

Lactase deficiency also can occur later in life. Intestinal lactase activity normally is downregulated by adulthood in most mammals and humans. A minority of humans (mostly those from the northern European gene pool) retain lactase activity into adult life, but even in this group, lactase activity often declines with age. The majority of people with lactose intolerance realize that lactose ingestion causes gassiness or diarrhea and avoid ingestion of dairy products. On the other hand, some individuals who retained lactase activity into adulthood may not recognize lactose ingestion as a cause for their symptoms, because they were always able to ingest milk and dairy products in the past.

The sugar alcohols, mannitol and sorbitol, are very sweet, but are poorly absorbed by the intestinal mucosa, making them ideal as non-nutritive sweeteners as long as they are ingested in limited amounts. If too much is ingested, gassiness and eventually diarrhea develop as the capacity of the flora in the colon to metabolize carbohydrate is exceeded. The threshold for symptoms may be as low as 10 grams and may be altered by the ingestion of antibiotics that affect the colonic flora. Common sources for sugar alcohols are dietetic candies, "sugarless" chewing gum, and medications, mainly syrups and suspensions.

Secretory diarrheas

Secretory diarrheas account for the vast majority of cases of watery diarrhea and for the largest differ-

Box 3.1 Differential diagnosis of chronic diarrhea

Chronic watery diarrhea
Osmotic diarrhea
    osmotic laxatives (e.g. Mg^{+2}, PO_4^{-3}, SO_4^{-2})
    carbohydrate malabsorption
Secretory diarrhea
    congenital syndromes (e.g. congenital chloridorrhea)
    bacterial toxins
    ileal bile-acid malabsorption
    inflammatory bowel disease
        ulcerative colitis
        Crohn's disease
        microscopic colitis
            lymphocytic colitis
            collagenous colitis
        diverticulitis
    vasculitis
    drugs and poisons
    laxative abuse (stimulant laxatives)
    disordered motility/regulation
        postvagotomy diarrhea
        postsympathectomy diarrhea
        diabetic autonomic neuropathy
        irritable bowel syndrome
Endocrine diarrhea
    hyperthyroidism
    Addison's disease
    gastrinoma
    VIPoma
    somatostatinoma
    carcinoid syndrome
    medullary carcinoma of the thyroid
    mastocytosis
Other tumors
    colon carcinoma
    lymphoma
    villous adenoma
Idiopathic secretory diarrhea
    epidemic secretory (Brainerd) diarrhea
    sporadic idiopathic secretory diarrhea

Chronic inflammatory diarrhea
Inflammatory bowel disease
    ulcerative colitis
    Crohn's disease
    diverticulitis
    ulcerative jejunoileitis
    infectious diseases
        pseudomembranous colitis (e.g. *Clostridium difficile*)
        invasive bacterial infections (e.g. tuberculosis, yersinosis)
        ulcerating viral infections (e.g. cytomegalovirus, herpes simplex virus)
        invasive parasitic infections (e.g. amebiasis, strongyloidiasis)
    ischemic colitis
    radiation colitis
    neoplasia
        colon cancer
        lymphoma

Chronic fatty diarrhea
Malabsorption syndromes
    mucosal diseases (e.g. celiac disease, Whipple's disease)
    short bowel syndrome
    small-bowel bacterial overgrowth
    mesenteric ischemia
Maldigestion
    Pancreatic exocrine insufficiency
    Inadequate luminal bile-acid concentration

---

ential diagnosis of any category of diarrheal diseases (Box 3.1).

Bacterial enterotoxins and immunological mediators, such as cytokines, reduce fluid and electrolyte absorption or promote their secretion by the intestine and are common causes of secretory diarrhea. Blood and pus in stools, findings characteristic of inflammatory diarrhea, are present only when bacteria or inflammation cause mucosal ulceration, accounting for the paradox that these "inflammatory" causes of diarrhea may produce a "secretory" diarrhea. This is often the case with microscopic colitis, a condition in which mucosal inflammation is responsible for diarrhea, but white blood cells are inconsistently found because ulceration is not present (see discussion below). Other forms of inflammation, such as vasculitis, may also produce a secretory diarrhea.

Many drugs and some poisons may produce chronic diarrhea. More than half of the approved drugs in the US Pharmacopeia list diarrhea as a potential side effect. While some, like lactulose, produce diarrhea by an osmotic mechanism, most produce a secretory diarrhea. A special category of drugs causing diarrhea are non-osmotic laxatives such as senna. These drugs may be ingested surreptitiously to produce factitious diarrhea (see below).

Another cause of secretory diarrhea is bile-acid malabsorption by the ileum. Each day bile acids cycle from the liver to the small intestine and back again to help with the solublization of dietary fat. If the terminal ileum is diseased or has been resected, bile acid spills into the colon and may reach a concentration of 3 to 5 mmol/L, the level at which colonic absorption is inhibited. The prevalence of bile-acid malabsorption as a cause of chronic diarrhea is controversial (see below).

An indisputably uncommon cause for chronic diarrhea is congenital absence of a mucosal electrolyte transporter. The best described of these is congenital chloridorrhea, an absence of the chloride–bicarbonate exchanger that is normally present in the ileum and colon. This defect makes it impossible to absorb chloride against a concentration gradient, and so chloride accumulates within the lumen obligating excretion of water. This can be treated by reducing dietary chloride ingestion and by reducing chloride secretion by the stomach by inhibition of gastric-acid secretion. Defects in sodium transporters have also been described.

Motility disorders may result in intestinal hurry, in which there may not be enough time for complete absorption to occur, resulting in watery diarrhea. These include surgeries in which the extrinsic innervation of the gut is interrupted, such as vagotomy and sympathectomy, diabetic autonomic neuropathy, hyperthyroidism, and some cases of irritable bowel syndrome. Less well-described syndromes such as idiopathic secretory diarrhea may also involve intestinal hurry.

Neuroendocrine tumors that produce secretagogues, such as gastrin, vasoactive intestinal polypeptide, calcitonin, serotonin, and kinins, may also cause a secretory diarrhea. While there has been a great emphasis on the effect of secretagogues on intestinal electrolyte transport, they may produce diarrhea mainly by intestinal hurry. These tumors are very rare and their diagnosis may be complicated (see below).

Other conditions that should be considered in the differential diagnosis of secretory diarrhea include colon cancer, which may rarely present with diarrhea, and Addison's disease. Patients with Addison's disease typically have nausea, vomiting, and fatigue along with watery diarrhea.

Patients with secretory diarrhea that has evaded diagnosis after a detailed evaluation are said to have "chronic idiopathic secretory diarrhea". This condition occurs in both sporadic and epidemic forms and has a remarkably consistent clinical course (see below).

Fatty diarrhea

Fatty diarrhea is the result of malabsorption or maldigestion. Malabsorption occurs in patients with mucosal diseases, such as celiac sprue, short-bowel syndrome due to extensive small-bowel resection, small-bowel bacterial overgrowth, and mesenteric ischemia. Maldigestion is the result of defective luminal digestion because of pancreatic exocrine insufficiency or bile-acid deficiency. Although many disorders can produce these defects (Box 3.1), it is usually possible to work through the differential diagnosis of fatty diarrhea successfully.

Inflammatory diarrhea

Idiopathic inflammatory bowel disease (ulcerative colitis and Crohn's disease) and invasive bacterial infections are the major causes of diarrhea with blood and pus. Since most bacterial infections run their courses within 4 weeks, invasive bacterial infection is a rare cause of chronic diarrhea. Other potential causes include chronic ulcerating viral colitis, such as that due to cytomegalovirus, ischemic colitis, radiation colitis, and cancers with ulcerated surfaces.

Initial evaluation and classification of patients with chronic diarrhea (Figure 3.1)

History

A careful history can go a long way toward making a diagnosis in patients with chronic diarrhea. Attention should focus initially on the onset of diarrhea. In some patients the onset is insidious, with a gradual change from their normal bowel habits to diarrhea. This pattern is often the case in slowly progressive systemic illnesses, such as diabetes. In others the onset is sudden with the patient able to specify the date of onset. This pattern is often the case with infections, with inflammatory bowel disease, and with chronic idiopathic secretory diarrhea. The course of diarrhea should also be reviewed; progressively increasing or decreasing diarrhea, or a stable course should be noted. The physician should also record whether the diarrhea has been intermittent or continuous since onset.

Epidemiological factors that should be explored include any travel history preceding the onset of

Initial evaluation and classification of patients with chronic diarrhea

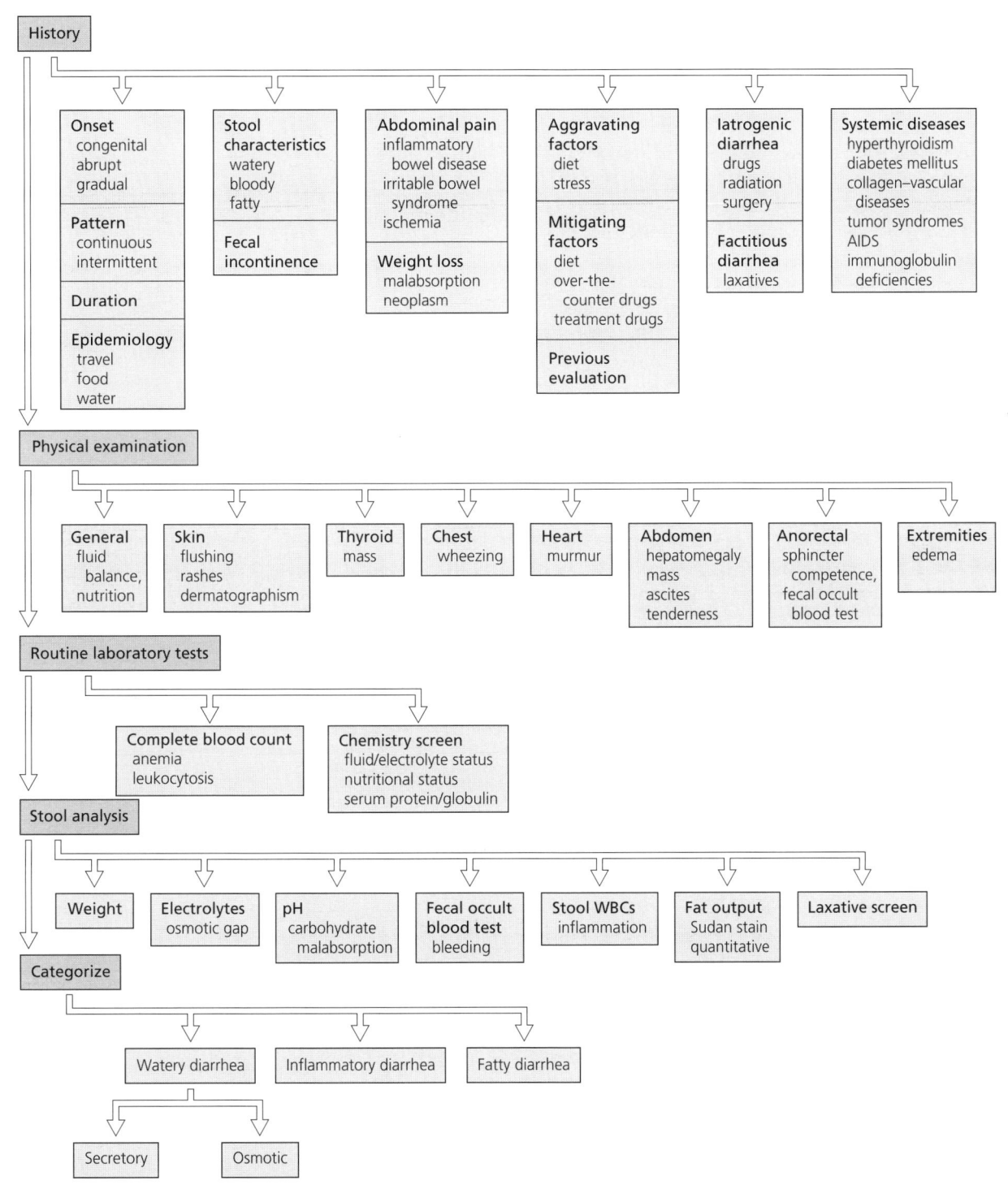

Figure 3.1 Flow chart, or "mind map", for the initial evaluation of chronic diarrhea. Efforts should be directed to the classification of chronic diarrhea based on history, physical examination, basic laboratory tests, and stool analysis (reproduced from Fine KD, Schiller LR. American Gastroenterological Association technical review on the evaluation and management of chronic diarrhea. *Gastroenterology* 1999; 116: 1464–1486).

diarrhea, living conditions and water source, occupation, sexual preference, and use of illicit drugs or alcohol. Patients living in rural areas may be exposed to farm animals that may harbor pathogenic bacteria such as *Salmonella*. Ingestion of well water or raw milk has been associated with epidemics of chronic diarrhea (e.g. Brainerd diarrhea). Health-care workers are at risk of acquiring nosocomial infections and having factitious diarrhea. Anal intercourse is a risk factor for proctitis associated with gonorrhea, herpes simplex, *Chlamydia*, syphilis, and amebiasis. Promiscuous or unprotected sex is a risk factor for acquired immunodeficiency syndrome (AIDS) and the many causes of diarrhea in that syndrome. It is also important to note details of contacts who may have had diarrhea starting at about the same time and their family history.

Some estimation of severity should be made. Frequency is only a rough guide to the severity of diarrhea; patients may have equal daily volumes of stool passed in two large bowel movements or twenty small bowel movements each day. Patients have at best a marginal concept of the volume of their bowel movements. The physician should try to ascertain whether individual stool volumes are "large" or "small" realizing that these estimates may not reflect reality. Better measurements of severity are the need for hospitalization for administration of fluids, and weight loss. Most patients with severe diarrhea realize that they can reduce stool frequency by fasting and consequently lose weight. Weight loss may be due to other factors of course such as food aversions, and neoplastic or inflammatory diseases.

Another feature often considered as a measure of severity by patients is the symptom of fecal incontinence. Incontinence can make a bad situation worse by adding social stigma to a difficult problem, but it is not due to voluminous diarrhea. If the continence mechanisms are intact, prodigious diarrhea can be passed in controlled circumstances. Incontinence almost always is the result of compromise of the neuromuscular machinery of continence and should be evaluated as a separate problem from the diarrhea.

The relationship of bowel movements to meals, fasting, and sleep should be identified. Most individuals with diarrhea have intact gastrocolic reflexes and will have bowel movements after any sort of meal. Specific foods may induce diarrhea in some people, but most patients do not recognize any relationship if diarrhea occurs more than 1 or 2 hours after ingestion of the inciting food. Changes in diet and any special diets should be noted. Intake of "sugar-free" foods (sometimes sweetened with poorly absorbable sugar alcohols) can cause diarrhea. The usual intake of potentially problematic foods, such as fiber, fruits and fruit juices, vegetables, dairy products and caffeinated beverages, should be estimated. Fasting decreases diarrhea due to almost any cause because there is less food to be absorbed, there is a reduced volume of meal-stimulated secretions which lessens the volume of intraluminal fluid, and the gastrocolic reflex is not triggered. Osmotic diarrheas are abolished by fasting because the poorly absorbed substance is no longer being ingested. Diarrhea that wakes the patient from sleep is likely to be due to a structural or metabolic cause rather than a functional illness such as irritable bowel syndrome.

The consistency, qualities, and content of stools should be noted. Stool consistency can be graded as formed, semi-formed (initially intact but readily disrupted), semi-liquid (unformed but not pourable), liquid (pourable but thick), and watery. These categories roughly correlate with increasing water content. The presence of blood, mucus, and pus suggests inflammatory diarrhea, and pasty, buttery stools with an oil layer in the commode indicate fatty diarrhea. Watery, voluminous stools suggest disorders of the small intestine or proximal colon, while frequent, small-volume stools are often associated with tenesmus, and mushy stools suggest left colon or rectal disorders.

Systemic symptoms, such as fever, fatigue, and weight loss, raise the possibility of inflammatory bowel disease, lymphoma, amebiasis, tuberculosis, Whipple's disease, and other infections and malignancies. Associated symptoms, such as abdominal pain or bloating, can also be illuminating. Periumbilical abdominal pain may be a symptom of mesenteric vascular insufficiency, small-bowel obstruction, or irritable bowel syndrome. Bloating and excess flatus may signal the presence of carbohydrate malabsorption.

Additional history that should be obtained includes a detailed review of previous medical problems, previous surgeries, previous radiation therapy, prescription medications, over-the-counter medications, and herbal and nutritional supplements. Medical problems and surgeries on the gastrointestinal tract may be complicated by diarrhea. Many drugs and supplements can produce diarrhea as a side effect. Patients should be asked about new medications, magnesium preparations, and any antibiotics taken within 2 months of the onset of diarrhea.

Risk factors for laxative abuse should be explored. Patients at risk include those who may have indicators of anorexia or bulimia, those with secondary gains from diarrhea (such as disability status), patients with many previous consultations raising the question of Munchausen's syndrome, and patients who are children or dependent adults who could be poisoned by a caregiver.

Physical examination

The most important signs to note are those that indicate the volume status and nutritional status of the patient, i.e. postural hypotension, skin turgor, hydration of mucous membranes, subcutaneous fat, muscle mass, and evidence of vitamin deficiencies. Examination of an old photograph (e.g. on a driver's license) can reveal subtle changes in appearance that may be of diagnostic value.

Occasionally, physical findings may be clues to a specific diagnosis. For example, flushing can be seen in carcinoid syndrome, medullary carcinoma of the thyroid, or pancreatic cholera syndrome (VIPoma). Necrotizing migratory erythema, a scaling red dermatitis, is characteristic of glucagonoma. Urticaria pigmentosa is seen with mastocytosis. Other physical findings that can be helpful include the presence of mouth ulcers, evidence of atherosclerosis, lymphadenopathy, and findings of peripheral edema or neuropathy.

Examination of the abdomen is usually of little direct value, although any abnormalities that are detected can be a great help with diagnosis. For example, hepatomegaly or abdominal mass may point toward a diagnosis of malignancy. Tenderness may indicate inflammatory disease. Patients put great emphasis on borborygmi as evidence of bowel dysfunction, but the pitch and loudness of bowel sounds is of little diagnostic help.

A careful rectal examination is indicated in all patients complaining of diarrhea. Findings of fissures, fistulas, fluctuance, and tenderness suggest inflammatory bowel disease. The examiner should ask the patient to contract the external anal sphincter as if to prevent evacuation and try to appreciate the strength of the anal sphincter mechanism. Weakness raises the possibility of fecal incontinence. Some patients with diarrhea have fecal incontinence complicating their condition and others complain of diarrhea, but only have incontinence with no real alteration in stool consistency. A fraction of patients complaining of diarrhea will have formed stool in the rectal vault, suggesting either intermittency of diarrhea or incontinence as the real problem. If stool is present, the examiner should appreciate its color and consistency and test it for occult blood.

Routine laboratory testing

A complete blood count looking for anemia or leukocytosis, and chemistry screening to assess fluid and electrolyte status, renal function, liver function, nutritional status, and thyroid function should be done in all patients with chronic diarrhea. These tests provide evidence of the impact of diarrhea on the patient and may provide clues to the diagnosis.

Stool analysis

Information critical to the classification of diarrhea as watery, fatty, or inflammatory is provided by stool analysis. All of the necessary information can be obtained from a spot stool sample, but quantitative information can be very helpful in assessing diarrhea, and so a timed stool collection is preferable. The duration of stool collection required to produce reproducible results depends on the intensity of diarrhea. The more voluminous the diarrhea, the shorter the stool collection need be to be representative. In general, a 48-hour stool collection is adequate for most patients with chronic diarrhea. Longer collections should be considered in patients with formed or semi-formed stools in whom stool weights are likely to be lower, or if greater precision is needed. Measurement of stool weight allows an assessment of the severity of diarrhea and calculation of quantitative output of fat and minerals which may be important in some circumstances.

In general, stools should be collected while the patient consumes his or her usual diet. If possible, a record of dietary intake during the collection should be made and analyzed later by a dietician to estimate fat and calorie intake. This can be used to calculate fractional fat absorption instead of mandating a 100 gram fat intake which many patients find problematic. If both secretory and malabsorptive processes are driving diarrhea, collection of a stool sample while fasting may be helpful in distinguishing the relative contributions of impaired fluid and electrolyte absorption and malabsorption to stool output. Diarrhea that persists while fasting is due to secretory mechanisms. On the other hand, diarrhea that ceases with fasting suggests that some ingested substance is causing the diarrhea.

Stool weight should be recorded and expressed as g/24 h. Stool weights are rarely, if ever, more than 500 g/24 h in irritable bowel syndrome and infrequently less than 1000 g/24 h in severe secretory diarrhea, such as pancreatic cholera syndrome. Stool weight can also be used as an indicator of the need for fluid repletion. Daily outputs of less than

1000 grams are unlikely to be associated with dehydration as long as the patient can eat and drink. Patients with stool weights more than 2000 g/24 h often require supplemental intravenous fluid or an intensive oral rehydration program. Normal stool weights (less than 200 g/24 h) in patients complaining of "severe" diarrhea raise the issue of fecal incontinence as the major problem.

Inspection of the collected stool is quite valuable. Watery stools are pourable and have little substance. Fatty stools tend to be sticky and buttery in consistency. Inflammatory diarrheas are characterized by stools that have mucus and gross blood mixed in.

Measurement of stool electrolytes (sodium and potassium) is quite useful in patients with watery diarrhea. If concentrations of these electrolytes are high, stool water is increased because of a defect in net electrolyte absorption (i.e. secretory diarrhea). If concentrations of electrolytes are low, excess stool water is retained intraluminally because some other osmotically active substance is present (i.e. osmotic diarrhea). This relationship can be quantified by calculating the fecal osmotic gap. For purposes of this calculation, intraluminal osmolality is taken as equal to body fluid osmolality (290 mOsm/kg or measured serum osmolality) and the contribution of electrolytes to that osmolality is taken to be twice the sum of the measured sodium and potassium concentrations in stool water to account for anions that are present. (Fecal anions include chloride, bicarbonate, and short chain fatty acids. Fermentation *in vitro* generates short chain fatty acids rapidly which then can react with bicarbonate in stool water and so measurement of these moieties in stool water is not an accurate reflection of their concentrations intraluminally.) The fecal osmotic gap is then calculated using the following equation.

Fecal osmotic gap = $290 - 2(Na + K)$

A value equal to or less than 50 mOsm/kg indicates that most of the stool water osmolality is due to electrolytes and hence a secretory diarrhea is present. A fecal osmotic gap greater than 100 mOsm/kg is consistent with low electrolyte concentrations in stool water and is the signature of an osmotic diarrhea. Intermediate values can be seen in mixed osmotic and secretory processes (e.g. short-bowel syndrome, celiac disease).

Although measured stool osmolality is not used to calculate the fecal osmotic gap for the reasons mentioned above, it may be useful if tampering with the stool collection is suspected. Unlike the nephron, the gut has no mechanisms that allow dilution of luminal contents below serum osmolality. Measured stool osmolality substantially less than 290 mOsm/kg therefore indicates addition of water or hypotonic urine to the specimen. This adulteration may be accidental or intentional, but needs explanation.

Fecal pH is another simple measurement with implications in the diagnosis of chronic diarrhea. In most secretory states, substantial bicarbonate remains in stool water and so fecal pH remains near neutral (pH 7.0). Patients ingesting calcium carbonate or magnesium oxide may have slightly alkaline stools. Low fecal pH is most useful in suggesting carbohydrate malabsorption. Because colonic bacteria ferment malabsorbed carbohydrate and dietary fiber into short chain fatty acids, luminal contents become more acid. This process may continue *in vitro* after stool collection, exaggerating acidification. A measured stool pH less than 5.3 is strongly suggestive of isolated carbohydrate malabsorption, whereas a value over 5.6 suggests that additional mechanisms of diarrhea are present. Patients with generalized malabsorption tend to have less acid stools because of buffering by proteins and amino acids. Carbohydrate excretion can be measured directly with anthrone reagent and reducing sugars can be identified by Clinitest tablets, but these tests are rarely used.

Fecal fat excretion can be estimated by qualitative testing or quantified by chemical testing. Carefully done qualitative testing (e.g. Sudan staining of a fecal smear) correlates well with quantitative analysis and may be adequate to identify steatorrhea, even on a random stool specimen. Quantitative analysis is preferable in order to get the most information from a timed stool collection. Steatorrhea is defined as excretion of over 7 g/24 h (or 7% of fat intake) by most laboratories. Values between 7 and 14 g/24 h may be due just to the presence of diarrhea, and the test is specific for primary defects in fat absorption only when fat output exceeds 14 g/day.

The concentration of fat in stools can provide a clue to the cause of steatorrhea. Because pancreatic and biliary causes of steatorrhea (e.g. pancreatic exocrine insufficiency, advanced primary biliary cirrhosis) do not interfere with mucosal fluid absorption, but do compromise fat absorption substantially, the concentration of fat in stools is high. Conversely, in diseases in which mucosal absorption is compromised (e.g. celiac disease), malabsorbed fat is "diluted" in a larger stool volume and fecal fat concentration is lower. Fecal fat concentrations over 9.5 g/100 g stool are typical of pancreatic or biliary steatorrhea and values less than 9.5 g/100 g stool are characteristic of small-intestinal problems.

Additional tests that may be valuable to do on an initial stool specimen include fecal occult blood testing, assessment for fecal leukocytes, and laxative screening. Detection of gastrointestinal bleeding points toward inflammatory and neoplastic causes of chronic diarrhea. Many patients with chronic diarrhea have hemorrhoids, and rectal bleeding or a positive fecal occult blood test may be attributed to them. This conclusion should not be accepted unless other causes for bleeding have been excluded. Fecal leukocytes are another marker of mucosal inflammation. Their presence can be detected by staining a fecal smear and examining it with a microscope, or by chemical testing for leukocyte-specific enzymes such as lactoferrin. Tests are available for most laxatives including magnesium, phosphate, sulfate, senna, and bisacodyl. Laxative testing can be considered in the initial evaluation of patients who are likely candidates for laxative abuse or it can be postponed until a later stage in the evaluation of undiagnosed patients with chronic diarrhea.

Classification of diarrhea

At this point in the evaluation of patients with chronic diarrhea, the diarrhea can be categorized as watery diarrhea (with the subtypes of osmotic and secretory diarrhea), inflammatory diarrhea, or fatty diarrhea. This classification has important implications in limiting the differential diagnosis (Box 3.1). The physician also can make an assessment of the severity of diarrhea and outline the further evaluation of the problem.

Further evaluation of chronic secretory diarrhea (Figure 3.2A)

Exclude infection

Although the definition of chronic diarrhea (4 weeks or longer in duration) is designed to exclude most infections, some pathogens may produce chronic diarrhea and so infection should be excluded early in the evaluation of chronic secretory diarrhea. A standard bacterial culture should be submitted. The laboratory should be alerted to look for unusual bacterial pathogens that may require special culture techniques, such as *Aeromonas*, *Plesiomonas*, *Yersinia*, and tuberculosis. Serologic testing for HIV and cytomegalovirus should be considered in patients at risk for these infections. Standard microscopic evaluation of stools for ova and parasites, special stains for detecting coccidia and *Microsporidia*, and ELISA for *Giardia* spp. antigen should be obtained. A stool specimen should be analyzed for the presence of *Clostridium difficile* toxin, since this pathogen can cause chronic and recurrent diarrhea.

Exclude structural disease

Computerized tomography (CT) of the abdomen and pelvis, especially with high-resolution techniques such as spiral CT, is useful in the diagnosis of pancreatic tumors, lymphoma, inflammatory bowel disease, and other conditions that may cause secretory diarrhea. Computed tomography should be considered early in the further evaluation of secretory diarrhea, particularly if other clues point to one of these diagnoses. Since many causes of chronic secretory diarrhea involve the small intestine, small-bowel radiography with either follow-through or enteroclysis methods can be helpful.

Endoscopy or push enteroscopy can be used to visualize the mucosal surface and to obtain biopsy specimens and aspirates of luminal contents for quantitative culture. The role of capsule enteroscopy has not been assessed in chronic diarrhea, but it is likely to be less helpful than traditional techniques because specimens cannot be obtained. It may be of value in visualizing mucosal abnormalities in the mid- or distal small bowel that are impossible to detect by other techniques.

Sigmoidoscopy or colonoscopy with biopsy are of benefit in the diagnosis of inflammatory conditions that produce secretory diarrhea, such as microscopic colitis (see pp. 34–35). Since many colonic conditions that produce secretory diarrhea are diffuse and involve the entire colon, sigmoidoscopy with biopsy may be adequate for the assessment of most patients. Conditions which can be diagnosed by inspection of the colonic mucosa include melanosis coli, ulceration, polyps, tumors, Crohn's disease, and ulcerative colitis. Some conditions, in which the mucosa appears normal endoscopically, can be diagnosed by examining colon biopsies microscopically, they include microscopic colitis, amyloidosis, Whipple's disease, granulomatous infections, and chronic schistosomiasis.

Patients in whom the diagnosis is still obscure should be screened for endocrine diarrheas such as those caused by peptide-secreting tumors, mast cell disease, hyperthyroidism, or Addison's disease.

Evaluation of Chronic Diarrhea

More esoteric diagnoses, such as amyloidosis or immune deficiencies, should be considered in appropriate patients and ought to be evaluated with appropriate tests.

One condition that causes secretory diarrhea for which adequate clinical testing is not available is "bile-acid diarrhea." This condition can be due to several problems which compromise ileal bile-acid reabsorption and result in delivery of excess bile acid to the colon where it has cathartic properties (see discussion on pp. 36, 47). For practical purposes an empiric trial of bile-acid binders (e.g. cholestyramine) may be needed for diagnosis. If this is done, a high dose of bile-acid binder should be used initially to "confirm" the clinical diagnosis. The dose can be lowered later to the least effective dose.

Further evaluation of chronic osmotic diarrhea (Figure 3.2B)

When the stool analysis of a patient with watery diarrhea suggests an osmotic diarrhea (fecal osmotic gap greater than 100 mOsm/kg), the physician's job is to discover what poorly absorbed substance is being ingested. Two important clues are available from the stool analysis – fecal pH and magnesium concentration. Stools with a low pH, less than 5.3, indicate that diarrhea is likely to be due to carbohydrate malabsorption. In patients with acid stools, dietary intake review, breath hydrogen testing with various sugars (e.g. lactose, fructose), or direct assay of jejunal biopsy for lactase activity can be used to identify the offending substance. Stools with high magnesium concentrations (or a high daily magnesium output, if collected quantitatively) indicate that excess magnesium is the driving force of osmotic diarrhea. This can be due to inadvertent ingestion (e.g., when calcium supplements also contain magnesium) or as part of a pattern of laxative abuse (see pp. 36, 47). Other osmotic laxatives (such as sodium phosphate, lactulose, or polyethylene glycol) have not been abused frequently, but chemical assays are available for them should the occasion arise.

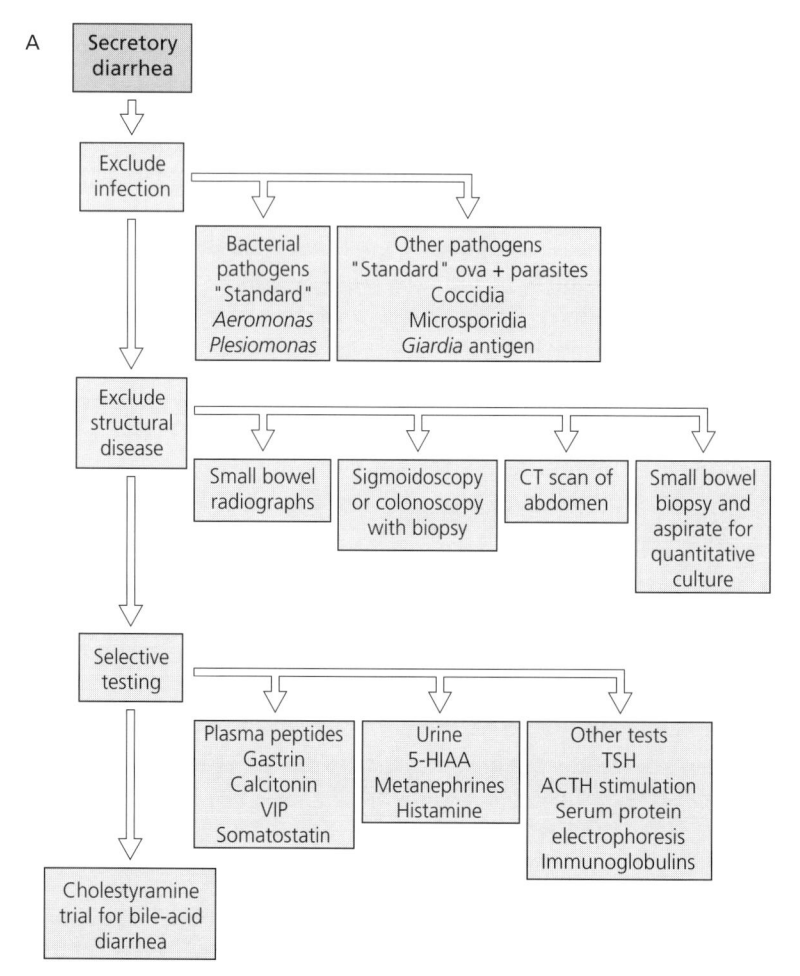

Figure 3.2 Flow charts, or "mind maps", for the further evaluation of chronic (A) secretory diarrhea, (see overleaf for figure 3.2, parts B, C and D)

Further evaluation of chronic inflammatory diarrhea

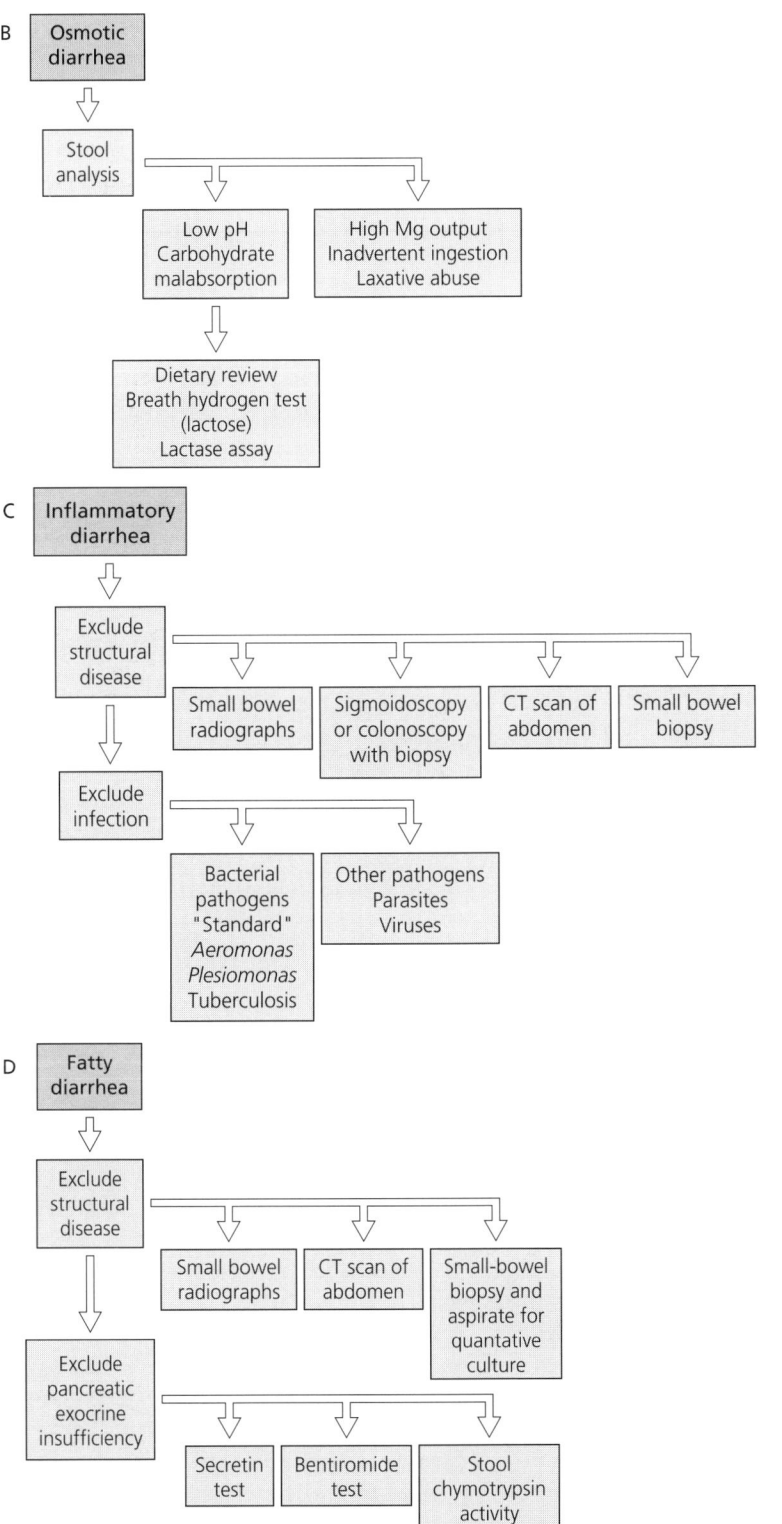

Figure 3.2 (continued) (B) osmotic diarrhea, (C) inflammatory diarrhea, and (D) fatty diarrhea. Every test in a given pathway need not be done once a diagnosis is reached (reproduced from Fine KD, Schiller LR. American Gastroenterological Association technical review on the evaluation and management of chronic diarrhea. *Gastroenterology* 1999; 116: 1464–1486).

B — Osmotic diarrhea → Stool analysis → Low pH / Carbohydrate malabsorption; High Mg output / Inadvertent ingestion / Laxative abuse → Dietary review / Breath hydrogen test (lactose) / Lactase assay

C — Inflammatory diarrhea → Exclude structural disease → Small bowel radiographs; Sigmoidoscopy or colonoscopy with biopsy; CT scan of abdomen; Small bowel biopsy → Exclude infection → Bacterial pathogens "Standard" *Aeromonas*, *Plesiomonas*, Tuberculosis; Other pathogens / Parasites / Viruses

D — Fatty diarrhea → Exclude structural disease → Small bowel radiographs; CT scan of abdomen; Small-bowel biopsy and aspirate for quantative culture → Exclude pancreatic exocrine insufficiency → Secretin test; Bentiromide test; Stool chymotrypsin activity

Further evaluation of chronic inflammatory diarrhea (Figure 3.2C)

When the initial evaluation of chronic diarrhea suggests an inflammatory process, a structural evaluation is most likely to lead to a diagnosis. Sigmoidoscopy or colonoscopy with biopsies and small-bowel radiographs are most often helpful. Properly interpreted biopsy specimens are the key to diagnosis in most of these conditions. Because the clinician knows the case best, personal consultation with the interpreting pathologist can help to reach a proper diagnosis. Computerized tomography of the abdomen and pelvis can provide useful information as to the presence of tumor, bowel-wall thickening, or complications of inflammatory bowel disease, and has assumed a more prominent role in the evaluation of these patients.

If evidence of enteritis or colitis is found, infection needs to be considered. "Standard" bacterial pathogens, such as *Shigella* or *Salmonella*, and less frequent infections, such as tuberculosis or yersinosis, should be sought. Other infections including amebiasis and cytomegalovirus can produce inflammatory diarrhea.

Further evaluation of chronic fatty diarrhea (Figure 3.2D)

Structural problems at a gross or microscopic level account for fatty diarrhea in many patients. Accordingly, evaluation of the small intestine by radiography, endoscopy and biopsy form the basis of the evaluation of steatorrhea. Most causes of malabsorption can be identified by mucosal biopsy and obtaining adequate samples is the key to diagnosis. During the course of endoscopy, it is worthwhile obtaining an aspirate of luminal contents for quantitative bacterial culture to test for bacterial overgrowth.

Pancreatic exocrine insufficiency is the most frequent cause of maldigestion. Formal testing for this condition is difficult. The secretin test is still the gold standard, but problems with the availability of the test limit its use. The bentiromide test, in which an artificial substrate that is hydrolyzed by chymotrypsin is given orally and recovery of the break-down product is measured in the urine, is no longer available commercially. Direct measurements of fecal chymotrypsin or elastase concentrations have been advocated, but probably serve at best as screening tests, because of their relatively low sensitivity, but adequate specificity. Breath tests for the diagnosis of pancreatic exocrine insufficiency have also been disappointing as definitive diagnostic tests. Perhaps the best approach to the diagnosis of pancreatic exocrine insufficiency is a therapeutic trial of pancreatic enzyme therapy. High doses of enzymes and careful documentation of the response of steatorrhea to enzyme supplementation is essential for an adequate interpretation of such a trial.

Rarely, bile-acid deficiency due to ileal resection or impaired bile excretion (e.g. primary biliary cirrhosis) produces maldigestion of fat. Measurement of the concentration of bile acid in the duodenum postprandially is the key to diagnosis. If an empiric, therapeutic trial of bile-acid supplementation is attempted, low doses should be used initially and then the dose should be titrated up in an effort to avoid bile-acid induced diarrhea.

Difficult-to-diagnose diarrheas

In most instances the cause of chronic diarrhea becomes evident as one works through the pathways outlined above. A small number of cases evade diagnosis and those patients are referred to centers specializing in chronic diarrhea. A review of patients referred to our center for difficult-to-diagnose diarrhea revealed that ten problems accounted for most of these cases: fecal incontinence, iatrogenic diarrhea, surreptitious laxative ingestion, microscopic colitis syndrome, bile-acid induced diarrhea, small-bowel bacterial overgrowth, pancreatic exocrine insufficiency, carbohydrate malabsorption, peptide-secreting tumors, and chronic idiopathic secretory diarrhea. This section will review the clinical presentation and diagnosis of these problems.

Fecal incontinence

Many patients do not distinguish between "diarrhea" and "fecal incontinence" and will not volunteer the complaint of incontinence unless prompted. Many physicians view incontinence as a complication of particularly severe diarrhea and not as an independent complaint. This results in overlooking this remediable problem. Every patient with diarrhea should be asked if they have fecal incontinence.

Incontinence is almost always due to defects in the nerves and muscles that regulate the passage of stool from the rectum. These defects can be latent and become evident only when stool consistency loosens. Typically, patients in whom incontinence is the major problem have relatively modest increases in stool weight. A good clue to the presence of incontinence is the patient's complaint of "severe" or "intolerable" diarrhea with a normal stool weight.

Physical examination can provide additional evidence that incontinence is a major problem. A careful digital rectal examination should be done in every patient complaining of diarrhea. The examiner should pay attention to anal tone and then ask the patient to squeeze as if to hold on to a bowel movement to assess external anal sphincter function. The puborectalis muscle should be palpated at rest and when the patient bears down as if defecating. The perineum should be observed during this maneuver to see whether it bulges out, a sign of pelvic floor weakness.

If incontinence is present, anorectal manometry can help to define what parts of the continence mechanism are defective and what parts are functional. This allows a rational treatment program to be developed. In some cases surgical repair of a torn muscle or biofeedback training can remedy the problem. In others the use of constipating drugs can reduce the frequency of episodes of incontinence.

Iatrogenic diarrhea

Diarrhea can be a side effect of drug treatment, surgery, or radiation therapy. While the connections seem obvious after recognition, the contribution of the treatment modality to chronic diarrhea may be missed in prospect. This is particularly true when there is a long gap between the therapy and the occurrence of diarrhea. For instance, it may be years before radiation therapy produces enough damage from progressive fibrosis to produce diarrhea. Likewise, post-surgical diarrhea may not become evident until some complication, such as bacterial overgrowth, occurs.

Drugs

Diarrhea is a side effect of many drugs (Box 3.2). It is important to obtain a complete listing of all medications, both prescribed and over the counter, that the patient is consuming. Particular emphasis should be placed on nutritional and herbal remedies, because these agents are not regulated closely, they may be mislabeled and contain drugs that may cause diarrhea. In general, diarrhea occurring as a result of drug ingestion begins shortly after starting the drug, but this may be masked by concomitant illness or therapy. Every drug that the patient is taking should be suspect and carefully considered as a contributing factor to the complaint of diarrhea.

Surgery

Abdominal surgery may also lead to diarrhea. Surgery for peptic ulcer disease or gastric exclusion for weight control (vagotomy, pyloroplasty, gastric resection, gastric partition with Roux-en-Y gastrojejunostomy) can be complicated by dumping syndrome. In this condition, unregulated emptying of nutrients from the stomach leads to release of humoral mediators and fluid shifts that result in flushing, weakness, hypotension, and diarrhea. This sort of surgery can also lead to bacterial overgrowth and diarrhea as a result of that mechanism. Small-intestinal surgery can also produce short-bowel syndrome, if enough surface area is removed.

Colonic resection produces its own set of problems. Resection of the distal ileum and right colon produces a special defect in the absorption of salt and water against an electrochemical gradient that is not well compensated for by remaining parts of the intestine. These patients often need anomalously high doses of opiates to control diarrhea.

Total colectomy with creation of an end ileostomy or ileoanal anastomosis results in high stool outputs since the function of the colon is absent. Under ideal circumstances, intestinal adaptation results in stool outputs averaging 750 mL daily. Stool output greater than 1250 mL daily is arbitrarily defined as ileostomy diarrhea and places the patient at risk for volume depletion. Ileostomy diarrhea can be due to partial small-bowel or stomal obstruction, stasis, and bacterial overgrowth, and uncovering small-bowel absorptive defects that had been masked by colon absorptive function.

Radiation therapy

Diarrhea resulting from radiation therapy can occur both acutely and a long time after radiation has been administered. Acute radiation enteritis or colitis is due to the immediate effects of radiation on the intestinal mucosa. Chronic radiation enteritis or colitis is thought to be due to ischemia produced by progressive vascular fibrosis. Diarrhea may be due to mucosal dysfunction or bile-acid malabsorption by the ileum leading to bile-acid diarrhea (see pp. 36, 47). Diagnosis is based on radiographic or endoscopic visualization of the gut.

Surreptitious laxative ingestion

Unlike most patients, those with surreptitious laxative ingestion are deceptive and seek medical attention reluctantly or without the expectation of cure. Laxative abusers fall into four categories

1. patients with anorexia or bulimia
2. patients with a secondary gain from illness

Evaluation of Chronic Diarrhea

Box 3.2 Drugs associated with diarrhea

Acetylcholinesterase inhibitors
   donepezil
   galantamine
   tacrine
Aminosalicylate drugs
   balsalazide
   mesalamine
   olsalazine
   sulfasalazine
Antacids and gastric-acid secretion inhibitors
   magnesium-containing antacids
   histamine$_2$-receptor antagonists
   proton pump inhibitors
Antibiotics and antivirals
Antidepressants
   selective serotonin re-uptake inhibitors
Anti-epileptics
   lamotrigine
   tiagabine
   valproic acid
   zonisamide
Anti-estrogens
   anastrozole
   letrozole
   tamoxifen
Anti-hypertensives
   ACE inhibitors
   angiotensin II-receptor antagonists
   beta-adrenergic receptor antagonists
Anti-inflammatory and arthritis drugs
   colchicine
   leflunomide
   non-steroidal anti-inflammatory drugs
Anti-neoplastic agents
   alemtuzumab
   bicalutamide
   capecitabine
   cis-platinum
   doxorubicin
   estramustine
   imatinib
   levamisole
   paclitaxel
   temozolomide
   vinorelbine
Anti-Parkinson's disease drugs and drugs used in neurological diseases
   entacapone
   glatiramer acetate
   riluzole
   tolcapone

Antiplatelet drugs
   anagrelide
   dipyridamole
   ticlopidine
Asthma preparations
   aminophyllin
   inhaled steroids
Biologicals
   erythropoietin analogs
   interferons
   oprelvekin
   vaccines
Chelation therapy
   penicillamine
   succimer
Cholesterol reducers
   gemfibrozil
   HMG-CoA reductase inhibitors
   niacin
Diabetes medications
   acarbose
   metformin
   oral hypoglycemics
   repaglinide
   rosiglitazone
Digoxin
Diuretics
   amiloride
Immunosuppressive drugs
   cyclosporine
   mycophenolate mofetil
   sirolimus
   tacrolimus
Laxatives
Megestrol
Modafinil
Osteoporosis treatment
   bisphosphonates
Pheochromocytoma therapy
   metyrosine
Phosphodiesterase inhibitors
   cilostazol
   sildenafil
Pilocarpine
Prostaglandin analog
   misoprostol
Quinidine
Sevelamer
Thalidomide
Tretinoin

3. patients with Munchausen's syndrome
4. patients with Polle syndrome (Munchausen's syndrome by proxy).

Patients with anorexia or bulimia are usually easy to identify. They are not always underweight, but conversation reveals a concern about excessive body weight that is out of proportion to body size. These patients are often reluctant to seek medical attention and are brought for evaluation by concerned relatives. Stimulant laxative use may result in hypokalemia and dehydration, which may prompt hospitalization.

Patients with secondary gain from factitious diarrhea are often anxious to cooperate with medical testing and may undergo multiple evaluations. Secondary gains from illness range from financial gains by collecting disability payments to strengthening interpersonal relationships by provoking caring behaviors in others. Patients who present disability papers for signature on their first visit or who are accompanied by an overly concerned relative should be suspected of laxative abuse.

Patients with Munchausen's syndrome may be difficult to recognize. The main clue is repeated visits to different physicians over time for evaluation of chronic diarrhea with no diagnosis being reached. These patients seem to make a career of their illnesses and seem resigned to their conditions. Nevertheless, they willingly pursue repeated extensive, expensive, and painful evaluations, even including laparotomy.

The most tragic group of laxative abusers are patients with Polle syndrome or Munchausen's syndrome by proxy who are poisoned with laxatives by their caregivers. These individuals are usually children or dependent adults. The motivation for the actions of the caregivers seems to be to show what good caregivers they can be. The caregivers are hovering and typically stay by the bedside day and night. Patients may be so ill that they are placed on total parenteral nutrition or have enteric feeding tubes placed. The only thing that may cause improvement is placement in an ICU setting where the caregiver cannot give the patient laxatives surreptitiously because access is limited.

In every case suspicion of laxative abuse should lead to analysis of the stool for laxatives. If positive, the test should be repeated on another sample to confirm the diagnosis before confronting the patient with the finding and obtaining psychiatric consultation. Patients who are confronted with the finding of laxative abuse are at risk of suicide and appropriate psychiatric care should be readily available. Patients with Polle syndrome need to be separated from their caregivers and police or other authorities should be involved once the diagnosis is made.

Microscopic colitis syndrome

In the past the existence of this condition has been controversial, but studies over the past 20 years have clarified the situation. Microscopic colitis syndrome is characterized by watery diarrhea with normal gross colonoscopic findings, but microscopic evidence of inflammation of the mucosa with crowding of the lamina propria with inflammatory cells and excess intraepithelial lymphocytes. In addition, some patients have thickening of the subepithelial collagen table while others do not. This differentiates the two subtypes of microscopic colitis – collagenous colitis and lymphocytic colitis. Most pathologists now readily recognize these findings and are less likely to interpret them as nonspecific colitis than in the past.

Patients with microscopic colitis often have other autoimmune conditions, such as arthritis, and it seems likely that the condition is due to dysregulation of the mucosal immune system, but the etiology is still not certain. It is a frequent diagnosis in patients with chronic watery diarrhea, comprising 10% to 20% of such patients in referral practices. The key to diagnosis is to biopsy normal–appearing mucosa in patients with chronic diarrhea. Biopsies can be obtained anywhere in the colon since very few patients have changes only in the right colon. Biopsies should be interpreted by pathologists familiar with the diagnosis.

Bismuth subsalicylate, bile-acid binding resins, and budesonide individually have been shown to be superior to placebo in symptom control. Bismuth subsalicylate seems to produce better regression of histological changes. Other therapies that have been used include 5-aminosalicylate drugs, prednisone, and immunosuppressive drugs, such as azathioprine. Symptoms usually can be controlled with opiate antidiarrheals alone.

Bile-acid induced diarrhea

A variety of conditions may result in entry of excessive bile acid into the colon and diarrhea. The best described of these conditions include ileal resection and disease in which the ileal bile-acid transporter is absent or inactive. Bile-acid malabsorption has also been implicated in the pathogenesis of post-cholecystectomy diarrhea, diarrhea in patients with microscopic colitis, and chronic idiopathic secretory diarrhea. The importance of bile-acid malabsorption in these conditions is moot; while bile-acid malabsorption has been documented, therapy aimed at this condition is not always successful.

Bile-acid malabsorption can be measured in two ways. First, the quantity of bile excreted during a quantitative stool collection can be measured directly by chemical testing. Second, radiolabeled bile-acid retention or excretion can be measured by nuclear medicine techniques. The most common of these methods is to measure whole-body retention of the synthetic bile acid, selena-homocholic acid conjugated with taurine (usually abbreviated as ^{75}Se-HCAT). This method has been widely used in Europe. An alternative is to administer ^{14}C-glycocholate during a 48- or 72-hour stool collection and then measuring fecal recovery.

Bile-acid malabsorption can occur as the result of diarrhea *per se* and therefore is not specific for bile-acid induced diarrhea. Even if bile-acid malabsorption is present, bile-acid concentrations within the colon may not reach the cathartic threshold of 3 to 5 mmol/L, especially if an unusually large volume of fluid enters the colon from the small intestine, and so diarrhea may not be aggravated by bile-acid malabsorption. Because of this, many clinicians use a therapeutic trial of a bile-acid binding resin, such as cholestyramine, as an indirect test for pathological bile-acid malabsorption. The validity of this approach has not been tested prospectively. If this approach is selected, a large dose of resin (e.g. 9 g q.i.d.) should be administered initially; it can be tapered to the least effective dose once an effect has been demonstrated.

Small-bowel bacterial overgrowth

The small intestine is not sterile but has a relatively sparse flora as compared to the lush bacterial flora in the colon. When bacteria build up in the small bowel, they can deconjugate bile acids and cause steatorrhea. It is likely that high concentrations of bacteria can also affect mucosal fluid and electrolyte absorption directly via toxins or immunological mechanisms.

Bacteria can build up in the small intestine under several different circumstances. First, structural problems, such as blind loops or diverticula, may allow build up of bacteria. Second, motility disorders, as seen with diabetes mellitus or scleroderma, may prevent normal clearance mechanisms, such as the migrating motor complex, from operating normally. Third, fistulas from the colon to the stomach or proximal intestine may seed bacteria into the upper intestine. Fourth, hypochlorhydria or achlorhydria may be present, particularly in the elderly or patients taking antisecretory agents, allowing colonization of the gut by ingested bacteria.

The gold standard for diagnosis is quantitative culture of an aspirate of fluid from the proximal intestine. More than 10^6 organisms/mL grown under aerobic or anaerobic conditions is the criterion for a positive culture. The methods of collection are not standardized and precautions must be taken to avoid contamination with oropharyngeal or gastric secretions.

Breath tests have been promoted as non-invasive alternatives to quantitative culture. In one test ^{14}C-glycocholate is given by mouth. If bacteria are present, the bile acid is deconjugated and radioactive carbon dioxide is released and measured in expired air. Another test uses ^{14}C-labeled xylose as the metabolizable substrate. However, xylose may be incompletely absorbed and may reach the colonic flora which will also produce radioactive carbon dioxide. Non-radioactive substrates, such as glucose or lactulose, have also been employed. With these substances, H_2 production by fermentation is detected in the expired air. All breath tests have limited sensitivity and specificity but can be helpful in screening patients for bacterial overgrowth.

Clues to the diagnosis of small-bowel bacterial overgrowth include variable severity of diarrhea and improvement with antibiotic therapy. Recurrence is common and near-continuous therapy with rotation of antibiotics may be needed.

Pancreatic exocrine insufficiency

One would think that the diagnosis of pancreatic exocrine insufficiency would not be readily overlooked, but this is not always the case. Steatorrhea may be relatively mild and inapparent clinically. Diagnostic testing may be difficult to obtain (see p. 44) and empiric trials may not have been conducted properly.

Non-invasive tests, including the bentiromide test, breath tests that assess the hydrolysis of radioactive triolein, the dual marker Schilling test, and measurement of pancreatic enzyme concentrations in the stool, have operating characteristics that make them more appropriate for screening rather than confirmation of a diagnosis of pancreatic exocrine insufficiency. The role of non-invasive pancreatic imaging with magnetic resonance pancreatography in this setting is uncertain.

The gold standard for diagnosis of pancreatic exocrine insufficiency is the secretin test (or the similar secretin–cholecystokinin test). In this test the duodenum is intubated for aspiration of pancreatic secretions and the stomach is intubated and aspirated to prevent gastric secretions from reaching the duodenum (and neutralizing pancreatic bicarbonate). After administration of secretin (or secretin and cholecystokinin) the aspirated fluid is collected and bicarbonate (and enzyme) excretion is measured. Because of the complexity of this test, therapeutic trials of enzyme replacement are often done instead. As pointed out before, an adequate trial requires the administration of a large dose of enzymes and evaluation of efficacy by measurement of stool fat excretion after treatment.

Carbohydrate malabsorption

Diarrhea due to isolated carbohydrate malabsorption (e.g. lactase deficiency) is quite variable, and depends upon the load of carbohydrate ingested. In the average adult the colonic flora is able to ferment approximately 80 g of carbohydrate daily. The products of fermentation include short chain fatty acids, carbon dioxide, and hydrogen gas. Short chain fatty acids are largely absorbed by the colonic mucosa, whereas the gases are only partially absorbed (and excreted in the breath). The clinical implications of this physiology are

1. usually more than 80 g of fermentable carbohydrate must be ingested to cause diarrhea
2. the severity of diarrhea is dependent on how much more than 80 g of carbohydrate is ingested
3. these patients often complain of excessive flatus (unlike patients with secretory diarrhea who are unlikely to be gassy).

These implications account for the finding that, while most adult humans manifest lactose intolerance with a breath hydrogen test, most will not develop diarrhea after ingesting only a glass of milk (containing about 12 g of lactose). When diarrhea occurs with carbohydrate malabsorption, large amounts of the offending substance or combinations of offending substances are ingested.

In addition to lactose, several other simple sugars or sugar alcohols may contribute to carbohydrate-induced diarrhea. Some individuals lack sucrase and malabsorb sucrose. Everyone has a finite capacity to absorb fructose; individuals who ingest large amounts of fruit, honey, or soda pop and other processed foods sweetened with high-fructose corn syrup may exceed their absorption capacity for this sugar. The sugar alcohols, mannitol and sorbitol, are poorly absorbed by the human intestine in spite of being similar in size to glucose. They are used commercially to sweeten "dietetic" candies, "sugar-free" gum, and medicines. Any of these substances can cause diarrhea if ingested in sufficient quantities.

Clinical clues to the presence of carbohydrate-induced diarrhea include intermittency of diarrhea, increased flatus, and production of acid stools with a pH less than 5.3. Analysis of a diet diary is the most useful way to determine what offending carbohydrate is being ingested. As an alternative, stool can be tested with Clinitest tablets or anthrone reagent. Reducing sugars, such as glucose, galactose, fructose, maltose, and lactose, give positive results with Clinitest tablets. Sucrose, lactulose, sorbitol, and mannitol do not react with Clinitest tablets. Anthrone reagent can be used to quantify carbohydrate excretion, but does not pick up mannitol or sorbitol. Eliminating the offending carbohydrate from the diet should cure the diarrhea and can be used as a confirmatory test.

Peptide-secreting tumors

Most physicians caring for a patient with chronic diarrhea consider the possibility that the patient has an endocrine tumor after an initial round of tests fails to yield a diagnosis. This is understandable since we are taught to avoid missing a diagnosis of cancer. The prevalence of these tumors is so low, however, that a peptide-secreting tumor is an unlikely diagnosis. For example, the estimated frequency of VIPoma is 1 per 10 000 000 population. If the annual incidence of chronic diarrhea is 3%, VIPoma will be encountered only once in every 300 000 patients with chronic diarrhea! This rarity affects the use of serum peptide assays to "screen" for endocrine tumors. Given such a low pre-test probability, false positive tests vastly outnumber true positive tests. Stated another way, the positive predictive value of serum peptide tests for tumor-associated diarrhea is very low (roughly 1%).

Strong consideration should be given to tumor-associated diarrhea in the setting of classical syndromes such as carcinoid syndrome, Zollinger–Ellison syndrome, pancreatic cholera syndrome, and multiple endocrine neoplasia. In such circumstances, measurement of serum peptide concentrations can confirm the clinical diagnosis. In everyone else, imaging studies, such as CT of the abdomen or radiolabeled octreotide scanning, should precede measurement of serum peptide levels. This makes sense because with the exception of gastrinoma which can produce symptoms when very small, most of these endocrine tumors have to be bulky or metastatic before producing diarrhea and other symptoms.

Chronic idiopathic secretory diarrhea

Some patients with chronic, continuous watery diarrhea complete a thorough evaluation without a specific diagnosis being made, other than the finding that they have a secretory diarrhea. They can be said to have "sporadic chronic idiopathic secretory diarrhea." While one might expect that these patients would have a variety of different conditions, they have remarkably similar clinical courses. They are in good health before the onset of illness. Typically diarrhea begins suddenly – most patients can recall the particular date of onset. There is often a history of travel to regional vacation areas, such as a state park or lake, just before the onset of illness. Family members are rarely ill. The diarrhea quickly reaches its maximum intensity and patients usually lose 10 to 20 pounds of body weight in the first months of illness. The diarrhea continues for 1 to 2 years and then gradually abates.

A similar pattern of illness can occur in large outbreaks. This is "epidemic chronic idiopathic secretory diarrhea" or Brainerd diarrhea, named after the town in Minnesota that had a well-described outbreak. These outbreaks have been linked to common sources such as water, raw milk, or specific restaurants with suboptimal standards of hygiene. This suggests an infectious etiology, but no recognized bowel pathogens have been isolated in any of these outbreaks.

The clinical similarity of the epidemic form to the sporadic cases suggests that those isolated cases might have an infectious etiology also, but this too is unproven. Antibiotics that are frequently successful against enteric pathogens have no effect in either type of chronic idiopathic secretory diarrhea. Treatment consists of the use of potent antidiarrheal drugs, such as opium or morphine, until spontaneous remission occurs. Patients often appreciate learning that a seemingly endless illness will eventually disappear. The disease does not seem to recur.

Functional diarrhea

The most common casual diagnosis made in patients with chronic diarrhea is irritable bowel syndrome. While this is sometimes appropriate, this diagnosis is a trap for the unwary. Irritable bowel syndrome has been defined as a condition characterized by pain associated with abnormal bowel function. Patients without substantial pain should not be labeled as having irritable bowel syndrome. Patients with continuous diarrhea, especially those without pain, are likely to have one of the other conditions discussed above rather than irritable bowel syndrome.

There may be conditions, for example one called the "painless diarrhea" form of irritable bowel syndrome, that should be labeled as functional diarrhea and criteria for this diagnosis have been promulgated by the Rome group. In my experience, functional diarrhea should be an infrequent diagnosis and should be reserved for patients who have intermittent diarrhea that does not prove to be due to carbohydrate malabsorption or other defined conditions.

Further reading

Donowitz M, Kokke FT, Saidi R. Evaluation of patients with chronic diarrhea. *N Engl J Med* 1995; 332:725–729.

Fernandez-Banares F, Esteve M, Salas A, *et al.* Bile acid malabsorption in microscopic colitis and in previously unexplained functional chronic diarrhea. *Dig Dis Sci* 2001; 46:2231–2238.

Fine KD, Schiller LR. American Gastroenterological Association technical review on the evaluation and management of chronic diarrhea. *Gastroenterology* 1999; 116:1464–1486.

Fine KD, Seidel RH, Do K. The prevalence, anatomic distribution, and diagnosis of colonic causes of chronic diarrhea. *Gastrointest Endosc* 2000; 51:318–326.

Jensen RT. Overview of chronic diarrhea caused by functional neuroendocrine neoplasms. *Semin Gastrointest Dis* 1999; 10:156–72.

Lee SD, Surawicz CM. Infectious causes of chronic diarrhea. *Gastroenterol Clin North Am* 2001; 30:679–692.

Potter GD. Bile acid diarrhea. *Dig Dis* 1998; 16:118–124.

Powell DW. Approach to the patient with diarrhea. In: *Textbook of Gastroenterology*, 3rd edn. Philadelphia: JB Lippincott, 1999:858–909.

Practice Economics Committee: American Gastroenterological Association medical position statement: Guidelines for

Further reading

the evaluation and management of chronic diarrhea. *Gastroenterology* 1999; 116:1461–1463.

Schiller LR, Hogan RB, Morawski SG, *et al*. Studies of the prevalence and significance of radiolabeled bile acid malabsorption in a group of patients with idiopathic chronic diarrhea. *Gastroenterology* 1997; 92:151–160.

Schiller LR, Sellin JH. Diarrhea. In: Feldman M, Friedman L, Sleisenger MH (eds) *Sleisenger and Fordtran's Gastrointestinal and Liver Disease: Pathophysiology, Diagnosis, Management*, 7th edn. Philadelphia, WB Saunders 2002; pp.131–153.

Schiller LR. Microscopic colitis syndrome: lymphocytic colitis and collagenous colitis. *Semin Gastrointest Dis* 1999; 10:145–155.

Sellin JH. Functional anatomy, fluid and electrolyte absorption. In: Feldman M, Friedman L, Sleisenger MH (eds) *Sleisenger and Fordtran's Gastrointestinal and Liver Disease: Pathophysiology, Diagnosis, Management*, 7th edn. Philadelphia, WB Saunders 2002; pp. 1693–1714

Shah RJ, Fenoglio-Preiser C, Bleau BL, Giannella RA. Usefulness of colonoscopy with biopsy in the evaluation of patients with chronic diarrhea. *Am J Gastroenterol* 2001; 96:1091–1095.

Wenzl HH, Fine KD, Schiller LR, Fordtran JS. Determinants of decreased fecal consistency in patients with diarrhea. *Gastroenterology* 1995; 108:1729–1738.

Chapter 4

Ulcerative Colitis

Jeffry A. Katz and Thomas A. Judge

CHAPTER OUTLINE

INTRODUCTION

PATHOPHYSIOLOGY

EPIDEMIOLOGY

GENETICS

ENVIRONMENTAL RISK FACTORS

CLINICAL SYMPTOMS AND SIGNS

Rectal bleeding

Diarrhea

Abdominal pain

Other symptoms

Physical signs

Laboratory results

ASSESSMENT OF DISEASE SEVERITY

DIAGNOSIS

Endoscopy

Radiology

Histology

DIFFERENTIAL DIAGNOSIS

DISEASE DISTRIBUTION AND NATURAL HISTORY

EXTRAINTESTINAL MANIFESTATIONS

GENERAL APPROACH TO TREATMENT

Medical therapies

Novel therapies

Surgical therapies

COMPLICATIONS OF ULCERATIVE COLITIS

Toxic megacolon, perforation, and colonic strictures

Dysplasia and carcinoma

ULCERATIVE COLITIS DURING PREGNANCY

FURTHER READING

Introduction

Ulcerative colitis is an inflammatory disorder which primarily affects the colon and rectum. Although relatively common, the etiology of ulcerative colitis remains unknown. The incidence of ulcerative colitis in the US is approximately 8 per 10^5 persons. The prevalence of ulcerative colitis is estimated at 200 per 10^5 persons. The clinical manifestations of ulcerative colitis derive from acute and chronic inflammation within the mucosa of the colon, or result from long-term complications of chronic colitis including the development of colorectal carcinoma. Ulcerative colitis is diagnosed most frequently in individuals in their second or third decade, but it has occasionally been diagnosed in individuals who are in their eighties. A wide spectrum of clinical manifestations occurs with ulcerative colitis, that are largely dependent on the extent and severity of the mucosal inflammation. Despite the relatively limited impact of ulcerative colitis on mortality, the disease results in significant morbidity and expense both directly and through loss of productivity of patients. In addition, potential complications of ulcerative colitis, including colorectal cancer, are an important consideration in the long-term management of these patients.

Pathophysiology

The etiology of ulcerative colitis is presently unknown. Its clinical and pathologic features are the manifestations of an immune response with acute and chronic inflammation damaging the colonic mucosa. The specific antigens initiating and promoting this pathologic inflammation have yet to be identified. A number of potential sources have been suggested but conclusive data in support of any one immunologic trigger has not been developed. These possible sources include pathogenic micro-organisms (as yet unidentified), dietary substrates, commensal bacterial and their metabolic by-products, and normal epithelial structures (i.e. autoimmune antigens).

Known bacterial and viral infections of the gastrointestinal tract may be accompanied by significant epithelial injury as well as pronounced mucosal inflammation. It is therefore possible that a micro-organism that is relatively resistant to an acute mucosal inflammatory response would elicit chronic colonic inflammation. However, although a number of possible viral and mycobacterial agents have been suggested as causes of inflammatory bowel disease (though more commonly Crohn's disease), there is a paucity of microbiologic and pathologic evidence in support of a single common infectious agent.

Similarly, although a number of anticolonic epithelial antibodies have been recognized in the sera of patients with ulcerative colitis, these antibodies have also been identified in patients with infectious colitis as well as in normal controls. One of the better characterized auto-antibodies present primarily in the sera of ulcerative colitis patients is an immunoglobulin G (IgG) isoform which recognize a 40 kD tropomyosin component of normal colon epithelium. This antibody has the potential to activate complement *in vitro*; however, no direct evidence of antibody-induced cytotoxicity has been observed *in vivo*. Nonetheless, while plasma cells in normal colonic mucosa express IgA-type antibody, the inflamed mucosa of ulcerative colitis patients is characterized by large numbers of activated B cells and plasma cells secreting IgG1-type antibodies suggesting a possible direct pathologic role for these autoantibodies.

At present, the commonly accepted stimulus for the abnormal colonic immune response associated with ulcerative colitis appears to be "normal" colonic luminal contents. Multiple animal models of chronic colitis are dependent on the presence of normal colonic bacteria to induce the observed inflammatory response. Interestingly, these animal models include not only deliberate disorders of immune regulation but also models of disrupted epithelium. These findings strongly suggest that a common pathologic phenotype (chronic mucosal inflammation) may arise from multiple potential etiologies.

The inflammatory response which characterizes ulcerative colitis includes both humoral and cell-mediated components. Normal colonic lamina propria is populated with plasma cells, macrophages, and lymphocytes which primarily support the production of secretory IgA. In contrast, the inflamed mucosa of ulcerative colitis patients exhibits not only expansion of activated mononuclear cells but also infiltration of substantial numbers of granulocytes in response to inflammatory mediators released by activated macrophages, lymphocytes, and colonic epithelial cells (see Figure 4.1). Enhanced expression of endothelial adhesion molecules in response to inflammatory mediators such as prostaglandins, leukotrienes, and chemokines direct circulating granulocytes and monocytes to the inflamed tissues thus perpetuating the inflammatory response. Release of cytolytic compounds from activated macrophages, infiltrating granulocytes, and stimulated mesenchymal cells results in direct tissue injury, vascular permeability, and epithelial dysfunction. These bioreactive compounds include reactive oxygen species, tissue-degrading metalloproteinases, and cytotoxic cytokines such as γ-IFN and TNFα. Release of soluble inflammatory mediators, in particular interleukin-1 (IL-1) and IL-6, results in many of the systemic signs associated with severe ulcerative colitis including fever, leukocytosis, and increased synthesis of acute-phase reactants.

Immune dysregulation also involves components of cell-mediated immunity. As noted previously, the mucosa of ulcerative colitis patients is characterized by increased numbers of IgG-secreting plasma cells. In addition, increased numbers of B lymphocytes isolated from resected colon specimens from ulcerative colitis patients exhibit signs of activation compared to B cells obtained from the colons of patients with malignancy or acute diverticulitis. Anticolonic epithelial antibodies have been identified in surgical specimens from patients with ulcerative colitis. Circulating antibodies to neu-

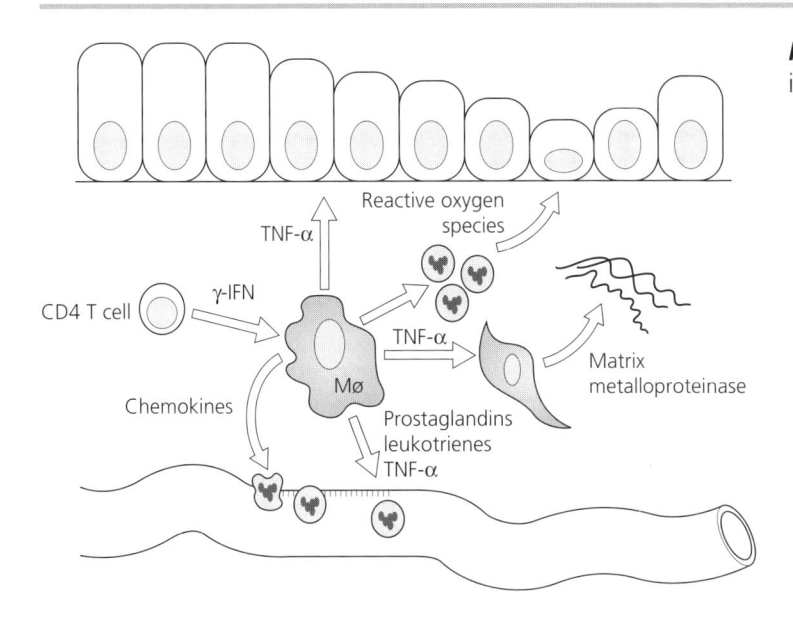

Figure 4.1 Soluble mediators of mucosal inflammation.

trophil cytoplasm (pANCA) can be identified in greater than 80% of ulcerative colitis patients. In ulcerative colitis pANCA do not appear to have a pathogenic role but rather serve as a useful marker for this disease. T-lymphocyte populations isolated from colonic mucosa of ulcerative colitis patients have an increase in the Th2 fraction. These CD4+ T helper lymphocytes express surface activation markers and secrete high levels of IL-4. Consistent with a Th2-type immune response in ulcerative colitis, the dominant IgG fraction identified in the mucosa of ulcerative colitis patients is IgG1. More recently, animal studies have suggested that an absence of regulatory T cells may play a role in the pathogenesis of chronic colitis. The precise role of these T-cell populations in regulating mucosal immune responses in general, and ulcerative colitis in particular, remains to be determined.

Epidemiology

As the etiology of both ulcerative colitis and Crohn's disease is unknown, epidemiologic features have been examined in an attempt to identify potential origins for these disorders. These studies have been limited to some extent by variations in the clinical manifestations of inflammatory bowel disease. It is not possible to distinguish ulcerative colitis from Crohn's disease distinctly in all cases. Moreover, the presentation of ulcerative colitis may vary with the severity and extent of disease. Studies of ulcerative colitis have also been limited by significant variability in health care systems worldwide, as well as by the ability of the systems to correctly identify and track the clinical characteristics of these patients in ambulatory settings. In fact, much of the available epidemiologic data on ulcerative colitis derives from large population studies conducted in northern Europe and North America or hospitalized patient pools particularly from tertiary referral centers.

Variations in the geographic distribution of inflammatory bowel disease are quite striking and have been documented in many studies. Ulcerative colitis has a higher prevalence in the populations of northern Europe and North America, in these regions, the age-adjusted annual incidence rates range from 10 to 13 per 10^5 population. The incidence rates in southern Europe, Asia, and South America are significantly reduced ranging from 0.5 to 6 per 10^5 population. Studies on time-dependent changes in incidence rates have been contradictory. The incidence rates in southern Europe appear to be increasing toward those in northern Europe while rates in the US, England, and Sweden have remained stable or shown modest declines. These changes in incidence rates are in contrast to Crohn's disease which has shown a progressive increase in incidence in all geographic regions examined. A relationship between the incidence of ulcerative colitis and western lifestyle has been suggested. Studies of immigrants to high-risk geographic regions have demonstrated increases in the incidence of ulcerative colitis in these populations. However, the incidence rate of ulcerative colitis in industrialized regions of Japan and Korea are similar to rates elsewhere in Asia. This would suggest that factors other than those accompanying highly developed industrial societies are involved in the pathogenesis of ulcerative colitis.

The peak incidence for ulcerative colitis occurs in the second and third decade of life. A second peak in ulcerative colitis incidence has been suggested between the ages of 60 and 70 years, though this is less pronounced than for Crohn's disease. No clear etiologic differences have been identified to explain the variation in the reported age of incidence. Although some studies have suggested a declining incidence in women after the age of 40 years, other studies have demonstrated that the male-to-female ratio is nearly one in all age groups examined. Diagnosis of ulcerative colitis before the age of 5 years or after 75 years is quite uncommon. In the US, initial studies of ulcerative colitis among African Americans reported an incidence rate of one third of American Caucasians. A more recent study utilizing HMO records suggested that the incidence rates for ulcerative colitis between African Americans and comparable white populations is equivalent. One ethnic group with increased incidence of ulcerative colitis appears to be Ashkenazi Jews. Within defined geographic regions, the incidence rates for inflammatory bowel disease among Jews of middle-European origin has been demonstrated to be 2- to 4-fold higher than the general population. These findings would suggest that environmental factors modulate a genetic predisposition to generate disease. Consistent with this, studies of immigrants to Israel demonstrate a higher incidence of ulcerative colitis in American and European Jews compared to emigrants from Africa and Asia.

Genetics

Genetic factors have also been linked to the development of ulcerative colitis. Family history of inflammatory bowel disease remains one of the principle risk factors. In families with a high incidence of ulcerative colitis, relatives are five times more likely to develop ulcerative colitis than Crohn's disease. The strongest evidence for a genetic influence is derived from twin studies. In three large European twin-pair studies reported to date, approximately 10% of monozygotic twin pairs had concordant ulcerative colitis, as compared with 3% of dizygotic twin pairs. Equally interesting, no twin pair demonstrated both ulcerative colitis and Crohn's disease. Studies of familial inflammatory bowel disease have also supported a genetic basis for ulcerative colitis. The relative risk of ulcerative colitis in a sibling of a patient with ulcerative colitis has been estimated as between 7 and 17 based on studies performed in North America and Europe. Parents, offspring, and second-degree relatives appear to have a much reduced risk for ulcerative colitis. As noted above, Jews appear to have an increased predisposition for inflammatory bowel disease. A 3-fold higher lifetime risk among first-degree relatives of Jewish patients as compared to relatives of non-Jewish patients has been documented. A similar increase in risk has been observed in relatives of patients with early onset of disease.

One potential area of genetic influence is the distribution of particular human leukocyte antigens (HLA) in populations at risk for inflammatory bowel disease. In fact, the HLA-DR2 allele is strongly associated with patients with pancolitis. Recently, a polymorphism in the IκBL gene, which lies within the HLA class III region, has been linked to extensive and intractable ulcerative colitis in a European cohort. Additionally, formal genetic linkage analysis using families with high incidence of ulcerative colitis has identified regions on chromosomes 2, 6, and 12 associated with ulcerative colitis. Although initially implicated in both Crohn's disease and ulcerative colitis, the IBD2 locus on chromosome 12 appears to have the strongest linkage demonstrated in datasets with large numbers of families with ulcerative colitis. No specific genes associated with ulcerative colitis have been delineated in these regions. In contrast, the recently identified NOD2/CARD15 gene mutations located on chromosome 16 associated with Crohn's disease are not expressed at higher levels in patients with ulcerative colitis.

Environmental risk factors

The best characterized environmental factor associated with the incidence of ulcerative colitis is cigarette smoking. Multiple studies have demonstrated a significantly reduced incidence of ulcerative colitis among current smokers compared to non-smokers. This effect is independent of genetic background and gender and a dose–response relationship has been suggested. Randomized studies using nicotine therapy have demonstrated improvement in clinical disease in patients treated with the highest dosage (25 mg/day) while lower doses were ineffective. Smokers also appear to have reduced rates of hospitalization for ulcerative colitis and reduced rates of pouchitis following colectomy. However, passive smoking by children does not appear to reduce the incidence of ulcerative colitis, in fact, children of smokers had twice the incidence of ulcerative colitis compared to children of non-smokers.

Other potential environmental risk factors examined in relation to the incidence of ulcerative colitis include oral contraceptives, high-carbohydrate diets, breast milk, and gastrointestinal infections. Although each has been associated with an increased risk for the development of Crohn's disease, none has been conclusively associated with alterations in the development of ulcerative colitis. However, a negative association between appendectomy and subsequent development of ulcerative colitis has been repeatedly demonstrated. Whether removal of appendiceal-associated lymphoid tissue abrogates a particular pathologic alteration in mucosal immune responses, or whether it merely characterizes an immune response distinct from ulcerative colitis remains to be determined. The absence of a protective effect from prophylactic appendectomy would suggest the latter.

Clinical symptoms and signs

Patients with ulcerative colitis may present with a variety of symptoms, commonly including diarrhea, rectal bleeding, passage of mucus per rectum, tenesmus, urgency, and abdominal pain (Table 4.1). In more severe cases, fever and weight loss may be prominent. Less often patients may have constipation as the predominant complaint. The presenting symptoms tend to differ according to the extent of disease. Patients with limited proctitis often have local symptoms of tenesmus, urgency, mucus, and bleeding, while patients with pancolitis may have more diarrhea, weight loss, fever, clinically significant blood loss, and abdominal pain. In general, symptom severity correlates best with the severity of the luminal disease, whether limited or extensive. Patients may, however, have endoscopic and histologic evidence of ulcerative colitis and yet remain entirely free of symptoms.

Patients typically present in a subacute manner, with symptoms present for weeks or months prior to diagnosis. Studies suggest that the interval between the onset of symptoms and diagnosis has not changed significantly in the last four decades, with a median interval of approximately 5 months. A minority of patients will present in a much more acute fashion with symptoms mimicking an infectious colitis. Indeed, it is not so uncommon to find a patient whose illness began with a documented infection, such as *Salmonella* spp. or *Clostridium difficile*, only to be diagnosed with ulcerative colitis after failing to improve. This raises the question as to whether the infection merely made obvious existing "silent" ulcerative colitis or was actually the triggering mechanism that initiated the disease.

Rectal bleeding

Rectal bleeding is very common in ulcerative colitis, with the characteristics of the bleeding being influenced by the location of the disease. Patients with ulcerative proctitis (i.e. inflammation limited to the rectum) typically complain of passing fresh blood either streaked onto the surface of the stool or passed separately from the stool. Often these symptoms are confused with bleeding hemorrhoids. Unlike most hemorrhoidal bleeding, however, patients with ulcerative proctitis commonly pass a mixture of blood and mucus. Patients with proctitis often complain of a frequent and urgent need to defecate, only to eliminate small quantities of bloody mucus without stool.

With extension of colitis beyond the rectum, blood is usually mixed with stool, or there may be grossly bloody diarrhea. When the disease is more severe, patients pass a liquid mixture of blood, mucus, pus, and stool. Active ulcerative colitis sufficient to cause diarrhea is almost always associated with visible blood in the stool, and the absence of visible blood brings into question the accuracy of the diagnosis. The passage of clots is uncommon, and suggests either very severe disease or an alternative diagnosis.

Table 4.1 Presenting symptoms in ulcerative colitis.

Symptoms	Percentage cases
Bloody diarrhea	75%
Blood per rectum without diarrhea	15%
Diarrhea without bleeding	5%
Abdominal pain or cramps	53%
Weight loss	43%
Fever	25%
Extraintestinal symptoms	13%

Diarrhea

Diarrhea is common, but not always present with ulcerative colitis. Up to 30% of patients with proctitis and proctosigmoiditis may actually complain of constipation. However, most patients with ulcerative colitis will complain of loose or liquid stools when their disease becomes active. Patients often note post-prandial and nocturnal diarrhea. Indeed, awakening from sleep with the urge to defecate and passing a loose bowel movement is one of the symptoms that can help distinguish irritable bowel syndrome from inflammatory bowel disease. Fecal urgency, a sense of incomplete evacuation, and fecal incontinence are common complaints, especially when the rectum is severely inflamed. The pathophysiology of diarrhea in ulcerative colitis is complex, but involves disordered absorption and secretion, abnormal motility, and loss of the normal mucosal barrier function.

Abdominal pain

Over half of ulcerative colitis patients complain of abdominal pain when the disease flares up. Patients typically complain of vague, lower abdominal discomfort, intermittent abdominal cramping preceding bowel movements and often persisting transiently after defecation, or a vague ache in the left iliac fossa. More severe unremitting cramping and abdominal pain can be seen in patients with severe disease flares.

Tenesmus, a painful spasm of the rectum associated with an urgent need to defecate is also common in ulcerative colitis, especially with proctitis. Tenesmus is often associated with painful straining and the passage of a scant amount of feces, typically mixed with mucus and blood.

Other symptoms

Systemic symptoms may be seen with disease of moderate or severe activity. Patients may become anorectic and nauseated, and weight loss may be noted in more than 40% of patients. Vomiting is uncommon and suggests very severe illness or an alternative diagnosis such as Crohn's disease. Fever is usually seen in more severe attacks and is usually of a moderate degree. A small number of patients will present with symptoms related to extraintestinal disease, typically an acute arthropathy, episcleritis, or erythema nodosum, all of which tend to parallel the activity of the colitis. Patients may also complain of symptoms of anemia and hypoproteinemia, including fatigue, dyspnea, and peripheral edema.

Physical signs

Patients with mild or even moderately severe disease generally have a normal physical examination. Indeed, both patient and physician may be frustrated by the burden of an illness with disabling clinical symptoms and complaints completely out of proportion to physical or laboratory abnormalities. These patients usually look well, are of normal weight, and show no obvious signs of a chronic illness. They may display some tenderness on palpation over the diseased colonic segments, but this is generally mild and not associated with rebound or guarding. Even digital rectal examination is often normal, though the rectal mucosa may feel edematous and boggy, and blood is often noted on the examining digit.

Patients with more severe attacks of disease may also look well, but more commonly will show signs of systemic illness, often with tachycardia, fever, and orthostasis. Weight loss is often noted. Bowel sounds may be hyperactive or normal, becoming less noticeable with progressive disease. Although the patient with severe ulcerative colitis typically complains of abdominal pain, the abdomen typically remains soft, with local or diffuse tenderness on examination. In fulminate colitis, the abdomen will often become distended and firm, with bowel sounds absent and peritoneal signs present. Clubbing of the fingernails may accompany chronic active disease.

Laboratory results

Laboratory findings in ulcerative colitis are non-specific and reflect the severity of the underlying disease. Patients with active proctitis and proctosigmoiditis often have normal laboratory results, as do patients with quiescent extensive colitis. Even though patients with limited disease extent frequently pass visible blood in the stool, the amount of blood lost is small and anemia is absent or mild. With worsening disease severity, laboratory abnormalities become more prominent. In patients with active extensive disease, anemia, leukocytosis, and thrombocytosis may be present. With dehydration, serum creatinine will rise and electrolyte abnormalities such as hypokalemia and acidosis may be noted. Hypoalbuminemia can be seen with both acute and chronic disease. Elevations of the erythrocyte sedimentation rate (ESR) and C-reactive protein (CRP) may be seen in more severe disease, but are usually normal or minimally elevated in more mild or moderate disease. The long half-life of proteins contributing to the ESR limits the sensitivity to distinguish rapid clinical changes; CRP has a shorter half-life and corresponds better with clinical and pathologic assessment of relapse, remission, and response to therapy. Though not specific for ulcerative colitis or even bowel inflammation, elevations of the ESR and CRP can be useful in clinical practice for assessing disease activity in individual patients, particularly if these values were normal during a time of disease quiescence.

Assessment of disease severity

Since symptoms, choice of treatment, and outcome are all influenced by disease severity, it is critically important to be able to accurately assess the severity of ulcerative colitis in each individual patient. Disease severity can be evaluated on clinical, endoscopic, and histologic characteristics. The criteria of Truelove and Witts are the most commonly used means of assessing disease activity in ulcerative colitis. This classification identifies patients as having mild, moderate, or severe disease based on a combination of clinical and laboratory findings (Table 4.2). Although this classification has never been formally validated, it is simple and easy to use in day-to-day clinical practice, widely accepted, and generally reliable. However, the Truelove and Witts criteria were designed for patients with extensive colitis, and may not adequately reflect disease severity in more limited disease. Furthermore, the criteria lack precision in the definition of severe disease, as it is not clear how many of the systemic feature must be present, and occasionally a patient with severe ulcerative colitis can be misclassified as having moderate disease.

In patients with limited extent of disease, the Ulcerative Colitis Disease Activity Index is commonly used. This simple four-part index includes evaluation of stool frequency, bleeding, sigmoidoscopic assessment, and physician global assessment. Though particularly popular in clinical trials of new therapies for ulcerative colitis, this scoring system has also never been formally validated.

Probably the best "bedside" guide to disease severity in the hospitalized patient is the early response to supportive and anti-inflammatory therapy. The absence of improvement within 48 to 72 hours is ominous. Indeed, more than eight stools per day and an elevated CRP greater than 45 mg/L after 72 hours of intensive in-patient treatment is associated with an 85% colectomy rate.

Sigmoidoscopic findings correlate loosely with clinical symptoms. Some patients can have severe symptoms with mild endoscopic disease, while other patients have mild symptoms with endoscopically severe disease. For an individual patient, however, correlations between clinical symptoms and macroscopic mucosal disease tend to be more consistent, and thus in clinical practice it is useful to follow sigmoidoscopic change over time. Because histologic features change more slowly than clinical symptoms or sigmoidoscopic findings, microscopic appearance is not useful in guiding decisions about therapy.

Diagnosis

The signs and symptoms of ulcerative colitis are non-specific and no single sensitive and specific diagnostic test exists. Rather, the diagnosis of ulcerative colitis relies upon the careful assimilation of clinical data, endoscopic findings, histopathology, and the elimination of potential infectious etiologies. Because the diagnosis of ulcerative colitis infers a lifelong chronic illness and increased colorectal cancer risk, it is important to be certain of the diagnosis. A diagnosis of ulcerative colitis

Table 4.2 Truelove and Witts classification of ulcerative colitis.

Mild	Moderate	Severe
Fewer than four bowel motions per day	Intermediate between mild and severe	More than six bowel motions per day
Small amounts of blood in the stool		Large amounts of blood in the stool
No fever		Fever (> 37.5 °C)
No tachycardia		Tachycardia (> 90 beats/min)
Mild anemia (> 75% of normal)		Anemia (< 75% of normal)
Erythrocyte sedimentation rate < 30		Erythrocyte sedimentation rate > 30

should be challenged if there is only a single episode of acute disease, a history of recent significant NSAID or antibiotic use, a history of recent hospitalization or travel, sudden acute onset (especially in the elderly), or if the pathologic findings are nonspecific.

Endoscopy

The endoscopic hallmark of ulcerative colitis is confluent inflammation beginning in the rectum and extending proximally without interruption (i.e. no "skip" areas) until the disease stops. In most cases, the diagnosis can be made by sigmoidoscopy. However, colonoscopy is necessary in all patients to establish the full extent of the colitis and to be certain that there are no skip areas, as seen in Crohn's disease. The earliest endoscopic sign of ulcerative colitis is distortion or loss of the normal vascular pattern. The affected blood vessels appear blunted and do not branch when compared to the normal blood vessels. It is unusual to see this minimal change in patients with active colitis, but loss of the normal vascular pattern may be the only endoscopic evidence of ulcerative colitis in remission.

More typically, the patient with mild ulcerative colitis will have erythematous, granular, and friable mucosa in association with loss of the normal vascular pattern. As the disease severity becomes more moderate, a loosely adherent, yellow-brown exudate is evident. This mucopurulent exudate is generally associated with ulceration of the mucosal surface. Mucosal ulcerations vary in size from 5 millimeters to several centimeters. Ulcerations may be punctate, annular, linear, serpiginous, or circinate, and appear in an area of already inflamed mucosa. In severe cases of ulcerative colitis there may be extensive loss of the mucosal surface from ulceration with marked edema, at times nearly obliterating the lumen, and exposure of the muscularis mucosa.

In active ulcerative colitis, inflammatory pseudopolyps, representing inflamed, regenerating epithelium between ulcerated areas may give the colonic mucosa a cobblestone appearance. In more chronic cases, as the ulcerations heal, inflammatory pseudopolyps are left behind. Pseudopolyps are usually small, pale, soft, fleshy, and friable, but may grow to be large sessile or pedunculated polyps several centimeters in size. Larger pseudopolyps often have an ulcerated surface. Although the colonic mucosa can heal and appear nearly normal in ulcerative colitis, pseudopolyps do not tend to regress with treatment. Occasionally, inflammatory pseudopolyps may be interconnected by bridging mucosal folds. These form in the wake of undermining ulcers and, on healing, leave an overlying latticework of bridging mucosal interconnections.

Over time longstanding inflammation may lead to the loss of the normal colonic architecture. Muscle hypertrophy, noted histologically as hypertrophy of the muscularis mucosa, causes loss of the normal haustral-fold pattern. Associated with muscle hypertrophy is a decrease in the overall luminal diameter of the colon. The overall appearance of the colon in chronic ulcerative colitis often resembles that of a long, featureless, narrow tube, the so-called "leaden pipe" noted on barium enema. In some cases of ulcerative colitis, muscular hypertrophy develops more focally than diffusely, appearing endoscopically and radiographically as a stricture. Strictures in ulcerative colitis are typically inflammatory and associated with mucosal ulcerations. Inflammatory strictures in ulcerative colitis are usually short and less than 2 to 3 cm in length. Longer strictures, and those without associated inflammation increase the concern for malignancy.

Radiology

Patients with ulcerative colitis must have a supine and upright film of the abdomen. Previously unsuspected inflammatory bowel disease may initially be diagnosed based on the loss of haustration of the air-filled colon. In severe disease, the mucosa becomes edematous and irregular, which can be detected radiographically as thickening of the bowel wall. The presence of marked colonic dilation may mean the patient has developed fulminant colitis or toxic megacolon. A plain abdominal radiograph may also detect unsuspected free air.

With the growth of endoscopy, barium studies of the colon have become less important in the diagnosis and management of ulcerative colitis. However, a barium contrast study can still provide information useful in the management and care of patients with ulcerative colitis. In particular, an air-contrast barium enema can show the precise diameter, location, and length of colonic strictures and chronic changes such as pseudopolyp formation, loss of haustra, shortening of the colon, and tubularization of the colon. In addition, barium enema and small bowel barium studies add important information about the terminal ileum and help in the differentiation of ulcerative colitis from Crohn's disease.

The earliest radiologic change of ulcerative colitis seen on barium examination of the colon is a fine mucosal granularity. With increasing severity, superficial ulcers appear. So-called "collar-button" ulcers represent deeper ulcerations through the mucosal surface (Figure 4.2). As the illness progresses, the haustral folds may become edematous and thickened, this can be seen on both barium contrast and plain studies. In long-standing disease, loss of haustration may become prominent, with the colon taking on a featureless, tubular appearance (Figure 4.3). Over time, the colon may also become shortened and widening of the presacral space may be seen on a lateral film of the rectum.

Histology

In most cases, ulcerative colitis is most severe distally and is progressively less severe in the more proximal colon. Orderly biopsies from multiple colonic sites will show this typical pattern. However, pathologic interpretation requires familiarity with all stages of the disease, since histologic appearance is affected by the duration and severity of the disease, as well as by the effects of medical therapy. For example, in acute, newly diagnosed ulcerative colitis, therapy may cause near complete healing of the mucosa in the rectum and distal sigmoid colon. Biopsies taken after therapy might then suggest relative sparing of the rectum by the inflammatory process, leading to a potentially erroneous diagnosis of Crohn's disease of the colon. Thus, it is important that the interpreting pathologist have enough biopsy material and enough clinical information to allow an accurate diagnosis. Similar findings can occur in patients treated with topical rectal medications.

Early ulcerative colitis is marked by mucosal edema and capillary and venule congestion, a stage rarely seen by the pathologist, followed by the development of an acute inflammatory cell infiltrate with formation of an exudate in association with epithelial cell necrosis. The infiltrate is primarily composed of neutrophils, though eosinophils and mast cells may be prominent in the early stages of disease. Depletion of goblet cells occurs, but is not specific for ulcerative colitis.

The classic pathologic findings of ulcerative colitis are that of a chronic active inflammatory process extending diffusely from the rectum proximally for variable extents. As well as evidence of ulceration and repair, the histologic features of note are a

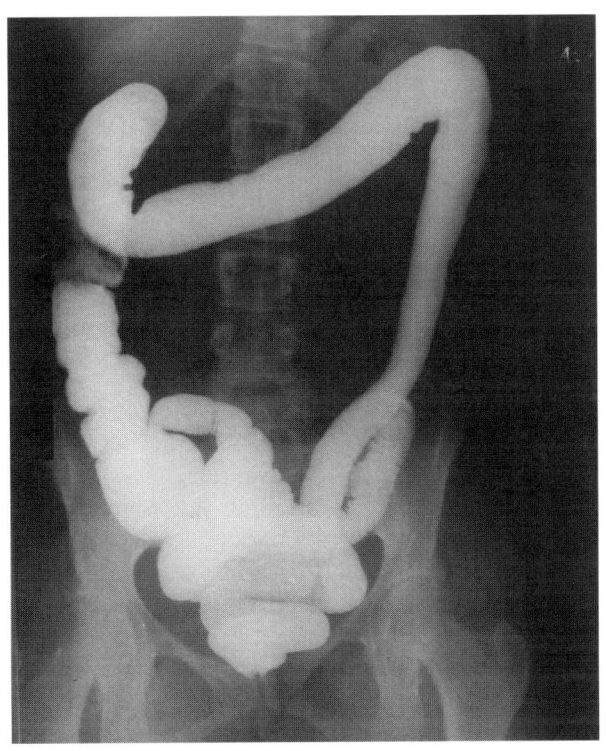

Figure 4.3 Loss of haustration and tubular appearance of the colon on air-contrast barium enema (reproduced with permission of Dr Dean Nakamoto).

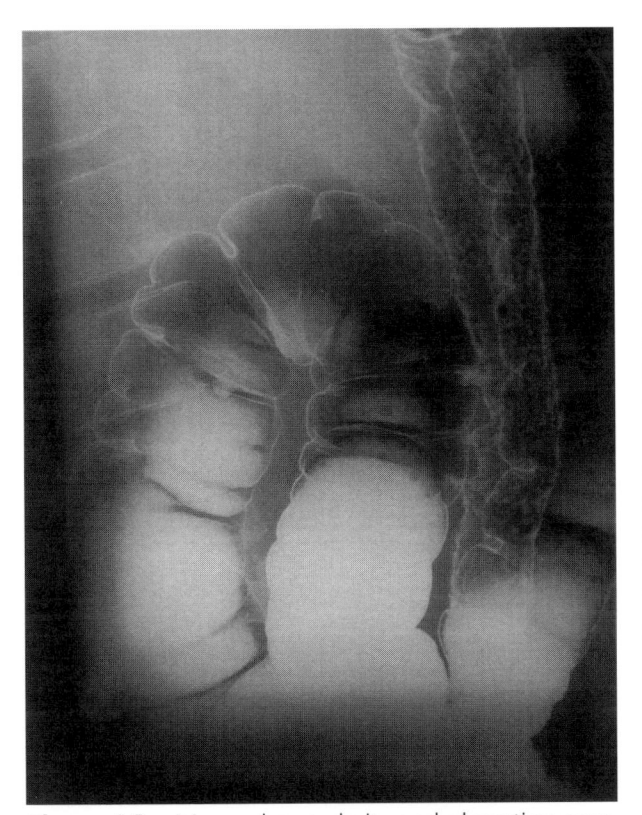

Figure 4.2 Mucosal granularity and ulceration seen in a case of left-sided ulcerative colitis (reproduced with permission of Dr Dean Nakamoto).

Ulcerative Colitis

dense lamina propria plasmacytosis often accompanied by marked eosinophilic infiltrate. The crypts typically show varying degrees of crypt distortion. Polymorphonuclear leukocyte infiltrate is centered on colonic crypts giving rise to acute cryptitis (neutrophilic infiltrate of colonic crypts) and crypt abscess formation (neutrophilic accumulations in crypt lumina) (Figure 4.4). Not uncommonly the inflammatory process will cause the crypts to rupture. A histiocytic response to crypt rupture, which may even contain giant cells, may be misinterpreted as evidence of Crohn's disease.

Inflammation in ulcerative colitis is characteristically limited to the lamina propria and inflammatory changes stop dramatically at the luminal aspect of the muscularis mucosa in most cases. However, as the disease becomes more severe and epithelial destruction progresses, the inflammatory infiltrate may descend into the submucosa, usually as a broad zone of inflammation. It is, however, only best appreciated in resection specimens (see Figure 4.5, this pattern is different to the fissuring type of transmural inflammation characteristic of Crohn's disease). In chronic, quiescent ulcerative colitis a thin band of mainly lymphocytic inflammation may be seen on both sides of the muscularis mucosa.

During the healing stages the mucosal inflammatory infiltrate lessens and epithelial regeneration occurs. Initially the healing mucosa is thin, with attenuated and flattened epithelial cells. The cells then become cuboidal and may have eccentric, large nuclei and prominent nucleoli. These regenerative changes can be confused with dysplasia. It must be emphasized, however, that a diagnosis of dysplasia in ulcerative colitis should be made with caution in the presence of significant acute inflammation.

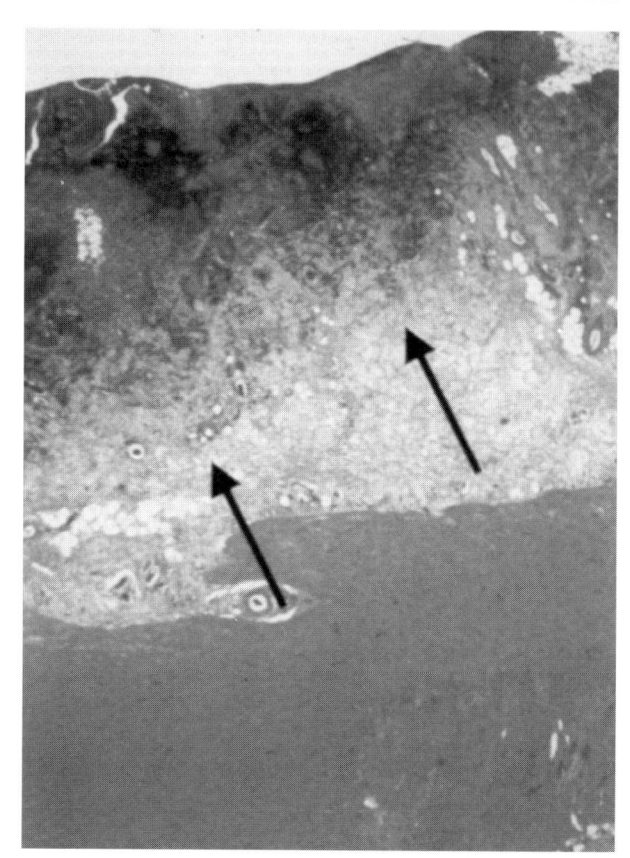

Figure 4.5 Low-power view of a completely denuded portion of colon with chronic inflammatory infiltrate extending to the level of the submucosa (arrows) (reproduced with permission of Dr Joseph Willis).

With continued healing crypt distortion and "drop-out" becomes evident and is a prominent feature of chronic quiescent ulcerative colitis. Crypts may be branched, widely separated from one another, and lose their usual close contact with the muscularis mucosa. A characteristic, but entirely non-diagnostic feature of healed ulcerative colitis is Paneth cell metaplasia of the colonic glands. Paneth cells do not typically occur beyond the hepatic flexure. Their presence in the distal colon indicates that re-epithelialization of the mucosa has occurred. A slight and irregular increase in collagen may be evident in the lamina propria of healed ulcerative colitis, but true fibrosis is uncommon. In chronic quiescent ulcerative colitis, varying degrees of acute and/or chronic inflammation of the lamina propria is present.

The severity of inflammation in inflammatory bowel disease does not necessarily correlate with a patient's symptomatology. Thus biopsies may be reported as demonstrating marked inflammatory changes in patients who are relatively symptom free.

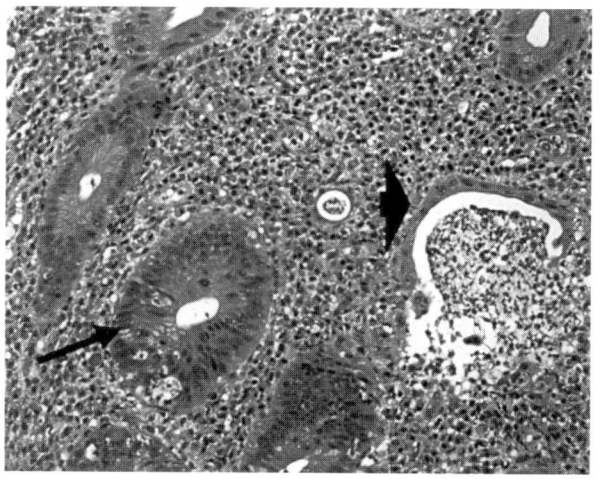

Figure 4.4 Ulcerative colitis characterized by marked lamina propria plasmacytosis, acute cryptitis (arrow), and crypt abscess (arrowhead) (reproduced with permission of Dr Joseph Willis).

Differential diagnosis

Crohn's disease of the colon, as well as a variety of other conditions, can mimic ulcerative colitis. These inflammatory bowel disease "impostors" fall into five broad categories: infectious, vascular, motility, inflammatory, and metabolic causes (Box 4.1). When Crohn's disease involves the rectum and no skip lesions or granulomas are present, it can be impossible to distinguish it from ulcerative colitis using clinical, endoscopic, and/or histologic criteria. This is especially true with newly diagnosed disease. Over time, the frequent development of small-bowel involvement or perianal complications makes a diagnosis of Crohn's disease obvious. However, in approximately 10% of patients a distinction between Crohn's disease and ulcerative colitis remains impossible and these patients are labeled as indeterminate colitis. Microscopic and collagenous colitis can present with symptoms similar to ulcerative colitis, but are distinguished by their normal endoscopic appearance and specific pathologic findings.

The infectious colitides are the most likely of the inflammatory bowel disease imposters to present with a picture clinically similar to ulcerative colitis. It is important to remember that patients with medically controlled inflammatory bowel disease can present with an acute infectious colitis masquerading as a flare of disease, or alternatively, an infectious colitis can serve as the trigger for a true flare of colitis, which persists after the infection has been cleared.

Salmonella, *Shigella*, *Escherichia coli* 0157:H7, *Campylobacter*, and *Yersinia* infections can all present with colitis. Other less common infections causing colitis include *Aeromonas hydrophilia*, usually acquired from drinking untreated water, and, rarely, *Listeria monocytogenes*. Clinical suspicion, appropriate cultures of the stool, and careful examination of pathology specimens will distinguish these infectious diseases from inflammatory bowel disease.

Cytomegalovirus (CMV) infection has been reported in up to 4.6% of ulcerative colitis patients. Abdominal pain and gastrointestinal bleeding are the most common presentations of CMV colitis, although occasionally patients will present with severe colitis requiring colectomy. The pathologic importance of CMV infection in cases of ulcerative colitis is debated. The virus may be a secondary infection in an otherwise diseased colon, however, the association with a relatively short duration of aggressive ulcerative colitis suggests that in some patients CMV infection may be the primary pathogenic event. Careful examination of biopsy samples confirms the diagnosis, and treatment with ganciclovir results in clinical improvement of the colitis and cure of the CMV infection.

Antibiotic-associated pseudomembranous colitis with *Clostridium difficile* may be confused with, or superimposed upon ulcerative colitis. Although *C. difficile* typically causes a watery diarrhea, it can cause a severe colitis and progress to bowel perforation because of toxic megacolon. *Clostridium difficile* toxin has been found in the stools of up to 20% of patients with inflammatory bowel disease, and *C. difficile* infection may be a factor in the relapse of inflammatory bowel disease in some patients. *Clostridium difficile* infection has been reported in inflammatory bowel disease patients who have not received antibiotics, but does not appear to be associated with sulfasalazine therapy. Since the infection can be transmitted among patients by hospital and nursing-home staff, it is especially important to carefully check for the toxin in the hospitalized

---

Box 4.1 Differential diagnosis of ulcerative colitis

Crohn's disease

Infectious causes
  Salmonella
  Shigella
  Ecsherichea coli
  Campylobacter
  Yersinia
  Entameba histolytica
  Clostridium difficile
  Aeromonas
  Listeria
  Cytomegalovirus

Inflammatory causes
  neutropenic colitis (typhlitis)
  microscopic/collagenous colitis
  eosinophilic colitis

Vascular causes
  ischemic colitis
  vasculitis (polyarteritis nodosa, Behçet's disease)
  radiation colitis

Drugs or toxins
  non-steroidal anti-inflammatory drugs
  gold
  hydroflouric acid

patient who is not responding to medical therapy as expected.

Less common causes of colitis mimicking ulcerative colitis include neutropenic colitis, or typhlitis, a rare complication of chemotherapy, eosinophilic colitis, parasitic infections, the use of medications, toxins, and ischemic colitis. Most of these processes can be distinguished from ulcerative colitis by careful history, stool examination, and endoscopic and histologic evaluation.

Disease distribution and natural history

At presentation approximately 30% of patients will have proctitis, 30% left-sided colitis, and 40% extensive colitis, of which 15% is pancolitis (Figure 4.6). The overall incidence of ulcerative colitis has not changed significantly over the past 30 years. However, surveys from different parts of the world have suggested that the number of patients with ulcerative proctitis at presentation is increasing, while that of more extensive ulcerative colitis is decreasing.

Most patients with ulcerative colitis (80%) have a disease course characterized by intermittent disease relapses and remissions, though fortunately over time, most patients spend more time in remission than with active disease. Unfortunately, the duration of the relapse-free interval varies greatly from patient to patient, and may be as brief as a few weeks or as long as several years. The likelihood of staying in remission for 1 year after a relapse has been estimated at 30%. However, if a patient does remain in remission for 1 year, the risk of relapse decreases to 20% for the next year. Analysis of patients followed over a 7-year period has shown that 40% of patients have more than one relapse a year, 50% have only one relapse a year, and 10% had no relapses during the follow-up period. A small number of patients (10%) will have chronic continuous symptoms without remission. Very rarely (1%) a patient will have only a single disease flare followed by a relapse-free course. The factors influencing disease relapse and remission are incompletely understood, but are known to include viral and bacterial infections, the use of NSAIDs and antibiotics, pregnancy and oral contraceptives, seasonal variation, cigarette smoking, and psychological stress.

The extent of ulcerative colitis significantly influences the severity of the disease and therefore the course of illness. A population-based study from Scandinavia suggests that in the first year after diagnosis, patients with pancolitis have a higher rate of colectomy compared to patients with left-sided disease. However, once the first year has passed, the subsequent disease course is similar for all patients regardless of disease extent, with a colectomy rate of approximately 1% per year. Thus, after 30 years of follow-up, roughly 30% of patients with ulcerative colitis will have required proctocolectomy.

At presentation, 5% to 15% of patients will have severe disease, according to the criteria of Truelove and Witts, and proceed to early colectomy within the first year. This number has varied little over decades, although the outcome of medical and surgical treatment for this group of patients has improved significantly and death from severe ulcerative colitis is now uncommon. The type of disease onset, whether sudden or gradual, has little bearing on short-term outcome. Older patients and those with significant comorbidities do worse.

Ulcerative colitis is not a static illness and limited disease may extend proximally over time. Likewise, though somewhat less common, extensive colitis may regress with treatment over time. Several studies suggest that 10% to 30% of patients with proctitis will have proximal extension of their colitis over 10 years, though the development of pancolitis appears to be uncommon. Population-based studies suggest that distal ulcerative colitis is not as benign a condition as originally thought, with up to 20% of patients requiring a colectomy after 20 years of disease. Left-sided colitis progresses over time in 20% to 30% of patients. The

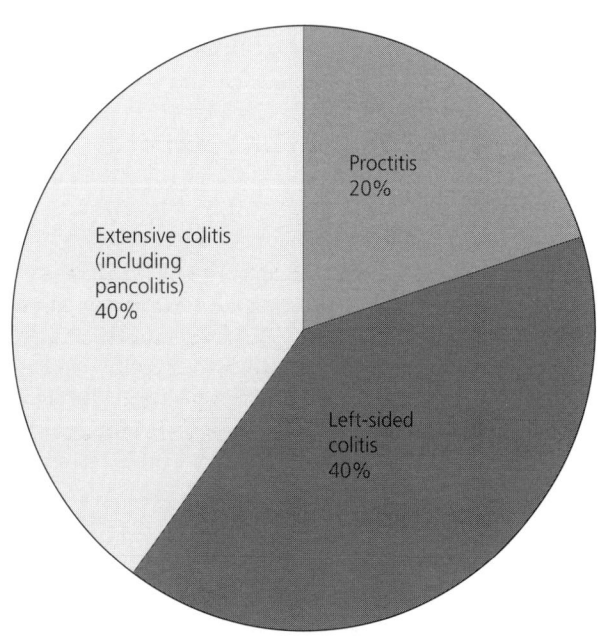

Figure 4.6 Distribution of ulcerative colitis at diagnosis.

factors associated with disease progression are poorly understood.

Although burdened by an unpredictable chronic illness, the majority of patients with ulcerative colitis (90%) are able to work and lead full and active lives. Nonetheless, ulcerative colitis adversely affects the quality of life to some degree for most patients, especially during disease flares. Not only do patients suffer the unpleasant physical symptoms associated with worsening disease, but also commonly experience difficulties at work and home. Many patients are embarrassed and stigmatized by their disease and its unpleasant and unsociable symptoms. Even when the disease is less active, patients often remain anxious and fearful, altering their lifestyle to accommodate the unpredictable nature of their illness.

Despite the morbidity of ulcerative colitis, mortality associated with the disease has dropped dramatically since the late 1950s and 1960s. The mortality for a severe attack of ulcerative colitis was approximately 35% before the introduction of steroid therapy and is now less than 2%. Long-term survival does not differ significantly from that expected from age-matched controls, even with the risk of colorectal cancer in long-standing colitis.

Extraintestinal manifestations

Ulcerative colitis is a systemic illness, and as such can be associated with a wide range of local and systemic symptoms that influence both the course of the disease and the complexity of treatment. Extraintestinal manifestations may occur before, during, or following episodes of clinical disease activity, and are generally divided into extraintestinal manifestations that are related to the activity of the colitis and those that are independent of colitis activity. The major organ systems affected by ulcerative colitis include the skin, eyes, mouth, joints, and liver.

Skin

Erythema nodosum occurs in 2% to 4% of patients with ulcerative colitis. Its activity parallels the activity of the colitis, though it can be seen as a drug reaction to sulfasalazine. Erythema nodosum typically presents as multiple, tender, raised, erythematous nodules on the anterior aspect of the lower legs.

A less common, but more clinically significant skin lesion is pyoderma gangrenosum, seen in 1% of patients. Although usually related to the activity of the colitis, pyoderma gangrenosum may present or persist despite quiescent bowel disease. The lesions may be single or multiple, and though usually appearing on the legs or trunk, may appear on the upper extremities or even the face. Pyoderma gangrenosum begins as small, tender, sterile pustules that rupture, ulcerate, and usually coalesce into large, tender ulcers. The ulcers are very painful and classically have a violaceous border. Treatment consists of controlling the activity of the bowel disease, intralesional steroid injection, and aggressive immunomodulatory treatment with cyclosporine or infliximab.

Probably the most common skin manifestations of ulcerative colitis are complications of drug treatment. Steroid therapy may commonly lead to pustular acne, a distressing side effect for adolescents and young adults. Hypersensitivity, photosensitivity, and urticarial reactions are commonly seen with sulfasalazine, and occasionally with the newer mesalamine compounds. Sweet's syndrome, an acute febrile neutrophilic dermatosis, may rarely complicate severe attacks of ulcerative colitis.

Eyes

Approximately 5% to 8% of patients will experience an ocular complication of ulcerative colitis. Episcleritis is associated with, and parallels, active colitis. The sclera and conjunctiva are moderately to markedly erythematous, but visual acuity is preserved. In contrast, anterior uveitis less closely follows the activity of the colitis. With uveitis, the eye is painful and visual acuity is compromised. Headache and photophobia are common. Treatment of the colitis and local steroid eye drops control the symptoms and inflammation.

Mouth

At least 10% of patients will develop shallow apthous ulcers on the buccal mucosa and oral palate with flares of colitis. These lesions rapidly resolve with control of the underlying bowel disease. Angular cheilitis and a sore tongue may be seen with iron and other micronutrient deficiencies.

Joints

An asymmetric, migratory, large-joint acute arthropathy will accompany attacks of ulcerative colitis in 15% of patients. The risk of arthropathy appears to increase with the extent of the colitis, although patients with limited proctitis may develop acute attacks. The arthropathy is non-destructive; the major symptoms are stiffness with limitation of movement and pain. The inflamed joint is swollen, erythematous, and hot. Treatment is control of the colitis, although tapping the joint to remove the effusion and intra-articular steroid injections may help to control symptoms.

Clinical sacroileitis occurs in 10% to 15% of patients, although up to 80% of patients will have findings on MRI. Low back pain is a typical symptom, but does not typically parallel the activity of the colitis. Most patients are HLA-B27 negative and do not develop ankylosing spondylitis. Ankylosing spondylitis ("bamboo spine") does develop in 1% to 2% of ulcerative colitis patients, and 80% of these are HLA-B27 positive. The course of ankylosing spondylitis is progressive and independent of the bowel disease. It leads to progressive fusion and stiffening of the axial skeleton.

Liver

The reported prevalence and incidence of hepatobiliary complications of inflammatory bowel disease ranges widely, although significant liver disease is estimated to be present in less than 10% of patients. Although minor elevations of liver enzymes are common with flares of acute colitis, most return to normal with resolution of the attack. These acute elevations appear to be related to a combination of factors, including fatty liver, sepsis, and malnutrition.

The most significant liver complication associated with ulcerative colitis is primary sclerosing cholangitis. Although this complication occurs in just 3% of inflammatory bowel disease patients, approximately 85% of all primary sclerosing cholangitis cases are seen in inflammatory bowel disease patients. Primary sclerosing cholangitis is a chronic, progressive, fibrosing disease of the biliary tract, that eventually leads to cirrhosis and liver failure. The inflammatory process may involve the extrahepatic, intrahepatic, or both, ductular systems, and the diagnosis is made cholangiographically. Although the histologic appearance may vary widely, the classic finding is one of concentric fibrosis around the bile ductules, associated with a variable chronic inflammatory infiltrate. No treatment to slow the progressive fibrosis has yet been found, and the disease is independent of the colitis activity. Although patients with ulcerative colitis and primary sclerosing cholangitis remain well for many years, the disease is progressive and patients developing end-stage liver disease require liver transplantation. Primary sclerosing cholangitis also carries a significantly increased risk of cholangiocarcinoma.

Other extraintestinal associations

Amyloidosis with progressive renal failure has been rarely reported with ulcerative colitis, but is more common in Crohn's disease. Inflammatory pulmonary disease and pericarditis have also been described.

General approach to treatment

The majority of patients with ulcerative colitis have a mild course of illness, which responds well to topical anti-inflammatory medications. In a recent longitudinal study of ulcerative colitis patients residing in Olmstead County, Minnesota from 1970 to 1993, more than 60% of patients did not require systemic corticosteroids or more aggressive medical and surgical treatment. Additionally, nearly 50% of ulcerative colitis patients treated with systemic corticosteroids remained in clinical remission without surgery or prolonged corticosteroid therapy during the following 12 months. Nonetheless, some 30% of patients with ulcerative colitis will require systemic therapy to control symptoms of ulcerative colitis and of these, approximately 10% to 15% will require colectomy because of refractory inflammation. Nutritional therapy is less frequently required in patients with ulcerative colitis than in Crohn's disease, in part because malabsorption of nutrients is seldom encountered in ulcerative colitis. Nonetheless, in patients with severe ulcerative colitis, weight loss and malnutrition may occur because of significant anorexia, the avoidance of food because of severe diarrhea, and increased catabolism associated with fever and inflammation. Total parenteral nutrition has been used to improve the overall nutritional status of individual patients prior to colectomy and has been demonstrated to reduce symptoms in patients with severe ulcerative colitis. However, total parenteral nutrition has not been demonstrated to improve colonic inflammation nor reduce the rate of colectomy in ulcerative colitis patients.

Medical therapies

5-aminosalicylic acid (5-ASA)

Sulfasalazine has been the mainstay of treatment for ulcerative colitis for more than 30 years. Sulfasalazine is composed of 5-aminosalicylic acid

(5-ASA), also known as mesalamine, that is diazo-bonded to sulfapyridine. The principle mucosal anti-inflammatory moeity is 5-ASA which is released in the colon by the action of bacterial azoreductase (Figure 4.7). 5-aminosalicylic acid acts topically by a variety of mechanisms, including the inhibition of synthesis of leukotriene B_4 (a potent chemotactic compound), impairment of phagocytosis, inhibition of IL-1 production, and scavenging of free oxygen radicals. A dose of 2 to 4 g/day is commonly used to treat mild to moderate ulcerative colitis (Table 4.3). Side effects limit its use in a large proportion of patients (approximately 25%). Common side effects include nausea, vomiting, headache, rash, and fever. Less-common side effects include anemia, hemolysis, epidermolysis, pancreatitis, pulmonary fibrosis, and sperm motility disorders. Sulfasalazine may limit the absorption of folate therefore patients undergoing long-term sulfasalazine therapy should also be given supplemental folate.

Nearly all of the side effects of sulfasalazine have been attributed to the sulfapyridine moiety. This has led to the introduction and ongoing development of a variety of compounds containing mesalamine. Taken in its native form, mesalamine is systemically absorbed in the proximal gastrointestinal tract and therefore is not topically active in the distal gastrointestinal tract. Delayed-release forms of mesalamine (Asacol®) are coated in pH-sensitive methylacrylate (Eudragit S). By varying the pH of dissolution, the level of release in the gastrointestinal tract also varies. Asacol®, adjusted to dissolve at a pH above 7, is designed to release mesalamine in the distal ileum and colon. Another type of delivery is mesalamine packaged in ethylcellulose microgranules (Pentasa®) with release activated by moisture resulting in a time-dependent sustained release. Given their substantially higher cost, the main role of these 5-ASA preparations is in the treatment of sulfasalazine-intolerant patients. It is also important to note that these pH- and time-dependent preparations have a more variable delivery of 5-ASA to the colon than diazo-bonded compounds. Both types of preparations usually have substantial release of 5-ASA in the small bowel (especially the time-dependent preparation). In addition, pH-dependent preparations may fail to adequately release active drug in the colon. One possible explanation for this is the reduced intraluminal colonic pH during an acute flare-up. This variability in release should be considered when patients fail to respond to treatment. Despite these limitations, these 5-ASA preparations are capable of delivering higher concentrations of 5-ASA than sulfasalazine, with minimal side effects even when used in high dosages. This will be especially true of the alternative diazo-bonded compounds. Renal function should be monitored periodically in patients treated with high-dose mesalamine compounds.

Two additional compounds containing ASA include olsalazine and balsalazide. Both agents are diazo-bonded and therefore have the same delivery characteristics as sulfasalazine. Olsalazine is a 5-ASA dimer, and balsalazide is 4-ASA that is

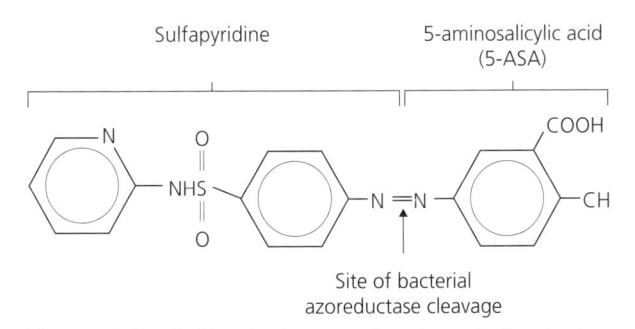

Figure 4.7 Sulfasalazine: mechanism of directed colonic delivery.

Table 4.3 Commonly available 5-aminosalicylic acid medications.

Medication	Form	Distribution	Dose (day)
Sulfasalazine	oral	colon	2–4 g in divided doses
Balsalazide (Colazal®)	oral	colon	6.75 g in divided doses
Mesalamine			
Asacol®	oral	ileum, colon	2.4–4.8 g in divided doses
Canasa®	suppository	rectum	500 mg twice a day
Pentasa®	oral	small bowel and colon	2–4 g in divided doses
Rowasa®	enema	left colon	4 g in 60 mL at bedtime
Olsalazine (Dipentum®)*	oral	colon	1.5–3.0 in divided doses

*Use solely as maintenance therapy

diazo-bonded to an inert carrier amino acid. Olsalazine is only approved for maintenance of remission in ulcerative colitis. A side effect unique to this agent is a secretory diarrhea in a small but significant minority of patients; this limits its usefulness in treating active ulcerative colitis. In general, these sulfasalazine analogs are well tolerated, with minimal side effects. Given the possibility of diarrhea as a side effect, use of olsalazine should be avoided in the treatment of acute colitis.

Patients with limited disease are good candidates for medication applied per rectum once or twice daily. Patients with disease limited to the rectum (the distal 10 cm) may be treated with 5-ASA suppositories. Patients with disease beyond the rectum but not beyond the descending colon may be treated with 5-ASA retention enemas (4 g/60 mL). It is important to consider that some patients with acute colitis may have difficulty retaining enemas. Nonetheless, the advantage of these preparations is the local delivery of high concentrations of mesalamine to the affected mucosa.

Corticosteroids

Despite appropriate administration of sulfasalzine and other 5-ASA medications, 20% to 30% of colitis patients will fail to respond and require systemic corticosteroid therapy. Prednisone, at doses of 40 to 60 mg/day orally, induces remission in 75% to 90% of patients with ulcerative colitis. Corticosteroids appear to act through a variety of mechanisms, including inihibition of T-cell function, impairment of chemotaxis and phagocytosis, and reduction of cytokine and eicosanoid synthesis. Most patients with moderate exacerbations of ulcerative colitis will achieve fairly prompt remission with oral prednisone. Severely ill patients and those who fail to respond to high-dose oral corticosteroids should be hospitalized for treatment with intravenous methylprednisolone at doses of 40 to 60 mg/day. Use of systemic corticosteroids has resulted in a substantial reduction in the mortality from fulminant colitis which prior to the use of corticosteroids exceeded 30%. Following induction of clinical remission, corticosteroids are tapered slowly over a 6 to 8-week period.

In fulminant colitis, the anti-inflammatory effects of corticosteroids may well be overwhelmed by excessive synthesis of pro-inflammatory cytokines because of enhanced degradation of inhibitory molecules such as IκB allowing transcription factors to bind to promotor elements in genes expressing inflammatory molecules. True steroid resistance is therefore more frequently encountered in patients presenting with severe colitis. In addition to steroid-resistant colitis, the spectrum of clinical presentations defined as "steroid-refractory colitis" includes partial clinical responses and control of symptoms only with persistent use of systemic corticosteroids (steroid dependence). Approximately 30% of patients requiring corticosteroids to induce remission become steroid dependent with recurrence of clinical symptoms on attempted steroid withdrawal. Long-term use of corticosteroids is complicated by potentially devastating side effects. These include, but are not limited to, a typical cushingoid appearance, osteoporosis, hypertension, diabetes mellitus, psychosis, aseptic necrosis of bone, neuropathy, and myopathy. Patients treated with corticosteroids should be treated concomitantly with 5-ASA preparations to take advantage of their potential "steroid-sparing" effects. Alternate-day dosing may be useful in some patients and may minimize side effects. Patients with aggressive and/or steroid-dependent disease should be given immunosuppressive medications early, rather than after a prolonged course of high-dosage corticosteroids.

Patients with limited disease who fail to respond to 5-ASA may be treated with hydrocortisone enemas (100 mg) once or twice daily. Corticosteroid foam and suppositories may be used for the treatment of ulcerative proctitis, though with less efficacy than comparable mesalamine preparations. There may be significant systemic absorption of these preparations particularly as the colonic epithelium heals. This may result in many of the systemic toxicities of corticosteroid therapy, including Cushing's syndrome, with long-term use. Topically active but rapidly metabolized corticosteroids such as budesonide (available as an enema preparation from compounding pharmacies) may avoid many of these long-term toxicities.

Immunosuppressive drugs

The purine analogs, azathioprine and 6-mercaptopurine, have an important place in the treatment of ulcerative colitis. They are the drugs of choice in the management of disease that is dependent on, or resistant to corticosteroids. 6-mercaptopurine and azathioprine, a prodrug which is non-enzymatically converted to 6-mercaptopurine, have been used interchangeably in most large studies examining the efficacy of these medications in inflammatory bowel disease therapy. However, 6-mercaptopurine is presently more expensive than azathioprine which is available in generic form in the US. Purine analogs inhibit nucleotide synthesis. Their mechanism of action in inflammatory bowel disease is uncertain but may be related to the inhibition of T-cell clonal expansion. There is some limited data suggesting additional immune modulating effects from azathioprine because of alterations in lymphocyte membrane structures and NK cell function. The main limitation to the purine analogs is their slow onset of action. The mean time to clinical response is 3 months, with full clinical response in some patients taking 6 to 9 months. Controlled studies have confirmed the efficacy of azathioprine in the maintenance of clinical remission induced by either corticosteroids or cyclosporine A. Evidence for an advantage to 6-mercaptopurine or azathioprine in the induction of clinical remission is less convincing, but both agents have demonstrated potent steroid-sparing effects. Approximately 75% of patients treated with 6-mercaptopurine or azathioprine are able to taper off or significantly reduce their steroid dose. 6-mercaptopurine undergoes extensive intracellular conversion to active 6-thioguanine metabolites. Three enzyme systems compete to metabolize 6-mercaptopurine. Xanthine oxidase converts 6-mercaptopurine to the inactive metabolite 6-thiouric acid, and thiopurine methyltransferase converts 6-mercaptopurine to the metabolite 6-methylmercaptopurine, whose immunomodulatory activity is unclear. 6-mercaptopurine is also converted to the active metabolites, the 6-thioguanine nucleotides, by a series of enzymatic steps involving hypoxanthine phosphoribosyl transferase, inosine monophosphate dehydrogenase and guanosine monophosphate synthetase. Differences in the enzymatic activities of these pathways result in considerable variation in the levels of both active metabolites and potentially toxic compounds. Polymorphisms in the thiopurine methyltransferase gene are associated with reduced activity of this gene. Absence of thiopurine methyltransferase activity is estimated to occur in 0.3% of the population; an additional 11% of patients have significantly reduced thiopurine methyltransferase activity. These patients are at pronounced risk for bone-marrow suppression. Conversely, excess production of 6-methylmercaptopurine has been correlated with hepatotoxicity. Recent studies have suggested that measurement of 6-thioguanine nucleotides may guide therapy; in particular levels of 6-thioguanine nucleotides over 235 pmol/10^8 erythrocytes have been associated with improved clinical outcomes. Patients should be fully informed of the toxicities, which include marrow suppression, pancreatitis, hepatitis, and infections. Complete blood counts should be monitored throughout treatment as unexpected marrow suppression has occurred months after initiating therapy. Pancreatitis occurs in 3% to 5% of patients, usually within the first month of therapy. Infections may occur in 5% to 10% of patients, but severe infections occur in less than 2%. Of special concern is the risk of cancer with long-term use of purine analogs. While lymphoma has been reported in renal transplantation patients taking azathioprine, there is little convincing evidence of an excessive risk in ulcerative colitis patients treated with azathioprine or 6-mercaptopurine. Teratogenicity is another concern. Although no excess birth defects have been reported in children of inflammatory bowel disease patients taking purine analogs, studies are limited in this population.

Two additional immunosuppressant medications have been used in the management of steroid-dependent and steroid-refractory ulcerative colitis. Methotrexate, an inhibitor of dihydrofolate reductase, has demonstrable steroid-sparing effects when used parenterally at a dose of 25 mg/week in the treatment of both Crohn's disease and ulcerative colitis. A single study using smaller doses of methotrexate administered orally failed to demonstrate efficacy. Methotrexate has a high incidence of side effects including bone-marrow suppression and hepatic toxicity. The incidence of significant hepatic fibrosis in ulcerative colitis patients receiving methotrexate therapy is unknown at present. Methotrexate is teratogenic and is therefore contraindicated in pregnant woman or those considering pregnancy including males within 3 months of conception. In practice, use of methotrexate has been limited to steroid-dependent patients refractory or intolerant to azathioprine and 6-mercaptopurine.

Cyclosporine A is a potent immunosuppressant medication most commonly utilized in solid-organ transplantation. Its mechanism of action results from binding to cyclophilin molecules within T lymphocytes resulting in blockade of T-cell activation, inhibition of IL-2 synthesis, and reduction in T-cell clonal proliferation. The onset of action is rapid relative to the purine analogs. Cyclosporine A has been most frequently used in medical management of steroid refractory severe ulcerative colitis in patients wishing to avoid urgent colectomy. A single placebo-controlled study of intravenous cyclosporine A in steroid-refractory ulcerative colitis demonstrated rapid induction of clinical remission in 80% of patients. Following induction of remission, patients are maintained with oral cyclosporine A for approximately 3 months while azathioprine or 6-mercaptopurine is instituted. Premature discontinuation of cyclosporine A or failure to maintain remission with azathioprine or 6-mercaptopurine is associated with an increased rate of colectomy within 1 year. Anecdotal evidence suggests a similar response rate for tacrolimus, an immunosuppressant agent with a mechanism of action similar to cyclosporine A. Both cyclosporine A and tacrolimus have significant potential toxicities. These include renal impairment, hypertension, and neurologic dysfunction of which peripheral neuropathies, seizure, and headache are most prominent. The incidence of these side effects appears to be increased in patients with pre-existing renal disease, advanced age, and low serum cholesterol levels.

Novel therapies

A number of biological and other novel agents have been used in small numbers of ulcerative colitis patients with variable success; these include nicotine, heparin, cytokines and growth factors, and most recently, infliximab, an anti-TNFα chimeric antibody. Nicotine has been demonstrated to be effective as a steroid-sparing agent in a number of controlled trials of mild to moderate ulcerative colitis. In general, former smokers have tolerated this medication better than non-smokers. Side effects have included pruritis, headaches, sleep disturbance, and nightmares. Heparin was suggested to be beneficial in mild to moderate ulcerative colitis in several case series and small controlled studies. However, recent large randomized placebo-controlled clinical trials of heparin therapy failed to demonstrate efficacy in ulcerative colitis patients. A variety of cytokines including IL-10, IL-11, and keratinocyte growth factor have been studied for efficacy in the treatment of inflammatory bowel disease. None of these agents has been demonstrated to be effective in treating ulcerative colitis to date. However, two recent small clinical trials utilizing either Bowman-Birk inhibitor or the PPARg agonist, rosiglitizaone, have demonstrated efficacy with improvement in clinical symptoms and colonic inflammation associated with moderate to severe ulcerative colitis. Larger randomized controlled trials of these agents are presently underway. In addition, several investigators have reported small uncontrolled case series with successful use of infliximab in the treatment of severe ulcerative colitis. Although an initial randomized trial of infliximab in severe ulcerative colitis was limited by recruitment problems, a large multi-center randomized controlled trial for moderate to severe ulcerative colitis is currently enrolling patients. As a result, recommendations regarding the use of infliximab and other anti-TNFα agents await the results of these studies.

Surgical therapies

The principle objectives of surgical therapy for ulcerative colitis are elimination of the diseased colon and the preservation of continence, if possible. The indications for surgical treatment of ulcerative colitis include perforation, severe hemorrhage, dysplasia or cancer, and disease refractory to medical therapy. The role of prophylactic proctocolectomy in patients with long-standing extensive ulcerative colitis is controversial. Most clinicians have believed that although the risk of colorectal cancer is increased it is not high enough to warrant prophylactic proctocolectomy. Nonetheless, currently available surveillance techniques have not been demonstrated to reliably diminish the risk of a cancer-related death. Patients with extensive ulcerative colitis for a long duration (more than 20 years) should be informed of the limitations of colonoscopic surveillance and given the option of prophylactic proctocolectomy.

Several surgical options are available including

- total proctocolectomy with a standard Brooke end ileostomy
- colectomy with ileorectal anastomosis
- proctocolectomy with continent ileostomy (Koch pouch)
- restorative proctocolectomy with ileopouch–anal anastomosis.

At present, restorative proctocolectomy with ileopouch–anal anastomosis is the procedure of choice for preservation of continence. The challenges presented by this operative procedure are not insignificant. Despite increased experience with this procedure, overall complication rates reported in large series range from 29% to 87%. Pouch-related septic complications and pouchitis are significant contributing factors to the morbidity and result in pouch failure in 3% to 13% of cases. Nocturnal seepage and fecal incontinence are reported in 10% to 25% of patients undergoing ileopouch–anal anastomosis, particularly in elderly patients and in those patients with pre-existing anal dysfunction. Sexual and urinary dysfunction also complicates ileopouch–anal anastomosis procedures. Despite a variety of technical modifications including the use of prophylactic antibiotics, stapled anastomosis, avoidance of mucosectomy, and the alterations in ileal pouch construction, prospective studies have failed to demonstrate significant improvement in surgical outcome. Patient characteristics, including age, malnutrition, toxic colitis and megacolon, and the use of high-dose corticosteroids remain the primary risk factors associated with increased complications following ileopouch–anal anastomosis.

A recent modification of this operation omits the rectal mucosectomy and instead anastomoses the ileal pouch to the distal rectum in close proximity to the dentate line (1 to 4 cm). This ileopouch–distal rectal anastomosis is technically easier to perform, is thought by some to have less risk for incontinence, and in some hands can be performed as a single-stage operation without a diverting ileostomy. Controversy regarding the ileopouch–distal rectal anastomosis is related to the fact that some "transitional" epithelium is left intact that may be a source of future cancer risk.

Despite these limitations, surgery is curative for ulcerative colitis. Resolution of some extraintestinal disorders associated with ulcerative colitis, including primary biliary cirrhosis, axial arthropathy, and pyoderma gangrenosum, has not been observed following proctocolectomy. Nonetheless, the majority of patients with refractory ulcerative colitis who undergo proctocolectomy experience significant improvement in their quality of life following surgery. Complications such as pouchitis, though experienced by 50% to 60% of ulcerative colitis patients following ileopouch–anal anastomosis, are frequently clinically mild and responsive to metronidazole therapy.

Complications of ulcerative colitis

Serious complications of ulcerative colitis are uncommon but can be life threatening. These include toxic megacolon, perforation, and the development of colonic strictures. These complications are more frequently associated with extensive ulcerative colitis and are usually heralded by a pronounced change in clinical signs and symptoms.

Toxic megacolon, perforation, and colonic strictures

Toxic megacolon results from extension of the inflammatory reaction beyond the mucosa to involve large segments of the underlying tissues including the muscularis mucosa. Loss of contractility results in the accumulation of gas and fluid within the lumen with resultant dilation of the colon. Clinical deterioration accompanies colonic dilation with the frequent development of fever, malaise, hypotension, and diffuse abdominal distension with associated tenderness. Clinical laboratory abnormalities, reflecting progressive severe systemic inflammation, fluid sequestration and bloody diarrhea, include marked neutrophilic leukocytosis, anemia, and electrolyte disturbances. Criteria for the clinical diagnosis of toxic megacolon include radiographic evidence of colonic distension (colon diameter greater than 6 cm) which is most frequently observed in the transverse colon.

Toxic megacolon is most frequently encountered early in the course of chronic ulcerative colitis and may be the initial presentation of the disease. Nearly 50% patients with toxic megacolon developed this complication within 3 months of their diagnosis in one series. Patients with extensive colitis appear to be most at risk for toxic megacolon, but this complication has also been reported in patients with disease limited to the left colon. Other risk factors for development of toxic megacolon include antimotility medications including anticholinergic drugs and narcotics as well as procedures such as barium enema or colonoscopy during a severe flare of ulcerative colitis. In these latter circumstances, distension of the inflamed colon appears to result in colonic ischemia and translocation of bacteria and fecal material into the walls of the colon.

Medical therapy for toxic megacolon is directed at prevention of free perforation and restoration of colonic motility. Reduction of fluid and air within the gastrointestinal tract may be achieved through a nothing-by-mouth status and nasogastric suction. Correction of fluid and electrolyte abnormalities (particularly hypokalemia) is frequently necessary and may improve colonic contractility. Patients are frequently treated with systemic antibiotics and intravenous corticosteroids, but these measures have not been proven to alter the clinical course in controlled clinical trials. The most critical feature of medical management is frequent observation for the development of impeding perforation. Patients with progressive abdominal distension, development of rebound tenderness, or cardiovascular instability should undergo colectomy. Similarly, a failure to improve after 48 hours of medical therapy should prompt surgical intervention. Mortality from toxic megacolon is directly correlated with perforation. Mortality following emergent colectomy was 44% in patients with perforation as compared to 2% in patients who underwent colectomy prior to colonic perforation. The development of toxic megacolon is also a poor prognostic sign even in patients who initially respond to medical therapy. In one series, nearly 50% of patients successfully treated for toxic megacolon ultimately required colectomy because of intractable disease.

Free perforation may also develop in the absence of toxic megacolon, albeit at a significantly reduced incidence. As with toxic megalcolon, patients with extensive colitis appear to be at greatest risk for this complication. In addition, this complication appears to occur most frequently early in the course of the disease. Case series of free perforations complicating ulcerative colitis indicate that the segment most at risk for perforation is the sigmoid colon. Although the role of high-dose corticosteroids has been suggested by some reviews, this has not been validated by results from other studies.

In contrast to toxic megacolon and free perforation, colonic strictures complicating ulcerative colitis occur late in the course of the disease. Although clinically significant strictures occur rarely, pathologic narrowing has been observed in over 10% of surgical specimens. As with other complications of ulcerative colitis, patients with extensive colitis, particularly those with intractable symptoms, appear to be at greatest risk. Clinically, strictures present with alterations in bowel habits including increased frequency of diarrhea and fecal incontinence. Pathologically, strictures associated with ulcerative colitis are short (2 to 3 cm in length) and result from hypertrophy and thickening of the muscularis mucosa rather than fibrosis. More worrisome, stricture in ulcerative colitis may result from malignancy which may not be identifiable on mucosal biopsy. As a result, the development of a colonic stricture, particularly in the setting of long-standing ulcerative colitis, should prompt surgical resection because of the risk of associated malignancy.

Dysplasia and carcinoma

Malignant transformation of the chronically inflamed epithelium is a well-recognized and much-feared complication of long-standing ulcerative colitis. The absolute risk for colorectal cancer in patients with ulcerative colitis has been subject to considerable debate. Estimates of the cumulative risk for all patients with ulcerative colitis range from 1.8% after 20 years of disease to 43% after 35 years of disease. These wide variances in risk estimates most likely reflect the effects of selection bias, loss of susceptible subjects, and limited control for other potential risk factors including age of disease onset and the anatomic extent of disease. The principle source of selection bias relates to the location in which the studies were performed. Studies conducted at large referral centers have reported a very high incidence of cancer which may reflect both patients with more severe inflammatory bowel disease and patients more likely to have cancer. Population-based studies are limited by the loss of susceptible subjects from population-based cohorts and may therefore underestimate the risk of cancer. Studies of ulcerative colitis-associated colorectal cancer, conducted in locations where colectomy is performed more frequently and earlier in the course of the disease, may be expected to have even lower cumulative risk estimates, particularly as colorectal cancer risk is strongly determined by duration of disease. Most large series have reported a lifetime risk for colorectal cancer of 5% to 15% in patients with greater than 20 years of disease. The incidence of colorectal cancer does not become appreciably increased until 8 to 10 years after the onset of ulcerative colitis.

A number of risk factors for colorectal cancer have been examined in these studies. These include duration of disease, extent of colitis, disease activity, age of onset, the presence of primary biliary sclerosis, and medical therapy. The strongest evidence for increased risk has been documented with the duration and anatomic extent of disease. As noted above, the cumulative risk of colorectal cancer increases dramatically after 10 years of disease with incidence rates of approximately 15% after 20 to 25 years. Most studies have documented a markedly increased colorectal cancer incidence in patients with extensive colitis as compared to disease limited to the left colon. Moreover, a 3-fold increase in colorectal cancer risk has recently been reported for patients with extensive colitis and "backwash ileitis" as compared with patients with extensive colitis in the absence of ileal inflammation. In one large population-based study, patients with extensive ulcerative colitis had a nearly 15-fold increased risk of colorectal cancer compared to the general population. Conversely, the increase in colorectal cancer risk in patients with disease limited to the rectum was only 1.7-fold.

Studies examining the impact of age of diagnosis on colorectal cancer incidence have reported conflicting results. While some investigators have documented an increased risk in patients with disease onset <15 years, other population-based studies have documented increased risk in patients >40 years. Other investigators have not identified any significant risk associated with age of diagnosis. These studies may have been confounded by difficulty establishing the time of disease onset in those patients who may have subclinical disease. Conversely, studies examining the role of disease activity have been hampered by the increased likelihood of colectomy in patients with more severe colitis. Nonetheless, no increased risk for colorectal cancer has been documented with increased disease activity.

The effect of primary sclerosing cholangitis on colorectal cancer risk in ulcerative colitis patients has also been subject to some controversy. Most studies of ulcerative colitis patients with concurrent primary sclerosing cholangitis have demonstrated a small increased incidence of colorectal cancer. The precise role of primary sclerosing cholangitis as an independent risk factor remains uncertain as these patients generally have quiescent ulcerative colitis. The increased risk of colorectal cancer may therefore reflect longer duration of disease.

The effect of medical therapy for ulcerative colitis on subsequent colorectal cancer risk is another area of controversy. Use of sulfasalazine and azathioprine has been reported to reduce the incidence of colorectal cancer in ulcerative colitis patients. Unfortunately, these results have not been replicated by other investigators to date. Similarly, it has been suggested that vitamin supplementation, in particular folic acid, decreases the incidence of colorectal cancer in ulcerative colitis patients. While several studies have indicated a decrease in sporadic colorectal cancer incidence with supplemental vitamins A, C, or E, there remains a paucity of data on vitamin supplementation in ulcerative colitis-associated colorectal cancer.

The biology of most sporadic colorectal cancer involves sequential mutations of numerous genes involved in epithelial proliferation and differentiation. These mutations result in a well-characterized, progressive development of adenomatous polyps and subsequently invasive cancer. In contrast, colorectal cancer developing in the background of ulcerative colitis typically does not develop along this adenoma-to-invasive cancer pathway. Rather, these cancers tend to arise in a background of flat dysplastic tissue. Genetic alterations identified in ulcerative colitis-associated colorectal cancer include DNA aneuploidy and microsatellite instability. Genomic instability, either directly or as a marker of impaired DNA repair mechanisms, may represent an early step in the carcinogenesis pathway within colonic tissue damaged by chronic inflammation. The specific pattern of genetic mutations associated with colorectal cancer also suggests a different mechanism of carcinogenesis in ulcerative colitis as compared to sporadic colorectal cancer (Figure 4.8). The APC gene is mutated in most sporadic colon cancers and is thought to be an early event in this carcinogenesis pathway. In contrast, the APC mutation is relatively rarely identified in ulcerative colitis-associated cancers. Conversely, mutations in p53, which typically occur late in the progression toward sporadic colon cancers, are detected at high frequency in ulcerative colitis-associated dysplasia and cancer.

The increased incidence of colorectal cancer has prompted the development of strategies to minimize the risk of invasive carcinoma in patients with long-standing ulcerative colitis. Prophylactic colectomy after 10 years of disease has been advocated by some clinicians for patients with extensive colitis. However, most clinicians have not embraced prophylactic colectomy in all patients with ulcerative

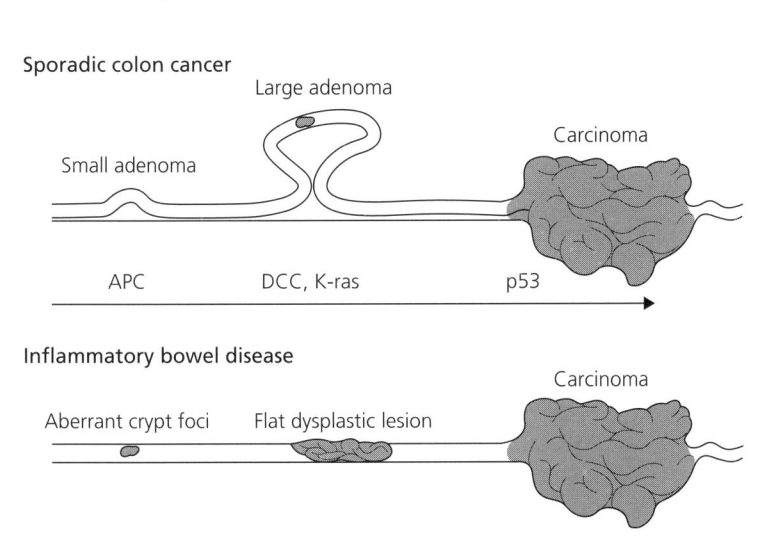

Figure 4.8 Differential patterns of genetic mutations associated with colitis-associated colon cancer as compared to sporadic colon cancer.

Ulcerative Colitis

colitis. Instead, strategies to identify ulcerative colitis patients at particularly high risk for colorectal cancer have been developed and implemented in most communities. Diagnostic colonoscopy at fixed time intervals with multiple mucosal biopsies to detect epithelial dysplasia is presently the surveillance strategy of choice for patients with ulcerative colitis of greater than 10 years' duration.

Dysplasia is believed to be a precursor lesion in the pathway towards the development of invasive carcinoma in patients with ulcerative colitis. Nearly 90% of colon specimens resected for malignancy in ulcerative colitis will have dysplasia located somewhere in the specimen. Although considered a precursor lesion, dysplasia is a neoplastic transformation of the colonic epithelium. Biopsy specimens are commonly classified as negative for dysplasia, indefinite for dysplasia, low-grade dysplasia, and high-grade dysplasia. When dysplasia is identified in macroscopically abnormal mucosa it is classified as a dysplasia associated lesion or mass. Identification of dysplasia in biopsy specimens obtained during surveillance colonoscopy has important prognostic implications. The presence of high-grade dysplasia has been associated with a 30% likelihood of concurrent colorectal cancer. Similarly, concurrent colorectal cancer has been reported in nearly 60% of patients with dysplasia associated lesions or mass lesions in some studies. The presence of low grade dysplasia is also associated with progression to high grade dysplasia and colorectal cancer, albeit at a reduced frequency.

Despite the widespread use of colon surveillance programs for patients with ulcerative colitis, no randomized controlled trial has been published demonstrating a reduction in mortality from ulcerative colitis-associated colorectal cancer as a result of participation in a colonoscopic surveillance program. Successful identification of Dukes A carcinomas have been reported by several large surveillance programs, but the absence of a control population limits the interpretation of these results. Some patients will develop invasive cancer despite recent negative surveillance colonoscopies. Failure to identify dysplasia during surveillance biopsies may result from sampling errors, as biopsies sample only a small fraction of the total mucosa. In addition, a significant number of advanced colorectal cancers have been identified even among patients enrolled in surveillance protocols. Improvements in diagnosis of epithelial dysplasia through the use of adjuctive diagnostic studies, including assessment for DNA aneuploidy, immunohistochemical staining for epithelial cell surface markers associated with dysplasia and colorectal cancer, and identification of dysplasia-associated genetic mutations are the focus of extensive clinical investigation. Presently, most algorithms for colorectal cancer surveillance in ulcerative colitis recommend initial screening colonoscopy after 10 years of disease in patients with disease proximal to the sigmoid colon followed by repeat colonoscopies at 2 to 3-year intervals (Figure 4.9). Multiple surveillance biopsies at 10 cm intervals utilizing jumbo forceps

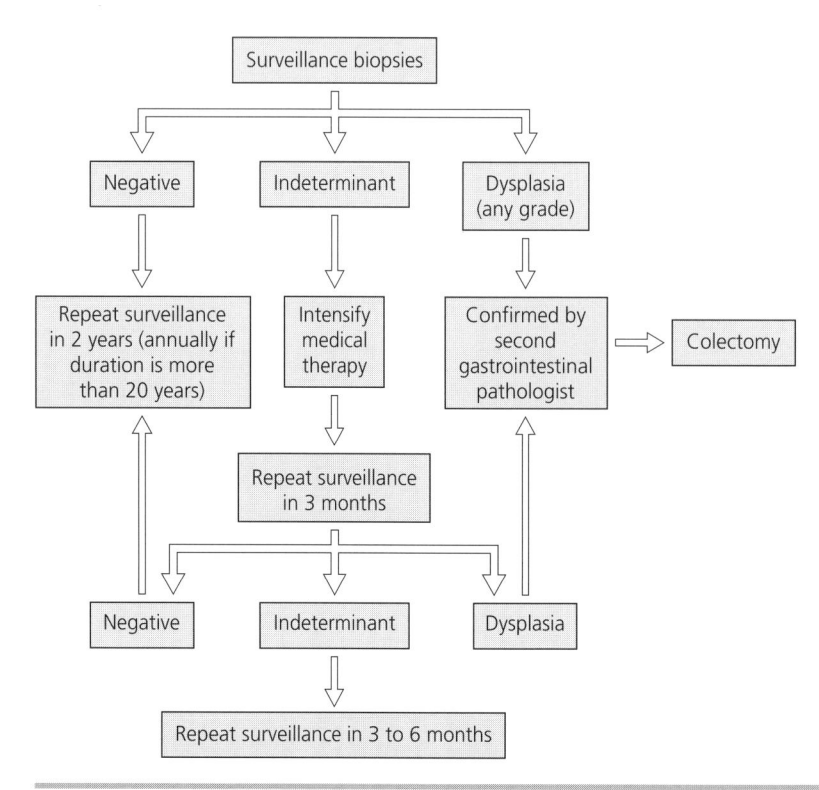

Figure 4.9 An approach to colon cancer surveillance in patients with chronic ulcerative colitis.

has been reported to identify dysplasia with a 95% confidence level in colon specimens with known colorectal cancer. Annual surveillance colonoscopy has been advocated for patients with extensive ulcerative colitis after 20 years duration.

Ulcerative colitis during pregnancy

Young patients with ulcerative colitis planning a family are obviously concerned about the effects of ulcerative colitis and drug treatment on the baby and the effects of pregnancy on disease activity in the female patient. Fortunately, most of the available data is reassuring. Retrospective studies have suggested no significant impact of ulcerative colitis on the outcome of pregnancy. Rates of healthy offspring between 76% to 97%, spontaneous abortions of 5% to 13%, stillbirths of 1% to 3%, and congenital abnormalities of 1% to 3%, do not differ significantly from those expected in the normal population. However, some population-based investigations have shown an increased risk of preterm birth, low birth weight and small size for gestational age. The risk of preterm birth appears to be particularly increased when the first hospitalization for ulcerative colitis occurred during pregnancy. The presence of ulcerative colitis has not influenced the mode of delivery or the incidence of eclampsia or pre-eclampsia.

The course of ulcerative colitis during pregnancy correlates with disease activity at the time of conception. Among pregnancies occurring in patients with inactive ulcerative colitis, approximately 34% will relapse during gestation and puerperium, this is similar to the relapse rate in non-pregnant ulcerative colitis patients. Most relapses occur during the first trimester; this may partially be related to patients stopping maintenance medications. Approximately two thirds of pregnant ulcerative colitis patients will have quiescent disease throughout the pregnancy.

Without drug therapy, active ulcerative colitis at conception is at risk of worsening during pregnancy. In women with active ulcerative colitis at the time of conception, the disease activity worsens in 45%, remains unchanged in 24%, and improves in 31% of individuals. Pregnancy will occasionally induce an improvement in disease activity or clinical remission, usually in the first trimester. Not infrequently, the first presentation of ulcerative colitis will coincide with pregnancy. Additionally, some patients will have symptomatic disease only when pregnant, with quiescence between pregnancies and exacerbations during subsequent pregnancies.

Maintenance therapy with sulfasalazine and mesalamine is safe throughout pregnancy. Steroids can be used for the control of acute flares of disease without ill effects on the fetus. Small reports suggest that azathioprine and 6-mercaptopurine may also be safe in patients where the potential benefits of controlling disease activity outweigh the potential small risks to the fetus of continued immunosuppression.

Further reading

Blam ME. Stein RB. Lichtenstein GR. Integrating anti-tumor necrosis factor therapy in inflammatory bowel disease: current and future perspectives. *Am J Gastroenterol*, 2001; 96(7):1977–97.

Farmer RG, Easley KA, Rankin GB. Clinical patterns, natural history and progression of ulcerative colitis: A long term follow-up of 1116 patients. *Dig Dis Sci* 1993;38:1137.

Farrell RJ, Peppercorn MA. Ulcerative colitis. *Lancet* 2002;359:331.

Faubion WA Jr, Loftus EV Jr, Harmsen WS, Zinsmeister AR, Sandborn WJ. The natural history of corticosteroid therapy for inflammatory bowel disease: a population-based study. *Gastroenterology* 2001; 121:255–60.

Fiocchi C. Inflammatory bowel disease: etiology and pathogenesis. *Gastroenterology* 1998;115:182–205.

Jewell, DP. Ulcerative colitis. In: Feldman M, Scharschmidt BF, Sleisenger MH (eds). *Gastrointestinal and Liver Disease*, 6th edn, vol 2. Philadelphia, WB Saunders 1998; p 1735.

Langholz E, Munkholm P, Davidsen M et al. Course of ulcerative colitis: Analysis of changes in disease activity over years. *Gastroenterology* 1994; 107:3.

Lewis JD, Deren JJ, Lichtenstein GR. Cancer risk in patients with inflammatory bowel disease. *Gastroenterol Clin North Am* 1999; 28(2):459–477.

Peeters M, Joossens S, Vermeire S, Vlietinck R, Bossuyt X, Rutgeerts P. Diagnostic value of anti-Saccharomyces cerevisiae and antineutrophil cytoplasmic autoantibodies in inflammatory bowel disease. *Am J Gastroenterol* 2001; 96:730–734.

Ritchie JK, Powell-Tuck J, Lennard-Jones JE. Clinical outcome of the first ten years of ulcerative colitis and proctitis. *Lancet* 1978;1:1140.

Sandborn WJ, Targan SR. Biologic therapy of inflammatory bowel disease. *Gastroenterology*, 2002;122(6):1592–608.

Surawicz CM, Belic L. Rectal biopsy helps to distinguish acute self-limited colitis from idiopathic inflammatory bowel disease. *Gastroenterology* 1984;86:104.

Sutherland LR. Clinical course and complications of ulcerative colitis and ulcerative proctitis. In: Targan SR, Shanahan F (eds). *Inflammatory Bowel Disease: From Bench to Bedside*. Baltimore, Williams and Wilkins, 1994; p 279.

Swidsinski A, Ladhoff A, Pernthaler A, *et al*. Mucosal flora in inflammatory bowel disease. *Gastroenterology* 2002; 122:44–54.

Tysk C, Lindberg E, Jarnerot G, Floderus-Myrhed B. Ulcerative colitis and Crohn's disease in an unselected population of monozygotic and dizygotic twins: a study of heritability and the influence of smoking. *Gut* 1988; 29:990–996.

Chapter 5

Crohn's Disease

Chinyu Su and Gary R. Lichtenstein

CHAPTER OUTLINE

INTRODUCTION

PATHOGENESIS
- Immunological mechanisms
- Genetics of Crohn's disease
- Environmental factors

CLINICAL FEATURES
- Clinical findings
- Radiographic and endoscopic findings
- Pathology
- Disease activity

DIAGNOSIS
- Differential diagnoses

MEDICAL THERAPY
- General principles
- Aminosalicylates
- Corticosteroids
- Antibiotics
- Immunomodulators
- Anti-tumor necrosis factor therapies
- Other biological therapies
- Additional novel therapies
- Nutritional therapy

SURGICAL THERAPY

EXTRAINTESTINAL COMPLICATIONS
- Musculoskeletal diseases
- Dermatologic diseases
- Ocular diseases
- Hematologic diseases
- Genitourinary and renal diseases
- Hepatobiliary diseases

APPROACHES TO THE MANAGEMENT OF CROHN'S DISEASE

MANAGEMENT OF SPECIFIC CLINICAL PROBLEMS AND COMPLICATIONS
- Abscesses and fistulas
- Obstructions
- Perianal disease
- Cancers
- Pregnancy

FURTHER READING

Introduction

Crohn's disease is a chronic inflammatory disorder of the gastrointestinal tract. It is characterized by exacerbations interposed between variable periods of remission and is associated with a wide spectrum of clinical features. Since the initial report of Crohn's disease by Dr Burrill Crohn, Dr Leon Ginzburg, and Dr Gordon Oppenheimer in 1932, significant advances have been made in our knowledge of the pathogenesis of Crohn's disease as well as in therapies for this potentially debilitating disorder. The incidence of Crohn's disease in the US is approximately 5 per 100 000 persons per year. There is evidence that the incidence of Crohn's disease has been increasing worldwide over the past several decades. The prevalence of Crohn's disease has been estimated at 90 per 100 000 persons. Although the incidence and prevalence of Crohn's disease remain relatively low compared to other more common gastrointestinal diseases, the total annual costs in the US have been estimated to be approximately 2 billion dollars. While medications account for only 10% of the total costs, hospitalizations and surgeries account for approximately half of the costs. It is unknown how the newer medical therapies will impact on the overall health-care costs, however it is clear that the health-care costs associated with Crohn's disease are substantial.

Pathogenesis

The pathogenesis of Crohn's disease is incompletely understood. There is increasing evidence suggesting that Crohn's disease is the result of the complex interaction of three elements – genetic susceptibility, host immunity, and environmental factors. In a normal individual, the gut exists in a constant low-grade inflammatory state in response to environmental stimuli such as bacterial products or endogenous factors. The currently prevailing hypothesis suggests that dysregulation of these physiological processes leads to inappropriate amplification of the enteric immune response and manifestations of mucosal injuries are seen in Crohn's disease in genetically predisposed individuals.

Immunological mechanisms

The currently held paradigm of the pathogenesis of Crohn's disease emphasizes the role of the enteric immune response. The initiation and regulation of this process involves a number of elements. Detection of immunogenic signals requires transduction by the epithelium and antigen sampling across the epithelium. One of the key regulators of this innate immune response is Toll-like receptors expressed by the intestinal epithelial cells.

Following antigen presentation, activated T-cells and macrophages elaborate cytokine mediators which differentially induce one of the two major immune phenotypes, T helper 1 and T helper 2. The T-helper-1 response is characterized by cell-mediated immunity and is associated with the production of interleukin (IL)-1, IL-2, IL-6, tumor necrosis factor alpha (TNFα), and interferon gamma. The differentiation of T cells along a T-helper-1 pathway is stimulated by IL-12 generated in response to exposure to bacteria. The T-helper-2 response is characterized by the production of cytokines IL-4, IL-5, and IL-10, which amplify the humoral immune response. In general, these cytokines can be broadly categorized as pro-inflammatory (TNFα, IL-1, IL-2, IL-6, IL-8, and IL-12) or anti-inflammatory (IL-4, IL-5, IL-10, IL-11, and transforming growth factor beta) cytokines based upon their ultimate effects. The induction of the T-helper-1 pathway and release of T-helper-1 cytokines result in tissue destruction by activated matrix metalloproteinase and further amplifies the inflammatory response by upregulating adhesion molecules and facilitating recruitment of other inflammatory mediators. Both T-helper-1 and T-helper-2 pathways can be regulated by specific suppressor T-cell ($T_H 3$, $T_R 1$) subsets, which produce IL-10 and transforming growth factor beta and downregulate inflammation. Termination of the immune response is also regulated by the apoptosis of mucosal T cells.

Although not strictly dichotomized, Crohn's disease is generally considered to be characterized by the T-helper-1 phenotype. Other defects at various levels of the mucosal immune response have also been noted in Crohn's disease, including alteration in the epithelial expression of Toll-like receptors and resistance of T cells to apoptosis. Thus, mucosal injury in most patients with Crohn's disease can be accounted for by the downstream effects of excessive T-helper-1 cytokine responses and/or failure to counter-regulate these responses.

Genetics of Crohn's disease

The evidence for genetic components for Crohn's disease is derived primarily from family and twin studies. The risk of developing Crohn's disease in a first-degree relative of a Crohn's disease patient is 5% to 8%. The concordance rates for monozygotic and dizygotic twins for Crohn's disease are approximately 67% and 8%, respectively. In contrast, there is no increased incidence of Crohn's disease in the spouse of a patient compared to the general population. This observation of relatively high concordance among monozygotic twins and discordance among spouses supports the notion of a genetic susceptibility of Crohn's disease. In addition, there are also ethnic variations in the prevalence of Crohn's disease, supporting the genetic contribution to this disorder. There is an increased prevalence of disease in the Jewish population compared to the non-Jewish population, and this high rate of disease is most prominent among the Ashkenazi Jews. The various genetically engineered animals which exhibit phenotypes resembling Crohn's disease further support the genetic heterogeneity of this disease. No single gene or genetic model can fully explain the development of Crohn's disease.

Several susceptibility gene loci have been identified for Crohn's disease. The first susceptibility locus is mapped to a region designated *IBD1* locus on chromosome 16. Additional susceptibility loci have also been mapped to other chromosomes, including *IBD2* (chromosome 12), *IBD3* (chromosome 6), and *IBD4* (chromosome 14). Although there are candidate genes within or near each of these loci that may have pathogenic importance, the exact nature of disease susceptibility for these genetic changes remains unknown. The best studied susceptibility locus is the *IBD1* locus. Mutations of the *NOD2* gene in this region have been shown to be associated with Crohn's disease. The *NOD2* gene is expressed primarily in monocytes. It encodes cytosolic Nod2 proteins which bind to bacterial lipopolysaccharides. The Nod2 proteins also activate nuclear factor kappa B, a key event in inflammatory processes. The activation of nuclear factor kappa B by Nod2 proteins is thought to be regulated by the lipopolysaccharide binding domain of the gene; deletion of this domain has been shown to stimulate the nuclear factor kappa B signaling pathway. Several mutations of the *NOD2* gene have been identified that are associated with Crohn's disease. The relative risk for developing Crohn's disease in homozygotes and compound heterozygotes for *NOD2* mutations is approximately forty-fold. It is important to note that *NOD2* variants account for less than 20% of Crohn's disease, thus additional gene variants or alternative loci contribute to disease susceptibility.

Environmental factors

There is strong evidence supporting the contribution of environmental factors to the development of Crohn's disease. The concordance rate of considerably less than 100% for Crohn's disease within monozygotic twins strongly suggests that genetic determinants alone cannot account for the development of Crohn's disease. The role of environmental factors is also supported by several epidemiological observations. The risk of disease varies among ethnic groups living in different geographical regions, and the disease is more common in developed than in less-developed countries, and more common in urban than in rural areas. It is postulated that environmental factors contribute to the development of disease by influencing the enteric immune system, the intestinal flora, or both.

The luminal bacterial flora plays a major role in the pathogenesis of Crohn's disease. The strongest evidence supporting the role of intestinal microflora comes from animal models where colitis does not develop in a germ-free environment. In patients with Crohn's disease, inflammation is present predominantly in regions of the bowel with the highest bacterial concentrations. Diversion of the fecal stream can ameliorate the disease, while restoration of the fecal stream results in disease relapses in patients with Crohn's disease. Patients with Crohn's disease also exhibit immune reactivity against enteric bacteria, with increased serum and secreted antibodies and the presence of mucosal T cells recognizing luminal bacteria. It has been postulated that both alterations of the normal luminal flora and excessive immune responses to the normal intestinal flora may be present in patients with Crohn's disease. Examples of some differences in the composition of the enteric flora of Crohn's patients compared to healthy individuals include increased concentrations of *Bacteroides*, *Eubacterium* and *Peptostreptococcus*, and decreased counts of *Bifidobacterium* in patients with Crohn's disease. Given the complexity of enteric flora and the host–flora interactions, no specific microorganism has been identified as an etiologic agent for Crohn's disease.

Clinical features

Crohn's disease may affect any portion of the gastrointestinal tract, but there are three common patterns of involvement

1. approximately 40% to 50% of patients have disease in the terminal ileum and the cecum at presentation
2. approximately 30% of patients have disease limited to the small bowel
3. 25% of patients have colonic-limited disease at presentation.

The rectum is typically spared. Less commonly, patients may have involvement of the upper gastrointestinal tract including the mouth, esophagus, stomach, and duodenum.

Given the heterogeneity of its clinical presentations, it is difficult to uniformly classify Crohn's disease. Disease classification has traditionally been based primarily on the anatomic location and the behavior of the disease, which are important in determining clinical outcomes. The disease behavior can generally be categorized into three patterns based on the predominant clinical feature – inflammatory, fibrostenotic (stricturing), or perforating (fistulizing) disease. A recently developed classification, the Vienna Classification, includes age at diagnosis as a variable in addition to the location and behavior of the disease (Table 5.1). In this classification system, age at diagnosis is defined as younger than 40 years, or equal to or greater than 40 years. Location of disease is classified as terminal ileum, colon, ileocolon, and upper gastrointestinal tract. Behavior of disease is categorized as stricturing, penetrating, and non-stricturing non-penetrating. Genetic markers may also supplement the phenotypic stratification in the future. For example, *NOD2* mutations have been found to be associated with ileal-only disease.

Another important feature of Crohn's disease is its variable clinical course. The majority of patients with Crohn's disease have intermittent exacerbations of disease interposed with variable periods of relatively quiescent disease or remission. The probability of a prolonged remission and a continuously active course after 10 years from the initial diagnosis are 12% and 1% based on a Swedish population-based study, respectively. Thus, the majority of patients have an intermittently relapsing course. Approximately 60% to 70% of patients will eventually require surgery over the course of their disease.

Table 5.1 Vienna Classification of Crohn's disease.

Age at diagnosis	A1 < 40 years
	A2 ≥ 40 years
Location	L1 terminal ileum
	L2 colon
	L3 ileocolon
	L4 upper gastrointestinal tract
Behavior	B1 non-stricturing non-penetrating
	B2 stricturing
	B3 penetrating

Clinical findings

The clinical manifestations of the disease vary depending on its location and pattern. The classical symptoms of Crohn's disease include right-lower-quadrant abdominal pain and diarrhea. Other common symptoms include low-grade fever, decreased appetite, fatigue, and weight loss. Patients with colonic disease may have symptoms of colitis, including hematochezia, fecal urgency, and tenesmus. Patients with a more diffuse inflammatory pattern of the small bowel have more prominent components of malabsorption such as diarrhea and weight loss. In contrast, patients with fibrostenotic disease usually present with symptoms of a partial small-bowel obstruction, including abdominal pain, bloating, nausea, and vomiting.

Findings on physical examination depend on the pattern and severity of the disease. The abdomen is typically tender to palpation over the region of active disease. Examination may reveal fullness or a palpable mass in the right lower quadrant, due to the presence of thickened and adherent loops of bowel or intra-abdominal abscess. Patients with long-standing severe disease may exhibit signs of malnutrition. A careful rectal examination is important in patients with Crohn's disease to identify fistulas, prominent skin tags, and evidence of a perianal abscess as suggested by induration, erythema, or tenderness in the perianal region.

Laboratory findings are generally non-specific. Mild leukocytosis and thrombocytosis may present with active disease. Marked leukocytosis should alert clinicians for the presence of suppurative complications such as abscesses. The erythrocyte sedimentation rate may be elevated in the presence of active disease, but it is also non-specific. Other laboratory abnormalities typically reflect chronic disease and malnutrition, including anemia and hypoalbuminemia. Deficiency in iron, folate, and vitamin B_{12} may all contribute to anemia, as well as gastrointestinal blood loss from active mucosal disease.

Radiographic and endoscopic findings

The radiological features of early Crohn's disease include a coarse granular pattern, mucosal nodularity, and fold thickening (Box 5.1). Aphthous ulceration is a common early finding, but it is non-specific for Crohn's disease. With progression of disease, large and coalescing ulcerations form. These ulcers tend to be deep, linear, and serpigi-

Clinical features

> **Box 5.1** Radiologic features of Crohn's disease
>
> Mucosal nodularity
> Fold thickening/bowel wall thickening
> Aphthous ulceration
> Linear longitudinal ulceration
> Cobblestoning
> Fistula formation
> Stricture formation
> Pseudopolyps
> Skip lesions
> Asymmetric involvement
> Small bowel involvement

nous. Additional features include cobblestoning, fistulas, pseudopolyps, and bowel-wall thickening. In Crohn's colitis, the disease involvement is patchy, asymmetric, and discontinuous, with normal mucosa intervening between lesions. This pattern results in the characteristic skip lesions. This is in sharp contrast to ulcerative colitis where the disease involvement is continuous, confluent, circumferential, and symmetrical.

The endoscopic appearance corresponds to radiographic findings (Box 5.2). The earliest endoscopic feature of Crohn's disease is the aphthous ulcer, which is characterized by a white depressed center surrounded by a halo of erythema, and may appear in an otherwise normal segment of bowel. It should be stressed that these are not specific for Crohn's disease, and may be seen in many other cases of infectious colitis such as *Yersinia*, *Shigella*, amebia-

> **Box 5.2** Endoscopic features of Crohn's disease
>
> Aphthous ulcerations
> Ulcers within normal mucosa in early disease
> Cobblestoning
> Pseudopolyps
> Loss of haustral folds
> Linear surface scars
> Bridging fibrosis
> Fistulas
> Fissures
> Skip lesions
> Asymmetric involvement
> Terminal ileitis
> Rectal sparing

sis, herpes simplex virus and cytomegalovirus colitis, and Behçet's colitis. Smaller ulcerations may coalesce to form larger ulcers, while the surrounding mucosa has a normal appearance. This is in sharp contrast to ulcerative colitis where ulcerations always occur within areas of active inflammation. Another important endoscopic feature of Crohn's disease is cobblestoning, characterized by a colonoscopic appearance that ranges from fairly uniform nodularity to criss-crossing furrowed ulceration. Because of the nature of "skip lesions", severe cobblestoning may be seen adjacent to normal-appearing mucosa, and is almost pathognomonic for Crohn's disease. Other colonoscopic features can be seen in both Crohn's disease and ulcerative colitis, including inflammatory pseudopolyps, loss of haustral folds, and linear surface scars. When Crohn's disease involves the proximal gastrointestinal tract, similar findings may be present on esophagogastroduodenoscopy, including aphthous ulcerations, inflammatory pseudopolyps, and cobblestoning. Upper endoscopy, however, commonly demonstrates only non-specific inflammation.

Pathology

In Crohn's disease the involved bowel is typically thickened and edematous on gross examination, and may adhere to the adjacent bowel or organ. The characteristic appearance of "creeping fat" occurs when mesenteric fat tissues spread over the serosal surface of the bowel. The mucosa of the involved bowel in the early stage of the disease may exhibit aphthous ulcers, which subsequently enlarge, deepen, and eventually coalesce to form transverse and longitudinal linear ulcers as the disease progresses. The mucosa may also exhibit a cobblestoned appearance. The transmural disease process may give rise to the formation of fissures, abscesses, or fistulas. With chronic inflammation and healing processes the involved bowel may become fibrotic and form a stricture.

The hallmark of the histological findings in Crohn's disease is transmural and patchy inflammation. This is in contrast to ulcerative colitis where the disease is limited to the mucosa and submucosa. There may be inflammatory cell infiltration in the lamina propria and lymphoid aggregates in the submucosa, occasionally extending to the muscularis propria. Crypt architectural distortion may be present in Crohn's colitis but is less common than in ulcerative colitis. The presence of non-caseating granulomas may allow distinction from ulcerative colitis, but they are present in up to only 40% of endoscopic biopsy specimens. Granulomas may also be seen in non-inflammatory bowel disease conditions, including tuberculosis, fungal infections, *Yersinia* infections, and sarcoidosis.

Disease activity

An accurate assessment of the disease activity in patients with Crohn's disease is often difficult because of the wide spectrum of clinical manifestations and the lack of a specific diagnostic test. Several numerical indices have been developed to allow standardized evaluation of disease activity for Crohn's disease. The most commonly used in clinical trials is the Crohn's Disease Activity Index. This is an index derived from eight weighted, subjective and objective components, including the number of diarrheal stools, abdominal pain, general well-being, extraintestinal or systemic manifestations, use of antidiarrheal medications, abdominal mass, hematocrit, and body weight. A patient is considered to be in remission if the Crohn's Disease Activity Index score is less than 150, have mild to moderate disease activity if the score is 200 to 450, and have severe disease activity if the score is greater than 450. However, this index requires the patient to keep a diary for 1 week and is inconvenient for daily practice. Its use has been primarily in the clinical-trial setting.

In clinical practice, patients who are asymptomatic or have no inflammatory sequelae are considered to be in remission. Patients are generally considered to have mildly to moderately active disease when they are ambulatory, able to tolerate oral diet, and manifest no signs of dehydration, toxicities, abdominal tenderness, painful mass, or obstruction (Table 5.2). Moderate to severe disease refers to patients refractory to treatment for mild to moderate disease or those with prominent symptoms of fever, significant weight loss, abdominal pain and tenderness, nausea and vomiting (without obstruction), or significant anemia. Severe or fulminant disease applies to patients with persistent symptoms despite corticosteroid therapy, or those exhibiting high fever, persistent vomiting, evidence of intestinal obstruction, rebound tenderness, cachexia, or evidence of an abscess.

Laboratory markers including erythrocyte sedimentation rate, C-reactive protein, and orosomucoid levels may be helpful but are non-specific. Recent studies suggest that fecal levels of neutrophil-specific proteins such as calprotectin and lactoferrin may correlate with disease activity and appear to be more sensitive and specific than the traditional serum erythrocyte sedimentation rate. Thus, stools assays of these proteins potentially may serve as a non-invasive tool of monitoring disease activity and predicting pending relapses.

Diagnosis

The diagnosis of Crohn's disease is based on a constellation of characteristic clinical presentations, radiographic and endoscopic appearances, and histological findings. Because the presentations can be variable and many associated symptoms and signs are non-specific, the interval between symptom onset and the diagnosis of Crohn's disease has been reported to be approximately 2 to 3 years. The two primary tools commonly used for diagnosing Crohn's disease are radiography and endoscopy. The choice of diagnostic tests is primarily guided by the patient's clinical presentations and the suspected location of disease involvement. In general, endoscopy is the preferred method for establishing the diagnosis whenever possible because it allows the direct inspection of luminal mucosa and provides biopsy specimens for histological analyses. In contrast, air-contrast luminal radiography provides information about the location, extent, and contiguity of disease throughout the gastrointestinal tract. It also allows examination of the bowel distensibility and the presence of strictures or fistulas.

Given that the majority of patients with Crohn's disease present with terminal ileum or colonic involvement or both, colonoscopy is an important tool for establishing the diagnosis. Intubation of the terminal ileum should be a routine part of the evaluation in cases of chronic diarrhea and suspected inflammatory bowel disease. An alternative to colonoscopy is a double-contrast barium study. In double-contrast studies, the mucosal surface is coated with a thin layer of barium, and the lumen is distended with air. Reflux into the terminal ileum at the time of barium enema examination may also provide double-contrast views of the terminal ileum.

Evaluation of the small bowel may be achieved by barium small-bowel follow-through or small-bowel enema, which is also known as small-bowel enteroclysis. In evaluating the small intestine, a single-contrast upper gastrointestinal series with small-bowel follow-through is most appropriate because it uses a lower density barium than a double-contrast upper gastrointestinal series, which

Table 5.2 Criteria for the severity of disease based on the American College of Gastroenterology Guidelines.

Mild to moderate disease	Moderate to severe disease	Severe disease

Ambulatory
Tolerance for oral diet
No evidence of any of the following
   dehydration
   high fever
   rigors
   abdominal tenderness
   painful mass
   obstruction
	Refractory to treatment for mild to moderate disease
	One or more of the following
	   fever
	   significant weight loss (>10%)
	   abdominal pain and tenderness
	   intermittent nausea and vomiting
	   significant anemia
		Disease progression despite corticosteroid therapy
		Persistent symptoms of the following
		   high fever
		   vomiting
		   rebound tenderness
		   cachexia
		   evidence of abscess
		   evidence of obstruction

visualizes, albeit inadequately, the small bowel. A supplemental technique to small-bowel follow-through is the peroral pneumocolon examination, which allows further evaluation of the terminal ileum and ileocecal junction. In performing a peroral pneumocolon, air is introduced into the colon via a rectal catheter after the orally administered barium reaches the cecum. Reflux of air into the distal ileum then provides air-contrast views of the terminal ileum. The small-bowel enema or enteroclysis permits a detailed examination of the jejunum and ileum. In this study, barium is injected through an enteroclysis catheter introduced into the proximal jejunum. In a double-contrast enteroclysis, barium instillation is followed by injection of methylcellulose solution or air. The small-bowel enema is particularly useful in evaluating fistulas and mass lesions in distal small bowel, but may be inferior to the small-bowel follow-through in assessing subtle mucosal lesions.

Occasionally, involvement of the esophagus, stomach, and duodenum coincides with or precedes the onset of ileal or colonic Crohn's disease. Either upper endoscopy or barium radiography can be used to evaluate the more proximal gastrointestinal tract. When using barium radiography to examine the proximal gastrointestinal tract, a double-contrast upper gastrointestinal series is preferred to a single-contrast barium study, because the former allows better delineation of fine mucosal details. Therefore, although a dedicated small-bowel follow-through also allows visualization of the stomach and duodenum, it is not sufficient for the evaluation of more proximal disease.

Cross-sectional imaging studies complement the luminal radiography in the diagnosis and management of Crohn's disease. In patients without a prior history of Crohn's disease presenting with acute abdominal symptoms, or in patients with known Crohn's disease presenting with symptoms suggesting exacerbation of their disease, CT scanning is an important tool in evaluating the disease activity of Crohn's disease and its complications, and excluding other processes. In particular, CT is useful in identifying inflammatory phlegmon, abscess, pylephlebitis, fistulas, or other unsuspected complications. It is also useful in assessing perianal disease and fistulas. However, magnetic resonance imaging (MRI) is preferred over CT for imaging complex perianal Crohn's disease. As with CT, MRI scanning also allows evaluation of intra-abdominal abscesses and inflammatory changes in the bowel.

Serological tests serve as an adjunct to the diagnosis of Crohn's disease. These serological tests detect the presence of antibodies that are typically absent in patients without inflammatory bowel disease, and may be helpful in differentiating Crohn's disease from ulcerative colitis. The anti-*Saccharomyces cerevisiae* antibodies (ASCA) are directed against cell wall components of *Saccharomyces cerevisiae*, a form of baker's yeast. Serum ASCA are present in 50% to 70% of patients with Crohn's disease, but in only 5% of patients with ulcerative colitis. In contrast, the perinuclear antineutrophil cytoplasmic antibodies (pANCA) are antibodies directed against the cytoplasmic components of neutrophils with perinuclear staining pattern. Serum pANCA are detectable in 50% to 80% of patients with ulcerative colitis and in only 10% to 25% of patients with Crohn's disease. Combining both ASCA and pANCA (positive ASCA and negative pANCA) yields a sensitivity and specificity of 49% and 97% for diagnosing Crohn's disease from ulcerative colitis.

These serological markers have recently been shown to correlate with specific disease patterns. Patients with Crohn's disease and a positive pANCA are more likely to have clinical and pathological features resembling those observed in ulcerative colitis, including left-sided colonic involvement and a higher rate of colectomy. In contrast, a high level of ASCA expression, especially with a negative pANCA, is associated with small-bowel disease complicated by fibrostenosing, internal fistulas or abscesses, and a higher rate of small-bowel surgery. The utility of these serological studies in disease stratification is currently being defined.

Laboratory studies in general are not useful in establishing the diagnosis, as there are few laboratory markers sufficiently sensitive or specific for detecting active disease. The role of laboratory studies in evaluating patients with Crohn's disease is to complete the assessment of the overall clinical status. As mentioned in the previous section, mild leukocytosis and thrombocytosis may be seen with active disease. However, significant leukocytosis should prompt a search for infectious complications, particularly the presence of abscesses. Stool studies should be obtained to rule out concurrent infections. These should include culture for bacteria, examination for ova and parasites, and testing for *Clostridium difficile* toxin.

Differential diagnoses

The symptoms of Crohn's disease can mimic many other entities (Box 5.3). One of the conditions that often needs to be differentiated from the initial episode of Crohn's disease is acute appendicitis, since ileocecal disease is the most common involvement at the initial presentation of Crohn's disease. These two entities can usually be distinguished by history, with more acute onset of symptoms for appendicitis and more chronic symptoms for Crohn's disease. Abdominal and pelvic CT is helpful in differentiating these two conditions. Other entities that should be considered in more acutely symptomatic patients include cecal diverticulitis and gynecological diseases such as pelvic inflammatory disease, ovarian torsion or ruptured ovarian cysts, and ectopic pregnancy.

Several infectious entities may resemble Crohn's disease. It is important to make this distinction because steroid therapy may exacerbate infections. *Yersinia* infection may cause an acute self-limited ileitis. Diagnosis can be made by stool culture or serologic studies. Intestinal tuberculosis can mimic Crohn's disease both clinically and pathologically. Ileocecal disease is the most common intestinal involvement in tuberculosis. Intestinal tuberculosis usually occurs with pulmonary involvement, but may also occur without pulmonary tuberculosis. Cytomegalovirus infection in immunosuppressed patients may result in ileocecal disease resembling Crohn's disease.

Another general class of differential diagnoses is neoplastic diseases. Intestinal lymphoma, cecal carcinoma, and gynecological cancers (such as ovarian cancer) need to be differentiated from Crohn's disease. Other inflammatory conditions including celiac sprue, eosinophilic gastroenteritis and microscopic colitis may also present with diarrhea. These can usually be readily differentiated from Crohn's disease by endoscopic and pathologic diagnoses. Ischemic disease of the small bowel may resemble Crohn's disease, and may be due to medications such as oral contraceptives or systemic vasculitis. Behçet's disease is a systemic vasculitis characterized by painful oral and genital ulcerations and uveitis. Gastrointestinal symptoms tend to be less prominent.

In patients with disease limited to the colon, the main differential diagnosis is ulcerative colitis. This distinction can be difficult, and a definitive diagnosis of Crohn's disease may not be possible. Endoscopic or radiographic studies and pathological findings usually allow this differentiation as discussed above in the section on Clinical Features. Other differential diagnoses of Crohn's colitis include infectious colitis from *Campylobacter*, *Salmonella*, *Shigella*, *Clostridium difficile*, cytomegalovirus, or ameba. Infections can be established on stool studies for bacterial culture, ova and parasites, and *Clostridium difficile* toxins. Giant-cell inclusion body can be seen on endoscopic biopsies in patients with cytomegalovirus infection. Non-infectious colitis, including ischemic colitis and radiation colitis, may also mimic Crohn's colitis, and require endoscopic and histological differentiation.

Medical therapy

General principles

Much of the management of patients with Crohn's disease involves the use of appropriate medical therapies. Based on our current understanding of the pathogenesis of inflammatory bowel disease, the principal therapy focuses on regimens that alter host response to decrease mucosal inflammation. Given the complexity of the inflammatory and immune processes involved in the pathophysiology of disease, therapies have been developed to target not only specific cytokines, but also other aspects of the

Box 5.3 Differential diagnoses for Crohn's disease
Ileal or ileocecal disease
appendicitis
cecal diverticulitis
pelvic inflammatory disease
ovarian torsion/ ruptured ovarian cysts
ectopic pregnancy
Yersinia infection
intestinal tuberculosis
CMV infection
intestinal lymphoma
cecal carcinoma
gynecological neoplasm
celiac disease
eosinophilic gastroenteritis
microscopic colitis
systemic vasculitis
Colonic disease
ulcerative colitis
infectious colitis (*Campylobacter, Salmonella, Shigella, Giardia, Clostridium difficile*, CMV, ameba, *Chlamydia*)
ischemic colitis
diverticulitis
radiation-induced colitis

once remission is achieved (to maintain remission). This concept of induction of remission and maintenance of remission forms the basis guiding our evaluation of the efficacy of specific therapy. Additionally, an ideal therapy for Crohn's disease should be able to modify the disease process, improve the patient's quality of life, and have a low toxicity profile, while being easy to administer. A wide range of therapeutic options is available for both treatment of active disease and maintenance of remission, from time-honored aminosalicylates to recently developed biological agents (Tables 5.3, 5.4).

Aminosalicylates

Sulfasalazine was initially designed for the treatment of rheumatoid arthritis. It is a combined drug, where an antibacterial component, sulfapyridine, is azo-bonded to a salicylate, 5-aminosalicylic acid (mesalamine). Its benefit in inflammatory bowel disease was first reported in 1942 by Nana Svartz of the Karolinska Institute, when it was observed that patients with inflammatory bowel disease who

inflammatory process. Additionally, the rationale for manipulating the enteric flora appears sound and may be the basis of additional future therapeutic strategies.

In general, therapeutic choice depends primarily on the type, location, and severity of disease. The current strategies used to manage patients with Crohn's disease can be broadly classified into therapies that treat active disease (to induce remission) and therapies that prevent recurrence of disease

Table 5.4 Medical options of maintenance therapy for Crohn's disease.

Remission	Prevention of postoperative recurrence
5-aminosalicylates	5-aminosalicylates
Metronidazole	Azathioprine or 6-mercaptopurine
Azathioprine or 6-mercaptopurine	
Methotrexate	
Infliximab	

Table 5.3 Medical options of induction therapies for Crohn's disease.

Mild to moderate disease	Severe disease	Perianal or fistulous disease	Steroid-dependent disease
Oral or topical 5-aminosalicylates*	Parenteral corticosteroids	Metronidazole ± ciprofloxacin	Azathioprine or 6-mercaptopurine
Metronidazole ± ciprofloxacin	Infliximab	Azathioprine or 6-mercaptopurine	Methotrexate
Oral corticosteroids	Total parenteral nutrition	Infliximab	Infliximab
Azathioprine or 6-mercaptopurine	? Cyclosporine	Cyclosporine	
Methotrexate			
Infliximab			
*topical 5-aminosalicyclates for distal colitis.			

received sulfasalazine for rheumatoid arthritis also had improvement of their intestinal symptoms. The determination of the active moiety of sulfasalazine for the treatment of inflammatory bowel disease first came to light in 1977 by Dr Azad Kahn when 5-aminosalicylic acid and sulfasalazine were found to be equally effective in patients with left-sided colitis in a study comparing enemas of sulfapyridine, 5-aminosalicylic acid, and sulfasalazine. There was no placebo arm in this study. Thus, it became clear that sulfapyridine serves as the inactive carrier to deliver 5-aminosalicylic acid, the principal therapeutic moiety, to the colon. Approximately 90% of the compound reaches the colon, and only a small amount is absorbed in the small bowel. Upon reaching the colon, the 5-aminosalicylic acid component is released by the action of the enzyme azoreductase produced by colonic bacteria. This enzyme cleaves the azo bond releasing the constituent moieties that comprise sulfasalazine, mesalamine, and sulfapyridine. Approximately 20% of the absorbed 5-aminosalicylic acid undergoes hepatic N-acetylation and is excreted in the urine. If 5-aminosalicylic acid is administered orally alone or uncoated, 5-aminosalicylic acid is rapidly absorbed in the small bowel, limiting the amount reaching the colon.

Various formulations of 5-aminosalicylic acid have been developed to deliver the active moiety to the target site of the gastrointestinal tract without the sulfapyridine molecule, which is thought to be responsible for many of the side effects discussed below (Figure 5.1, Table 5.5). Olsalazine (Dipentum®) is composed of two 5-aminosalicylic acid molecules linked by an azo bond. Two identical 5-aminosalicylic acid compounds are delivered to the colon after being released by the action of bacterial azoreductase enzyme. Approximately 98% of the material is delivered to the colon intact. Balsalazide (Colazal®) is another formulation that consists of a 5-aminosalicylic acid molecule azo-bonded to a benzoic acid derivative, 4-aminobenzyol beta alanine. Similar to sulfasalazine and olsalazine, balsalazide releases 5-aminosalicylic acid via bacterial azoreductase in the colon. Approximately 99% of the drug is delivered intact to the colon, and thus provides potential advantage of greater potency for colonic disease. For patients with small-bowel disease, other formulations are needed to allow delivery of 5-aminosalicylic acid to the small bowel. Asacol® is a Eudragit-S-coated mesalamine tablet that is released at pH above 7 in the distal ileum and the colon. Approximately 75% to 80% of Asacol® reaches the colon. Pentasa® uses ethylcellulose-coated mesalamine microgranules that release mesalamine after the molecules are dissolved by water absorbed into the small beads. The release of mesalamine from Pentasa® is time dependent, and occurs from the duodenum throughout the remainder of the small bowel and the colon. Approximately 50% of mesalamine enters the colon intact in patients ingesting Pentasa®.

The exact mechanism by which 5-aminosalicylic acid exerts its anti-inflammatory properties is unknown. Many hypotheses have been proposed. These include inhibition of the cyclooxygenase and 5′-lipoxygenase pathways, platelet-activating factor, oxidants, and free radicals. In addition, 5-aminosal-

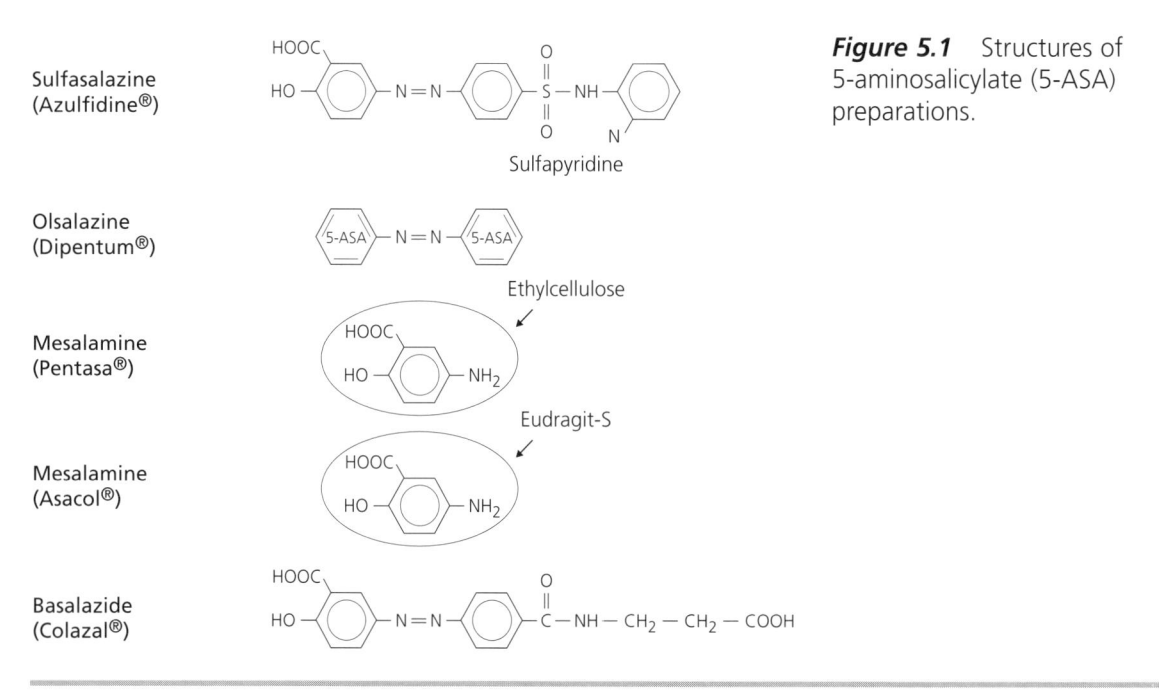

Figure 5.1 Structures of 5-aminosalicylate (5-ASA) preparations.

Table 5.5 Formulation, sites of release, and recommended doses of 5-aminosalicylate (5-ASA) preparations available in the US.

Drug	Formulation	Site of release	Dose Active disease	Remission
Oral				
Sulfasalazine				
Azulfidine®	Tablets, 500 mg	Colon	4–6 g/day	2–4 g/day
Olsalazine				
Dipentum®	Gelatin capsules, 250 mg	Colon	–*	1.5–3 g/day
Mesalamine				
Asacol®	Tablets, 400 mg	Distal ileum, colon	2.4–4.8 g/day	1.2–4.8 g/day
Pentasa®	Capsules, 250 mg or 500 mg	Duodenum to colon	2–4 g/day	1.5–4 g/day
Balsalazide				
Colazal®	Capsules, 750 mg	Colon	–*	–*
Topical				
Mesalamine				
Canasa®	Suppository, 500 mg	Rectum	500 mg–1 g/day	500 mg–1 g/day
Rowasa®	Enema, 4 g	Distal colon	2–4 g/day	2–4 g/day

*insufficient data or of questionable benefit.

icylic acid decreases the production of IL-1 and immunoglobulins, thus altering humoral immunity. Also 5-aminosalicylic acid impairs the function of lymphocytes, macrophages, and monocytes. Sulfasalazine has also been shown to inhibit activation and production of nuclear factor kappa B, mitogen-activated protein kinase, and TNF.

Efficacy The initial discovery of the potential benefit of sulfasalazine in patients with inflammatory bowel disease led to studies evaluating its efficacy in the treatment of ulcerative colitis. The acceptance of sulfasalazine as a therapy for Crohn's disease did not occur until the 1970s. The first controlled trial reporting the benefit of sulfasalazine for Crohn's disease was the National Cooperative Crohn's Disease Study. This landmark study and the subsequent European Cooperative Crohn's Disease Study demonstrated that sulfasalazine at a dose of 3 to 5 g/day is effective in the treatment of active Crohn's disease. This benefit appears to be limited to patients with ileocolonic and colonic disease, as sulfasalazine is only comparable to placebo in patients with isolated ileal disease. However, this benefit of sulfasalazine for active Crohn's disease is inferior to that of corticosteroids.

Studies evaluating the newer mesalamine preparations for the treatment of active Crohn's disease have not consistently demonstrated positive results, although mesalamine preparations at high doses appear to be effective in some studies. Pentasa® at 4 g/day, but not lower doses, is effective in inducing remission in patients with active Crohn's disease. In a meta-analysis of three placebo-controlled studies, the mean reduction of the disease activity instrument scores, the Crohn's Disease Activity Index, from baseline to 16 weeks was 63 points in Pentasa-treated patients compared to a 45-point reduction in placebo patients ($P = 0.04$). Although the difference in the reduction of Crohn's Disease Activity Index is statistically significant, the clinical significance of an 18-point difference is unclear given the 45-point within-patient variations over time for the Crohn's Disease Activity Index. Additionally, it is unknown that if patients with isolated ileal disease may achieve a greater benefit with Pentasa® in such an analysis. Asacol® at 4 g/day has been shown to be comparable to methylprednisone at 40 mg/day in inducing remission in patients with mildly to moderately active Crohn's ileitis. Although no controlled trial has evaluated the utility of mesalamine in doses higher than 4 grams daily, anectodal evidence suggests its benefit for the treatment of active Crohn's disease, and active research is ongoing to address this question.

The efficacy of 5-aminosalicylic acid compounds for the maintenance of remission in patients with Crohn's disease remains controversial. The best evidence supports its use as maintenance therapy for surgically induced remission. Early large randomized controlled trials from the National Cooperative Crohn's Disease Study and European Cooperative Crohn's Disease Study failed to show a maintenance benefit of sulfasalazine. Subsequent studies reported conflicting data with

5-aminosalicylic acid compounds. Although meta-analyses have shown that the 5-aminosalicylic acid compounds are effective in maintaning remission in patients with quiescent disease, the effective dose is uncertain given the wide range of dosages in the studies. Mesalamine (Pentasa®) at 4 g/day appears to have a limited role in facilitating steroid withdrawal and decreasing steroid dependency following steroid-induced remission. Both sulfasalazine and mesalamine have been shown to be beneficial in preventing postoperative recurrence, although the benefit with the latter appears to be limited to patients with isolated small-bowel disease.

Patients with Crohn's disease involving the distal colon may benefit from topical mesalamines through suppositories or enemas, although no controlled study has evaluated its efficacy in Crohn's disease. These topical agents may be used alone or in conjunction with oral agents. Distribution of the enemas has been shown to reach as high as the splenic flexure, while suppositories provide medications primarily to the rectum.

Side effects Sulfasalazine therapy is associated with a number of common and significant side effects that lead to the discontinuation of medications in approximately 10% to 20% of patients (Table 5.6). Many of the side effects are related to the sulfapyridine molecule. Since the metabolism of 5-aminosalicylic acid involves acetylation by the liver, individuals with slow acetylation as genetically determined have an increased incidence of side effects from sulfapyridine. Common side effects include headache, nausea, vomiting, anorexia, dyspepsia, and fatigue. These are dose dependent and usually improve with a reduction in dose. Idiosyncratic reactions include fever, rash,

Table 5.6 Adverse events of standard medical therapies for Crohn's disease.

Drug	Common adverse events	Rare serious adverse events
Sulfasalazine	Anorexia Headache Gastrointestinal symptoms (nausea, vomiting, dyspepsia) Sperm abnormalities Rash Fever Folic acid malabsorption Urine discoloration and skin discoloration	Hypersensitivity reactions Hemolytic anemia Agranulocytosis/aplastic anemia Hepatitis Fibrosing alveolitis Worsening of colitis Pancreatitis
5-aminosalicylates	Headache Gastrointestinal symptoms (nausea, vomiting, abdominal pain, diarrhea, dyspepsia) Back pain Rash, pruritis	Hypersensitivity reactions Renal insufficiency Pericarditis/myocarditis Bone marrow suppression
Corticosteroids	Acne, cushingoid state Fat redistribution Fluid retention, electrolyteabnormality, hypertension Weight gain Mood changes Hyperglycemia/glucose intolerance Cataracts, glaucoma Infection Impaired wound healing, petechiae, thin fragile skin Growth retardation in children	Striae Osteoporosis, osteonecrosis, fracture, myopathy
Metronidazole	Gastrointestinal symptoms (dyspepsia, nausea, abdominal pain) Metallic taste Headache Disulfuram-like reaction with alcohol Peripheral neuropathy	Seizures

Medical therapy

Table 5.6 Adverse events of standard medical therapies for Crohn's disease. — Cont'd

Drug	Common adverse events	Rare serious adverse events
Ciprofloxacin	Gastrointestinal symptoms (nausea, vomiting, abdominal pain, diarrhea) Headache Rash	Seizure Toxic psychosis Hypersensitivity reaction Spontaneous Achilles tendon ruptures Abnormal liver chemistry Anosmia, taste loss, visual abnormality, and hearing loss
Azathioprine/ 6-mercaptopurine	Bone marrow suppression Abnormal liver chemistry Gastrointestinal symptoms (nausea, abdominal pain, diarrhea) Infections	Hypersensitivity reactions Malignancy Pancreatitis
Cyclosporine	Hypertension Tremor Renal insufficiency Electrolyte abnormalities Headache Hirsutism Gingival hyperplasia Paresthesia Gastrointestinal symptoms (nausea, vomiting, diarrhea) Hepatotoxicity Infections	Seizure Anaphylaxis Opportunistic infections
Methotrexate	Gastrointestinal symptoms (nausea, vomiting, diarrhea) Bone marrow suppression Folate malabsorption Rash/pruritis Stomatitis Abnormal liver enzymes Opportunistic infection	Hepatic fibrosis Pneumonitis Hypersensitivity Teratogenicity
Infliximab	Gastrointestinal symptoms (nausea, vomiting, abdominal pain) Upper respiratory tract infections Headache Myalgias Infusion-related reactions (acute and delayed) Autoantibodies	Serious infections (fungal, tuberculosis) Exacerbation of heart failure Malignancy/lymphoproliferative disorder

agranulocytosis, hemolytic anemia, hepatitis, pancreatitis, and pneumonitis. Up to 80% of males on sulfasalazine have reversible sperm abnormalities (abnormal motility and dysmorphic sperm) and the issue of potential infertility should be discussed with patients prior to initiating the medication. Sulfasalazine also impairs folate absorption and folate supplementation is recommended. A primary advantage of the mesalamine derivatives over sulfasalazine is the reduced number of side effects. Up to 90% of patients who are intolerant to sulfasalazine can tolerate 5-aminosalicylic acid. Rare hypersensitivity reactions, including pneumonititis, pancreatitis, hepatitis, nephritis, and worsening of colitis have all been reported. Male sperm abnormality is not seen with these newer mesalamine preparations.

Corticosteroids

Corticosteroids have long been the mainstay of therapy for moderately to severely active Crohn's disease. Despite their widespread use, the exact mechanism of action of corticosteroids in Crohn's disease remains elusive. The potent anti-inflammatory effect of corticosteroids appears to result from a multitude of properties. Corticosteroids block the arachidonic acid pathway via inhibition of phospholipase A2. In addition, corticosteroids also suppress the production of a host of proinflammatory cytokines, chemokines, and adhesion molecules. On a cellular level, corticosteroids interfere with intercellular interaction and trafficking of immune cells, impair phagocytic and degranulation function, and suppress intestinal mucosal natural killer cell activity. Corticosteroids have also recently been shown to inhibit nuclear factor kappa B and activating protein-1, two key transcription factors involved in inflammatory cascade and cellular growth and differentiation.

Efficacy Both oral and parenteral corticosteroids are effective for the treatment of active luminal Crohn's disease, regardless of disease distribution. In moderate to severe flares of Crohn's disease, corticosteroids, in doses equivalent to 40 to 60 mg/day (or 0.5 to 0.75 mg kg^{-1} day^{-1}) of prednisone, are an effective first-line therapy for the induction of remission. The use of higher doses is not recommended given the increased side effects without an appreciable clinical benefit. In moderate to severely active Crohn's colitis, the addition of sulfasalazine to corticosteroids does not result in additional benefit. Although intravenous administration has not been shown to be superior to the oral route, patients with severe or fulminant disease, or small-bowel obstruction should be hospitalized and receive intravenous corticosteroid therapy. In patients with Crohn's disease involving the distal colon, topical corticosteroids can also be used alone or in conjunction with oral agents.

Long-term use of corticosteroids is not recommended given their lack of efficacy in maintaining remission and the associated increase in side effects. Additionally, steroid use does not appear to alter the disease course. At 1 year following steroid therapy for active Crohn's disease, 56% of patients are either steroid resistant or steroid dependent, and only 44% have a prolonged response to corticosteroids.

Newer corticosteroid preparations such as oral budesonide have been developed to minimize the side effects of traditional steroids. Budesonide is different from prednisone in the basic hydrocortisone molecule (16α-hydroxyprednisolone). This structural alteration results in greater topical anti-inflammatory activity and affinity for glucocorticoid receptors than prednisone. Its high first-pass metabolism (approximately 90%) in the liver and erythrocytes lends to its low systemic bioavailability and fewer side effects. Oral budesonide has been shown, in clinical trials, to be superior to placebo or mesalamine, and comparable to traditional corticosteroids (approximately equivalent to prednisolone 40 mg/day) in the treatment of mildly to moderately active Crohn's disease. The optimal dose is 9 mg/day. Oral budesonide is also associated with fewer side effects and less adrenal suppression compared to traditional steroids. The controlled ileal release oral budesonide, Entocort®, consists of eudragit-L-coated microgranules with an internal ethylcellulose component that release budesonide at pH above 5.5. Approximately 50% to 80% of budesonide is absorbed in the ileocecal region. Accordingly, studies with Entocort® demonstrate the greatest efficacy in patients with ileal and right-sided colonic Crohn's disease.

The benefit of budesonide in maintaining remission remains unsettled. The initial report that oral budesonide prolonged time to relapse in patients with quiescent Crohn's disease has not been confirmed in subsequent studies. Long-term therapy with oral budesonide does not appear to offer significant benefit for preventing relapses in most studies. However, it may decrease endoscopic recurrence in the subgroup of patients with remission induced following surgery for active, non-fibrostenotic Crohn's disease.

Side effects Corticosteroids are associated with myriad side effects involving virtually all organ systems – musculoskeletal, endocrine, metabolic, neurological, psychiatric, gastrointestinal, dermatological, ophthalmological, immunological, cardiovascular, and hematologic systems (Table 5.6). Common side effects include moon face, acne, mood changes, insomnia, fluid retention, increased appetite, weight gain, amenorrhea, hyperglycemia, hypertension, hirsutism, impaired wound healing, and striae. Osteoporosis is an important musculoskeletal complication of chronic steroid use. Corticosteroid therapy at an average daily dose of 7.5 mg prednisone is associated with a five-fold increased risk of fracture compared to non-users. Other important toxicities of corticosteroids include avascular osteonecrosis, cataracts, myopathy, growth retardation in children, and suppression of the hypothalamic–pituitary–adrenal axis. Particular caution also needs to be taken with corticosteroid therapy in patients with Crohn's disease because of the increased risk of infection and the potential for intestinal perforation or masking of its presence.

Side effects of corticosteroids are usually related to dosage, duration of therapy, and route of administration. A short-term course of corticosteroids is generally safe. Although topical steroids are associated with less systemic absorption compared to oral or intravenous forms, prolonged therapy with topical corticosteroids may still be associated with steroid-related side effects. Alternate-day therapy may decrease suppression of the hypothalamus–pituitary–adrenal axis and other side effects, except possibly osteoporosis and cataracts. Since patients with Crohn's disease are at an increased risk of osteoporosis, even in the absence of corticosteroid therapy, bone densitometry studies should be obtained at baseline and follow-up. In addition, patients with Crohn's disease treated with corticosteroids should receive daily calcium (1200 to 1500 mg/day) and vitamin D (400 to 800 IU/day). Hormone replacement and bisphosphonates may be beneficial in preventing corticosteroid-induced osteoporosis.

Antibiotics

Abundant evidence from experimental and clinical observations supports the microbial participation in the pathogenesis of inflammatory bowel disease. First, patients with Crohn's disease have been found to have abnormal intestinal flora compared to individuals without Crohn's disease. The bowel wall and mesenteric lymph nodes of patients with Crohn's disease have been shown to contain intestinal bacteria, and the disease usually arises primarily in regions of the bowel with the highest concentrations of luminal bacteria. Additional evidence comes from *in vivo* observations. Diversion of the fecal stream delays postoperative relapse of Crohn's disease, while restoration of the fecal stream is associated with disease recurrence. Although many infectious organisms have been implicated, no specific causative agent has yet been identified. Thus, based on this hypothesis that bacterial flora plays a role in the pathogenesis of inflammatory bowel disease and their potential immunosuppressive properties, various antimicrobial agents have been used for Crohn's disease. In addition, antibiotics are important in managing Crohn's disease patients with suppurative complications.

Efficacy The two most widely used and studied antibiotics are metronidazole and ciprofloxacin. Metronidazole, at doses of 10 to 20 mg kg^{-1} day^{-1}, is effective as primary therapy and is as effective as 3 gm/day of sulfasalazine for the treatment of mildly to moderately active ileocolonic and colonic Crohn's disease. Ciprofloxacin at 1 gm/day has also been shown to be as effective as mesalamine at 4 gm/day for patients with mildly to moderately active disease. It is unknown if the combination therapy is superior to either agent alone, but the combination of metronidazole and ciprofloxacin has been shown to have equal efficacy to standard dose of intravenous corticosteroids.

The use of antibiotics for maintaining medically induced remission has not been evaluated in any controlled fashion, but antibiotics appear to be beneficial in preventing postoperative recurrence of Crohn's disease. Metronidazole for 3 months postoperatively is associated with a trend toward reduced recurrences in the short term but not in the long term. The nitroimidazole antibiotic ornidazol, a compound similar to metronidazole but with fewer side effects (currently unavailable in the US), has shown long-term efficacy in a randomized controlled trial for maintaining remission following surgical resection for active disease. Both endoscopic and clinical recurrence rates at 1 year postoperatively are significantly reduced with ornidazole at 1 gm/day for 12 months. Another broad spectrum antimicrobial agent, clarithromycin, has also demonstrated potential benefit for both induction and maintenance of remission in one open-label study.

Antibiotics may be particularly useful in the management of perineal disease. Therapy with metronidazole at 20 mg kg^{-1} day^{-1} results in complete closure of perianal fistulas in 34% to 50% of patients in five open-label studies. Ciprofloxacin similarly may be beneficial in treating fistulas and perineal disease in patients with Crohn's disease. There is currently no randomized controlled data comparing these antibiotics with a placebo in patients with perineal Crohn's disease.

Side effects The use of antibiotics is associated with a number of side effects (Table 5.6). Long-term therapy with metronidazole can lead to the development of peripheral neuropathy, which is usually reversible upon discontinuation of the medication. Patients receiving metronidazole should abstain from alcohol because of the potential disulfiram-like reaction. In patients intolerant of metronidazole, ciprofloxacin is a useful alternative. The long-term use of ciprofloxacin has been linked to spontaneous tendon ruptures.

Immunomodulators

Given the pivotal role of the inflammatory and immune processes in the pathogenesis of inflammatory bowel disease, immunomodulators have become important therapeutic options in the management of patients with inflammatory bowel disease. Among the various agents in this category of medications, azathioprine and 6-mercaptopurine are the first to be used in patients with Crohn's disease. Other immune modifiers used for Crohn's disease include methotrexate and, less commonly, cyclosporine.

Azathioprine and 6-mercaptopurine

Azathioprine and 6-mercaptopurine are thiopurine analogs that modulate the immune response via a number of mechanisms. They inhibit purine biosynthesis, interfere with the cytotoxicity of natural killer cells and T cells, and decrease suppressor T-cell function and thus cell-mediated immunity. Azathioprine is a prodrug for 6-mercaptopurine, which is converted to several metabolites via competing enzymatic pathways (Figure 5.2). The primary active metabolites are 6-thioguanine nucleotides. Two additional pathways competitively convert 6-mercaptopurine to inactive metabolites, 6-thiouric acid via xanthine oxidase, and 6-methylmercaptopurine via thiopurine methyltransferase.

Efficacy Azathioprine and 6-mercaptopurine are effective as primary therapy in patients with active Crohn's disease, with a response rate of approximately 54%. This benefit corresponds to a number needed to treat of five to observe an effect of therapy in one patient. The benefit of azathioprine and 6-mercaptopurine is dose dependent. The optimal dose is generally considered to be 2.0 to 2.5 mg kg^{-1} day^{-1} for azathioprine and 1.0 to 1.5 mg kg^{-1} day^{-1} for 6-mercaptopurine. In patients with steroid-dependent Crohn's disease, these agents may offer a steroid-sparing benefit. Approximately 65% of patients receiving azathioprine or 6-mercaptopurine are able to taper their corticosteroids to less than 10 mg/day (prednisone equivalent) compared to 35% of patients receiving placebo. This difference corresponds to a minimum of three patients needed to be treated to obtain a steroid-sparing benefit (to a dose less than 10 mg of prednisone) in one patient. Studies have also suggested potential benefit of 6-mercaptopurine in patients with fistulas and perineal Crohn's disease. Therapy with azathioprine or 6-mercaptopurine results in partial or complete healing of fistulas in approximately 55% of patients.

Once remission is achieved, azathioprine or 6-mercaptopurine allow maintenance of remission in approximately 67% of patients. Whether the maintenance benefit of azathioprine and 6-mercaptopurine persists with long-term therapy is unclear. In one randomized controlled trial of Crohn's patients in clinical remission for at least 3 years on azathioprine, medication withdrawal resulted in a significantly greater relapse rate at 18 months compared to continued azathioprine therapy for an additional 18 months. Controlled and uncontrolled data suggest that these agents continue to provide a maintenance benefit for up to 5 years. In a statistical model analyzing the risks and benefits of therapy with azathioprine or 6-mercaptopurine in patients with active Crohn's disease, the effect of maintenance of remission extends to a 10-year period. In patients with surgically induced remission, 6-mercaptopurine at 50 mg/day appears to be superior to placebo and mesalamine (Pentasa®)

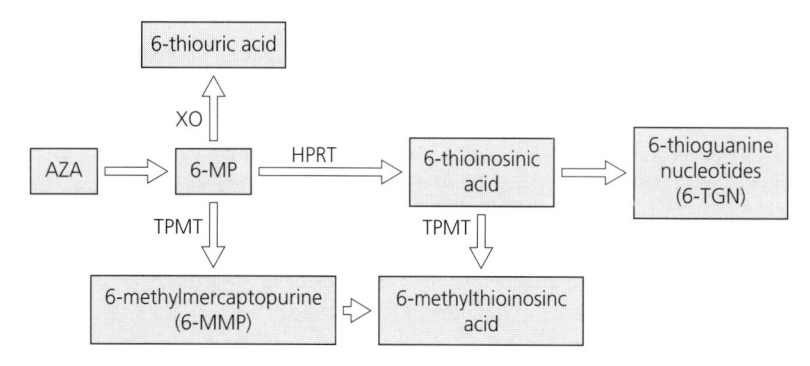

Figure 5.2 Metabolism of azathioprine and 6-mercaptopurine.

AZA = azathioprine
6-MP = 6-mercaptopurine
XO = xanthine oxidase
TPMT = thiopurine methyltransferase
HPRT = hypoxanthine phosphoribosyltransferase

in preventing postoperative recurrence of Crohn's disease.

Concurrent therapy with sulfasalazine (and other mesalamine derivatives) may augment the efficacy of azathioprine or 6-mercaptopurine via the inhibition of thiopurine methyltransferase enzyme activity. However, the true clinical extent of this potential benefit requires further evaluation in a prospective manner.

Side effects Side effects of azathioprine and 6-mercaptopurine include nausea, vomiting, bone-marrow suppression, elevated liver enzymes, and infections (Table 5.6). Idiosyncratic, dose-independent toxicities such as pancreatitis and allergic reactions with fever, rash, or arthralgia may also develop with azathioprine or 6-mercaptopurine therapy. Pancreatitis most commonly occurs during the first month of therapy, and is usually reversible on discontinuation of the medication. Although the development of allergic reactions requires prompt medication withdrawal, there are reports of individuals who develop allergic reactions with 6-mercaptopurine but are able to tolerate subsequent challenge with azathioprine. Bone-marrow suppression, primarily leukopenia, occurs in 2% to 5% of patients treated with azathioprine or 6-mercaptopurine. This toxicity is dose-dependent, and may increase with concurrent use of allopurinol, sulfasalazine agents, or antibiotics. Some studies suggest that therapy with azathioprine or 6-mercaptopurine is associated with an increased risk of hematological malignancy such as lymphoma. This potential adverse effect of azathioprine and 6-mercaptopurine remains controversial in patients with inflammatory bowel disease. Most recent data fail to demonstrate an increased risk of malignancy with azathioprine or 6-mercaptopurine therapy in patients with Crohn's disease. Cases of lymphoma that develop in such a setting appear to be associated with Epstein–Barr virus.

Baseline studies of complete blood counts and liver-associated enzymes should be obtained prior to initiating azathioprine or 6-mercaptopurine. For the duration of therapy with these agents, patients should receive periodic complete blood counts and liver-associated enzyme studies to monitor for bone marrow and hepatic toxicities, as they can occur as long as 10 years after the initiation of medication. It is recommended that a complete blood count be obtained frequently; a sample regimen might be weekly for 4 weeks, biweekly for 4 weeks, and then every 1 to 2 months for the duration of therapy.

Special considerations in dosing and monitoring A major limiting factor in the clinical utility of azathioprine and 6-mercaptopurine in patients with active Crohn's disease is their delayed onset of action. It takes 3 to 6 months of therapy to achieve the effect of these agents. The administration of an intravenous loading dose does not shorten the time to response.

The effective dosages for azathioprine and 6-mercaptopurine appear to be 2.0 to 2.5 mg kg^{-1} day^{-1} and 1.0 to 1.5 mg kg^{-1} day^{-1}, respectively. However, the optimal dose of these agents in an individual is unclear, and there is currently no formal dose-ranging study in the literature. Retrospective data suggest that erythrocyte 6-thioguanine nucleotide levels greater than 235 to 250 pmol/8 × 10^8 erythrocytes correlate with a clinical response in patients with Crohn's disease. This is similar to the observation in children with acute lymphoblastic leukemia where 6-thioguanine nucleotide levels are inversely correlated with the risk of relapse. In contrast, induction of leukopenia (white blood cell count less than 5000/mm^3) has been shown to increase the likelihood of the therapeutic response in some but not all studies. Although leukopenia is associated with higher 6-thioguanine nucleotide levels, it is not a reliable marker of therapeutic response and is definitely not required for induction of remission in patients with active disease.

The recommended starting dose of azathioprine or 6-mercaptopurine is controversial. The medication can be initiated at 50 mg/day and increased by 25 mg every 1 to 2 weeks. Alternatively, the medication may be initiated at the anticipated optimal dose by weight. In either case, monitoring of blood counts is necessary as previously outlined. The incorporation of 6-thioguanine nucleotide metabolite measurement for dose adjustment has yet to be confirmed. In addition, monitoring for levels of 6-thioguanine nucleotides and 6-methylmercaptopurine may minimize toxicities, since 6-thioguanine nucleotide levels above 450 pmol/8 × 10^8 erythrocytes appear to be associated with an increased risk of myelotoxicity, while 6-methylmercaptopurine levels greater than 5700 pmol/8 × 10^8 erythrocytes appear to be associated with hepatotoxicity. The use of 6-methylmercaptopurine for the assessment of hepatotoxicity needs further prospective evaluation to define its role, if any, in the management of patients. If the metabolite assays for 6-thioguanine nucleotides and 6-methylmercaptopurine are to be utilized, the test should be performed at least 2 weeks following any dose change to allow the steady state to be reached.

The thiopurine methyltransferase enzyme exhibits polymorphism in the population. Approximately 11% of the population has mutant thiopurine methyltransferase genotypes and consequent low or absent thiopurine methyltransferase enzyme activity. Azathioprine or 6-mercaptopurine therapy in these individuals is associated with an increased bone-marrow toxicity because of the shunting of 6-mercaptopurine metabolism toward the excessive production of 6-thioguanine nucleotides. The determination of thiopurine methyltransferase genotype or enzyme activity prior to initiation of medications may allow appropriate dosing and minimize potential toxicities. The utility of such a practice for all patients with Crohn's disease has yet to be confirmed, since most patients with cytopenia while receiving azathioprine have no thiopurine methyltransferase mutations.

Methotrexate

Methotrexate is a folate analog and has a similar structure to sulfasalazine, another folic-acid antagonist. Methotrexate and its intracellular metabolite, methotrexate polyglutamate, inhibit dihydrofolate reductase, thymidine synthase, and other folate-dependent enzymes. This results in the inhibition of DNA synthesis by interfering with purine synthesis. In addition, methotrexate also decreases the production of proinflammatory cytokines including IL-1, IL-2, and leukotriene B_4.

Efficacy Intramuscular methotrexate at 25 mg/week for 16 weeks results in withdrawl of corticosteroids and remission in 39% of patients with active Crohn's disease compared to 19% of patients receiving placebo ($P = 0.025$). In addition, methotrexate therapy is associated with reduced steroid requirement. Oral administration of methotrexate at a lower dose of 15 mg/week or 12.5 mg/week, however, has not been shown to be effective for inducing remission in patients with active Crohn's disease. The use of higher doses of methotrexate administered orally or lower doses given intramuscularly or subcutaneously has not been examined in patients with active Crohn's disease.

In contrast to treating patients with active disease, intramuscular methotrexate at the lower dose, 15 mg/week, allows remission to be maintained up to 40 weeks in 65% of patients with methotrexate-induced remission, compared to 39% of patients receiving placebo ($P = 0.04$). This maintenance benefit with low-dose intramuscular methotrexate is not observed with oral administration; oral methotrexate at 12.5 mg/week does not decrease the rate of relapses compared to placebo therapy in patients achieving remission following methotrexate therapy at the same dose.

Side effects Common side effects of methotrexate include nausea, vomiting, diarrhea, headache, and stomatitis (Table 5.6). Dose-limiting nausea may be more common with oral administration. Less common but more serious potential toxicities include hypersensitivity reaction, bone-marrow suppression, hypersensitivity pneumonitis, lymphoma, and hepatotoxicity. Hepatic fibrosis is a major concern of long-term therapy with methotrexate. The risk of significant hepatic fibrosis or cirrhosis is approximately 7% in patients receiving methotrexate for psoriasis and 1% for rheumatoid arthritis. Factors that appear to increase the risk of hepatotoxicity include abnormal baseline liver-associated enzymes, a history of excessive alcohol consumption, obesity, diabetes, a cumulative dose of methotrexate in excess of 1.5 gm, and daily dosing of methotrexate. The precise risk of hepatic injury from methotrexate in patients with inflammatory bowel disease is unknown, although preliminary data suggest that the risk is low. At present, pretreatment liver-associated enzymes and complete blood counts should be determined in all patients. A liver biopsy is recommended prior to initiation of methotrexate in individuals with at least one of the above-mentioned risk factors for hepatotoxicity or concurrent infection with hepatitis B or C. Liver-associated enzymes and complete blood counts should be obtained every 2 to 4 weeks during the initial phase of induction therapy and every 4 to 6 weeks during the maintenance therapy. A follow-up liver biopsy may be considered after every 1.5 gm of methotrexate therapy, although this practice has not been validated.

Cyclosporine

Cyclosporine A is a lipophilic peptide extracted from the soil fungus Tolypocladium *Infatum gams*. It binds to an endogenous peptide (cyclophilin) to inhibit the production of IL-2 by T-helper lymphocytes. Other immunomodulatory properties of cyclosporine A include inhibition of the production of other cytokines, such as IL-3, IL-4, TNFα, and interferon gamma. It may also alter B-cell function by inhibiting T-helper cells. The bioavailability of oral cyclosporine A is variable, ranging from 12% to 35%. In general, 4 mg kg^{-1} day^{-1} of intravenous cyclosporine A is equivalent to approximately 16 mg kg^{-1} day^{-1} of oral cyclosporine A. Various factors can also affect the absorption of oral cyclosporine A, including gut motility, bowel length, intact mucosa, and the presence of bile. Thus, bowel dysmotility, diseased mucosa, small-bowel resection, and bile diversion can all interfere with its bioavailability.

Efficacy Studies have not shown a clear benefit of long-term therapy with oral cyclosporine A in patients with chronic active Crohn's disease. Large randomized controlled trials have failed to show any benefit of low-dose oral cyclosporine A (5 mg kg^{-1} day^{-1}) over placebo in patients with chronic active and quiescent disease. In contrast, oral cyclosporine A at a higher dose (7.5 mg kg^{-1} day^{-1}) for 3 months has demonstrated efficacy in one study. The lack of sustained benefit following cyclosporine A withdrawal and the potential toxicities associated with long-term therapy of high-dose cyclosporine A, however, limit its utility for the treatment of chronic active Crohn's disease. Uncontrolled data suggest that intravenous cyclosporine A may be beneficial for the treatment of active inflammatory Crohn's disease. In patients with fistulizing Crohn's disease, intravenous cyclosporine A at 4 mg kg^{-1} day^{-1} results in improved symptoms in 88% to 100%, and complete closure in 44% to 83% of patients. On conversion to oral cyclosporine A, approximately 33% to 36% of patients relapse.

Side effects Cyclosporine A therapy is associated with various side effects including hypertension, seizures, paresthesias, tremor, headache, gingival hyperplasia, hypertrichosis, electrolyte and liver enzyme abnormalities, opportunistic infections, nephrotoxicity, and anaphylaxis (Table 5.6). These usually occur with high-dose cyclosporine A therapy, while the incidence of adverse events is relatively low with low-dose oral cyclosporine A for Crohn's disease. Some of the toxicities are potentially life-threatening and therefore careful monitoring for side effects is critical during cyclosporine A therapy. Serum electrolytes, creatinine, cholesterol, and liver chemistry values should be measured prior to initiation of cyclosporine A therapy. Patients with an impaired creatinine clearance and a serum cholesterol less than 120 mg/dL at baseline should not receive cyclosporine A, to minimize severe nephrotoxicity and risk of seizures, respectively. Serum levels of cyclosporine A should be monitored regularly while on therapy. Patients receiving intravenous cyclosporine A should have a cyclosporine A concentration (as performed by high performance liquid chromatography) and serum electrolytes determined daily, while patients receiving oral cyclosporine A should have these studies weekly. The cyclosporine A dose should be adjusted to achieve a concentration that allows maximal efficacy and safety. This optimal concentration ranges between 200 and 400 ng/mL. The dose should also be decreased when the serum creatinine increases by 30% from the baseline. When long-term cyclosporine A is used, the maximal duration of therapy should be 6 months, and patients should receive *Pneumocystis carinii* pneumonia prophylaxis with trimethoprim sulfamethoxazole.

Other immunomodulators

Mycophenolate mofetil is an immunosuppressant with pharmacodynamic properties comparable to azathioprine and 6-mercaptopurine. It inhibits inosine monophosphate dehydrogenase leading to the impairment of lymphocyte proliferation. Mycophenolate mofetil also inhibits the *de nova* pathway of purine synthesis. It has a more rapid onset of action than azathioprine or 6-mercaptopurine. Studies of mycophenolate mofetil have primarily explored its use as an alternative immunosuppressive therapy for patients with chronic active Crohn's disease who do not tolerate or have failed azathioprine or 6-mercaptopurine therapy. The only randomized controlled trial published to date showed the combination of mycophenolate mofetil (15 mg kg^{-1} day^{-1}) and corticosteroid taper is as effective as the combination of azathioprine (1.5 mg kg^{-1} day^{-1}) and corticosteroid taper for the treatment of chronic active Crohn's disease. In the subgroup of patients with severely active Crohn's disease, however, the benefit of mycophenolate mofetil appears to occur earlier than azathioprine therapy. Based on experience with transplant patients, side effects of mycophenolate mofetil include diarrhea, vomiting, leukopenia or thrombocytopenia, drug exanthema, and invasive cytomegalovirus infection. In the limited data from patients with Crohn's disease, mycophenolate mofetil therapy appears to be well tolerated and has fewer side effects than azathioprine. Depression and migraine necessitating drug withdrawal have been reported in two patients.

Tacrolimus is another immunosuppressant with actions similar to cyclosporine A. It decreases the production of IL-2 by T-helper lymphocytes. In contrast, tacrolimus has a 100-fold greater potency and more rapid onset of action compared to cyclosporine A. Its bioavailability is also less dependent on intact gut mucosa and bile flow. Thus, it can be an alternative to oral cyclosporine A in patients with complicated proximal small-bowel and fistulizing Crohn's disease. Limited data suggest that combination therapy with oral tacrolimus and azathioprine/6-mercaptopurine may be effective treatment for Crohn's disease complicated by perianal fistulas. The initial dose of tacrolimus ranges from 0.15 to 0.31 mg kg^{-1} day^{-1} and the duration of therapy varies from 5 to 47 weeks.

A recent randomized controlled trial showed that therapy with oral tacrolimus at 0.2 mg kg^{-1} day^{-1} for 10 weeks is associated with a significant improvement in fistulous disease, as defined by closure of at least half of all fistulas. However, tacrolimus therapy is not associated with a greater remission rate compared to placebo, as defined by complete closure of all fistulas. In addition to fistulizing disease, tacrolimus therapy at 0.1 to 0.2 mg kg^{-1} day^{-1} may also have both short-term and long-term benefits in treating active Crohn's disease refractory to conventional medical therapy. Side effects of tacrolimus are similar to cyclosporine A, and include nephrotoxicity, electrolyte abnormalities, nausea, diarrhea, headache, tremor, paresthesias, insomnia, alopecia, hirsutism, and gingival hyperplasia.

Anti-tumor necrosis factor therapies

Infliximab

Anti-tumor necrosis factor therapies emerge as a result of our improved understanding of the pathogenesis of inflammatory bowel disease. Tumor necrosis factor is a key cytokine of the inflammatory pathways involved in the development of inflammatory bowel disease. Among this class of therapies, infliximab is an engineered chimeric monoclonal antibody directed against TNFα. It is constructed by linking the constant regions of the human immunoglobulin G (IgG subclass 1) to the variable regions of a murine anti-human TNFα antibody. Thus, it consists of 75% human and 25% murine proteins. Infliximab is thought to be effective via a multitude of mechanisms. It binds to both soluble and membrane-bound TNFα, and thus directly antagonizes its activity. In addition, it is cytotoxic on immune cells and induces apoptosis of T-cells and monocytes.

Efficacy Multiple clinical trials have demonstrated the efficacy of infliximab in the treatment of patients with Crohn's disease. A single infusion of infliximab at 5, 10, or 20 mg/kg is superior to placebo therapy in patients with moderately to severely active Crohn's disease. The 5 mg/kg dose has the best results, with an 81% response rate and 48% remission rate at 4 weeks. The response to infliximab typically occurs within 2 weeks of therapy, and the duration of response is 8 to 12 weeks. A three-dose induction regimen, consisting of infusions at weeks 0, 2, and 6, has been shown to be more effective than the single-infusion regimen for treating active disease. Long-term therapy with infliximab is effective at maintaining remission for up to 1 year. Following response to initial infusions, repeated infliximab therapy every 8 weeks allows remission to be maintained in 28% to 38% of patients at 1 year. In contrast to the study of single infusions, maintenance therapy with infliximab at 10 mg/kg appears to have a slight advantage over the 5 mg/kg dose.

Infliximab is also effective for the treatment of enterocutaneous fistulas associated with Crohn's disease. Three infusions of 5 mg/kg of infliximab at weeks 0, 2, and 6, result in complete closure of over half of fistulas in 68% of patients and complete closure of all fistulas in 55% of patients. Similar to therapy with active inflammatory disease, the effect of infliximab is rapid, and occurs within 2 weeks of the first infusion. The benefit persists with re-infusions at 8-week intervals. Maintenance therapy with infliximab at 5 mg/kg significantly prolongs the time to loss of the initial response compared to patients receiving placebo maintenance therapy, with 36% of infliximab-treated patients maintaining complete closure of all fistulas at 1 year.

Another important benefit of infliximab is its steroid-sparing properties. Single infusions of infliximab have been shown to allow successful steroid withdrawal. Once steroid is discontinued, repeated infliximab therapy at 8-week intervals is more effective than a single infusion for maintaining remission.

Side effects Most patients tolerate infliximab infusions well, but data on its long-term safety is limited. Common side effects include headache, myalgia, upper respiratory tract infections, fatigue, nausea, abdominal pain, and diarrhea (Table 5.6). Antibodies against infliximab (formerly known as human anti-chimeric antibodies) develop in 13% of patients, although the clinical significance of this immune response is unclear. Acute infusion reactions occur in approximately 6% to 16% of the patients and are usually mild. They are more common in patients who develop antibodies against infliximab and in patients who have received more than one infusion. Delayed hypersensitivity-like reactions can develop following a lapse of 2 to 4 years between infusions. This type of reaction is characterized by the onset of myalgia, polyarthritis, fever, rash, and leukocytosis approximately 3 to 12 days after infusion. Delayed hypersensitivity-like reactions appear to be associated with the presence of antibodies against infliximab. Autoantibodies, including antinuclear and double-stranded DNA antibodies may develop following infliximab therapy, but their clinical significance in this setting is unclear.

Serious infections such as pneumonia, sepsis, abscess, peritonitis, meningitis, and systemic fungal infections can develop but are rare. Development of active tuberculosis has been reported in patients receiving infliximab for rheumatoid arthritis and Crohn's disease. Most of these cases manifest extrapulmonary disease. The majority of reported cases also occur in patients from countries with a low incidence of tuberculosis. The exact risk of active tuberculosis associated with infliximab therapy is currently unknown. All patients should be screened for latent or active tuberculosis prior to initiating infliximab. Exacerbation of pre-existing heart failure has also been reported in patients receiving infliximab for congestive heart failure. Patients with New York Heart Association class III or IV heart failure should not receive infliximab therapy. Diagnosis of malignancy has been reported in patients following infliximab therapy. The two cases of lymphoma reported to date include one patient with long-standing Crohn's disease and another patient with lymphoma diagnosed 3 weeks after an infliximab infusion for Crohn's disease. The precise risk of malignancy associated with infliximab therapy is unknown, but is generally thought to be no greater than the general population. Demyelinating neurological disorders can rarely develop with anti-TNF therapies; at least one case of multiple sclerosis has been reported in patients receiving infliximab for Crohn's disease.

Other anti-tumor necrosis factor therapies

CDP571 Another engineered 'humanized' chimeric antibody directed against TNFα is CDP571. It is derived from the IgG_4 subclass and consists of 95% human constant region and 5% murine variable region. Similar to infliximab, CDP571 binds to both soluble and membrane-bound TNFα, but is thought not have complement-fixation properties.

Therapy with CDP571 at 10 mg/kg is effective in achieving a clinical response (54%) at 2 weeks after infusion in patients with moderately to severely active Crohn's disease. There is a trend toward higher rates of clinical remission with CDP571 compared to placebo therapy, but the benefit is not statistically significant. Repeat infusions of 10 mg/kg dose every 8 or 12 weeks may also be beneficial over 24 weeks, but the remission rate with CDP571 retreatment is not significantly superior to placebo therapy. Similar to infliximab, CDP571 may have both steroid-sparing properties and particular benefit for fistulizing disease. In clinical trials of CDP571, antibodies against CDP571 developed in 3% to 9% of patients and anti-double stranded DNA antibodies in 7% of patients. There has been no direct comparison between CDP571 and infliximab to date. A recent trial has been completed, however, evaluating the efficacy of CDP571 in patients who have experienced adverse events related to infliximab.

Etanercept Etanercept is another product of molecular engineering techniques. It is a recombinant human fusion protein linking the soluble portion of the human TNF receptor (TNFR, p75) with the C-terminal portion of the immunoglobulin heavy chain (Fc portion) of the human IgG_1. The resultant fusion protein antagonizes the action of TNFα by competitively binding to TNFα and thus preventing TNFα from binding to its cell-surface receptors. Such a design of fusion protein is thought to be potentially less immunogenic than the humanized chimeric antibodies. Limited data is available on the use of etanercept for Crohn's disease. In the only randomized controlled trial reported to date, subcutaneous etanercept at 25 mg twice weekly for 8 weeks failed to demonstrate efficacy in patients with moderately to severely active Crohn's disease. It is unknown if a different dosing regimen may be beneficial.

Thalidomide Thalidomide is an oral agent initially used as a hypnotic and sedative agent. Its potent teratogenicity led to limited use of this drug for decades. The resurgence of interest in thalidomide followed the discovery that inhibition of TNFα is one of its modes of action. It should be pointed out that thalidomide also has other anti-inflammatory properties, including downregulation of integrins and IL-12 and inhibition of angiogenesis and leukocyte migration. Preliminary studies suggest potential benefit of thalidomide in the treatment of luminal and fistulizing Crohn's disease refractory to conventional therapies. At doses ranging from 50 mg/day to 300 mg/day in patients with active inflammatory Crohn's disease, thalidomide results in a response rate of 56% to 70%, a remission rate of 20% to 33%, and complete steroid withdrawal in approximately 40% of patients. The rate of complete fistulous closure is 38% in patients with fistulizing Crohn's disease. The use of thalidomide as a maintenance therapy has also been reported in pediatric patients. In clinical trials of thalidomide in Crohn's disease, the major side effects are sedation and peripheral neuropathy. Additional studies are required to further assess the utility of thalidomide in the management of Crohn's disease. There are now second and third generation agents that are similar to thalidomide but lack its adverse effects.

Other biological therapies

Anti-inflammatory cytokine therapies

Interleukin-10 is a classic T-helper-2 response mediator, with both anti-inflammatory and immunosuppressive properties. Interleukin-10 inhibits macrophage expression of class I major histocompatibility complex, and decreases cytokine production by T lymphocytes and activated monocytes. In two randomized controlled studies of active Crohn's disease, subcutaneous recombinant human IL-10 failed to demonstrate significant superiority over placebo therapy at various dosages – 1, 4, 5, 10, and 20 $\mu g\ kg^{-1}\ day^{-1}$. There was a trend toward a higher rate of clinical response with subcutaneous recombinant human IL-10 at $8\mu g\ kg^{-1}\ day^{-1}$. A preliminary study suggests potential benefit of intravenous recombinant human IL-10 in patients with steroid-resistant Crohn's disease, although its efficacy has not been formally evaluated. Therapy with recombinant human IL-10 is associated with anemia and thrombocytopenia. These adverse events are usually dose related, mild to moderate, and reversible on discontinuation of the medication.

Interleukin-11 is a pleiotropic cytokine with thrombocytopoietic properties and protective effects on intestinal mucosa. In a randomized controlled trial, therapy with subcutaneous recombinant human IL-11 at various dosing regimens resulted in improvement of disease activity in patients with active Crohn's disease. Patients receiving 16 $\mu g\ kg^{-1}\ week^{-1}$ of recombinant human IL-11, both the twice and five-times weekly schedules had the best results, with response rates of 33% to 42% and remission rates of 17% to 33%. Adverse events include dose-dependent thrombocytosis and hyperfibrinogenemia, without requiring discontinuation of medications.

Biological therapies directed at cytokine manipulation continue to evolve. Humanized monoclonal antibody against interferon alpha is another agent in this class that has failed to demonstrate benefit in a recent study. Given the currently available efficacy data and side effect profiles, further investigations are necessary to define a safe and effective dosing regimen for these cytokine therapies in patients with Crohn's disease.

Adhesion molecule antagonists

Adhesion molecules are transmembrane proteins that function in recruiting inflammatory cells from the systemic intravascular space into sites of inflammation in response to inflammatory stimuli. In the intestinal tract, they are present on mucosal endothelial and lamina propria mononuclear cells. Their expressions are upregulated in inflammation. These cell adhesion molecules include intercellular adhesion molecule 1, vascular cell adhesion molecule 1, integrins, and selectins.

ISIS-2302 is an antisense oligonucleotide that selectively inhibits cytokine-induced expression of intercellular adhesion molecule 1 in a variety of cells. In addition to cell trafficking, intercellular adhesion molecule 1 may play a role in activating T cells. Despite initial promise in a preliminary study, ISIS-2302 failed to demonstrate efficacy in patients with chronic active Crohn's disease in two large, randomized controlled trials.

Antegren is a humanized monoclonal antibody directed against alpha 4 integrin, which is expressed in the gut-associated lymphoid tissues and mediates the selective homing of lymphocytes to intestinal tissues. Preliminary data suggest a potential benefit of antegren in the treatment of active Crohn's disease, but its efficacy awaits the completion of a large controlled trial.

Granulocyte and granulocyte– macrophage colony stimulating factors

One hypothesis for the pathogenesis of Crohn's disease is that some patients with this condition have impaired neutrophil and/or monocyte functions. The use of colony-stimulating factors is thought to modulate such an innate immune defect in patients with Crohn's disease. Preliminary data suggest potential benefit of granulocyte colony-stimulating factors in the treatment of active Crohn's disease and maintenance of surgically induced remission. One pilot study also reported encouraging results with granulocyte–monocyte colony-stimulating factors in patients with active Crohn's disease. Randomized controlled trials are necessary to confirm the efficacy of these novel therapies for the treatment of Crohn's disease.

Additional novel therapies

Probiotics

Although most medical therapies are directed toward altering the host immune response, probiotics have been used in recent years to manipulate the enteric flora, which is known to be altered in patients with Crohn's disease. Two probiotic therapies that have been investigated for the treatment of Crohn's disease are *Lactobacillus GG* and *Saccharomyces boulardii*. *Lactobacillus GG* is a probiotic bacterium known to transiently colonize the human intestine. In four children with active Crohn's disease, *Lactobacillus GG* therapy decreased disease activity starting at 1 week, and the benefit sustained with continued therapy for 6 months. Another preliminary study in adult Crohn's patients suggested benefit of *Saccharomyces boulardii* as a maintenance therapy in conjunction with mesalamine. Additional data is needed to determine the efficacy of probiotics in the treatment of Crohn's disease. It is conceivable that probiotic agents may emerge as an important adjunctive therapy to conventional treatments in patients with Crohn's disease.

Growth hormone

The use of intestinal growth factors in patients with Crohn's disease is based on their effects on intestinal growth and repair, particularly in patients with short-bowel syndrome. Growth hormone has been shown to have pleiotropic properties in the intestinal tract in both *in vitro* and *in vivo* studies. Growth hormone increases the trophic activity of the small-intestinal mucosa, enhances proliferation and morphological adaptation of the remaining bowel, and promotes wound healing following intestinal resection. In addition, growth hormone enhances the intestinal uptake of amino acids and electrolytes, and increases intestinal protein synthesis in animal models. It has also been shown to decrease mucosal permeability and intestinal secretions. The precise mechanism of the therapeutic action of growth hormone in Crohn's disease is unknown. In a small controlled study, growth hormone (somatotropin) in combination with nutritional therapy appeared to be beneficial in patients with active Crohn's disease. In this study, patients who received growth hormone at a dose of 5 mg/day subcutaneously for 1 week followed by a maintenance dose of 1.5 mg/day for 4 months had a significant reduction in their disease severity compared to patients receiving placebo therapy. All patients in the study increased their protein intake to more than than 2 grams per kilogram of body weight per day. Growth hormone has also been shown to be of particular benefit in children with steroid-dependent disease, with positive changes in body composition, bone metabolism, and linear growth. The clinical efficacy of growth hormone in Crohn's disease is currently being evaluated in a randomized controlled trial.

Nutritional therapy

The role of nutritional therapy as a primary therapy for Crohn's disease is controversial, but it is an important adjunct in the management of Crohn's disease. The mechanism of its potential benefit as a primary therapy remains unknown. In addition to the improved nutritional status, the primary beneficial effect of nutritional therapy is thought to derive from the elimination of dietary antigenic exposure to the inflamed bowel. In addition, nutritional therapy may also modulate intestinal inflammation and improve intestinal permeability. Certain nutrients such as glutamine have been shown to be important in maintaining intestinal metabolism, structure, and function. Dietary factors such as omega-3 fatty acids, or fish oils, have also been shown to possess anti-inflammatory properties.

Various forms of enteral nutrition are available. In general, these diets are classified by the nitrogen source derived from the amino acid or protein components of the formula. The elemental diets consist of single amino acids and are thus antigen-free. The non-elemental diets include semi-elemental (oligopeptide-based) and polymeric (derived from whole proteins) formula. Although there are many studies evaluating the efficacy of nutritional therapy in Crohn's disease, there has been no placebo-controlled trial of enteral nutrition reported in the literature. Several meta-analyses have failed to show equivalence of enteral nutrition compared to corticosteroids in inducing remission in patients with Crohn's disease. There is also no difference in efficacy between elemental and non-elemental diets.

Although the efficacy of enteral diets as the primary therapy for inducing remission has not been clearly demonstrated, enteral nutrition continues to be an important adjunct in managing patients with Crohn's disease, particularly in children or adolescents, to ensure adequate nutrition and appropriate growth. Further research is needed to determine if nutritional therapy is superior to placebo, and if there is an optimal enteral formulation.

Parenteral nutrition should be reserved only for patients in whom enteral nutrition cannot be administered, including those with a high-output fistula or obstructive disease. There is currently no evidence that elimination of particular dietary components is necessary, although lactose restriction may be beneficial in some, but not all, patients. Patients with symptomatic fibrostenotic disease should also be placed on a low-residue diet to minimize potential obstruction.

Surgical therapy

In general, medical therapy is the mainstay of therapy for Crohn's disease. However, approximately 60% of patients will have undergone surgery for Crohn's disease after 10 years of diagnosis. Given the high postoperative recurrence rate, the potential complication of short-bowel syndrome, and the myriad of options available for medical therapy, surgery should be reserved for failure of medical therapy or complications of Crohn's disease (Table 5.7). Failure of medical therapy includes refractoriness to medical therapy, intolerance or toxicities from medical therapy, and avoidance of potential toxicities as in the case of steroid-dependent disease. Complications of Crohn's disease that may require surgical interventions include obstruction, fistulas and abscess.

One important point that needs to be considered prior to recommending surgical therapy is that many of the symptoms in Crohn's disease may be the sequelae of chronic disease rather than manifestations of active inflammation. For example, diarrhea and weight loss are common symptoms of Crohn's disease, but they may also be the consequence of fatty acid malabsorption, bile-salt induced diarrhea, or small-bowel bacterial overgrowth. Identification of the problems and optimal medical therapy should be undertaken. Conversely, obstructive symptoms may occur from strictures secondary to prior inflammation. These fibrotic strictures that have minimal active inflammatory components usually do not respond to our current medical therapy, and should be managed with surgery.

Surgical approaches for Crohn's disease depend on the reason for surgery and the location of bowel involved. Surgery for active small-bowel disease requires resection. The general principle for small-bowel resection is to minimize the segment of bowel to be removed, as the disease will likely progress in the long term. The incidence of recurrence at the anastomotic site is high. Clinical relapses within 1 year after ileal or ileocecal resection for Crohn's disease occur in approximately 20% to 40% of patients. This rate increases to up to 86% at 3 years after surgical resection. Endoscopic recurrences can be present preceding clinical symptoms of disease; endoscopic evidence of disease at the anastomotic site has been reported to be present in up to 73% of patients at 12 months in one report (24% and 93% in two further reports) and 100% at 3 years postoperatively. Approximately 50% of patients will ultimately require reoperation for recurrent disease within 10 years after the initial surgical resection.

An alternative to resection for small-bowel stricture caused by fibrosis is stricturoplasty. The most commonly used method of stricturoplasty is the Heineke–Mikulicz type, which involves a longitudinal incision of the narrowed segment followed by transverse closure, thereby relieving the stricture.

Table 5.7 Indications for surgery in patients with Crohn's disease.

Indications	Surgical options
Medically refractory or steroid-dependent disease	
small bowel disease	Segmental small bowel resection
limited colonic disease	Segmental colonic resection
extensive colonic disease	Subtotal colectomy, ileostomy
Stricture	Segmental resection
	Stricturoplasty
	Balloon dilatation
Intra-abdominal fistula or abscess	Drainage, subsequent resection
Simple perianal disease	Drainage of abscess, seton placement
	Fistulotomy
Complex perianal disease	Ileostomy

One advantage of stricturoplasty is that it preserves the bowel and minimizes potential short-gut syndrome. There are several surgical approaches for Crohn's colitis, depending on the extent of disease involvement. Segmental resection is preferred if only a relatively short segment of colon is involved. More extensive colitis may require subtotal colectomy or total proctocolectomy with ileostomy. In contrast to ulcerative colitis, total colectomy with ileoanal anastomosis is not appropriate for Crohn's colitis, because the potential recurrence of Crohn's disease in the ileal portion of the pouch would require reoperation and additional resection of a long segment of ileum. In appropriate patients, hand-assisted laparoscopic techniques may present a desirable alternative to the traditional open surgery by minimizing the length of hospital stay and the time to full recovery.

Extraintestinal complications

A variety of extraintestinal manifestations can occur in patients with Crohn's disease (Box 5.4). These disorders can be broadly classified into three groups. The first group includes disorders involving the skin, eye, joints, and mouth, and usually occurs in patients with colonic disease. The activity of these colitis-related manifestations may or may not parallel the activity of the underlying bowel disease. The second group of manifestations is secondary to complications of direct extension of bowel disease, and includes nephrolithiasis, obstructive uropathy, and gallstones. Manifestations in the third group cannot be clearly categorized as being of one type, and include osteoporosis, hepatic diseases, and amyloidosis.

Musculoskeletal diseases

The most common extraintestinal manifestations are musculoskeletal diseases, and these include rheumatologic and metabolic bone disorders. The rheumatologic manifestations can be broadly classified as peripheral and axial arthropathy.

Peripheral arthropathy occurs in 10% to 20% of patients with Crohn's disease. In general, the risk of developing peripheral arthropathy increases with the extent of colonic disease, and the presence of complications such as abscesses, perianal disease, and other extraintestinal manifestations (erythema

---

Box 5.4 Extra-intestinal manifestations of Crohn's disease in more commonly involved organ systems

Musculoskeletal
  peripheral arthropathy
  ankylosing spondylitis
  sacroiliitis
  osteopenia
  osteoporosis
  osteomalacia
  osteonecrosis
Cutaneous
  erythema nodosum
  pyoderma gangrenosum
  angular stomatitis
  aphthous stomatitis
  Sweet's syndrome
  pyostomatitis vegetans
  erythema multiforme
  epidermolysis bullosa acquisita
  psoriasis
  metastatic Crohn's disease
Ophthalmologic
  episcleritis
  uveitis/iritis
  retinal vascular disease
Hematologic
  anemia
  leukocytosis/leukopenia
  thrombocytosis/thrmobocytopenia
  thromboembolic disease
Genitourinary
  nephrolithiasis
  obstructive uropathy
  fistulas
  amyloidosis
  glomerulonephritis
Hepatobiliary
  primary sclerosing cholangitis
  pericholangitis
  cholangiocarcinoma
  hepatic steatosis
  granulomatous hepatitis
  autoimmune hepatitis
  portal vein thrombosis
  cholelithiasis

nodosum, stomatitis, uveitis, and pyoderma gangrenosum). Approximately 20% to 25% of Crohn's disease patients with peripheral arthropathy have human leukocyte antigen B27. The arthropathy manifests in an asymmetric and migratory pattern, and mainly involves large joints – with decreasing frequency of involvement these joints are knee, ankle, shoulder, elbow, wrist, and metacarpophalangeal joints. This peripheral arthropathy has also been further subclassified into two distinct types

1. type 1 is pauciarticular arthropathy affecting less than five joints, it usually involves the large joints (knees, elbows, ankles) and manifests as acute, self-limited episodes
2. type 2 is polyarticular arthropathy affecting at least five joints, it typically involves small joints and presents with persisting symptoms lasting for years.

While type 1 arthropathy usually parallels the activity of the underlying bowel disease, type 2 is usually independent of the bowel disease activity.

Axial arthropathy occurs less frequently than peripheral arthropathy and does not parallel the activity of the underlying bowel disease. The spondylitis associated with inflammatory bowel disease is generally considered one of the spondyloarthropathies. Patients with ankylosing spondylitis often experience severe onset of back pain associated with morning stiffness or exacerbated by periods of rest. The course is typically progressive, resulting in permanent skeletal damage. Isolated sacroiliitis, in contrast, may be asymptomatic and does not progress to ankylosing spondylitis. While the majority of patients with spondylitis are human leukocyte antigen B27 positive, most patients with sacroiliitis are negative for human leukocyte antigen B27.

In general, peripheral arthropathy usually responds to treatment of colitis. The progressive nature of the axial arthropathy, however, is not altered by treatment of the underlying bowel disease. Other treatment modalities include rest, physical therapy, and intra-articular steroid injections.

Metabolic bone disorders, including osteoporosis and osteopenia, are common in patients with Crohn's disease. The bone loss occurs in both trabecular and cortical bone. Factors contributing to these complications in patients with Crohn's disease include corticosteroid therapy, low physical activity, inflammatory cytokines, small-bowel disease or resection, and vitamin D deficiency. Patients with Crohn's disease should receive a baseline bond densitometry. Repeat evaluations at 1- to 2-year intervals are recommended for patients with additional risk factor for osteoporosis, including low calcium diet, family history of osteoporosis, and corticosteroid therapy (greater than 7.5 mg of prednisone daily for 6 months). Patients with Crohn's disease should also receive calcium and vitamin D supplementation. The use of bisphosphonates may decrease bone loss, but has not been adequately evaluated.

A less common metabolic bone disorder is osteomalacia, which is characterized by accumulation of improperly mineralized bone matrix. The resultant fragile bone leads to deformities and pseudofractures. Osteonecrosis (avascular or aseptic necrosis of bone, or osteochondritis dissecans) is a serious complication of Crohn's disease. Patients usually present with joint swelling and pain associated with motion. The most commonly involved sites are the hips, followed by the knees and shoulders. Corticosteroid therapy, particularly a high dose of corticosteroids, is an important risk factor for osteonecrosis. Treatment with prednisone at 25 mg/day for at least 1 month is generally considered the minimum for predisposing a patient to developing osteonecrosis, although the complication can occur with a significantly lower amount of steroid therapy.

Dermatologic diseases

Erythema nodosum and pyoderma gangrenosum are the two most commonly encountered cutaneous manifestations of Crohn's disease. Erythema nodosum occurs in 10% to 20% of patients with Crohn's disease, and is characterized by tender, red nodules typically on the extensor surface of the lower extremities. It usually correlates well with the activity of the bowel disease, and responds to treatment of the underlying colitis. Severe lesions may require systemic corticosteroid or immunosuppressive therapy. Pyoderma gangrenosum is less common in Crohn's disease, and usually begins as an erythematous pustule or nodule that spreads to adjacent skin and develops into a burrowing, sterile ulcer with irregular, violaceous edges. These lesions usually occur on the extensor surface of the lower extremities or sites of trauma. In contrast to erythema nodosum, most cases of pyoderma gangrenosum, except the pustular variant, are usually independent of the underlying bowel-disease activity, but may resolve with treatment of the underlying colitis. Mild cases may be managed by local therapy alone, including topical cromolyn sodium and topical 5-aminosalicylic acid. Other local therapies include intralesional corticosteroids and topical tacrolimus. Effective systemic therapies include oral sulfasalazine, dapsone, corticosteroids, various immunomodulators (azathioprine, cyclophosphamide, cyclosporine, methotrexate, tacrolimus, and mycophenolate mofetil), and anti-TNF therapy (infliximab and thalidomide).

A variety of oral lesions may be associated with Crohn's disease. The most common ones are aphthous and angular stomatitis. Pyostomatitis (pyoderma) vegetans manifests with pustular lesions of the oral mucosa, often with a cobblestone appearance. Sweet's syndrome, or acute febrile neutrophilic dermatosis, can manifest with cutaneous lesions as tender, erythematous plaques or nodules on the extremities, torso, or face. This rare condition is also characterized by leukocytosis, fever, arthritis, and conjunctivitis. Other rare dermatological manifestations include epidermolysis bullosa acquisita and erytherma multiforme. Psoriasis is also more common in patients with Crohn's disease.

Ocular diseases

Episcleritis and uveitis are the most common ophthalmologic disorders associated with Crohn's disease. Episcleritis is characterized by painless hyperemia of the sclera and conjunctiva without loss of vision, while uveitis presents with painful eye, blurring vision, photophobia, headache, and iridospasm. Despite the visual blurring, there is usually no significant impairment in visual acuity unless the posterior uveal structures or the retina is involved. Episcleritis usually parallels the underlying bowel-disease course, while uveitis does not. Prompt treatment with topical or systemic corticosteroids is necessary for uveitis to prevent progression to blindness. Posterior subcapsular cataracts are potential complications of corticosteroid therapy in patients with Crohn's disease. The risk of developing posterior subcapsular cataracts increases with the dose and duration of steroids. Thus, annual opthalmological examination is recommended in patients with Crohn's disease receiving corticosteroids.

Hematologic diseases

Anemia is commonly present in patients with Crohn's disease, and may be multifactorial. Factors contributing to anemia in patients with Crohn's disease include chronic disease, acute or chronic gastrointestinal blood loss, deficiency of nutrients including iron, folate, and vitamin B_{12}, and autoimmune hemolysis. Nutritional deficiency may be secondary to inadequate dietary intake or malabsorption of iron, malabsorption of vitamin B_{12} because of terminal ileal disease or resection, and folate deficiency from proximal small-bowel disease or medications (sulfasalazine, methotrexate). Leukocytosis and thrombocytosis are usually associated with active disease, while leukopenia and thrombocytopenia are usually secondary to medications such as immunosuppressants and sulfasalazine. Patients with inflammatory bowel disease have been suggested, although not proven, to have an increased risk of developing thromboembolic events, including deep venous thrombosis, pulmonary embolism, renal artery thrombosis, cerebrovascular accidents, coronary artery thrombosis, and venous thrombosis of mesenteric, portal, and hepatic vessels.

Genitourinary and renal diseases

Nephrolithiasis occurs in up to 10% of patients with Crohn's disease. The two most common types of stones are uric acid and calcium oxalate. Calcium oxalate stones result from hyperoxaluria associated with distal ileal Crohn's disease or ileal resection. The fat malabsorption in these patients results in increased luminal fatty acids which compete with oxalate to bind to calcium. Thus, oxalate remains in the soluble sodium form and is readily absorbed in the colon, leading to hyperoxaluria. Since the absorption of sodium oxalate occurs in the colon, calcium oxalate stones are seen primarily in patients with intact colon, and not in patients with colectomy. In contrast, patients with an ileostomy may become volume depleted, thus predisposing them to develop uric acid stones. Management of nephrolithiasis is similar to that for patients without Crohn's disease, and consists of analgesia, hydration, alkalinization of urine for uric acid stones, lithotripsy, and surgery. In patients with Crohn's disease, calcium supplementation may decrease the risk of calcium oxalate stones by allowing luminal oxalate to bind to calcium, which is then excreted in the stools.

Obstructive uropathy may occur as a result of extrinsic compression of the ureter by the enteric inflammation. Fistulizing disease complicating the urinary tract may present with pneumaturia or recurrent urinary tract infections. Surgery may be necessary if medical therapies fail to heal the fistulas. Secondary systemic amyloidosis is rare in patients with Crohn's disease, but often involves the kidney, with nephritic syndrome and renal insufficiency.

Hepatobiliary diseases

Pericholangitis is one of the most common hepatobiliary complications of Crohn's disease. It is thought to be part of the spectrum of sclerosing cholangitis. Patients with pericholangitis have elevated alkaline phosphatase levels and histological evidence of non-specific portal tract inflammation. Sclerosing cholangitis is characterized by fibrosing inflammation of the intrahepatic and extrahepatic bile duct. It is diagnosed by endoscopic retrograde cholangiopancreatography. Although it is much less common in Crohn's disease than in ulcerative colitis, the high prevalence of inflammatory bowel disease in patients with sclerosing cholangitis mandates the need for colonoscopy even in patients without intestinal symptoms. Biliary strictures are common problems of sclerosing cholangitis and must be differentiated from cholangiocarcinoma, which can also occur in patients with sclerosing cholangitis. Other hepatic diseases associated with Crohn's disease include fatty liver, chronic hepatitis, and cirrhosis. Cholesterol gallstones may form secondary to bile-salt malabsorption and the decrease in bile-salt pool in patients with ileal disease or ileal resection.

Approaches to the management of Crohn's disease

As noted previously, management of patients with Crohn's disease depends on the type, location, and severity of disease. In general, the choice of medical therapies follows the paradigm of a disease-activity-based pyramid (Figure 5.3), and there are general management guidelines that may be applied to patients with either mild to moderate disease or severe disease (Figures 5.4, 5.5). Management of specific clinical problems and complications are discussed in the following section.

For patients with mildly to moderately active disease, oral aminosalicylate therapy may be one of the first line agents (Figure 5.4). The choice of aminosalicylate depends on the location of the disease (Table 5.5). Patient tolerance and compliance can be enhanced by starting aminosalicylates at a moderate dose and increasing gradually to maximal doses. Oral aminosalicylates can be used alone or in combination with oral corticosteroids or antibiotics. In general, if patients do not respond to aminosalicylates and/or antibiotics, or the disease progresses to increasing severity, oral corticosteroids should be initiated. Corticosteroid therapy should be tapered off once a good response is achieved. The rate of steroid taper has never been formally evaluated in clinical trials. One common algorithm for steroid taper consists of decreasing corticosteroids by the equivalent of 5 mg of prednisone every 1 to 2 weeks. If patients do not respond to oral corticosteroids, experience disease exacerbation upon steroid withdrawal, or become steroid dependent, other standard medical therapies may be used, including infliximab, azathioprine or 6-mercaptopurine, and methotrexate. With our increasing experience with these agents and the desire to minimize steroid-related complications, use of medications such as infliximab and azathioprine or 6-mercaptopurine are likely to enter our therapeutic pyramid at an early stage of the disease severity.

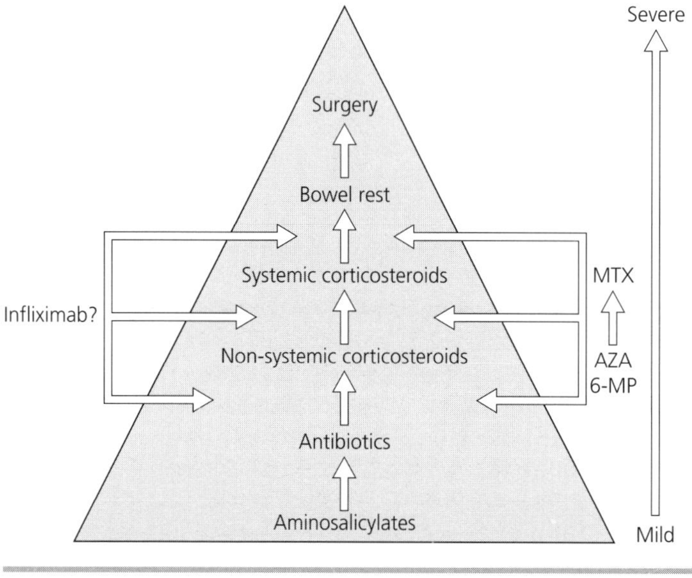

Figure 5.3 Therapeutic pyramid for Crohn's disease.

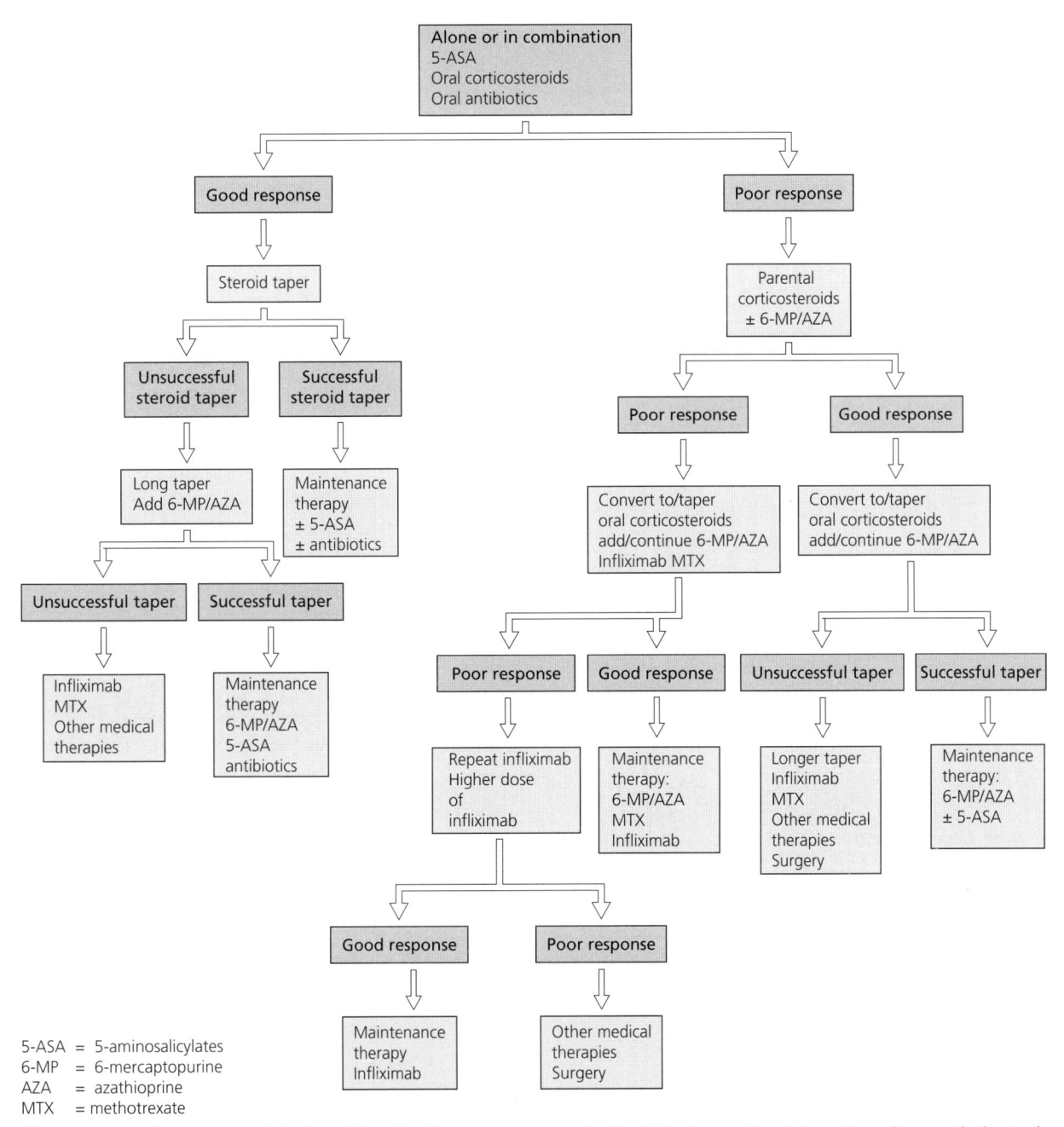

Figure 5.4 Recommended algorithm for the management of mildly to moderately active disease (adapted with permission from Hecht TEH, Su CG, Lichtenstein GR. Medical therapy of inflammatory bowel disease. In Cohen R (ed.) *Inflammatory Bowel Disease: Diagnosis and Therapeutics*. Totowa NJ, Humana Press, 2002).

5-ASA = 5-aminosalicylates
6-MP = 6-mercaptopurine
AZA = azathioprine
MTX = methotrexate

If patients fail regimens for mild to moderate disease, including oral corticosteroids, or if they demonstrate severely active disease, parenteral corticosteroids should be initiated (Figure 5.5). Severely ill patients with systemic symptoms should be hospitalized and receive both parenteral corticosteroids and bowel rest. Infliximab may be used in patients who do not respond to this regimen. Azathioprine/6-mercaptopurine or methotrexate may be initiated concurrently, but the time to onset of action for these agents precludes their use as a single primary therapy in patients with severely active disease. In patients who respond to parenteral corticosteroids, the medication should be converted to the oral form followed by a slow taper. If the symptoms exacerbate on

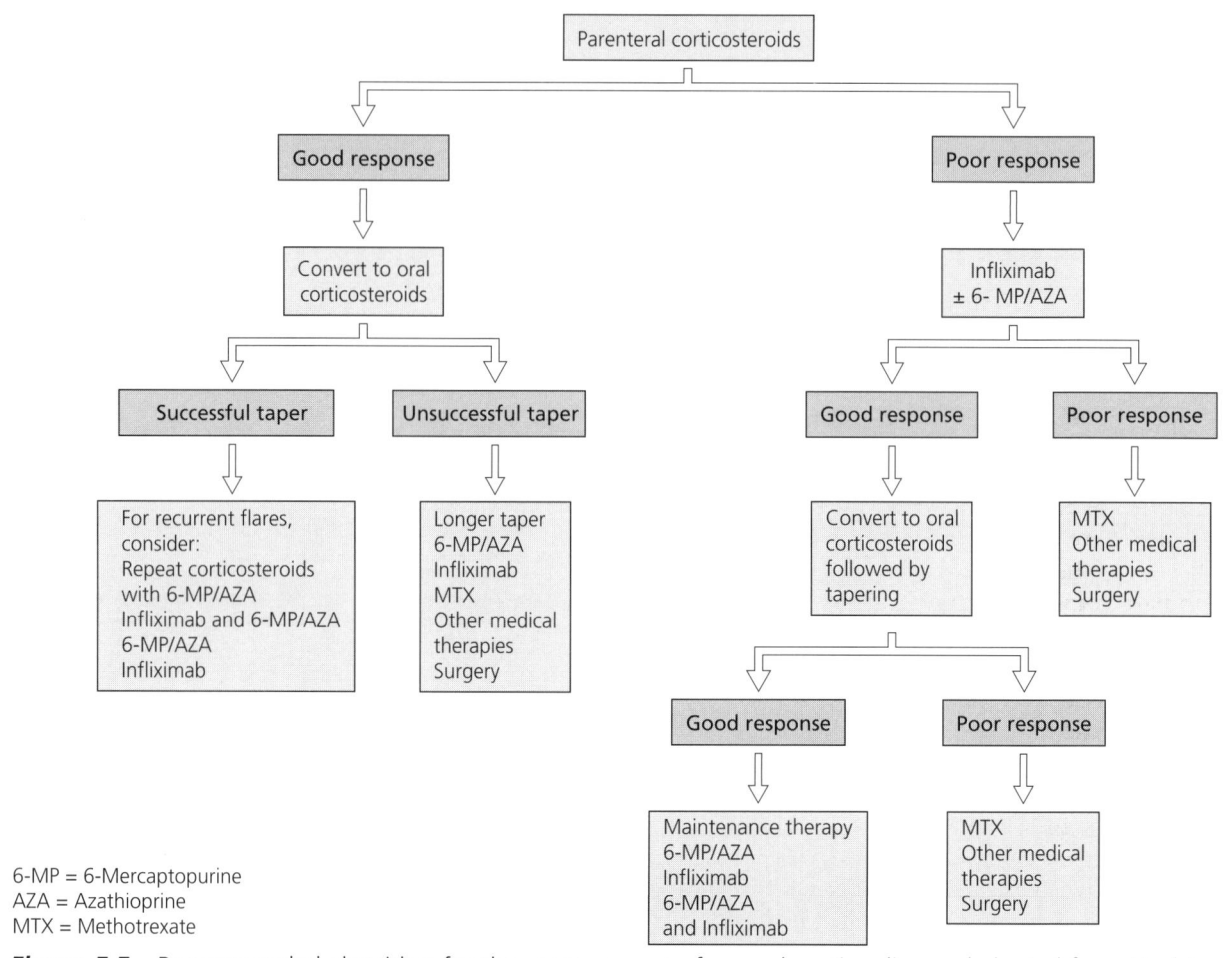

Figure 5.5 Recommended algorithm for the management of severely active disease (adapted from Hecht TEH, Su CG, Lichtenstein GR. Medical therapy of inflammatory bowel disease. In Cohen R (ed.) *Inflammatory Bowel Disease: Diagnosis and Therapeutics*. Totowa NJ, Humana Press, 2002).

6-MP = 6-Mercaptopurine
AZA = Azathioprine
MTX = Methotrexate

steroid withdrawal, infliximab, azathioprine/ 6-mercaptopurine, or methotrexate may be used for steroid sparing.

Management of specific clinical problems and complications

Abscesses and fistulas

The major complications of perforating disease are abscesses and fistulas. Abscesses develop when intestinal contents leak into the peritoneal cavity as a result of perforating disease. Fistulas form when there is a direct communication between the gastrointestinal tract and the adjacent organ or abdominal wall.

Abscesses complicating Crohn's disease are usually intra-abdominal and most commonly arise from the diseased ileum. Extension into the retroperitoneal region can also occur. Intra-abdominal abscesses typically present with fever and abdominal pain. Physical examination may reveal tenderness and abdominal mass at the site of the abscess. The most common laboratory abnormality is leukocytosis. Diagnosis is usually made on CT scan. When an abscess is suspected or identified, the patient should be placed on broad-spectrum antibiotics and bowel rest. If possible, percutaneous aspiration and drainage of the abscess should be performed under CT guidance. Oral diet may be initiated when the drainage output diminishes. However, a prolonged course of total parental nutrition may be necessary if the drainage output increases with re-institution of oral diet. Ultimately, patients with an abscess are likely to require surgery, as simple drainage usually results in the formation of enterocutaneous fistulas. Definitive surgery preferably should be postponed until the abscess is completely drained and the underlying disease is controlled on medications. Early surgery is necessary if CT-guided drainage is not possible or if there is evidence of peritonitis.

Approximately 20% to 40% of patients with Crohn's disease have at least one fistula. The majority of fistulas are either enterocutaneous or enteroenteric. Enterovaginal and enterovesical fistulas comprise only a small proportion of the cases. Fistulas develop when the disease is active, but often persist even after the inflammation becomes quiescent. Clinical presentations depend on the type of fistulas. When enteroenteric fistulas are of significant size, patients usually present with malabsorption with diarrhea and weight loss. Enterocutaneous fistulas are often problematic because the drainage can be intolerable. Rectovaginal fistulas may present with a feculent vaginal discharge or the passage of gas through the vagina. Similarly, enterovesicular fistulas may present with pneumaturia or recurrent urinary tract infections. Diagnosis of fistulas usually requires barium studies, depending on the location of the fistulas. Symptomatic fistulas can be managed either medically or surgically. The use of medications must be weighted against their long-term efficacy, including antibiotics, immune modifiers (azathioprine and 6-mercaptopurine) and anti-TNF therapy as discussed in more details in the previous section on medical therapy (pp. 84–99). A course of bowel rest and total parenteral nutrition may be necessary. Surgery with resection of the involved bowel is indicated for symptomatic fistulas refractory to medical therapy and complex fistulas associated with abscesses.

Obstructions

Obstruction is a common complication of Crohn's disease, typically in the small bowel. Obstruction may be due to bowel-wall thickening from active inflammation, scarring and fibrosis from prior disease, or adhesion. It may be difficult to differentiate whether the bowel narrowing is the result of active inflammation or fibrosis, and both processes may co-exist. Patients typically present with episodes of crampy abdominal pain, diarrhea, nausea, and vomiting that worsen after a meal. Location of the obstruction and length, diameter, and mucosal appearance of the stricture may be evaluated by contrast studies or endoscopy, depending on the location and degree of obstruction. Conservative therapy should be the first-line therapy, including bowel rest, nasogastric decompression, and intravenous hydration. In the presence of active disease, medical therapy should be initiated as well. Patients who fail to respond to medical therapy likely have a significant fibrotic component to their stricture and require surgical therapy. Either resection of the strictured segment or stricturoplasty can be performed. Occasionally, endoscopic balloon dilation may be attempted if the fibrotic stricture is short and accessible by endoscope, although most will eventually require surgery.

Perianal disease

Perianal disease can be particularly problematic in patients with Crohn's disease. In addition to anal fissures and hemorrhoids, perianal complications of Crohn's disease usually present with perirectal fistulas or abscesses. These complications arise from disease in the rectum and anal canal, and a single ulcer can give rise to multiple fistulous tracts. The external openings of the perianal fistulas are usually in the perianal skin, but can be in the adjacent genital areas.

Perianal fistulas usually present with drainage of serous, mucous, or even feculent materials. When the fistula is not drained adequately, pus accumulates and forms an abscess. Perirectal abscesses typically present with fever, pain, and induration at the perianal region. The pain worsens on defecation, sitting, or walking, and digital rectal examination elicits significant tenderness. However, there may be no local signs of abscess depending on its location.

The gold-standard for evaluating perianal disease is surgical examination under anesthesia. Alternatives include MRI and rectal endoscopic ultrasound. Both techniques have been shown to achieve good accuracy. Rectal endoscopic ultrasound may be technically more difficult as patients with perianal disease usually have significant discomfort precluding an adequate examination. Surgical examination under anesthesia has the advantage of allowing therapeutic intervention if necessary. Barium enema may be used as an adjunct to assess the course of fistulas. Computed tompgraphy scans may also be useful in evaluating perianal abscesses, although MRI is preferred over CT scan.

Management of perianal complications can be difficult. The goal of therapy is to relieve symptoms while preserving the anatomy, specifically the anal sphincter. Local therapy with sitz baths should be the initial step. Active bowel disease should be aggressively controlled with medical therapy.

Fistulas may be closed with medications, including antibiotics, immunomodulators (e.g. azathioprine and 6-mercaptopurine), and anti-TNF therapy. Placement of setons or drains in the fistulous tracts allows continued drainage while fistulas heal. This is particularly important with infliximab therapy that has a relatively rapid onset of action, as abscesses may form if the fistulous tracts close before complete drainage of pus. Abscesses require drainage and antibiotics. In refractory cases, bowel rest with total parenteral nutrition or surgeries may be necessary. Fecal diversion by colostomy usually results in symptomatic improvement, but disease usually recurs when the bowel continuity is re-established. In severe cases where there is significant destruction of the anal sphincter, proctectomy may be required.

Cancers

There is an increased risk of adenocarcinoma of the small bowel and colon in patients with Crohn's disease. These cancers typically arise in areas of chronic active disease. Given that small-bowel adenocarcinoma in the general population is rare, its absolute risk in patients with Crohn's disease is still very low even with an increased risk of up to 100-fold in one report. The magnitude of risk of colorectal cancer in patients with Crohn's disease varies among studies. It is generally accepted that patients with Crohn's colitis are at an increased risk of colorectal cancer. Most cases of cancer develop in the presence of macroscopic colitis. The biology of colorectal cancer in Crohn's disease is thought to be similar to that in ulcerative colitis. One landmark study has found that all the colorectal cancers associated with Crohn's disease were contiguous with the presence of high-grade dysplasia. In general, patients with Crohn's colitis have an increased risk of colorectal cancer similar to that in ulcerative colitis patients with comparable duration and extent of disease. It has been estimated that the cumulative incidence of colorectal cancers was 8% in patients with extensive Crohn's colitis for approximately 20 years. It is unknown whether patients with Crohn's disease limited to the small bowel have an increased risk for colon cancers. In contrast to ulcerative colitis, there is currently no definite consensus on a colorectal cancer surveillance program in patients with Crohn's disease. However, it is generally agreed that patients with long-standing, extensive Crohn's colitis should undergo a surveillance program, which can be similar to the one recommended for patients with ulcerative colitis.

Pregnancy

The issue of pregnancy in inflammatory bowel disease is a question that is frequently encountered by gastroenterologists because the peak age of onset of the disease corresponds to the child-bearing age. There is limited data on pregnancy in patients with Crohn's disease. Although some studies suggest that patients with Crohn's disease may have decreased fertility, it is difficult to ascertain to what extent the problem is due to the disease itself. Many factors may impact on conception in patients with Crohn's disease. Certain medications commonly used for Crohn's disease may impair fertility or are contraindicated during pregnancy. The disease may also impact on the patient's willingness to conceive. Additionally, pelvic adhesions and scarring from prior surgery or disease may impair fertility.

Once conceived, the outcome of pregnancy in patients with Crohn's disease is most dependent on the disease activity. Patients with active disease at conception and during the course of pregnancy are more likely to have spontaneous abortions and prematurity. The outcome of pregnancy in patients with inactive disease is thought to be similar to the general population. One limited population-based study suggested that infants born to mothers with Crohn's disease are more likely to be pre-term infants and have low birth weight and smallness for gestational age. Thus, efforts to maintain the patients in remission before conception and throughout the pregnancy are critical to optimize both maternal and fetal outcomes of the pregnancy. The mode of delivery is controversial. Episiotomy is contraindicated in women with Crohn's disease associated with perianal complications. Cesarean section is probably indicated in most patients with Crohn's colitis.

The effect of pregnancy on the disease activity is thought to depend on the trimester of the pregnancy. There may be a slight increase in recurrence during the first trimester and postpartum period, but overall there is no increased incidence of exacerbation during the entire pregnancy course. However, when the disease flares during the pregnancy, the exacerbation tends to be more severe. The majority of patients who entered the pregnancy with quiescent disease will remain in remission throughout the course of pregnancy.

Table 5.8 Safety of medications for Crohn's disease during pregnancy and breast-feeding.

Drug	FDA pregnancy category	Safety in nursing mothers
Sulfasalazine 5-aminosalicylates	B	Probably safe
Asacol	B	Probably safe
Pentasa	B	Probably safe
Dipentum	C	Unknown
Colazal	B	Unknown
Corticosteroids	C	Safe
Metronidazole	B*	Probably safe
Ciprofloxacin	C	Unknown
Azathioprine/6-Mercaptopurine	D	Probably unsafe
Cyclosporine	C	Unsafe
Methotrexate	X	Unsafe
Infliximab	C	Unknown

Food and Drug Administration (FDA) categories for pregnancy:
A = well-controlled studies fail to demonstrate risk to the fetus.
B = animal studies fail to demonstrate risk to the fetus (B1) or animal studies show some risk to the fetus but this is not confirmed in human studies (B2).
C = animal studies show risk to the fetus but no human studies are available (C1) or animal and human studies are unavailable (C2).
D = drugs associated with birth defects but with potential benefits that may outweigh known risks.
X = drugs associated with birth defects and with potential risks that clearly outweigh potential benefit.
* contraindicated in the first trimester.

Management of patients with Crohn's disease during pregnancy should involve judicious use of diagnostic tests and efforts at maintaining remission which should already be achieved at the onset of pregnancy. Colonoscopy and radiologic studies such as barium contrast studies and CT should be avoided if possible. The approach to medical therapy during pregnancy is similar to that in the general population. The majority of the medications are safe in pregnancy and nursing, and they should be used when indicated (Table 5.8). In general, sulfasalazine and 5-aminosalicylic acid agents are considered safe. Folate supplement should be given with sulfasalazine. Corticosteroids are also considered safe and the dosages are the same as for nonpregnant patients. The safety of azathioprine and 6-mercaptopurine during pregnancy is controversial, with limited human data available. Its use is generally considered safe during pregnancy in renal transplant patients and patients with systemic lupus erythematosus. While some studies have reported that exposure to these agents during pregnancy may be associated with a small risk of congenital or developmental abnormalities in the newborns, others have shown no appreciable risk of complications except for a possibly higher incidence of spontaneous abortion. Paternal use of 6-mercaptopurine within 3 months preceding conception may be associated with an increased risk of spontaneous abortions and congenital anomalies. At the present time, the use of azathioprine or 6-mercaptopurine in patients planning to conceive, or during pregnancy, should be individualized and based on informed discussions between patients and physicians. Methotrexate and metronidazole are both contraindicated during pregnancy and nursing. Limited data suggest that infliximab appears to be safe during pregnancy; however, adverse pregnancy outcomes have been reported. Additional data will be helpful in this regard as our experience with this agent accumulates with time.

Further reading

Achkar JP, Hanauer SB. Medical therapy to reduce postoperative Crohn's disease recurrence. *Am J Gastroenterol* 2000; 95(5): 1139–1146.

Blam ME, Stein RB, Lichtenstein GR. Integrating anti tumor necrosis factor-alpha therapy in inflammatory bowel disease: current and future perspectives. *Am J Gastroenterol* 2001; 96(7): 1977–1997.

Cho JH. The Nod2 gene in Crohn's disease: implications for future research into the genetics and immunology of Crohn's disease. *Inflamm Bowel Dis* 2001;7(3): 271–275.

Hanauer SB, Feagan BG, Lichtenstein GR, *et al.* Maintenance infliximab for Crohn's disease: the ACCENT I randomised trial. *Lancet* 2002; 359(9317): 1541–1549.

Hanauer SB, Sandborn W. The Practice Parameters Committee of the American College of Gastroenterology. Management of Crohn's disease in adults. *Am J Gastroenterol* 2001; 96(3): 635–643.

Lewis JD, Schwartz JS, Lichtenstein GR. Azathioprine for maintenance of remission in Crohn's disease: benefits outweigh the risk of lymphoma. *Gastroenterol* 2000; 118(6): 1018–1024.

Lichtenstein GR. Approach to corticosteroid-dependent and corticosteroid-refractory Crohn's disease. *Inflamm Bowel Dis* 2001; 7(Suppl 1):S23–29.

Lichtenstein GR. Treatment of fistulizing Crohn's disease. *Gastroenterology* 2000; 119(4):1132–1147.

Present DH, Rutgeerts P, Targan S, *et al*. Infliximab for the treatment of fistulas in patients with Crohn's disease. *N Engl J Med* 1999; 340(18):1398–1405.

Sandborn W, Sutherland L, Pearson D, May G, Modigliani R, Prantera C. Azathioprine or 6-mercaptopurine for inducing remission of Crohn's disease. *Cochrane Database Syst Rev* 2000; (2):CD000545.

Sandborn WJ. A review of immune modifier therapy for inflammatory bowel disease: azathioprine, 6-mercaptopurine, cyclosporine, and methotrexate. *Am J Gastroenterol* 1996; 91(3):423–33.

Sands BE. Therapy of inflammatory bowel disease. *Gastroenterology* 2000; 118(2 Suppl 1):S68–82.

Stein RB, Lichtenstein GR. Medical therapy for Crohn's disease: the state of the art. *Surg Clin North Am* 2001; 81(1):71–101.

Su CG, Judge TA, Lichtenstein GR. Extraintestinal manifestations of inflammatory bowel disease. *Gastroenterol Clin North Am* 2002; 31

Su CG, Stein RB, Lewis JD, Lichtenstein GR. Azathioprine or 6-mercaptopurine for inflammatory bowel disease: Do risks outweigh benefits? *Dig Liver Dis* 2000; 32(6):518–531.

Yang YX, Lichtenstein GR. Corticosteroids in Crohn's disease. *Am J Gastroenterol* 2002; 97(4):803–23.

Chapter 6

Evaluation of Malabsorption and Maldigestion

Melissa Teitelman and Julius J. Deren

CHAPTER OUTLINE

MECHANISMS OF MALABSORPTION
- Carbohydrate absorption
- Protein absorption
- Fat absorption
- Cobalamin absorption
- Iron absorption
- Folate absorption

TESTS FOR MALABSORPTION
- Anatomic investigations
- Tests for carbohydrate malabsorption
- Tests for fat malabsorption
- Tests for protein malabsorption
- Schilling test
- Tests for bacterial overgrowth
- Tests for pancreatic exocrine function
- Tests for bile acid malabsorption

EVALUATION OF THE PATIENT WITH SUSPECTED MALABSORPTION
- The physical examination
- Laboratory investigation
- Anatomic analysis
- Malabsorption in special circumstances:

MANAGEMENT OF THE PATIENT WITH MALABSORPTION

FURTHER READING

Mechanisms of malabsorption

When we refer to the term "malabsorption" we often mean either malabsorption or maldigestion. Technically, it is important to differentiate malabsorption from maldigestion since each has specific connotations and treatments that differ. When we evaluate the etiology of "malabsorption", we first determine if the patient's symptoms are due to a mucosal defect which is referred to as malabsorption, as opposed to an intraluminal defect which is referred to as maldigestion. One must also have a clear understanding of normal absorption prior to undertaking an investigation into the etiology of the malabsorption. The following section is a review of carbohydrate, protein, fat, water, vitamin, and mineral absorption. In addition, the disease entities associated with the presence of malabsorption of these nutrients will be discussed.

Carbohydrate absorption

Carbohydrates are consumed in the form of polysaccharides, sugars, and oligosaccharides. Sugars and oligosaccharides are quite soluble in water whereas polysaccharides demonstrate a range of solubilities. The sugars, especially sucrose, may be effectively dissolved in the water in the food. Upon ingestion, the food mixes with salivary amylase which initiates hydrolysis of the starch and produces a wide range of molecular fragments. The action of salivary amylase is terminated in the stomach and the starches subsequently become hydrated by gastric contents. The mixing process of the stomach further disperses the soluble carbohydrates, and the peristaltic movements of the stomach drive the contents toward the pylorus and small intestine. Hydrolysis of starches is completed in the duodenum and jejunum with the introduction of pancreatic α-amylase which hydrolyzes starches to oligosaccharides and disaccharides. In the absorptive phase, disaccharides are too large to cross the mucosal cell membrane. The disaccharidases are enzymes responsible for hydrolysis of disaccharides to absorbable monosaccharides. The disaccharidases are not present in the pancreatic secretions and are instead located at the brush border of the intestinal membrane.

The major brush border enzymes are lactase, sucrase, and maltase. Lactase hydrolyzes lactose to the monosaccharides glucose and galactose, sucrase hydrolyzes sucrose to the monosaccharides fructose and glucose, and isomaltase and maltase hydrolyze isomaltose and maltose into two glucose molecules. The glucose is then absorbed by active transport via a sodium dependent cotransport system. The concentration of these cotransporter sites is the highest in the duodenum and upper jejunum. The absorption of fructose is felt to be carrier-mediated facilitated diffusion. Interestingly, it appears that fructose is more effectively absorbed in the presence of glucose or from sucrose than absorbed as fructose alone. In many adults, lactase activity is low. Levels of lactase are high at birth and increase with the suckling of milk. Lactase activity then decreases rapidly after weaning. The rate-limiting step in the absorption of lactose is the rate of hydrolysis of lactase. Caucasian populations maintain significant lactase activity into adult life but in other ethnic and racial groups, variable enzyme activity persists throughout life. Once the monosaccharides have been effectively absorbed into the enterocyte, they traverse the enterocyte by diffusion and are then thought to cross the basolateral membrane by sodium independent carriers into the portal circulation.

Now that normal carbohydrate absorption has been reviewed, it will be easier to illustrate the mechanisms of carbohydrate malabsorption. Carbohydrate malabsorption occurs in pancreatic exocrine insufficiency, as in chronic pancreatitis or cystic fibrosis due to lack of pancreatic α-amylase. Adding to carbohydrate malabsorption in pancreatic insufficiency, the intestinal transit time is significantly accelerated in pancreatic insufficiency to approximately 50% of normal transit time. Brush border enzyme deficiencies, such as lactase deficiency, also result in carbohydrate malabsorption, from either intestinal injury or, more commonly, from alterations in the genetic expression of lactase-phlorizin hydrolase which is the etiology of lactose intolerance in much of the world's adult population. Carbohydrate malabsorption can also occur with disruption of brush border and enterocyte function as with celiac sprue and regional enteritis. In celiac sprue, there is a T-cell mediated immune response to ingested wheat gluten, rye, or barley resulting in an inflammation injury of the mucosa of the small intestine. It usually manifests clinically with significant diarrhea most notably in children with celiac sprue. In addition, regional enteropathies resulting in mucosal inflammation, probably occurring from a variety of etiologies, can also lead to carbohydrate malabsorption which appears clinically similar to celiac sprue. Lastly, there can also be loss of mucosal surface area as with short bowel syndrome. Short bowel syndrome occurs in individuals who have 200 cm or less of jejunum-ileum remaining after intestinal resection. This length of small bowel usually results in insufficient mucosal surface area to effectively absorb adequate carbohydrates as well as other nutrients.

Protein absorption

In the normal adult, the recommended dietary protein intake is $0.75 \text{ g kg}^{-1} \text{ day}^{-1}$. Protein digestion begins in the stomach with proteolysis by gastric pepsins. The pepsins are released as proenzymes and are autocatalytically activated at an acidic pH. Dietary protein is subsequently hydrolyzed into polypeptides, oligopeptides and few free amino acids. The degree to which proteolysis occurs in the stomach depends on the other food products present in the stomach as well as the pH and the gastric motility. It appears that the gastric phase of protein digestion is not critical since patients who have undergone gastrectomy, have achlorhydria, or who have poorly controlled gastric emptying can nevertheless digest and absorb adequate protein to meet their daily requirements. However, the protein products of gastric digestion help stimulate cholecystokinin release from duodenal and jejunal epithelial cells. One released, cholecystokinin then stimulates the release of pancreatic enzymes.

The pancreatic phase of protein digestion involves inactive zymogens or proenzymes secreted by the pancreas. One of these zymogens is trypsinogen which is converted to the enzyme, trypsin by enteropeptidase, an enzyme on the brush border of duodenal enterocytes. Trypsin then hydrolyzes the other zymogens which results in the fully activated chymotrypsin, elastase, carboxypeptidase A and B as well as trypsin. The products of luminal proteolysis are free amino acids and small peptides with chain length of two to six amino acids.

In the final phase of protein digestion, dietary protein is reduced by peptidases in the intestinal mucosal cells located in the brush border to free amino acids, dipeptides and tripeptides. The free amino acids and peptides are then transported by sodium – potassium dependant ATPase pump at the brush border membrane. These transporters are specific for acidic, basic or neutral amino acids. In addition to active transport, amino acids can also be transported by facilitated or simple diffusion when concentrations are high in the lumen. Di- and tripeptides that are absorbed are then hydrolyzed by peptidase in the cytoplasm of the enterocytes. The free amino acids are then transferred from the enterocyte across the basolateral membrane into the portal blood flow by facilitated and simple diffusion. The above processes are efficient as evidenced by the fact that approximately 6 to 12 grams of protein are secreted daily in the feces. Most of the protein is absorbed by the jejunum.

There are, of course, diseases that lead to protein malabsorption. Pancreatic insufficiency as with chronic pancreatitis, cystic fibrosis or pancreatic resection causes pancreatic enzyme deficiencies and protein maldigestion and malabsorption. Amino acid transport deficiencies such as Hartnup disease or cystinuria which affect the brush border transport system results in defective protein assimilation. Finally, diseases that cause loss of absorptive surface area including celiac disease, enteritis, tropical sprue, Crohn's disease or short bowel syndrome result in protein malabsorption. It has also been shown that patients with HIV – related conditions including cytomegalovirus enteritis, bacterial enteritis and Kaposis sarcoma have exhibited increased fecal protein excretion.

Fat absorption

Dietary fat is ingested in the form of triglycerides with three long chain fatty acids on a glycerol backbone. Hydrolysis of dietary fat begins in the stomach. Lingual lipase is activated at the gastric pH and liberalizes some of the fatty acids without requiring the activity of bile salts. The released fatty acids along with ingested proteins, aid in stimulating the release of cholecystokinin from the duodenal mucosa. The cholecystokinin then stimulates the release of pancreatic secretions and causes gallbladder contraction with relaxation of the sphincter of oddi which allows bile salt secretion. For the most part, triglyceride lipolysis occurs in the duodenum. It is in the duodenum that an emulsion is formed. An emulsion is a suspension of fat in water that allows a large surface area of dietary lipids to be exposed to lipase. The formation of the emulsion begins with the activity of lingual lipase and the liberalization of free fatty acids which facilitates the binding of colipase in the duodenum. Colipase is a low molecular weight protein that binds to bile salt–lipid surfaces and facilitates the interaction of pancreatic lipase with di- and triglycerides, thus permitting effective hydrolysis. Lastly, hydrogen ions in gastric acid cause secretin release which, along with cholecystokinin, stimulates pancreatic fluid and bicarbonate secretion. The bicarbonate and water present in pancreatic secretions also act to further emulsify the water-insoluble triglyceride and the increased pH in the duodenal lumen facilitates effective lipase activity. As will be discussed below (pp. 112–113), abnormalities in duodenal pH, cholecystokinin, pancreatic secretion, or loss of bile salts will all lead to some degree of lipid malabsorption.

Bile acids and phospholipids secreted by the liver in response to cholecystokinin combine with cholesterol, free fatty acids, and monoglycerides to form water soluble macromolecules called micelles. Absorption of fatty acids was once believed to be by passive diffusion. Recently, it has been discovered that a fatty acid transport protein called FATP4 is expressed at high levels on the apical side of the mature enterocytes in the small intestine. Once inside the enterocyte, fatty acids are transported into the smooth endoplasmic reticulum and triglycerides are resynthesized. The triglycerides, cholesterol esters, phospholipids, and apoproteins are packaged into a chylomicron which is then transported into the lymphatic system.

Absorption of lipids occurs in the proximal two thirds of the jejunum. The ileum does not participate in lipid absorption unless there is diseased jejunum. In this case, the ileum is capable of adapting to absorb fat in order to limit steatorrhea.

There are many steps that can malfunction during the process of lipid digestion and absorption and result in lipid malabsorption. First, there are many conditions associated with impaired lipolysis.

Zollinger–Ellison syndrome involves a gastrinoma or gastrin-secreting tumor which causes gastric-acid hypersecretion. The increased acid dramatically lowers the duodenal pH and inhibits the effectiveness of lipase, precipitates bile salts, and damages the jejunal mucosa leading to malabsorption and diarrhea. In addition, post-gastrectomy syndromes and post-vagotomy diarrhea can often result in rapid transit and fat malabsorption. There can also be decreased cholecystokinin release with severe intestinal mucosal destruction as with celiac sprue and regional enteritis. Pancreatic insufficiency leads to decreased secretion of lipase and subsequent maldigestion of ingested lipids. In addition, with pancreatic insufficiency, there is markedly decreased intestinal transit time causing the site of digestion and absorption to be the ileum as opposed to the duodenum and proximal jejunum resulting in malabsorption and diarrhea.

There are also conditions associated with impaired micelle formation. There can be decreased hepatic synthesis of bile salts as in severe liver disease, or decreased availability of bile salts in the intestinal lumen as with biliary obstruction or cholestasis. There can also be increased intestinal loss of bile salts as occurs with ileal disease or resection. This phenomenon is seen with Crohn's disease and in patients with AIDS.

Cobalamin absorption

The primary source of ingested cobalamin is foods that contain animal protein. Vitamin B_{12} is released from the food by gastric acid and pepsin. In the stomach, vitamin B_{12} combines with intrinsic factor which is manufactured and secreted by the gastric parietal cells. The vitamin B_{12}– intrinsic factor complex is then absorbed in the ileum. Vitamin B_{12} also binds to R-proteins in intestinal secretions the R-protein–B_{12} complex can not be absorbed by the ileum. The pancreatic proteases cleave this bond making B_{12} available to bind with intrinsic factor and enabling subsequent absorption.

Malabsorption of B_{12} occurs in a variety of conditions, pernicious anemia due to lack of intrinsic factor has recently been shown to constitute approximately 6% to 17% of cases of vitamin B_{12} malabsorption and deficiency. Pancreatic insufficiency can lead to vitamin B_{12} deficiency if the pancreatic enzymes are unavailable to cleave the R-protein–B_{12} bond. Vitamin B_{12} deficiency was also found to be common in patients with untreated celiac disease but it does resolve when patients comply with a gluten-free diet. In addition, it has been shown that malabsorption of vitamin B_{12} is highly prevalent in HIV-infected patients with chronic diarrhea and there is evidence that vitamin B_{12} deficiency becomes increasingly more common as the HIV disease progresses. It is also established that vitamin B_{12} malabsorption is more common in the elderly and in those with *Helicobacter pylori* infection. Atrophic gastritis leads to low serum vitamin B_{12} concentrations secondary to lack of intrinsic factor. Lastly, diseases that involve the terminal ileum, such as Crohn's disease, or resection of the terminal ileum, lead to vitamin B_{12} malabsorption. Bacterial overgrowth can also lead to cobalamin malabsorption and deficiency because the bacteria consume the dietary vitamin B_{12}.

Iron absorption

Iron is essential for multiple human metabolic processes including DNA synthesis and oxygen transport. The absorption of iron occurs in the proximal small intestine and must be tightly regulated as humans do not have a physiologic pathway for excretion of iron. Dietary iron is largely ingested in one of two forms; as either heme or ferric iron. Ferric iron must be solubilized and chelated to ferrous iron in the stomach at a pH above 3 to be available for absorption in the duodenum. In order for ferrous iron to remain in the reduced state it requires continuous chelation or reduction to prevent exposure to oxygen. The best known reducing agent in the diet is ascorbic acid. Ferrous iron is then transferred across the apical membrane of the enterocytes by the divalent metal transporter 1. In contrast, heme iron is freed from myoglobin and hemoglobin by pancreatic enzymes. It enters the intestinal absorptive cells as an intact metalloporphyrin and then is either stored as ferritin or transported across the basolateral membrane into the plasma. The mucosal uptake of iron is regulated by the concentration of iron in the absorptive cells. Inadequate absorption is a significant cause of iron deficiency. Etiologies of malabsorption of iron include poor bioavailability, loss or dysfunction of the absorptive enterocytes, short bowel syndrome, irritable bowel disease, and celiac disease. In addition, dietary intake of phytates, carbonates, phosphates, oxalates, and tannates causes ferric iron to precipitate and become unavailable for absorption. Likewise, achlorhydria can cause iron deficiency because ferric iron will not be solubilized and chelation can not occur. Lastly, the divalent metal transporter 1 is not specific to iron and also transports manganese, cobalt, copper, zinc, cadmium, and lead. Excess intake of these divalent cations can lead to decreased iron absorption.

Folate absorption

Humans cannot synthesize folate and therefore depend on dietary sources of this vitamin. Folate is ingested as polyglutamates and enters the small intestine unchanged. It is then hydrolyzed to monoglutamates by folate deconjugase at the brush border membrane. Folate is then avidly taken up by the enterocytes by a saturable folate transporter which is driven by a transmembrane pH gradient. Absorption can occur throughout the small intestine, although it is more efficient proximally. Diseases of the jejunal mucosa and drugs are the most common etiologies of folate malabsorption. Once again, celiac disease with disruption of the jejunal mucosa can lead to folate malabsorption. Alcohol also interferes with absorption of folate, transport to tissues, and storage and release by the liver.

Tests for malabsorption

The clinical manifestations of malabsorption are myriad. Global malabsorption usually presents with greasy, voluminous, foul-smelling stool in addition to weight loss in the absence of anorexia. The presentation of malabsorption can also be more subtle and present with only anemia, as with vitamin B_{12} or folate malabsorption. With carbohydrate malabsorption, patients usually will have watery diarrhea and flatulence. After taking a thorough history, performing a complete physical examination, and carrying out routine blood tests, the next step is usually to pursue an anatomic investigation. If imaging or endoscopy is unrevealing, or if the history points to a specific type of malabsorption, dedicated tests can be performed. Gold standards to diagnose specific etiologies of malabsorption have been established although novel tests are continually being devised to further facilitate an accurate diagnosis.

Anatomic investigations

The search for the cause of malabsorptive symptoms often begins with imaging studies such as barium studies or endoscopy. The initial test often performed is an upper gastrointestinal series with a small-bowel follow through or an enteroclysis. Enteroclysis is a double contrast study in which a tube is passed into the small bowel, and barium and methylcellulose are injected. The findings of malabsorption on small-bowel follow through are nonspecific and consist of flocculation and segmentation of barium, thickening of mucosal folds, and dilatation of intestinal loops. In celiac disease, the diagnosis can usually be reliably made with jejunal biopsy but enteroclysis can be helpful in differentiating celiac disease from other conditions with similar histology. In celiac disease, enteroclysis often demonstrates a reversal of the jejunal and ileal folds with an increased amount of ileal folds and a decreased amount of jejunal folds. Enteroclysis can also help identify malignant complications of celiac disease and can be helpful in those with an atypical presentation. In diagnosing bacterial overgrowth, enteroclysis can demonstrate anatomic abnormalities that predispose to bacterial overgrowth, such as blind loops and jejunal diverticulosis. A micronodular mucosal pattern can be observed in diffuse disorders such as Whipple's disease, amyloidosis and lymphangiectasia.

In chronic pancreatitis, MRI and CT scan are effective diagnostic methods used for imaging inflammatory and neoplastic pancreatic disease. Endoscopic ultrasound is also an acceptable means for diagnosing chronic pancreatitis and is recommended as an adjunct to endoscopic retrograde pancreatography or CT scan. Although these imaging studies are reliable ways to diagnose chronic pancreatitis, they will not necessarily provide information as to the functional capacity of the pancreas or degree of malabsorption.

Endoscopy

Malabsorption due to small-bowel disease commonly involves the duodenum. The use of upper endoscopy with duodenal biopsies can provide vital information to help elucidate the etiology of malabsorption. In celiac disease, the endoscopic markers are scalloped folds, mosaic pattern of the mucosa, decreased number of duodenal folds, and visible underlying blood vessels. These findings have a sensitivity of 94% and specificity of 92% and positive predictive value of 84% in diagnosing celiac disease. Use of magnification endoscopy with dye spraying can also be helpful in diagnosing celiac disease especially in patients with partial or patchy villous atrophy as the duodenum may appear normal in these patients. This procedure, using indigo carmine dye, has a sensitivity of 94% and a specificity of 88% in identifying patients with villous atrophy. In Crohn's disease, one would expect to see scalloping of the mucosa on standard endoscopy, thus reinforcing the concept that these endoscopic findings are not specific for diagnosing celiac sprue.

The small-bowel biopsy is a safe procedure and often paramount to establishing the diagnosis. The biopsy can be obtained by passing forceps through the gastroscope or enteroscope. The biopsies should be taken distal to the ampulla of Vater in order to increase the diagnostic yield. At least four random biopsies should be taken. The classic histologic appearance of the mucosa in a patient with untreated celiac disease is villous atrophy and crypt hyperplasia.

In chronic pancreatitis, the gold standard imaging procedure is endoscopic retrograde cholangiopancreatography. This can identify pancreatic ductal changes as mild, moderate, or severe although the changes in the appearance of the ducts may not fully correlate with the degree of pancreatic functional impairment.

Tests for carbohydrate malabsorption

Carbohydrate malabsorption is usually due to enzyme defects such as lactase deficiency or global malabsorption. The tests for carbohydrate malabsorption rely on fermentation of carbohydrates by bacteria or measurement of specific nutrients after ingestion of a test dose.

Lactose tolerance test

There are two forms of the lactose tolerance test. First, the serum test consists of an oral test dose of 50 grams of lactose with subsequent measurements of blood glucose levels at 0, 60, and 120 minutes. An increase of blood glucose less than 20 mg/dL and development of symptoms (e.g. diarrhea, abdominal cramping, flatulence) is diagnostic of lactose intolerance. Second, it is also possible to measure breath hydrogen following a lactose challenge. This test relies on colonic bacterial fermentation of malabsorbed lactose. An increase in breath hydrogen of more than 20 ppm is diagnostic of lactose intolerance. This has been considered the most reliable, non-invasive, and economical technique to make the diagnosis. Studies have shown that simply looking at hydrogen values at 0 and 120 minutes after the lactose challenge is sufficient to determine lactose malabsorption. Other investigators have noted that gastrointestinal symptoms after a lactose challenge are more strongly associated with hydrogen excretion than with glucose concentration. False positive results occur with the breath hydrogen test when patients have bacterial overgrowth. The other problem that occurs with the execution of this diagnostic test is that it can be fundamentally difficult to perform.

D-xylose

The D-xylose test measures the absorptive capacity of the small intestine. D-xylose is a pentose found in plants that is absorbed unchanged from the small intestine. The liver metabolizes 30% of ingested D-xylose to carbon dioxide and threitol, 5% is excreted in bile and undergoes enterohepatic cycling, the rest is excreted in the urine. Given the reliability of the metabolism of D-xylose, it is an ideal compound to use to assess intestinal malabsorption, specifically carbohydrate malabsorption.

The standard D-xylose test requires that the patient fasts overnight. The patient should fast because in addition to passive absorption, there is facilitated absorption of D-xylose which may be hindered with the ingestion of meat or fiber. Antimotility and promotility agents should also be avoided prior to the test. The patient ingests 25 grams of D-xylose, the urine is then collected for the next 5 hours and a serum sample is drawn at 1 hour post-ingestion. A urine excretion of less than 6 grams, or a serum concentration of less than 20 mg/dL is considered to indicate abnormal absorption.

There have been some attempts to investigate variations on the standard D-xylose test. One study attempted to improve the accuracy of the D-xylose test by combining a 1-hour and a 3-hour serum D-xylose level. They found the 1-hour D-xylose concentration of less than 20 mg/dL to have a sensitivity of 71% and specificity of 100%, but when a 3-hour D-xylose serum level of less than 22.5 mg/dL was measured instead of the 5-hour level, the sensitivity improved to 90% with a specificity of 95%.

Some researchers have determined that the 5-hour urine collection more accurately reflects the extent of intestinal malabsorption as opposed to the 1-hour serum value. However, the amount of D-xylose in the urine depends on renal function and is therefore difficult to interpret in the setting of renal insufficiency. The urine measurement is also prone to false positive results in the elderly who can also have depressed urinary values because of a decreased glomerular filtration rate. In addition, urine can also be difficult to collect, for example with children. False positive results can also occur with decreased gastric emptying, ascites, urinary retention, dehydration, and bacterial overgrowth. Drugs, such as non-steroidal anti-inflammatory agents and glipizide, can also interfere with the urinary excretion of D-xylose. Of note, the D-xylose test should be normal in those with pancreatic insufficiency as there is no loss of small intestine absorptive capacity in this disease.

The D-xylose breath test

The principle on which this test was based is that when a carbohydrate load is given to a patient with small-intestine malabsorption, it will reach the colon and be metabolized by colonic bacteria which in turn will produce excessive amounts of breath hydrogen. Alveolar breath samples can then be measured for hydrogen in 30-minute intervals for the 5 hours after ingestion of 25 grams of D-xylose. The hydrogen breath test with D-xylose has been shown to be as valid as the traditional urine test. In fact, some have reported that it may identify patients who would otherwise have a false negative result with the urine test. In addition, investigators have found that the D-xylose breath test can be used, not only for the diagnosis of malabsorption, but also for follow-up of diseases such as celiac disease once treatment is ongoing. Finally, it also appears that the D-xylose breath test is an accurate way to diagnose small-intestinal malabsorption in the elderly.

Tests for fat malabsorption

Fecal-fat determination

Fecal-fat determination is the gold standard for the diagnosis of steatorrhea. The normal daily fecal-fat excretion is 6 g/day and usually more than 7 to 10 g/day of stool fat is considered to be abnormal. For best determination of the degree of steatorrhea, patients must consume 70 to 100 grams of fat per day and stool should be collected for 3 days (72 hours). A stool weight can also aide diagnosis with a stool output of more than 200 g/day indicating diarrhea. Once the stool is collected the percentage fat absorbed, i.e. the ratio of fat intake to fat output, can be determined; more than 94% fat absorption is considered normal. Patients should also avoid fat substitutes, such as olestra or the ingestion of mineral oil, as they have been shown to cause false positive results in fecal-fat estimation. In addition, medications that cause fat malabsorption such as orlistat should be avoided for the same reason. Studies have also shown that diarrhea itself increases fecal fat and mild abnormalities (up to 14 g/day) are not specific for a primary defect in fat digestion or absorption. Despite the fact that there have been multiple other tests designed to estimate the degree of fat malabsorption, the 72-hour stool collection and measurement of fecal fat remains the gold standard.

Sudan stain

The sudan stain test is based on the affinity of the stain for triglycerides. This test for fecal fat lacks specificity and is a qualitative, as opposed to quantitative, assessment of fat malabsorption. It appears that fecal-fat sudan microscopy, which involves a dedicated approach to counting and measuring the maximal diameter of fat globules, may offer increased sensitivity with similar specificity to the traditional method of fecal-fat collection and analysis.

The acid steatocrit

The acid steatocrit is another method used to quantitatively assess the presence and degree of steatorrhea. It can be done on random stools and studies have shown it to be highly sensitive and specific in the detection of steatorrhea. It can estimate the quantitative fecal fat with a positive predictive value of 90%. This method uses a small amount of stool that is microcentrifuged and the ratio of the fat and the solid layer is then determined. Multiple studies, done mostly on children, have confirmed the sensitivity and specificity of this test and have also demonstrated that the steatocrit is a simple test to use to follow response to therapy.

^{14}C-triolein breath test

The ^{14}C-triolein breath test requires the ingestion of radiolabeled triglyceride triolein which is then hydrolyzed with the subsequent release of carbon dioxide. The measurement of breath carbon dioxide correlates with fat absorption. Although this test and the similar ^{13}C-triglyceride breath test are reported to have a high sensitivity and specificity and are practical in the elderly, there are some inherent limitations to these studies. First, the study takes 6 hours to perform and requires the administration of radioisotopes and laboratory tests for determination are not readily available and are expensive. Second, although this study is meant to be a measurement of fat absorption, fatty acid oxidation is altered in some disease states including diabetes mellitus, thyroid disease, obesity, and fever. Any of these conditions may lead to an unreliable test result. In addition, diseases such as pulmonary disease that manifests as carbon dioxide retention can lead to measurement inaccuracies. Finally, when compared to the fecal-fat excretion, the ^{14}C-triolein breath test had low specificity in patients with chronic liver disease.

Near infrared reflectance analysis

Near infrared reflectance analysis has been shown to be a sensitive and specific method to evaluate the amount of fat in feces. It appears to be as accurate and less cumbersome than fecal-fat collection. It also allows for simultaneous measurement of fecal protein and carbohydrates. This method is not widely available in the US at present and therefore the 72-hour fecal-fat collection remains the gold standard.

Tests for protein malabsorption

Tests for protein malabsorption are inherently difficult to perform because they require balance studies. They are also hard to interpret as protein malabsorption and hypoproteinemia may commonly occur secondary to a protein-losing enteropathy or bacterial overgrowth. Most of the techniques used to evaluate protein malabsorption are restricted to research. Enteral protein loss can be evaluated by fecal alpha-1-antitrypsin clearance. Studies have shown that in celiac disease, there is a significant relationship between alpha-1-antitrypsin clearance and the degree of alteration of jejunal histologic structure and activity of disease. The alpha-1-antitrypsin clearance may also be a reliable method for following response to treatment in celiac disease as well. There are also a variety of HIV-related conditions such as cytomegalovirus infection, bacterial enteritis, and Kaposi's sarcoma that have increased protein excretion as measured by fecal alpha-1-antitrypsin levels. Alpha-1-antitrypsin in the stool can be measured by either nephelometry or radial immunodiffusion. Fecal nitrogen can also be directly measured in the stool by near infrared spectroscopy. Lastly, studies have also demonstrated that post-absorptive citrulline concentration is a marker of functional absorptive capacity in short-bowel syndrome.

Schilling test

The Schilling test identifies the cause of vitamin B_{12} malabsorption. As previously discussed, vitamin B_{12} requires intrinsic factor secreted by the gastric parietal cells and is then absorbed by the terminal ileum. There are two parts of the Schilling test. Stage one involves the ingestion of radiolabeled cobalamin and then during a subsequent 24-hour urine collection, the percentage of radiolabeled cobalamin is measured. If the result of stage one is abnormal, the second stage is performed 3 to 7 days later. At this point, the patient ingests labeled cobalamin and intrinsic factor. In patients with vitamin B_{12} deficiency and normal stage one of the Schilling test, the deficiency is likely to be secondary to dietary deficiency, hypochlorhydria, or gastrectomy. If stage one is abnormal and stage 2 is normal, the differential diagnosis includes pernicious anemia, absence of intrinsic factor, gastrectomy, or gastric bypass. Both stages are abnormal in the presence of ileal disease, renal insufficiency, bacterial overgrowth, or pancreatic insufficiency. It is actually a rare instance that requires the Schilling test to identify the cause of vitamin B_{12} deficiency. Often the result of the Schilling test does not alter clinical management and the patient will be receiving vitamin B_{12} supplementation regardless of the result.

Tests for bacterial overgrowth

A quantitative bacterial count and/or a culture of an intestinal aspirate are the gold standard for diagnosis of bacterial overgrowth. Normal counts are less than 10^4/mL in the jejunum and less than 10^5/mL in the ileum. This is a technically difficult and invasive test. Several indirect measurements have been proposed including hydrogen breath tests after the ingestion of glucose or lactulose. These tests have a reported sensitivity of 60% to 95% and a specificity of approximately 90%. Nevertheless, there is no single ideal test for the diagnosis.

Tests for pancreatic exocrine function

Pancreatic disease is usually evident on imaging studies such as abdominal plain films, CT scans, endoscopic retrograde cholangiopancreatography and abdominal ultrasound. In diagnosing exocrine pancreatic insufficiency, the gold standard is a quantitative pancreatic stimulation test. This requires intubation and stimulation of pancreatic secretion with secretogogues such as a Lundh test meal (standardized composition of nutrients), secretin, and pancreozymin (cholecystokinin). The duodenal contents are then collected and analyzed. This test is invasive, technically difficult, and expensive and rarely done in clinical practice but instead is limited to research centers.

The secretin stimulation test is based on the principle that secretin will cause secretion of amylase and bicarbonate from the pancreas. The patient swallows a catheter and secretin is administered, the duodenal contents are then sampled via the catheter. Pancreatic exocrine insufficiency is diagnosed if the bicarbonate concentration is less than 80 mEq/L or there is decreased amylase output.

There are also multiple non-invasive tests that have been developed to evaluate pancreatic exocrine function. First, the pancreolauryl test in which fluorescein dilaurate is administered and fluorescein is then released by the pancreatic esterases. Fluorescein is conjugated by the liver and excreted in the urine where it can be measured. The sensitivity of this test was found to be 90% and the specificity is 97.6%. The bentiromide test is similar to the pancreolauryl test using a different substrate. N-benzoyl-L-tyrosyl-p-aminobenzoic acid is cleaved by chymotrypsin to p-aminobenzoic acid which can also be measured in the urine. For both of these tests, liver disease, renal insufficiency, and intestinal malabsorption can lead to false positive results. Both tests are of limited usefulness in mild to moderate pancreatic insufficiency and require a specialized laboratory. Fecal chymotrypsin has been used as a marker of pancreatic exocrine function. It has a lower sensitivity than the pancreolauryl or bentiromide tests in diagnosing mild to moderate insufficiency and only appears useful in diagnosing advanced disease. Finally, fecal elastase measurement has been shown to be more sensitive and specific than fecal chymotrypsin in diagnosing pancreatic insufficiency. It appears that this test is the most sensitive and specific early in the course of pancreatic insufficiency and can be performed despite pancreatic replacement therapy. In a study comparing fecal elastase to the secretin–caurulein test (used as the gold standard), fecal elastase was found to have a sensitivity and specificity of 93%.

Tests for bile-acid malabsorption

Bile-salt malabsorption has been shown to occur with either resection of the terminal ileum or diseases of the terminal ileum such as Crohn's disease and HIV infection. As many as one third of patients with diarrhea of unknown origin are thought to have bile-acid malabsorption,

The usual course of treatment in patients with suspected bile-acid malabsorption is a trial of cholestyramine therapy. If this therapy is unsuccessful, it is often necessary to further investigate the etiology of the diarrhea. There are two tests that have shown merit in detecting bile-acid malabsorption. First, the measurement of ^{99m}technetium labeled selenium-75-homocholic acid taurine (^{75}SeHCAT) which is a synthetic analog of the conjugated bile acid taurine. It is ingested and the disappearance of the radioactivity is measured. It has proved useful in differentiating bile-acid malabsorption from other causes of diarrhea in patients with HIV-related diarrhea and Crohn's disease. It has also proved useful in following therapy in these diseases. Nevertheless, there are some drawbacks to this diagnostic test. First, the use of radioactivity with a long half life (180 days) limits its use and the results may be affected by liver disease.

In an attempt to devise a diagnostic tool that does not employ radioactivity, a test measuring serum 7 alpha-hydroxy-4-cholesten-3-one (HCO) was devised. Bile acids returning from the intestine to the liver inhibit their own synthesis, HCO is a marker of hepatic cholesterol 7α-hydroxylase activity which has increased activity with impaired bile-acid absorption. It was found to correlate well with the ^{75}SeHCAT test and has a sensitivity of 90% and a specificity of 79% when compared to the ^{75}SeHCAT test.

Evaluation of the patient with suspected malabsorption

In attempting to evaluate the patient with suspected malabsorption the first step, and often the key to diagnosis, is an exhaustive history and a complete physical examination. When taking the patient's history, the interviewer should be mindful to ask about family history. Inflammatory bowel disease, celiac disease, and cystic fibrosis are just a few of the genetic diseases that can manifest as malabsorption. It is important to ask about autoimmune diseases and weight loss especially unintentional weight loss. A history of recurrent peptic ulcer disease can be a clue to the diagnosis of Zollinger–Ellison syndrome. Since Zollinger–Ellison syndrome can also be part of the multiple endocrine neoplasia type 1 syndrome a careful history, including a serum calcium level and family history, is important. A history of anemia can also be helpful as iron deficiency anemia is now the most common presentation of celiac disease in adults. Anemia can also lead to the diagnosis of vitamin B_{12}, folate, or iron malabsorption. Neurologic findings such as ataxia and dementia will often differentiate vitamin B_{12} deficiency causing macrocytic anemia from folate deficiency. It takes 10 to 20 years for pancreatic insufficiency to develop in alcoholics and therefore a detailed history of substance abuse is obviously necessary. The interviewer must also ask about abdominal surgery as this may lead to the diagnosis of bacterial overgrowth, bile-acid malabsorption, blind loop syndrome, short-bowel syndrome or dumping syndrome. Lastly, a history of radiation, specifically to the pelvis in the setting of bloody diarrhea, may be a clue to radiation enteritis or radiation colitis.

When asking about a patient's symptoms, the appearance of the stool is critical. Steatorrhea usually presents with greasy, foul-smelling, voluminous stools although this classic presentation is also uncommon. Carbohydrate malabsorption usually presents with watery stools, flatulence, and abdominal distension. These symptoms usually occur within 60 to 90 minutes of carbohydrate ingestion. The presence or absence of abdominal pain can also be a clue to etiology as most of the causes of malabsorption do not present with abdominal pain except for pancreatitis and Crohn's disease. Intestinal ischemia can also lead to severe abdominal pain usually occurring in the immediate post-prandial period. It is important to remember that the symptoms of malabsorption may be extremely subtle and may present only with weakness secondary to anemia. Thus, it is clear that an accurate and thorough medical history is imperative to discovering the diagnosis.

The physical examination

Table 6.1 lists the signs and symptoms of malabsorption of selected nutrients and Table 6.2 lists the features of common diseases that present with malabsorption. Malabsorption again may be as subtle

Table 6.1 Signs and symptoms of malabsorption.

Nutrient	Clinical features	Laboratory findings
Fat	Greasy, foul-smelling, voluminous stool, steatorrhea.	6 g/day of stool fat.
Carbohydrates	Flatulence, abdominal distension, watery diarrhea.	Increased breath hydrogen. Possible abnormal lactose tolerance test. Increased stool osmotic gap.
Protein	Edema, amenorrhea.	Hypoalbuminemia. Hypoproteinemia.
Vitamin B_{12}	Anemia, peripheral neuropathy, impairment of posterior columns, dementia, neuropsychiatric changes.	Macrocytic anemia. Macro-ovalocytes and hypersegmented neutrophils on peripheral smear. Decreased serum vitamin B_{12} level. Abnormal Schilling test.
Folate	Anemia, *no* neurologic findings.	Macrocytic anemia. Normal vitamin B_{12} levels. Decreased folate levels in serum or red blood cells. Macro-ovalocytes and hypersegmented neutrophils on peripheral smear.
Iron	Anemia with tachycardia, fatigue, tachypnea on exertion, glossitis, cheilosis, brittle nails.	Iron deficiency anemia. Decreased serum iron. Decreased serum ferritin. Increased total iron-binding capacity.
Calcium/Vitamin D	Tetany, positive Chvostek and Trousseau's signs, pathologic fractures, osteomalacia.	Hypocalcemia. Decreased vitamin D levels. Increased serum alkaline phosphatase.
Vitamin K	Hematomas, increased bleeding.	Decreased vitamin K-dependent clotting factors. Increased prothrombin time. Rapid correction with vitamin K replacement.

Table 6.2 Presentation of common diseases causing malabsorption.

Disease	Common clinical features	Laboratory findings
Celiac disease in children	Impaired growth, diarrhea, abdominal, distension, short stature, pubertal delay, iron/folate deficiency with anemia, rickets, apthous stomatitis, arthralgias, behavioural disturbances.	Antiendomysial antibodies. Immunoglobulin A and immunoglobulin G antigliadin antibodies. Iron deficiency. Hypocalcemia. Decreased vitamin D. Abnormal small-bowel biopsy with loss of villi and hypertrophic crypts.
Celiac disease in adults	Iron deficiency anemia, macrocytic anemia, diarrhea, flatulence, weight loss, lactose intolerance, abdominal discomfort/bloating, apthous stomatitis, vitamin D deficiency with decreased serum calcium, vitamin K deficiency, bone fractures, infertility, peripheral neuropathy, ataxia, seizures.	Same as above.
Chronic pancreatitis	Abdominal pain radiating to mid-back and scapula, nausea and vomiting associated with abdominal pain, diabetes, jaundice, weight loss, diarrhea.	Increased amylase and lipase. Increased fecal fat excretion. Increased total bilirubin and alkaline phosphatase with compression of bile duct with edema or fibrosis of the pancreas.
Crohn's disease	Abdominal mass, abdominal pain, usually right lower quadrant, fever, weight loss, non-bloody intermittent diarrhea, fistulas, perianal disease, oral apthous ulcers, nephrolithiasis, cholecystitis.	Laboratory findings are non-specific including increased erythrocyte sedimentation rate, C-reactive protein, white blood cell count. Strictures, fistulas, ulcerations on upper gastrointestinal series with small-bowel follow-through. Apthous ulcers, strictures, segmental involvement on colonoscopy
Lactose intolerance	Bloating, abdominal cramps, flatulence, osmotic diarrhea with large lactose ingestion.	Stool osmotic gap/stool pH < 6.0. Abnormal breath hydrogen test.
Zollinger-Ellison syndrome	Recurrent peptic ulcer disease, esophagitis, diarrhea, weight loss, liver metastasis.	Increased fasting serum gastrin. Abnormal secretin stimulation of gastrin secretion.
Bacterial overgrowth	Can be asymptomatic, distension, weight loss, steatorrhea, watery diarrhea, macrocytic anemia due to vitamin B_{12} deficiency.	Abnormal fecal-fat excretion. Abnormal D-xylose test.
Whipple's disease	Arthralgias or migratory arthritis, abdominal pain, diarrhea, distension, flatulence, steatorrhea, weight loss, myocardial/valvular abnormalities, ocular findings, fever, lymphadenopathy.	Duodenal biopsy revealing PAS-positive macrophages containing gram negative bacilli and dilation of the lacteals.

as with celiac disease and present only with anemia. The physical examination should focus on the general appearance and overall nourishment of the patient. The neurologic, abdominal, and skin examinations will often yield important insight as to the cause of malabsorptive symptoms. In addition, information obtained with the history taking should also guide a focused physical examination.

If a patient describes diarrhea consistent with steatorrhea without abdominal pain, a diagnosis of celiac disease, Whipple's disease, or pancreatic insufficiency should be considered. Patients who complain primarily of flatulence, abdominal distension, and watery diarrhea may have lactose intolerance or other less common disaccharidase deficiencies. If the presenting symptoms are consistent with anemia with tachypnea on exertion, tachycardia, and fatigue, this may be due to celiac disease but a peripheral blood smear as well as iron studies will help sort out whether the anemia is secondary to iron, folate, or vitamin B_{12} deficiency.

Neurologic manifestations such as dementia, impaired proprioception, and neuropsychiatric symptoms are all consistent with a diagnosis of vitamin B_{12} deficiency whereas tetany is associated with hypocalcemia. When investigating neurologic symptoms, it is has been noted that some cases of Whipple's disease also have central nervous system involvement and may occur without intestinal involvement. Peripheral neuropathy, ataxia, and seizures have all been associated with celiac disease. Skin manifestations such as dermatitis herpetiformis occurs in patients with celiac disease. Erythema nodosum, pyoderma gangrenosum, episcleritis, perianal disease, and apthous ulcers are all prevalent with Crohn's disease. Bruising, easy bleeding, and hematomas should cause concern for vitamin K deficiency which can occur in any disease with malabsorption of fat and fat soluble vitamins such as celiac disease. Arthralgias and arthritis may be apparent with Crohn's disease and Whipple's disease whereas osteomalacia or osteoporosis is seen in hypocalcemia and protein malabsorption. Ocular findings also occur with Whipple's disease and Crohn's disease.

Laboratory investigation

The etiology of the malabsorption may be evident after taking a thorough history and performing a complete physical examination. A laboratory investigation remains essential not only to make an accurate diagnosis but also to evaluate for possible complications of malabsorption.

Hematologic workup

As previously stated, it is common for the presentation of malabsorption to be subtle and present only with anemia. A complete blood count should be obtained on any patient with suspected malabsorption. If anemia is present, a peripheral smear should be examined. Hypersegmented neutrophils and macro-ovalocytes are consistent with both vitamin B_{12} and folate deficiencies and serum levels of both should be drawn. Vitamin B_{12} deficiency can be seen with decreased absorption as with blind loop syndrome, bacterial overgrowth, and surgical resection of the ileum or ileal Crohn's disease. It can also be seen with decreased production of intrinsic factor as with gastrectomy or pernicious anemia. Decreased absorption of folate occurs with celiac disease as well as with certain drugs such as phenytoin, sulfasalazine, and trimethoprim-sulfamethoxazole. If both vitamin B_{12} and folate are decreased, the diagnosis of protein-losing enteropathy should be considered and if vitamin B_{12} is decreased but folate is increased, bacterial overgrowth is more likely.

Microcytosis and hypochromatic red blood cells are consistent with iron deficiency anemia or anemia of chronic disease. Iron deficiency can be caused by blood loss, as with Crohn's disease, or decreased absorption as is seen with gastric surgery or celiac disease. At this point, it is prudent to check ferritin, total iron binding capacity and serum iron levels.

Leukocytosis is a non-specific finding but can be seen in Crohn's disease, an acute bout of pancreatitis or Whipple's disease. A depressed white blood cell count should bring to mind the possible diagnosis of HIV and HIV-associated causes of malabsorption. In addition, lymphocytopenia with decreased serum cholesterol and decreased gamma globulins may be secondary to lymphatic obstruction leading to a protein-losing enteropathy.

Serum biochemical analysis

In addition to the usual set of chemistries, zinc, magnesium, calcium, albumin, alkaline phosphatase, and a prothrombin time should be drawn in any patient with suspected malabsorption. Severe diarrhea may result in a non-anion gap metabolic acidosis and hypokalemia. With severely depressed albumin (less than 2.5 g/dL) in the absence of nephrotic syndrome or hepatic disease, the diagnosis of protein-losing enteropathy must be entertained and it is prudent to pursue a fecal alpha-1-antitrypsin level . The different causes of protein-losing enteropathy are multiple. Causes include damage to the gut mucosa as with lymphoma, gastric carcinoma, chronic gastric ulcer, or inflammatory bowel disease. Lymphatic obstruction secondary to infections such as tuberculosis, Whipple's disease, sarcoidosis, neoplasms, cardiac disease, or primary intestinal lymphangectasia will also cause a protein-losing enteropathy. Finally, an idiopathic transudation is also possible with Zollinger–Ellison syndrome, amyloidosis, combined variable immunodeficiency, systemic lupus erythematosis, eosinophilic gastroenteritis, celiac disease, or allergic protein-losing enteropathy. Laboratory work-up of protein-losing enteropathy includes serum protein electrophoresis, antinuclear antibody, C3, lymphocyte count as well as serologic tests if a particular diagnosis appears likely.

It is important to obtain a calcium level along with an alkaline phosphatase level to check for osteomalacia, although this has a poor negative predictive value. One should be suspicious of osteomalacia with a patient who complains of bone pain and tenderness and proximal muscle weakness especially the pelvic girdle muscles. The causes of osteomalacia may be due to calcium deficiency but also may be secondary to malabsorption of vitamin D or phosphorus. The correct diagnosis will also guide the appropriate therapy.

Serologic evaluation

Serologic tests have proved important screening tools as well as effective means for following therapy for certain diseases. Positive antinuclear antibody is seen in celiac disease as well as autoimmune enteropathy. More importantly, when entertaining the diagnosis of celiac disease, antigliadin IgA has a specificity of 67% to 100% and a sensitivity of 89% to 100% whereas antigliadin IgG has a specificity of 47% to 70% and a sensitivity of 89% to 100%. Immunoglobulin A is also a convenient tool to monitor compliance; the IgA levels decrease after 1 to 3 months of a gluten-free diet and levels are undetectable by 6 to 12 months. This pattern is not seen with the IgG antibody levels. A more sensitive serologic test for celiac disease is an antiendomysial antibody level. This test has a sensitivity and correlation with villous atrophy in untreated patients of 100%. When investigating patients with partial as opposed to global villous atrophy, the sensitivity of antiendomysial antibody drops as low as 31%. When combined with IgA antigliadin levels, the sensitivity rises to 76%. Therefore, if the serology is negative but suspicion remains high for celiac disease, jejunal tissue should be obtained with pursuit of a histologic diagnosis.

Erythrocyte sedimentation rate and C reactive protein are non-specific markers of inflammation but are valuable for follow-up and response to treatment in Crohn's disease.

It is also prudent to check an HIV antibody level in patients with unexplained malabsorption, especially if they are at high risk of infection, have lymphopenia or a decreased CD4 count. Lastly, in patients with diarrhea secondary to chronic infections such as giardia, a quantitative immunoglobulin screen may reveal an immunodeficiency syndrome such as common variable immunodeficiency or selective IgA deficiency.

Stool examination

The stool examination is invaluable when investigating the etiology of malabsorption. The first step is often an examination for fecal fat. The fecal sudan stain will provide a qualitative examination for fat while the stool collection is underway for the quantitative evaluation of fecal-fat excretion. If the fecal-fat excretion is abnormal, the differential diagnosis includes Whipple's disease, celiac disease, bile-salt malabsorption, pancreatic insufficiency, and bacterial overgrowth. If the fecal fat is normal, then a diagnosis of protein malabsorption can be evaluated with a fecal alpha-1-antitrypsin level and an investigation of the small intestine. In addition, with a normal fecal fat, a diagnosis of carbohydrate malabsorption should also be considered. If an infectious cause is suspected, the stool should also be sent for routine culture as well as culture for ova and parasites.

Anatomic analysis

If the stool examination is suspicious for pancreatic insufficiency, pancreatic function tests can then be performed along with an anatomic investigation including a possible endoscopic retrograde cholangiopancreatography or endoscopic ultrasound in addition to abdominal CT or ultrasound. Patients may simply have chronic pancreatitis leading to pancreatic exocrine insufficiency but it is important to identify those with symptoms suggestive of chronic pancreatitis that is masking pancreatic cancer. When patients have evidence of chronic inflammatory diarrhea with white blood cells or blood in the stools, they may have irritable bowel disease or infectious diarrhea and an evaluation should start with stool studies and a search for structural abnormalities by sigmoidoscopy or colonoscopy in addition to small-bowel radiographs. A small-bowel biopsy is also helpful in diagnosing or confirming the diagnosis of diseases such as celiac disease, Whipple's disease, lymphangectasia, and amyloidosis. Giardia and cryptosporidiosis can also be diagnosed by small-bowel biopsy which would clearly be helpful in directing treatment in a patient with HIV-associated malabsorption.

Malabsorption in special circumstances

Malabsorption in AIDS

Multiple infectious causes of diarrhea have been associated with HIV and AIDS. Opportunistic infections include cytomegalovirus, *Mycobacterium avium-intracellulare*, Kaposi's sarcoma, and herpes simplex virus proctitis. Other potential pathogens include *Giardia*, *Campylobacter*, *Salmonella*, *Cryptosporidium*, and *Microsporidium*. Studies have also found that patients with HIV-associated chronic diarrhea have abnormal parameters of absorption and malnutrition and that malabsorption is likely to be a large contributor to the AID wasting syndrome. They also observed that those with diarrhea-associated microsporidia demonstrated more severe malabsorption. There is no known optimal diagnostic investigation. Up to 83% of patients with AIDS have at least one gut pathogen. The pathogen can usually be identified by stool analysis and light-microscopy evaluation of duodenal and rectal biopsies. Some experts believe that some pathogens will be missed unless all of these investigations are done on all such patients. Finally, malabsorption has also been known to occur in the absence of infectious causes. One study found that up to 50% of patients with HIV have qualitative fecal-fat studies consistent with steatorrhea and the authors felt that the primary defect in these patients is a primary defect in fat malabsorption independent of detectable pathogens.

Malabsorption in the elderly

There is actually little clinical evidence of digestive problems due purely to age, and also malabsorption is not a common finding in the elderly. Any disease that causes malabsorption in the young can occur in the elderly, although older individuals may have more subtle signs and symptoms. The populations most at risk for complications of diarrhea or malabsorption are those at the extremes of age. Some common causes of malabsorption in the elderly include celiac disease, pancreatic disease, diarrhea due to gastrectomy, and bacterial overgrowth due to hypochlorhydria or altered intestinal motility. A common infectious cause of diarrhea and malabsorption in the elderly is *Clostridium difficile* most often seen in the setting of antibiotics. Most patients will not complain of overt symptoms of malabsorption and instead may present with vitamin B_{12} deficiency, decreased serum folate, a decreased prothrombin time, osteopenia, or non-specific gastrointestinal symptoms. Therefore, there needs to be a high index of suspicion for malabsorption when evaluating an elderly patient with non-specific symptoms of gastrointestinal disease.

Management of the patient with malabsorption

Prior to a brief discussion of the treatment of specific diseases associated with malabsorption, a few basic principles of the management of malabsorption will be discussed. Treatment of malabsorption requires not only the treatment of the underlying disorder but management of the macro- and micronutrient deficiencies that accompany the disorder. In patients with steatorrhea, a low-fat high-protein diet that contains adequate calories is recommended to maintain nutritional status. Medium chain triglycerides do not require lipase for hydrolysis, or micelle formation for absorption and can be used as fat substitutes. In addition, in all patients with steatorrhea, vitamin and mineral deficiencies such as fat soluble vitamins, vitamin B_{12}, calcium, folate, and zinc are common and should be actively sought and corrected.

In patients with celiac disease, treatment of the underlying disorder requires total elimination of wheat, rye, and barley from the diet. Patients with celiac disease and dermatitis herpetiformis require a gluten-free diet permanently. Steroids are rarely needed in the treatment of celiac disease. Seventy percent of patients with celiac disease have an improvement within 2 weeks of starting the gluten-free diet. Patients must also avoid lactose initially as some patients with untreated celiac disease have secondary lactose deficiency. In addition, patients often need to avoid oats initially as they may have been contaminated by small amounts of wheat during processing. Patients with malabsorption should also receive a multivitamin, iron, and folate supplement. If they have hypocalcemia and osteopenia, calcium and vitamin D supplements should be started as well. In celiac disease, vitamin B_{12} levels usually normalize on a gluten-free diet alone although symptomatic patients may need supplementation .

In patients with chronic pancreatitis, steatorrhea and diabetes are the dominant symptoms. If a patient exhibits malabsorption, it is likely that more than 90% of the exocrine pancreatic function is lost. Pancreatic enzyme replacement therapy before meals is the primary treatment for pancreatic steatorrhea. A low-fat diet and medium chain triglycerides may be used because they minimize the need for enzymes. Acid suppressants or enteric coating of the enzymes can be used to minimize gastric-acid degradation. Dosages and strengths of the preparations should be carefully considered.

Fecal fat should also be examined repeatedly to measure response to treatment. Patients may also need fat soluble vitamins until the steatorrhea is under control.

The treatment for Crohn's disease is primarily medical with surgery used only for treatment failures or emergencies. The treatment of Crohn's disease is outlined in detail in Chapter 5. Nutritional support has limited use as a primary therapy. Parenteral and enteral nutrition may induce a remission but relapse occurs with resumption of regular food intake. There is a role for parenteral therapy in patients with short-bowel syndrome due to extensive small-bowel resection. There is also likely to be a role for preoperative nutrition support to improve nutritional status and subsequent wound healing and recovery. Patients will need a multivitamin supplement and those with ileal Crohn's disease should be evaluated for vitamin B_{12} deficiency and supplemented when appropriate.

For patients with HIV or AIDS-associated diarrhea and malabsorption, the treatment is directed toward the underlying cause. As previously reviewed, an extensive search for a potential pathogen should be undertaken with directed treatment of the culprit pathogen. If no pathogen or etiology is found, therapy should be directed at preventing malnutrition by providing adequate calories and protein and correcting any vitamin or mineral deficiencies. There have been reports of decreased fat and nitrogen losses in patients with AIDS receiving medium chain as opposed to long chain triglyceride-containing formulas although medium chain triglycerides are expensive.

Patients with malabsorption due to short-bowel syndrome usually have resolution of these symptoms as the small bowel adapts to increased absorptive surface area. Studies have examined the effect of growth hormone with glutamine on intestinal absorption without success. In patients with significant loss of small bowel and ongoing malabsorption, short- or long-term parenteral nutrition may be necessary.

Further reading

Amann ST, Josephson SA, Toskes PP. Acid steatocrit: a simple, rapid gravimetric method to determine steatorrhea. *Am J Gastroenterol* 1997; 92(12):2280–4.

Andrews NC. Disorders of iron metabolism. *N Engl J Med* 1999; 341(26):1986–5.

Carlson S, Craig RM. D-xylose hydrogen breath tests compared to absorption kinetics in human patients with and without malabsorption. *Dig Diseases & Sciences* 1995; 40(10):2259–67.

Carmel R. Cobalamin, the stomach, and aging. *Am J Clin Nutrition*, 1997; 66(4):750–9.

Carvajal SH, Mulvihill SJ. Postgastrectomy syndromes: dumping and diarrhea. *Gastroenterol Clinics North Am* 1994; 23(2):261–79.

Craig RM, Ehrenpreis ED. D-xylose testing. *J Clin Gastroenterol* 1999; 29(2):143–50.

Erickson RH, Kim YS. Digestion and absorption of dietary protein. *Ann Rev Medicine* 1990; 41:133–9.

Farrell RJ, Kelly CP. Celiac sprue. *N Engl J Medicine* 2002; 346(3):180–8.

Fine KD, Schiller LR. AGA technical review on the evaluation and management of chronic diarrhea. *Gastroenterology* 1999; 116(6):1464–86.

Holt PR. Diarrhea and malabsorption in the elderly. *Gastroenterol Clinics North Am* 2001; 30(2):427–44.

Lucock M. Folic acid: nutritional biochemistry, molecular biology, and role in disease processes. *Molecular Genetics & Metabol* 2000; 71(1–2):121–38.

Rostami K, Kerckhaert J, et al. Sensitivity of antiendomysium and antigliadin antibodies in untreated celiac disease: disappointing in clinical practice. *Am J Gastroenterol* 1999; 94(4):888–94.

Shaw AD, Davies GJ. Lactose intolerance: problems in diagnosis and treatment. *J Clinical Gastroenterol* 1999; 28(3):208–16.

Southgate DA. Digestion and metabolism of sugars. *Am J Clinical Nutrition* 1995; 62(1 Suppl):203S–210S; discussion 211S.

Steer ML, Waxman I, Freedman S. Chronic pancreatitis. *N Engl J Medicine* 1995; 332(22):1482–90.

Chapter 7

Diverticular Disease
James D. Lewis and Howard M. Ross

CHAPTER OUTLINE

INTRODUCTION

EPIDEMIOLOGY OF DIVERTICULOSIS

PATHOLOGY OF DIVERTICULOSIS

ETIOLOGY OF DIVERTICULOSIS

    Role of colonic motility

    Role of colonic fiber

SYMPTOMATIC DIVERTICULAR DISEASE

    Acute diverticulitis

    Diverticular stricture

    Diverticular hemorrhage

    Chronic abdominal pain

SURGICAL CONSIDERATIONS IN DIVERTICULAR DISEASE

    Diverticulitis

    Perforated diverticulitis

    Diverticular hemorrhage

    Diverticular stricture

CONCLUSIONS

FURTHER READING

Introduction

Diverticulosis of the colon (heretofore referred to as diverticulosis) refers to herniation of the colonic mucosa and submucosa through the muscle layers. Diverticulosis is a common condition in western societies. While most people with diverticulosis never experience symptoms attributable to the diverticulosis, symptomatic diverticular disease remains relatively common. This chapter discusses the etiology of diverticulosis, the hypothesized causes of complicated diverticular disease, and management of these complications.

Epidemiology of diverticulosis

Diverticulosis is relatively uncommon prior to the age of 40 years, but the prevalence increases with increasing age. Estimates suggest that more than 50% of adults have colonic diverticuli by their ninth decade of life. Furthermore, the number of diverticula within the colon appears to increase with age.

Studies of the prevalence of diverticular disease in different geographic regions and across different time periods lend some insight to the etiology of this condition. The prevalence of diverticular disease differs across geographic regions. Colonic diverticulosis is extremely common in adults living in the US and other developed countries. In contrast, diverticulosis is relatively uncommon among people living in less developed regions within Africa and Asia. It has been hypothesized that this difference may be related to differences in fiber intake between more and less industrialized nations.

Further support to the fiber hypothesis comes from studies of the prevalence of diverticulosis across time within a single region. Such studies have documented rising rates of death from diverticular disease during the first half of the 1900s. Again, this was hypothesized to be related to changing dietary habits among western culture during this time. However, it is important to realize that studies of secular trends of disease can be influenced by numerous factors. Importantly, it is possible that physicians were better able to diagnose diverticulosis and diverticular diseases as technology improved. Furthermore, as life expectancy increases, the prevalence of diverticulosis would also be expected to increase.

Pathology of diverticulosis

Diverticulosis of the colon is truly a condition of pseudodiverticula, with herniation of the colonic mucosa and submucosa through the muscle layers. In general, the diverticula are more common in the left colon, with some studies demonstrating diverticula in the sigmoid colon in more than 90% of patients with diverticular disease. Interestingly, studies from Japan have not observed the same pattern. In Japan, there appears to be a much higher rate of right-sided diverticular disease.

Several pathological features are routinely seen in patients with diverticulosis. Massive thickening of the colonic-wall muscle layers is very common among patients with diverticulosis. The potential role of this finding in the etiology of diverticulosis is discussed further (see below). In addition, diverticula tend to occur at areas of weakness in the colonic-wall muscle layers. These herniations of the most superficial wall layers occur between the mesenteric and lateral tenia, particularly at the point were the vasa recta penetrate the circular muscle layer.

Etiology of diverticulosis

The cause of colonic diverticulosis is likely to be multifactorial. Hypothesized factors contributing to the etiology of diverticulosis have included abnormal colonic motor activity, dietary fiber intake, changes in the structure and function of the colonic wall with aging, and increased cross-linking of collagen.

Role of colonic motility

Colonic diverticulosis is believed to result from excessive intracolonic pressure leading to outpouching of the colonic wall. Painter has demonstrated that during colonic contractions, the pressure within the colonic lumen increases. This pressure can be transmitted either to the fecal content or to the colonic wall, thus increasing colonic-wall tension. When the intracolonic pressure is greater than the pressure of the colonic musculature, herniation occurs. With repeated episodes of herniation, permanent diverticuli can form.

A common observation in patients with sigmoid diverticulosis is the presence of markedly thickened colonic muscle layers and shortening of the tenia. It is hypothesized that the thickened muscle layers may actually contribute to the etiology of the diverticulosis. The thickened muscle layers allow for complete obliteration of the colonic lumen during muscle contraction, allowing for the colon to be separated into unique compartments. Maximal intraluminal pressure is attained within these compartments. This hypothesis is consistent with the finding of high prevalence of diverticuli within the sigmoid colon, the region of the colon with the narrowest lumen. Thus, within the sigmoid colon, the intraluminal pressures during contraction are higher than in other parts of the colon.

Role of colonic fiber

Increased contraction pressures could result from increased stimuli for colonic contraction or as a result of the need for greater contraction to propel the solid feces through the colon. This latter mechanism applies to conditions in which there the stool bulk is reduced.

Both animal and human data support an etiologic role for fiber in the development of colonic diverticulosis. Insoluble fiber, such as psyllium, plays an important role in determining stool bulk and colonic transit time. Higher concentrations of fiber in the diet result in greater stool bulk and reduced colonic transit time. The greater stool bulk is believed to result in more efficient propulsion of the fecal bolus with less contraction of the colonic wall. This in turn leads to lower intracolonic pressures. Diets high in fiber would be expected to protect against the development of high intracolonic pressures and as such protect against the development of diverticulosis.

Support for this hypothesis has been suggested by numerous observations, both in humans and in experimental animals. First, both rats and rabbits fed a diet deficient in fiber have been shown to develop diverticulosis more often than those fed high-fiber diets. In humans, diverticulosis and diverticulitis are much more prevalent in industrialized nations where there is lower fiber intake. Furthermore, there has been an increase in the prevalence of diverticular disease concurrent with the decline in fiber intake in industrialized countries. These ecological studies and analyses of secular trends have subsequently been confirmed using cohort and case-control methodology with patient level data on patients with symptomatic diverticular disease. Finally, vegetarians have been found to have a lower incidence of diverticulitis than nonvegetarians living in the same geographic region. Based on these observations, it is likely that diets high in dietary fiber protect against the development of diverticulosis and, as a result, protect against symptomatic diverticular disease.

Symptomatic diverticular disease

Diverticulosis is an asymptomatic condition in most people. However, several complications of diverticulosis can occur (Box 7.1). Among these are acute diverticulitis, diverticular stricture formation, diverticular hemorrhage, and chronic pain syndromes. It is estimated that 10% to 25% of patients with diverticulosis will develop diverticulitis, and that approximately 5% will experience diverticular hemorrhage. Thus, more than 70% of patients with diverticulosis would be expected to have no complications from the condition.

Acute diverticulitis

Acute diverticulitis is believed to result from obstruction of the diverticular orifice with fecal material. This concept is similar to the proposed etiology of acute appendicitis. With the lumen of the diverticulum obstructed, secretion of mucus and proliferation of bacteria can lead to increased intradiverticular pressure. Eventually this pressure is sufficiently high to allow for ischemic necrosis of the diverticula resulting in perforation. Often this is a micro-perforation with walling off of the periverticular abscess. Interestingly, however, studies have shown that the colonic mucosa within areas of acute diverticulitis can be microscopically normal.

While the mechanical obstruction theory for diverticular disease is appealing, it is unclear why certain diverticula become obstructed and develop diverticulitis while others do not. In general, epidemiological studies of risk factors for acute diverticulitis are lacking. Certainly, dietary patterns may influence this condition. Cohort and case-control studies of patients with symptomatic diverticular disease have identified an association with low fiber diet and symptomatic diverticular disease, however, these studies have generally not focused on the select group of patients with acute diverticulitis.

A few studies have suggested that consumption of non-steroidal anti-inflammatory drugs (NSAIDs) may be related to the development of diverticulitis. Again, however, these studies have either combined acute diverticulitis with other types of symptomatic diverticular disease or have been limited by small sample sizes and potential methodological problems. Thus, the exact relationship between NSAID consumption and diverticulitis remains uncertain.

Similarly there are limited data on the role corticosteroids play in promoting acute diverticulitis. However, it seems evident that patients consuming corticosteroids at the time of onset of acute diverticulitis are more likely to develop septic complications such as peritonitis or large intra-abdominal abscesses.

Age and obesity may also be related to the development of diverticulitis. Because diverticulosis is more common among older adults, it is not surprising that diverticulitis is also more common among this group. Interestingly, however, in young patients, particularly those less than 40 years of age, obesity appears to be a potential risk factor for acute diverticulitis. Whether this is related to dietary habits or to some other factor has not been

---

Box 7.1 Possible sequealae of diverticulosis

Acute diverticulitis
    peritonitis
    abscess
Diverticular stricture
Diverticular hemorrhage
Chronic abdominal pain

Box 7.2 Proposed risk factors for symptomatic diverticular disease

Diets low in fiber
Diets containing seeds
Non-steroidal anti-inflammatory drugs
Obesity
Increasing age
Decreased exercise

Diverticular Disease

well characterized. This could potentially be related to decreased physical activity among obese subjects.

Clinical manifestations of acute diverticulitis

Patients with acute diverticulitis generally present with non-specific symptoms (Box 7.3). Pain in the lower abdomen, particularly in the left lower quadrant is extremely common. Patients will often complain of a change in bowel habits, including both diarrhea and constipation. Likewise, urinary symptoms can be seen. On physical examination, left lower quadrant tenderness is common. The presence of occult blood in the stool is not uncommon, however frank hematochezia in the setting of acute diverticulitis is rare. Patients with more severe diverticulitis may have a palpable abdominal mass. In the setting of free perforation and peritonitis, guarding and rebound tenderness may be elicited.

Diagnostic tests for acute diverticulitis

Diagnosis of acute diverticulitis is generally established with radiographic studies. Computed tomography has become a standard test for diagnosing acute diverticulitis. Computed tomography evidence of diverticulitis includes evidence of pericolonic fat inflammation, bowel-wall thickening, or pericolonic abscess in a region of the colon with identifiable diverticula (Figure 7.1). Computed tomography has several advantages over barium enema and colonoscopy in the diagnosis of acute diverticulitis, and, most importantly, it is safer than either of these techniques since there is no need to insufflate the colon. Computed tomography is a highly sensitive test, although relatively high false negative rates have been reported in some small studies. In addition, CT scanning has the advantage of being able to assess for large intra-abdominal abscess collections. When an abscess is identified, CT can be used to guide drainage of the collections.

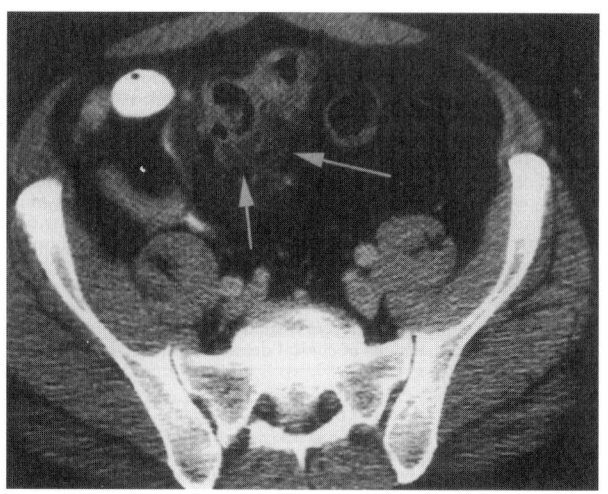

Figure 7.1 Computed tomography scan of the abdomen demonstrating sigmoid diverticulitis. Note the diverticuli and thickened wall of the sigmoid colon with stranding of the pericolic fat planes (reproduced from Farrel JR, Farrell JJ, Morrin MM. Diverticular disease in the elderly. *Gastroenterol Clin North Am* 2001; 30(2): 475–496).

Ultrasonography has been suggested by some authors as an alternative to CT scanning for the diagnosis of acute diverticulitis. Advantages of ultrasonography are its widespread availability and low cost. In appropriate hands, ultrasound has been shown to perform as well as CT scan for patients with suspected diverticulitis. However, this technique is very much operator dependent. In addition, it is less good at identifying alternative diagnoses in patients without diverticulitis. As such, the role of ultrasonography in diagnosing acute diverticulitis depends on the patient population, the suspicion for extracolonic complications, and the experience of the ultrasonographer.

Diverticular stricture

Colonic strictures can occur as a complication of diverticular disease and can present with non-specific symptoms such as abdominal pain or a change in bowel habits. Diagnosis is generally made with barium enema and colonoscopy. The differential diagnosis of a colonic stricture is between a benign and a malignant stricture. However, because of uncertainty in the diagnosis as well as persistent symptoms, most patients with significant colonic strictures secondary to diverticular disease ultimately require surgery.

Box 7.3 Common signs and symptoms of acute diverticulitis

Lower abdominal pain, particularly in the left lower quadrant
Alteration in bowel habits
Tenderness on palpitation in the left lower quadrant
Abdominal mass
Rebound tenderness
Guarding

Diverticular hemorrhage

Diverticular hemorrhage is another common complication of diverticulosis. Small-volume, non-hemodynamically significant bleeding is extremely common in western societies. This bleeding generally is a result of hemorrhoids. The frequency in which diverticula result in small-volume hematochiezia is not well established. In contrast, large-volume hematochezia is a well-described complication of diverticulosis.

Overall lower gastrointestinal bleeding of sufficient severity to warrant hospitalization occurs in approximately 20 per 100 000 persons annually. This is slightly more common among men and it increases dramatically with increasing age. Among patients admitted to hospital for lower gastrointestinal bleeding, diverticular hemorrhage is believed to account for more than 40% of the cases. In the past, diverticular hemorrhage was generally assumed to be the etiology of bleeding when no other source could be identified. More recently, both angiographic and colonoscopic evidence have confirmed that diverticuli are a common source of major lower gastrointestinal bleeding.

Chronic abdominal pain

An important question is whether diverticulosis, in the absence of diverticulitis, is a cause of chronic abdominal pain. The difficulty in establishing a causal relation between diverticulosis and abdominal pain relates to the high prevalence of irritable bowel syndrome in the US. Because both irritable bowel syndrome and diverticulosis are extremely common, distinguishing which is the cause of chronic abdominal symptoms can be difficult. Evidence that uncomplicated diverticulosis may not cause symptoms comes from several lines of research. One study has demonstrated that the natural history of patients with irritable bowel syndrome is not influenced by the presence or absence of diverticulosis. The role of fiber supplementation in these two conditions provides additional evidence that uncomplicated diverticulosis may not cause abdominal pain. Although fiber supplementation improves colonic transit, it has not convincingly been shown to improve symptoms of irritable bowel syndrome. Similarly, several studies of fiber supplementation in patients with "symptomatic diverticulosis" have shown a reduction in constipation, however a reduction in pain has not been a consistent finding. Thus, while further research into this question is needed, the current evidence does not strongly support the idea that uncomplicated diverticulosis is a cause of chronic abdominal pain. Clearly, before attributing symptoms of chronic abdominal pain to diverticulosis, it is imperative to rule out other potential diseases.

Surgical considerations in diverticular disease

Diverticulitis

Patients with mild diverticulitis are often managed without hospitalization and are generally treated with oral antibiotics to cover routine bowel flora. Clear liquid diet is often prescribed until symptoms begin to improve. Symptomatic improvement is expected within 2 to 3 days. Outpatient management should be limited to patients without peritoneal signs, who are able to take in sufficient oral hydration, and who have minimal comorbid illnesses. Patients not meeting these criteria or who have evidence of more severe diverticulitis require hospitalization.

The goal of the surgeon caring for patients with diverticular disease is to minimize patient suffering and intervene operatively before the complications of diverticulitis occur. There complications include perforation, fistula formation, and obstruction. The natural history of diverticulitis dictates its treatment. Multiple studies suggest that medical management will enable approximately 70% of patients to avoid hospitalization over 5 to 10 years after their initial uncomplicated attack.

The course of complicated diverticulitis is very different. Non-operative management of these patients is discouraged because medical management almost uniformly fails to return the patients to health. Elective sigmoid colon resection is considered after two attacks as the rate of complicated disease begins to rise after a recurrence of diverticulitis.

It is our treatment paradigm to allow patients who are hospitalized with their first bout of diverticulitis to be treated with antibiotics until they are pain free. Patients are restricted from oral intake until this pain-free state occurs. Diet advancement follows the resolution of pain. Hospital discharge follows shortly as long as diet is tolerated. Colonoscopy is performed 4 to 6 weeks after the bout resolves to evaluate other entities which can mimic diverticulitis. Cancer and Crohn's disease are two of the most common and important conditions. Postoperative diet is not restricted to either low residue or high fiber.

Perforated diverticulitis

The surgical treatment of a patient presenting with diffuse peritonitis secondary to a perforated diverticulum consists of resecting the diseased segment of colon and leaving the rectum as a Hartmann pouch. An end colostomy is created from non-diseased colon proximal to the area that was resected. When a resection for diverticular disease is performed, the distal resection margin must be at the top of the rectum. At operation, the top of the rectum is defined as that point at which the tenia becomes confluent. Anastomosis to the top of the rectum greatly minimizes the chance of recurrent diverticulitis, as the rectum does not contain diverticuli. The risk of recurrent diverticulitis is generally less than 5% and rarely requires further surgical intervention.

The temporary colostomy can be considered for closure after 3 months. This time interval allows intra-abdominal adhesions to become softer and less vascular. Colostomy closure can be performed in standard open fashion or laparoscopically. It is critical for the surgeon to pay careful attention to the creation of the ostomy, as a proportion of ostomies created as "temporary", are never reversed. The surgeon or enterostomal therapist should mark the ostomy site preoperatively.

Diverticulitis presenting with focal peritonitis and a CT scan revealing only minimal extraluminal air, in a non-immunocompromised individual, can be treated without immediate resection and ostomy formation. The patient must be hospitalized, placed on intravenous antibiotics, restricted from oral intake, and monitored carefully. Peritonitis should resolve within approximately 48 hours. If there is any sign of disease progression the patient should undergo an operation.

Hinchey created a diverticulitis staging system to help guide therapy (Box 7.4). Hinchey grades III and IV describe situations of gross contamination, which prevent primary anastomosis, and are currently managed with two-stage operative treatment. Three-stage operative treatment of diverticulitis involved temporary fecal diversion at an initial operation. At a second operation, resection of the diseased sigmoid colon occurred. This was followed by a third operation to restore intestinal continuity. Such three-stage paradigms are relegated to history.

Box 7.4 Hinchey's grading system for perforated diverticular disease

Stage I	confined pericolic abscess
Stage II	distant abscess (retroperitoneal or pelvic)
Stage III	generalized peritonitis caused by the rupture of a pericolic or pelvic abscess, non-communicating with the bowel lumen because of obliteration of the diverticular neck by inflammation
Stage IV	fecal peritonitis caused by free perforation of a diverticulum (communicating)

Such treatment resulted in higher morbidity and prolonged patient suffering.

Intra-abdominal abscess formation is the most common complication of diverticulitis. Percutaneous drainage of abscesses often speeds recovery and minimizes morbidity. Most abscesses are diagnosed with CT. Drainage catheters are placed under ultrasound or CT guidance. Abscess drainage can act as a bridge to facilitate a one-stage elective operation. Once the pericolic abscess is drained, weeks are allowed to pass to allow residual colon inflammation to resolve. Patients with diminished immune function may be better off with prompt resection of the diseased colon and colostomy formation. The health of this patient subgroup may depend on the most rapid removal of the septic focus. Delaying the operation to permit the phloegmous component of the diverticulits to resolve can be dangerous. Collections less than 5 cm in size can occasionally be managed medically. Fecal fistula formation may accompany catheter drainage but is not of great detriment as the diseased segment responsible for the fistula will be excised at the time of definitive resection.

Diverticular disease in patients younger than 50 years is an area of debate. One study revealed that only one third of patients under 50 years old, hospitalized with their first bout of uncomplicated diverticulitis underwent an operation within a follow-up period of up to 9 years. Two thirds of patients did not require surgery during the follow-up period. These authors assert that young patients should be treated like older patients, requiring colon resection after a second bout of diverticulitis or for complicated disease. Others counter that 30% of patients requiring operations within 5 years is a significant incidence, and that the true follow-up time in most studies is too short to reach a strong conclusion. Patients requiring a more aggressive surgical approach are those with immunocompromise or people who travel to areas where there is no access to medical and surgical care.

Laparoscopic approaches for the surgical treatment of diverticulitis are rapidly developing. Such approaches generally diminish the hospital stay by 2 to 3 days compared to open operations. A laparoscopic operation allows an earlier return to the full preoperative functional state. With techniques such as hand-assisted laparoscopy even complex phlegmonous disease and fistulas can be tackled. Over the 18-month period from October 2000 to April 2002 we, at the University of Pennsylvania, performed hand-assisted laparoscopic sigmoid colon resection in 20 patients with diverticulitis. The mean length of stay was 3 days. There were no anastomotic leaks and two wound infections. Three patients had active colovaginal fistulas.

Ureteral stenting preoperatively can be helpful if there is concern about the inflammatory process in the retroperitoneum. Ureteral stenting helps the surgeon identify the ureters and prevents their inadvertent injury.

Diverticular hemorrhage

Diverticular hemorrhage can be life threatening. Fortunately bleeding from diverticulae is usually self-limited. Bleeding will stop spontaneously in 80% to 90% of cases, returning in only approximately 20% of patients. Critical to the treatment of lower gastrointestinal bleeding is recognition of the potential severity of the disease. Appropriate fluid and blood product support is tantamount.

Diagnosis of diverticular hemorrhage is made using a combination of endoscopy, bleeding scan, and angiography. Each modality has benefits and limitations. Endoscopy allows visualization of the colonic mucosa and permits differentiation from other sources of bleeding. In the presence of significant bleeding, endoscopy can be difficult or impossible. If the bleeding has stopped endoscopy may not accurately identify the source of the hemorrhage. Bleeding scans are extremely sensitive for identifying bleeding when extravagation is 0.1 cc/min or greater. However, localization of the bleeding site can be inaccurate because of retrograde peristalsis. Likewise, bleeding scans provide no opportunity for therapy. Thus, bleeding scans are largely utilized to determine whether bleeding is ongoing and at a sufficiently high rate to warrant the use of angiography.

Angiography provides outstanding visualization of the bleeding site. However, angiography requires bleeding rates of 0.5 cc/mm to reveal bleeding. Importantly, with the advent of angioembolization, the active bleeding can be stopped with angiographic intervention. However, angiography is associated with several potential disadvantages. First, angiography is invasive. Exposure to intravenous contrast can result in renal injury. Although relatively rare, angiographic therapy can cause bowel ischemia. Finally, facilities and staff may not always be immediately available to perform angiography.

Our treatment paradigm is tailored to the rate of bleeding. If bleeding is massive an attempt is made to proceed immediately to angiography. This allows for the most accurate identification of the bleeding site and provides the opportunity for therapeutic intervention. Further, if embolization was not successful and surgery was required, the resection would be focused on the well-identified segment. Ischemia and necrosis after embolization is rare. Overall therapeutic success with this technique is in the range of 60% to 70%. For bleeding that has stopped we recommend colonoscopy. This allows the differentiation of other important entities.

Performing a segmental colectomy for bleeding that is not accurately identified leads to recurrent bleeding rates of approximately 30%. Non-localized bleeding should be treated with subtotal colectomy. We discourage segmental colectomy for bleeding based soley on the result of a bleeding scan.

Diverticular stricture

A colonic stricture significant enough to cause obstruction can result from repeated bouts of diverticulitis. Surgery to resect the colon segment containing the stricture is indicated to relieve obstruction and to exclude malignancy. The technique of on-table colonic lavage can be employed to allow primary anastomosis, if the obstruction prevented the patient from having a mechanical bowel preparation.

Conclusions

Diverticulosis is extremely common in industrialized societies. With the aging population, complications of diverticular disease are likely to become increasingly more common. Management of symptomatic diverticular disease needs to be tailored to the severity of the condition and the patient's underlying risk factors for recurrent disease. Collaboration between the primary care physician, gastroenterologists, radiologists, and surgeons are paramount for the optimal management of diverticular disease.

Further reading

Aldoori WH, Giovannucci EL, Rockett HR, Sampson L, Rimm EB, Willett WC. A prospective study of dietary fiber types and symptomatic diverticular disease in men. *J Nutrition* 1998; 128:714–719.

Bell AM, Wolff BG. Progression and recurrence after resection for diverticulitis. *Semin Colon Rectal Surg* 1990; 1:99–102.

Birnbaum BA, Balthazar EJ. CT of appendicitis and diverticulitis. *Radiologic Clinics North Am* 1994; 32:885–898.

Burkitt DP, Walker AR, Painter NS. Dietary fiber and disease. JAMA 1974; 229:1068–1074.

Ferzoco LB, Raptopoulos V, Silen W. Acute diverticulitis. *N Engl J Med* 1998; 338:1521–1526.

Formatis N, Tudor RG, Keighley MR. The 5 year natural history of complicated diverticulitis disease. *Brit J Surg* 1994; 81:733–735.

Guy GE, Shetty PC, Sharma RP. Acute lower gastrointestinal hemorrhage: treatment by superselective embolization with polyvinyl alcohol particles. *Am J Roentgenol* 1992; 159: 521–526.

Hinchey ES, Schaal PG, Richards GK. Treatment of perforated diverticular disease of the colon. *Adv Surg* 1978; 12:85–109.

Jensen DM, Machicado GA, Jutabha R, Kovacs TO. Urgent colonoscopy for the diagnosis and treatment of severe diverticular hemorrhage. *N Engl J Medicine* 2000; 342:78–82.

Kohler L, Saverland S, Neugebauer E. Diagnosis and treatment of diverticulitis disease: results of a consensus development conference. *Surg Endoscopy* 1999; 13:430–436.

Larson DM, Masters SS, Spiro HM. Medical and surgical therapy in diverticular disease. A comparative study. *Gastroenterology* 1976; 71:734–737.

Painter NS, Burkitt DP. Diverticular disease of the colon: a deficiency disease of Western civilization. *Brit Med J* 1971; 2:450–454.

Parts TG, Connell AM. The outcome of 455 patients admitted for treatment of diverticular disease of the colon. *Brit J Surg* 1970; 57:775–778.

Pradel JA, Adell JF, Taourel P, Djafari M, Monnin-Delhom E, Bruel JM. Acute colonic diverticulitis: prospective comparative evaluation with US and CT. *Radiology* 1997; 205:503–512.

Schauer PR, Ramos R, Ghiatas AA, Sirinek KR. Virulent diverticular disease in young obese men. *Am J Surg* 1992; 164: 443–446; discussion 446–448.

Chapter 8

Intestinal Polyposis Syndromes and Hereditary Colorectal Cancer

Jonathan P. Terdiman

CHAPTER OUTLINE

INTRODUCTION

POLYPOSIS SYNDROMES

Familial adenomatous polyposis

Hereditary hamartomatous polyp syndromes

Hereditary neural polyposis syndromes

Sporadic polyposis syndromes

Inflammatory polyposis

Lymphomatous polyposis

HEREDITARY NON-POLYPOSIS COLORECTAL CANCER

COMMON FAMILIAL COLORECTAL CANCER

GENETIC TESTING FOR HEREDITARY COLORECTAL CANCER

Available tests

Methods of mutation detection

Microsatellite instability testing and protein immunohistochemistry in hereditary non-polyposis colorectal cancer

Genetic counseling and informed consent

Indications and strategy for genetic testing in hereditary colorectal cancer

Familial adenomatous polyposis

Hereditary non-polyposis colorectal cancer

FURTHER READING

Introduction

Colorectal cancer is the second leading cause of cancer death in the US. Each year approximately 130 000 Americans are diagnosed with the disease and 50 000 of them will die of it. The cumulative lifetime risks of colorectal cancer, and mortality from colorectal cancer are approximately 3% to 6% and 2%, respectively. The majority of colorectal cancers occur in individuals over 60 years old, who have no previous personal or family history of the disease. Although the major risk factors for these sporadic cases are advancing age and environmental exposures, most importantly diet, approximately 20% to 25% of colorectal cancers are in younger individuals or in those with a personal or family history of cancer, suggesting a heritable susceptibility.

The genetic predisposition to colorectal cancer falls into two major groups

- common familial colorectal cancer – 15% to 20% of colorectal cancers
- hereditary colorectal cancer – 5% of colorectal cancers (Figure 8.1).

In common familial colorectal cancer, first-degree relatives of persons with colorectal cancer, or adenomatous polyps, have an approximately two-fold risk of developing colorectal cancer, and the risk increases with the number of relatives affected and the earlier the age of onset in the family. A family history of extracolonic cancers (e.g. uterine), or the presence in individual family members of multiple colorectal or other cancers, also increases the risk. The increased risk for colorectal cancer in common familial colorectal cancer is conveyed by the inheritance of one or, more likely, many possible, low

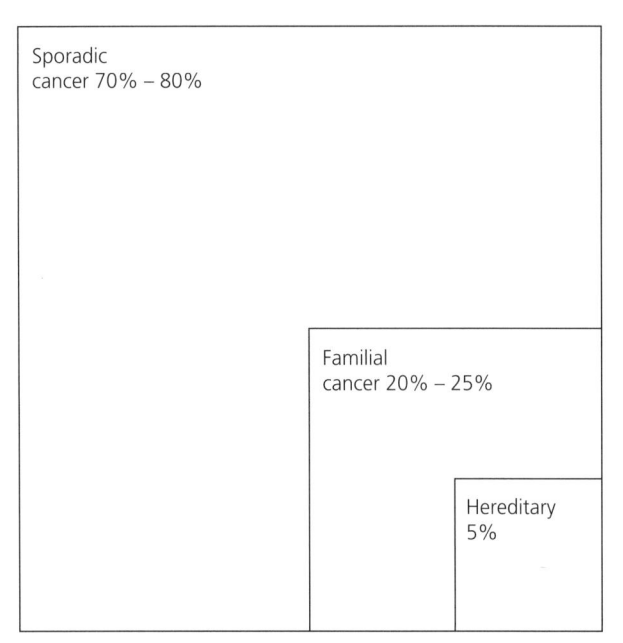

Figure 8.1 Frequency of sporadic, familial, and hereditary colorectal cancer.

Box 8.1 Classification of hereditary colorectal cancer syndromes

Polyposis syndromes (1% of all colorectal cancers)
Adenomatous polyposis syndromes
    Familial adenomatous polyposis (< 1% of all colorectal cancers)
        Gardner syndrome
        Turcot syndrome
        attenuated adenomatous polyposis coli
Hamartomatous polyposis syndromes (<< 1% of all colorectal cancers)
    Peutz–Jeghers syndrome
    Juvenile polyposis
        hereditary mixed polyposis syndrome
    Cowden syndrome
        Bannayan–Riley–Ruvalcaba syndrome
        Ruvulcaba–Myhre syndrome
        Bannayan–Zonana syndrome
    Soto syndrome
    Lhermitte–Duclos disease
Gorlin syndrome
Hereditary non-polyposis colorectal cancer (3% to 5% of all colorectal cancers)
    Lynch syndrome
    Muir–Torre syndrome
    Turcot syndrome

penetrance susceptibility alleles, most of which have yet to be identified. Carriage of these susceptibility alleles increases the risk of acquiring colorectal cancer, but by no means makes certain the development of colorectal cancer. In fact, in the large majority of allele carriers, colorectal cancer does not occur. Common familial colorectal cancer will be discussed in greater detail at the end of the chapter (pp. 149–150).

More than 5% of colorectal cancers are hereditary in etiology, meaning that they are caused by the carriage of a highly penetrant, dominantly inherited, susceptibility allele. Hereditary colorectal cancer is conventionally divided between the polyposis syndromes and hereditary non-polyposis colorectal cancer (Box 8.1). The polyposis syndromes are defined by the presence of multiple polyps in the gut lumen. The polyposis syndromes have conventionally been categorized by polyp histology. The most common and important of the polyposis syndromes is familial adenomatous polyposis. Familial adenomatous polyposis carries a lifetime risk of colorectal cancer approaching 100% if the colon is not removed. The other major category of hereditary polyposes are the hamartomatous polyposis syndromes, most importantly Peutz–Jeghers syndrome, hereditary juvenile polyposis and Cowden syndrome. There are a number of other very rare hereditary polyposis syndromes, as well as several non-hereditary polyposis syndromes.

Significantly more common than any of the polyposis syndromes is hereditary non-polyposis rectal cancer. At least 2% to 3% of all colorectal cancer is secondary to hereditary non-polyposis rectal cancer. The lifetime risk of colorectal cancer in patients with hereditary non-polyposis rectal cancer, approaches 70% to 80%, but not as a consequence of an increased number of colorectal adenomas.

The primary importance of familial and hereditary colorectal cancer is the increased risk of colorectal cancer, and often other cancers, for individuals with these conditions. Failure to recognize common familial colorectal cancer, or more importantly, one of the hereditary syndromes, will lead to inadequate cancer screening and surveillance in individuals at risk, with subsequent premature loss of life. Recently, the elucidation of the genes responsible for many of these syndromes has revolutionized the care of at-risk individuals and families. Genetic testing has the potential to greatly improve the efficiency and reduce the costs and morbidity of cancer screening and surveillance. Genetic testing is commercially available and is the standard of care of individuals and families with, or suspected of having, familial adenomatous polyposis or hereditary non-polyposis rectal cancer. Genetic testing may ultimately make an impact on the management of individuals at risk for common familial colorectal cancer as well. However, genetic testing raises a number of vexing clinical, ethical, legal, and psychosocial questions.

This chapter will discuss the clinical features, genetics and management of common familial and hereditary colorectal cancer, both the polyposis syndromes and hereditary non-polyposis rectal cancer. Special attention will be paid to the appropriate indications and methods for genetic testing in hereditary colorectal cancer.

Polyposis syndromes

Familial adenomatous polyposis

Clinical features: intestinal

Familial adenomatous polyposis is an autosomal dominant disorder that affects about 1 in 10 000 individuals and accounts for approximately 0.5% to 1% of colorectal cancers. In classic familial adenomatous polyposis, affected individuals develop hundreds to thousands of colonic adenomas by the mid to late teens, with over 95% of affected individuals demonstrating polyposis by the age of 35 years. Colorectal cancer is inevitable in the untreated individual, the majority of cancers appearing by age 40 years, and over 90% by age 45 years. Variants of familial adenomatous polyposis are now recognized in which polyps are greatly reduced in number, are predominantly or exclusively located in the right colon, and occur approximately a decade later than in classic familial adenomatous polyposis. This latter condition has been termed attenuated adenomatous polyposis coli or attenuated familial adenomatous polyposis.

In addition to colonic polyps, up to 90% of individuals with familial adenomatous polyposis will develop small-bowel adenomas, most commonly at or near the ampulla of Vater. These lesions are usually multiple and sessile, often forming carpet-like lesions. Because the ampulla of Vater is almost invariably involved, to assess the full extent of duodenal polyposis, duodenoscopy, in addition to routine upper endoscopy, is required. The burden of duodenal polyposis can be rated by the Spiegelman classification (Table 8.1). The lifetime risk for small-bowel carcinoma is approximately 5%, and duodenal cancer is the leading cause of cancer deaths in familial adenomatous polyposis patients that have undergone a colectomy. Individuals with stage III or IV polyposis are at greatest risk for periampullary/duodenal carcinoma.

Most familial adenomatous polyposis patients will also develop gastric polyposis. Gastric polyps are usually of the fundic-gland histological type, but adenomas rarely do occur. Gastric carcinoma risk is not much increased in western families, but is reported to be increased three- to four-fold in Japanese and Korean families with familial adenomatous polyposis. Overall the lifetime risk of gastric cancer in individuals with familial adenomatous polyposis has been reported at 0.5%. The gastric adenoma is felt to be the precursor lesion for gastric cancer as fundic gland polyps are considered to have almost no malignant potential. There has, however, been a case reported of gastric cancer arising in an area of fundic gland polyposis.

Table 8.1 Spiegelman classification for duodenal polyposis in familial adenomatous polyposis.

	Grade (points)		
	1	2	3
Number of polyps	1–4	5–20	> 20
Size of polyps (mm)	1–4	5–10	> 10
Histology	tubular	tubulovillous	villous
Dysplasia	mild	moderate	severe

Stage 0: 0 points
Stage 1: 1–4 points
Stage II: 5–6 points
Stage III: 7–8 points
Stage IV: 9–12 points

Clinical features: extraintestinal

Approximately two thirds of familial adenomatous polyposis patients will have congenital hypertrophy of the retinal pigment epithelium. These lesions typically are flat, oval, and pigmented, and are best detected by opthalmoscopy after pupillary dilation. In familial adenomatous polyposis the lesions are usually multiple (four or more), bilateral, or large. While congenital hypertrophy of the retinal pigment epithelium does not affect vision or have any malignant potential, it is important. In congenital hypertrophy of the retinal pigment epithelium-positive families all, or nearly all, individuals in the family with familial adenomatous polyposis will have congenital hypertrophy of the retinal pigment epithelium, and, because it can be detected at birth, examination of the fundus can identify susceptible family members at a young age.

Other benign extraintestinal manifestations of familial adenomatous polyposis include dental abnormalities, osteomas, lipomas, epidermoid cysts, and desmoid tumors. Desmoids develop in about

10% to 15% of individuals with familial adenomatous polyposis, the majority involving the small-bowel mesentery or incision sites. Over 70% are in women aged 20 to 40 years, suggesting a hormonal role in their development, and 80% are in those who have had prior abdominal surgery. Though desmoids are not malignant they cause considerable morbidity and mortality by local invasion. Familial adenomatous polyposis in conjunction with soft-tissue tumors, osteomas, and dental abnormalities is often referred to as the Gardner syndrome.

Individuals with familial adenomatous polyposis are at increased risk for cancer at sites other than the colorectum and small bowel. Malignancies associated with familial adenomatous polyposis include hepatoblastoma in young children, medulloblastoma, papillary carcinoma of the thyroid, and pancreatic cancer (Figure 8.2). The association of familial adenomatous polyposis and central nervous system tumors, primarily medulloblastoma, has been termed Turcot syndrome.

Genetics

Normally each individual has two functional copies of *APC* in all cells. Familial adenomatous polyposis is caused by a germline mutation of the tumor supressor *APC* gene located on chromosome 5q21. A minority of cases may be caused by biallelic mutation in the base-excision repair gene, MYH. Somatic mutation or loss of the second APC gene copy (allele) leads to loss of APC function in the cell. Since the colonic epithelial cells of familial adenomatous polyposis patients have only one functional copy of *APC*, initiation of colonic neoplasia is far more likely to occur, resulting in a dramatic increase in the number of colorectal adenomas and cancers. Data suggest that in some circumstances mutation of one gene copy alone may be enough to eliminate *APC* function in a cell because the mutant *APC* gene product can interfere with the function of the wild-type gene product.

APC is a large gene containing 15 exons and 2843 codons. The APC protein is involved in the control of cellular proliferation and apoptosis, and also in cellular adhesion. APC mutations are most commonly single base pair substitutions or short deletions or insertions that result in a truncated protein that loses all but one or two of seven β-catenin binding/ degradation sites. Without this functional domain, APC cannot participate in the regulation of cytoplasmic β-catenin levels via APC-mediated degradation (in coordination with axin/conductin and glycogen synthase kinase 3β). Degradation of β-catenin prevents its translocation into the nucleus where it binds one of the T-cell factors to initiate transcription of genes that promote cellular proliferation and prevent cell death such as *cyclin D* and *c-myc*.

The specific location of a germline mutation in *APC* may determine in part the disease phenotype. Mutations at either end of the gene (for example proximal to codon 158 or distal to codon 1900) are associated with an attenuated variant of the familial adenomatous polyposis characterized by sparse polyposis, though phenotypic variation occurs in these families, with some family members still demonstrating a classic phenotype. Mutations between codons 1250 and 1330 are linked with profuse polyposis. Congenital hypertrophy of the retinal pigment epithelium is present in patients in whom the mutation lies downstream to codon 463 but proximal to codon 1444. Severe periampullary polyposis is associated with mutations downstream from codon 1051, and desmoid tumors tend to occur with mutations between codons 1445 and 1578. Such genotype–phenotype correlation will prove useful in increasing the accuracy and effectiveness of screening, surveillance, and treatment.

Genetic testing for familial adenomatous polyposis is commercially available, and is the standard of care for families suspected of having the syndrome (see below). Testing starts with a family member suspected of having familial adenomatous polyposis, based on clinical presentation. If the disease-causing mutation can be identified, non-affected family members can then be tested to determine if they too carry the mutation. Family members proven not to have inherited the family mutation are spared burdensome screening and surveillance.

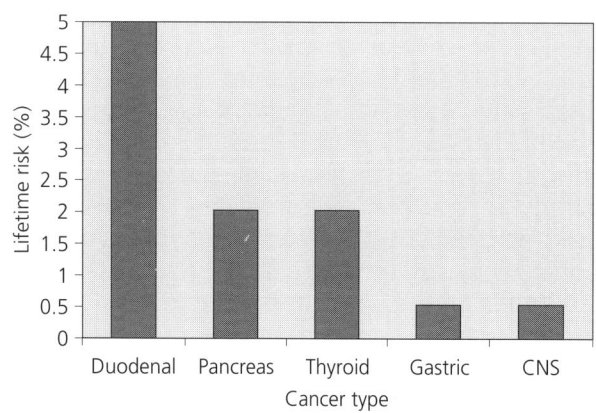

Figure 8.2 Frequencies of malignancies associated with familial adenomatous polyposis.

Screening, surveillance, and treatment

Colonic and extracolonic screening and surveillance recommendations for familial adenomatous

> **Box 8.2** Options for cancer prevention in familial adenomatous polyposis for known or suspected gene mutation carriers
>
> Primary recommendations
> - Annual flexible sigmoidoscopy beginning by age 10 to 12 years.
> - Annual colonoscopy, beginning by age 20 years, when attenuated familial adenomatous polyposis is suspected.
> - Prophylactic colectomy in teen years or when polyps are detected at colonoscopy.
> - Endoscopic surveillance every 4 to 6 months after ileorectal anastomosis and annually after ileoanal anastomosis.
> - Upper endoscopy, including duodenoscopy, every 6 months to 3 years starting by age 20 to 25 years.
>
> Secondary recommendations
> - Annual thyroid examination beginning by age 10 to 12 years.
> - Annual palpation of liver during first decade of life (consider annual hepatic ultrasound and measure of alpha fetoprotein).
> - Consider serial MRI of brain in families with Turcot syndrome.
> - Consider serial MRCP or endoscopic ultrasound in families with multiple pancreatic cancers.
> - Consider use of sulindac or celecoxib chemoprevention in individuals with colorectal adenomas.

polyposis are summarized in Box 8.2. Individuals at risk for familial adenomatous polyposis should undergo annual flexible sigmoidoscopy beginning at age 10 to 12 years. Once adenomas have been identified, yearly colonscopy is required. Colectomy should be undertaken once any of the polyps is 5 mm or larger in size, or if any polyp biopsies demonstrate villous features or high-grade dysplasia. If the polyp burden in the rectum is not great, then total abdominal colectomy with ileorectal anastomosis may be performed. However, much more commonly because of rectal polyposis, a total proctocolectomy is undertaken, usually with the creation of an ileal pouch anal anastomosis. In families with suspected attenuated adenomatous polyposis coli, screening should be undertaken with complete colonoscopy, rather than sigmoidoscopy. Because of the later onset of polyposis in these families, some experts recommend that screening can sometimes be safely deferred until approximately age 20 years. However, in the author's opinion, delaying the onset of screening in attenuated adenomatous polyposis coli families can be problematic because of the phenotypic variability in these families.

Screening for upper-tract adenomas is needed in familial adenomatous polyposis as well. Upper gastrointestinal endoscopy and duodenoscopy, with biopsy of the ampulla of Vater, should start once colonic adenomas have been identifed, and no later than age 25 years. Enteroscopy and/or enteroclysis also are advocated by some experts to exclude small-bowel adenomas distal to the duodenum. Thankfully, however, significant lesions in the middle or distal small bowel are rare. The upper gastrointestinal screening interval remains empirical, but generally screening should be undertaken every 1 to 3 years depending on the polyp burden encountered. Once detected, upper-tract adenomas can be removed or ablated by a variety of methods, if technically possible, though there are no data that this will improve long-term outcomes. If invasive cancer or high-risk adenomas are encountered (Spiegelman stage IV) then operative resection is indicated.

After colectomy ongoing surveillance is required. If the rectum is retained, endoscopic examination should be performed approximately every 6 to 12 months to remove or ablate any adenomas found. The risk of rectal cancer in individuals with familial adenomatous polyposis with an ileorectal anastomosis exceeds 10%, and upwards of 20% of patients that undergo a colectomy with ileorectal anastomosis will ultimately require completion proctectomy. Even after ileal pouch anal anastomosis, a substantial risk of the development of pouch adenomas exists, although the risk of developing invasive cancer appears to be low. Therefore, endoscopic examination of the ileal pouch is recommended every 1 to 2 years.

In addition to endoscopic screening, cancer prevention efforts in familial adenomatous polyposis may be augmented by chemoprevention with use of NSAIDs or cyclooxygenase 2 inhibitors. Both the NSAID, sulindac, and the cyclooxygenase 2 inhibitor, celecoxib, have been demonstrated to reduce the size and number of adenomas in individuals with familial adenomatous polyposis. Unfortunately, in a recent study, use of sulindac did not prevent the development of adenomas, but sulindac, celecoxib, and like drugs, may slow polyp progression. They are unlikely to obviate the need for surgery in patients, but may serve to delay the timing or prevent the need for a second operation in those with retained rectums. The exact role of these medications in the management of familial adenomatous polyposis remains to be elucidated.

Hereditary hamartomatous polyp syndromes

Peutz–Jeghers syndrome

Clinical features Peutz–Jeghers syndrome is an autosomal dominantly inherited cancer predisposition syndrome characterized by the presence of numerous hamartomatous polyps in the gastrointestinal tract and mucocutaneous pigmentation. The syndrome is rare, occurring in approximately 1 in 200 000 births. The classic mucocutaneous melanin pigment spots occur on the lips and buccal mucosa, but can also be found on other areas of the skin such as the dorsal and volar aspects of the hands and feet. The spots are often most obvious among affected caucasians with dark hair and skin tones, though Peutz–Jeghers syndrome occurs among all races and skin types. Pigment spots can be identified in 95% of patients with Peutz–Jeghers syndrome, often from birth or early infancy. However, the spots can fade with age, and therefore the absence of typical pigmentation does not exclude the diagnosis. No malignant potential has been ascribed to the hyperpigmentation of Peutz–Jeghers syndrome.

The predominant clinical feature of Peutz–Jeghers syndrome is the presence of numerous gastrointestinal harmartomatous polyps. The polyps have a distinctive histology with an arborizing pattern of smooth muscle in the lamina propria that distinguishes them from the hamartomas seen in juvenile polyposis or Cowden syndrome. The polyps can be pedunculated or sessile, and they range in size from several millimeters to giant polyps, 3 to 4 cm in size. The polyps occur throughout the gastrointestinal tract from the esophagus to the rectum. They are seen in the stomach in approximately 40% of cases, in the small bowel, especially the jejunum, in 80% of cases, and in the colorectum in 40% of cases. The polyps occur at a young age, and the typical age of diagnosis of Peutz–Jeghers syndrome secondary to polyp complications is in the mid-twenties. One third of patients with Peutz–Jeghers syndrome will experience polyp-related symptoms by the age of 10 years, and 50% to 60% will have symptoms before the age of 20 years. The major complications related to Peutz–Jeghers syndrome polyps are recurrent gastrointestinal bleeding and obstruction, often secondary to intussusception. Upwards of 40% to 50% of patients with Peutz–Jeghers syndrome will require operation for polyp-related bowel obstruction at some point in time.

Though the typical Peutz–Jeghers syndrome polyp is benign and without dysplasia, there is no doubt that Peutz–Jeghers syndrome is associated with very high rates of intestinal and extraintestinal cancer. The majority of deaths related to Peutz–Jeghers syndrome after the age of 30 years are secondary to malignancy, and the lifetime risk of cancer in Peutz–Jeghers syndrome approaches 90%. Intestinal cancers may be secondary to the malignant degeneration of the hamartomatous polyps, and foci of dysplasia can sometimes be found in large Peutz–Jeghers syndrome polyps. The majority of intestinal cancers are adenocarcinomas, though an increased risk for malignant gastrointestinal stromal tumors, such as leiomyosarcoma, exists as well. Extraintestinal cancers also are very common in Peutz–Jeghers syndrome, and in fact are more common than intestinal cancers. The most common extraintestinal cancer is cancer of the pancreas. Increased risk for cancer of the breast, ovary, lung, cervix, uterus, and testes has been documented (Table 8.2), as well as others. In addition to the more common intestinal and extraintestinal cancers, Peutz–Jeghers syndrome is associated with an increased frequency of unusual neoplastic and non-neoplastic tumors of the genital tract. Most of these lesions occur in women, and they are often small, bilateral, multifocal, and frequently benign. The lesions include ovarian sex cord tumors with annular tubules, mucinous neoplasms of the ovary, mucinous metaplasia of the fallopian tube, and extremely well-differentiated adenocarcinoma (adenoma malignum) of the cervix. Like women, men

Table 8.2 Cancer risk in patients with Peutz–Jeghers syndrome.

Cancer site	Approximate lifetime risk
All cancers	93%
Gastrointestinal cancers	
Colorectal	39%
Pancreas	36%
Stomach	29%
Small bowel	13%
Esophagus	0.5%
Non-gastrointestinal cancers	
Breast	54%
Ovary	21%
Lung	15%
Cervix	10%
Uterus	9%
Testes	9%

can also develop rare Sertoli cell or testicular tumors of the seminiferous tubules.

Genetics Peutz–Jeghers syndrome is caused by a germline mutation in the tumor-supressor *STK11* gene (also called *LKB1*) located on 19p. The *STK11* gene product is a serine threonine kinase involved in the transduction of intracellular growth signals. Mutations in *STK11* can be documented in about one half of the families with Peutz–Jeghers syndrome. Some mutations may not be readily detectable by the methods generally employed, but it also is possible that some families with Peutz–Jeghers syndrome may be the consequence of germline mutations in other genes, possibly one or more of those in the STK11 molecular pathway. As with familial adenomatous polyposis testing, if a pathogenic gene alteration can be detected in an affected family member, non-affected family members can then be tested with essentially 100% accuracy.

Screening, surveillance, and treatment

Though the lifetime risk of cancer in Peutz–Jeghers syndrome is extremely high, the ability to reduce cancer incidence and cancer-related mortality in patients with Peutz–Jeghers syndrome through intensive screening and surveillance remains unproven. Surveillance guidelines for Peutz–Jeghers syndrome remain empirical and have not been formally adopted by any of the major professional organizations (Box 8.3). However, most experts recommend surveillance and they further recommend that any intestinal polyps encountered, especially those greater than 1 to 1.5 cm in size be removed, even if that requires laparotomy and intraoperative endoscopy.

Juvenile polyposis

Clinical features Juvenile polyps are common, occurring in about 2% of children. Typically, the polyps are few in number. Juvenile polyposis is defined as the presence of 10 or more juvenile polyps. Approximately one third of cases of juvenile polyposis have a hereditary etiology, while the others are sporadic. Hereditary juvenile polyposis is rare (1 in 100 000 individuals). Histologically juvenile polyps are hamartomas with a characteristic hyperplastic appearance of the surface epithelium, expansion of the lamina propria and frequent cyst formation with mucus engorgement. The characteristic cystically dilated glands have led these polyps also to be termed juvenile retention polyps. The polyps can range in size from several millimeters to several centimeters, and they may be sessile

Box 8.3 Cancer prevention options in Peutz–Jeghers syndrome

Upper endoscopy every 2 years starting at age 10 to 15 years.
Enteroscopy/small-bowel X-ray (small bowel follow-through or enteroclysis) every 2 years starting at age 10 to 15 years.
Colonoscopy every 3 years starting at age 15 to 20 years.
Removal of all polyps found larger than 1 to 1.5 cm (either by endoscopy methods or at laparatomy with intra-operative endoscopy).
Endoscopic ultrasound or MRCP every 1 to 2 years starting at age 30 years.
Annual breast examination and mammography starting at age 25 years.
Annual pelvic examination, pap smear, transvaginal ultrasound and CA-125 levels starting at age 20 to 25 years.
Annual testicular examination starting at age 10 years, with testicular ultrasound for onset of feminizing features.

or pedunculated, more often the latter. Juvenile polyps are most commonly found in the colorectum, but in hereditary juvenile polyposis, they can be found throughout the gastrointestinal tract as well as in the colorectum. In contrast to individuals with sporadic juvenile polyps, those with hereditary juvenile polyposis will continue to form polyps throughout their lifetime.

The primary clinical manifestation of juvenile polyposis is colorectal bleeding. The blood loss may be occult, with subsequent development of iron deficiency anemia, or overt gastrointestinal bleeding may occur. Bleeding from juvenile polyps is one of the leading causes of lower gastrointestinal hemorrhage among children.

As with the other hereditary hamartomatous polyp syndromes, juvenile polyposis is associated with an increased risk for colorectal cancer. Increased cancer risk is not seen among individuals with sporadic juvenile polyps. The exact magnitude of the risk in hereditary juvenile polyposis remains uncertain, but may approach that seen in familial adenomatous polyposis. Cancer risk is certainly increased many-fold. Colorectal cancer occurs in juvenile polyposis patients at a young age, often in their mid-thirties. Cancer will arise from a juvenile polyp that has developed dysplastic/adenomatous features, and therefore, increased cancer risk can extend to other segments of the bowel involved with polyps. Individuals with many polyps with mixed histological features of juvenile polyps and adenomas are termed as having hereditary mixed polyposis sydrome. However, colorectal cancer can occur in individuals with no prior evidence of dysplastic polyps. What is not entirely certain is if there is an increased risk for extracolonic cancer in the absence of polyps in that segment of bowel, or if there is an increased risk of extraintestinal cancer, such as pancreatic cancer.

Genetics Hereditary juvenile polyposis is an autosomal dominant disorder, and disease-causing germline mutations can be found in about 50% of patients. The majority of mutations are found in *SMAD4*, located on 18q, and commercial genetic testing is available. *SMAD4* is a tumor suppressor gene of importance in the development of sporadic pancreatic and colorectal cancer, among others. *SMAD4* is a critical component of the growth inhibitory *TGF* signaling pathway. Some juvenile polyposis families are found to have disease-causing mutations in the *PTEN* gene (see below), or in the bone morphogenetic protein receptor 1A *(BMPR1A)* gene. *BMPR1A* is a serine-threonine kinase type receptor belonging to the superfamily of *TGF* receptors involved in growth inhibitory signaling.

Screening, surveillance, and treatment No formal screening or surveillance recommendations exist for hereditary juvenile polyposis. In asymptomatic children from families with the syndrome, complete colonoscopy should commence in the early teen years and should be repeated every 1 to 3 years depending on the size and number of polyps found. Polyps found should be removed. In hereditary juvenile polyposis, as with all the hereditary polyposis syndromes, polyps will continue to recur throughout the patient's lifetime. If the number of polyps is great, especially if polyps with dysplastic features are encountered, colectomy is indicated. At the time that colonic polyps are detected, upper endoscopy and small-bowel contrast X-rays should be performed to look for extracolonic polyps. If none is found, repeat upper gastrointestinal screening examinations may be performed approximately every 3 years.

Cowden syndrome

Clinical features Cowden syndrome, also termed the gingival multiple hamartoma syndrome, is a rare syndrome (1 in 200 000 individuals) characterized by skin lesions, intestinal hamartomas, and an increased risk of cancer. The syndrome is hereditary with an autosomal dominant means of transmission. The syndrome is most widely recognized on the basis of characteristic mucocutaneous lesions that include facial trichilemmomas, acral keratoses, café-au-lait spots, and verrucous papules of the oral mucosa, gingiva, and tongue. Subcutaneous lipomas and fibromas are common, as are benign thyroid nodules, uterine leiomyomas, and fibrocystic disease of the breast. The characteristic cutaneous lesions are found in approximately 85% of patients with Cowden syndrome. Sixty per cent of patients with Cowden syndrome develop hamartomatous polyps of the gastrointestinal tract. The gastrointestinal polyps most often resemble juvenile polyps, but other benign gastrointestinal-tract polyps can occur as well, including lipomas, ganglioneuromas, inflammatory polyps, and lymphoid hyperplasia. Juvenile-type polyps that contain some neural elements are particularly characteristic of the syndrome.

The syndrome is often associated with congenital abnormalities (50% of cases) that include craniomegaly and mental retardation. Families with macrocephaly, lipomas, and pigmentation of the glans penis belong to the Bannayan–Ruvalcaba–Riley syndrome (syndrome variations have been termed the Soto syndrome, the Ruvalcaba–Myhre sydrome, and the Bannyan–Zonana syndrome), while those with glial mass in the cerebellum leading to altered gait and seizures belong to the sub-syndrome called Lhermitte–Duclos disease.

Cowden syndrome is a cancer susceptibility syndrome, and cancer is the primary cause of morbidity and mortality among affected individuals. The lifetime incidence of breast cancer among women with Cowden syndrome is 25% to 50%, the cancer is often bilateral and has an early age of onset (median age 41 years). Individuals with Cowden syndrome also have a lifetime risk of follicular carcinoma of the thyroid that approaches 10%. Though many affected individuals have gastrointestinal-tract hamartomas, an excess of gastrointestinal cancer risk has not been clearly described. There is probably a modest increased risk for colorectal cancer among individuals with colorectal hamartomas. An increased risk of other cancers is also likely, including skin, ovary, uterus, lung, and kidney.

Criteria for the diagnosis of Cowden syndrome are listed in Box 8.4.

Genetics Cowden syndrome, and its associated sub-syndromes, are caused by a germline mutation in the tumor supressor gene *PTEN* on 10q. *PTEN* is an intracellular tyrosine phosphatase that has been shown to be mutated in a significant percentage of sporadic tumors, including glioblastomas and

> **Box 8.4** International Cowden syndrome consortium operational criteria for the diagnosis of the syndrome
>
> Pathognomonic criteria
>   Mucocutaneous lesions
>   facial trichilemmomas
>   acral keratoses
>   papillomatous papules
>   mucosal lesions.
>   Major criteria
>   breast carcinoma
>   thyroid carcinoma, especially follicular type
>   macrocephaly (≤ 97 percentile)
>   Lhermitte–Duclos disease.
>   Minor criteria
>   other thyroid lesions (adenoma, multinodular goiter)
>   mental retardation (IQ ≤ 75)
>   gastrointestinal hamartomas
>   fibrocystic breast disease
>   lipomas
>   fibromas
>   genitourinary tumors.
>
> Operational diagnosis in an individual
>   Mucocutaneous lesions alone if any of the following are present
>   six or more facial papules, of which at least three must be trichilemmomas
>   cutaneous facial papules and oral mucosal papillomatosis
>   oral mucosal papillomatosis and acral keratoses
>   six or more palmoplantar keratoses.
>   Two major criteria, but one must include macrocephaly or Lhermitte–Duclos disease.
>   One major and three minor criteria.
>   Four minor criteria.
> Operational diagnosis in a family where one individual is already diagnostic for Cowden syndrome
>   Any of pathognomonic criteria.
>   Any major criterion.
>   Two minor criteria.

prostate, thyroid, and kidney cancers. *PTEN*-mutation testing is commercially available, and mutations can be detected in about 90% of affected individuals. Principles of clinical genetic testing would mirror those in familial adenomatous polyposis, Peutz–Jeghers syndrome, and hereditary juvenile polyposis.

Screening, surveillance, and treatment The major cancer morbidity from Cowden syndrome is secondary to breast cancer. Breast cancer surveillance should commence at the age of 20 years (monthly self examination and yearly physician examination and mammography). Annual thyroid examinations are recommended to start in the teens. No guidelines regarding gastrointestinal screening or surveillance have been established. Upon diagnosis, it makes sense to perform upper and lower gastrointestinal endoscopy to look for gastrointestinal polyps. Among individuals with gastrointestinal polyps, regular surveillance and polypectomy is wise. Those without polyps initially might undergo screening colonoscopy starting at age 40 years, with repeat examinations every 3 to 5 years.

Gorlin syndrome

Gorlin syndrome is a rare autosomal dominantly inherited condition (1 in 55 000 people) characterized by multiple basal cell nevi and carcinomas. The condition is also called the basal cell nevus syndrome and accounts for about 0.5% of individuals with basal cell carcinoma. The carcinomas often first occur before 30 years of age, with 90% of affected individuals with cancer by the age of 40 years. Other features of the syndrome include odontogenic or polyostotic bone cysts, facial congenital defects including macrocephaly, cleft lip, or palate, congenital skeletal abnormalities of the ribs and/or spine, ectopic calcification of the falx cerebri, cardiac or ovarian fibromas, medulloblastoma, and characteristic pits of the skin of the palms and soles (three or more pits). Rarely, gastrointestinal hamartomas occur. The syndrome is caused by a germline mutation in the *PTC* gene on 9q. Spontaneous germline mutations of *PTC* are the cause of Gorlin syndrome in greater than 50% of cases.

Hereditary neural polyposis syndromes

Neurofibromatosis type 1

Neurofibromatosis type 1, also called von Recklinghsausen disease, is defined by the presence of café-au-lait spots (five or more greater than 0.5 cm), multiple cutaneous or subcutaneuos neurofibromas, multiple axillary or inguinal freckles, bilateral optic nerve gliomas, multiple hamartomas of the iris, and congenital abnormalities of the long bones (bowing or thinning of the cortex). Seizures are reported in 3% to 5% of affected individuals, and learning disabilities in 25% to 40%. This condition is caused by the autosomal dominant inheritance of a mutated *NF1* gene located on 17q. *NF1* encodes a guanosine triphosphatase-activating protein. Approximately 25% of patients with *NF1* have intestinal polypoid neurofibromas or ganglioneuromas. The polyps are most commonly found in the small bowel, but can occur in the stomach and colon as well. In most cases, the polyps are clinically silent, but rarely they cause abdominal pain or hemorrhage.

Multiple endocrine neoplasia type 2

Multiple endocrine neoplasia type 2 is characterized by the presence of medullary carcinoma of the thyroid, pheochromocytoma, parathyroid hyperplasia or adenomas, marfanoid habitus, and ganglioneuromas of the gastrointestinal tract. The ganglioneuromas occur in nearly all patients with multiple endocrine neoplasia type 2B, they occur throughout the gastrointestinal tract but are most common in the colorectum. The polyps are often clinically silent. However, generalized dysmotility of the gastrointestinal tract is often associated with the disease, and may be in part secondary to the intestinal ganglioneuromas. Multiple endocrine neoplasia type 2 is caused by a germline mutation in the *RET* proto-oncogene. The condition is transmitted in autosomal dominant fashion, though about 50% of cases are secondary to a spontaneous, new, germline mutation.

Sporadic polyposis syndromes

Hyperplastic polyposis

Hyperplastic polyposis is defined as the presence of ten or more typical colorectal hyperplastic polyps. Most cases of hyperplastic polyposis involve the occurrence of diminutive (one to several millimeters) polyps located in the rectum and left colon. This phenomenon is likely to be sporadic in etiology and not associated with an increased risk for colorectal cancer. Rarely patients may have tens to hundreds of diminutive hyperplastic polyps throughout the colon, simulating familial adenomatous polyposis. Whether or not cancer risk is increased in these patients is unclear. Very rarely, patients with hyperplastic polyposis have giant (up to 2 to 3 cm) polyps, often found in the proximal colon. In this circumstance an increased risk for colorectal cancer is likely, though the magnitude of the risk remains uncertain. Some experts recommend polypectomy for these large hyperplastic polyps and increased colonic surveillance in these patients. However, the risks and benefits of this approach are uncertain and such recommendations remain controversial. If the hyperplastic polyps have a mixed hyperpastic/adenomatous histology, the polyps are properly classified as being serrated adenomas. When serrated polyposis is present, the increased risk for colorectal cancer is clear, and the polyps must be removed, if possible by endoscopy, or by colectomy. The genetic basis of hyperplastic or serrated polyposis is uncertain. The molecular pathway to the giant hyperplastic polyp and/or serrated adenoma may be the consequence of the CpG island methylator phenotype, with promoter methylation and inactivation of the hyperplastic polyposis 1 gene (*HPP1*) on 2q. Whether or not some cases of hyperplastic polyposis are hereditary is unclear. Most cases appear to be sporadic. However, the hyperplastic/serrated polyposis has been described in families, suggesting a hereditary component in a minority of cases.

Cronkhite–Canada syndrome

Cronkhite–Canada syndrome is not a hereditary disease but rather is an acquired condition with onset occurring on average during the sixth to seventh decade of life. No familial occurrences of Cronkhite–Canada syndrome have been reported. The syndrome is extremely rare, with a worldwide distribution, and it has no known cause. Cronkhite–Canada syndrome is more common in men (60%) than in women, and is characterized by the onset of generalized gastrointestestinal polyposis, with esophageal sparing, in association with cutaneous hyperpigmentation, hair loss, nail atrophy, and hypogeusia. The polyps are sessile and innumerable, and they range in size from several millimeters to several centimeters. On histological examination the polyps resemble juvenile polyps, though dysplastic changes do rarely occur.

Cronkhite–Canada syndrome has an acute onset and is progressive, though symptomatic remission does occur in a minority of cases. The primary clinical manifestations are that of progressive diarrhea, often with significant malabsorption and protein losing enteropathy. Malnutrition is common, and the condition can be fatal. For those with a more protracted course of illness, the lifetime incidence of colorectal cancer exceeds 10%. The primary therapy is supportive care. Patients often require nutritional support and may require total parenteral nutrition to prevent severe dehydration and malnutrition. If a particular segment of the gastrointestinal tract is heavily involved with polyps, then operative resection may be helpful. Other interventions that have been tried with uncertain efficacy include administration of corticosteroids and antibiotics.

Inflammatory polyposis

Inflammatory polyposis, often called pseudopolyps, can occur during the healing phase of any inflammatory-type injury to the gastrointestinal tract. Inflammatory polyps are most commonly seen among individuals with ulcerative colitis or Crohn's disease affecting the colon. They can also occur during the healing phase of other colitides, such as ischemic colitis. The polyps have a characteristic filiform appearance and on histological examination they represent tissues with inflammatory elements that persist during healing. Inflammatory polyps may be few in number, or they may be innumerable, and their size ranges from several millimeters to several centimters. The polyps have no malignant potential themselves, though they are often associated with longstanding chronic colitis and its attendant risk of colitis-related dysplasia and cancer.

Inflammatory polyposis is an acquired condition. However, a case of familial inflammatory intestinal polyposis has been described and termed Devon polyposis.

Lymphomatous polyposis

Multiple lyphomatous polyposis is a rare manifestation of intestinal lymphoma. It is a non-Hodgkin B-cell lymphoma that appears to be the gastrointestinal counterpart of mantle cell lymphoma, and extraintestinal lymphoma is often present. Multiple nodular/ polypoid lesions of the gastrointestinal tract also may be seen in Mediterranean-type lymphoma. Mediterranean-type lymphoma of the gut begins as an intense proliferation of plasma cells in the lamina propria, with eventual malignant transformation. This lymphoma is almost always associated with production of an abnormal immunoglobulin A paraprotein.

Hereditary non-polyposis colorectal cancer

Clinical features Hereditary non-polyposis colorectal cancer, like familial adenomatous polyposis is an autosomal dominant disorder characterized by the occurrence of multiple colorectal cancers in a family. Hereditary non-polyposis colorectal cancer is also called the Lynch syndrome after Henry Lynch, MD, a pioneer in the field of familial cancer, who has devoted much of his career to the description of the syndrome and the care of affected families. Hereditary non-polyposis colorectal cancer accounts for approximately 1% to 5% of all colorectal cancer cases. Hereditary non-polyposis colorectal cancer is a misnomer because adenomatous polyps are the precursor of colorectal cancer in the syndrome. Unlike familial adenomatous polyposis, the number of polyps appears no greater than in the general population, but the polyps are far more likely to have villous features or high-grade dysplasia and, more importantly, to grow rapidly and progress to invasive cancer. Population-based data on hereditary non-polyposis colorectal cancer gene carriers are few, but individuals with this condition appear to have a lifetime risk of colorectal cancer of about 80%. The mean age of onset of colorectal cancer in hereditary non-polyposis colorectal cancer is approximately 45 years, but it may appear in the teens. Furthermore, synchronous and metachronous colorectal cancer is far more common in hereditary non-polyposis colorectal cancer than in sporadic colorectal cancer. Synchronous cancers present in 5% to 20% of patients and the rate of metachronous cancers approaches 1% to 3% per year, depending on the length of colon remaining after initial resection. This represents a five- to ten-fold increase in the rate of metachronous cancers compared with the sporadic colorectal cancer. Also, compared with sporadic colorectal cancer, hereditary non-polyposis colorectal cancers are more commonly on the right side of the colon, more poorly differentiated, and have other unusual histological characteristics, such as abundant extracellular mucin or lymphoid host response to the tumor. None the less, several studies have found that survival is better than in sporadic cancer when matched for stage.

The risk for other cancers in hereditary non-polyposis colorectal cancer is greatly increased. For example, endometrial cancer will occur in 20% to 60% of women with hereditary non-polyposis colorectal cancer, as compared with 3% in the general population. Individuals with hereditary non-polyposis colorectal cancer, are also at an increased risk of gastric, ovarian, small-bowel, transitional cell (renal pelvis, ureter), sebaceous, central nervous system, and possibly other cancers (Table 8.3). When hereditary non-polyposis colorectal cancer was first described in the 1920s, gastric cancer was the primary malignancy. The decreasing frequency of gastric cancers and increasing frequency of colorectal cancers in hereditary non-polyposis colorectal cancer kindred has mirrored this change in the general population. The occurrence of sebaceous adenomas, carcinomas, and keratoacanthomas in conjunction with hereditary non-polyposis colorectal cancer-related visceral malignancies define the Muir–Torre syndrome, a variant of hereditary non-polyposis colorectal cancer. Some cases of Turcot syndrome are also variants of hereditary non-polyposis colorectal cancer, with glioblastoma as the associated central nervous system cancer.

Diagnostic criteria Obtaining a personal and family cancer history from all patients is critical, and a high index of suspicion needs to be maintained if individuals with hereditary non-polyposis colorectal cancer are to be detected. Many diagnostic criteria have been proposed for hereditary non-polyposis colorectal cancer, the best known of which are the Amsterdam criteria

1. histologically verified colorectal cancer in three or more relatives, one of whom is a first-degree relative of the other two, having excluded familial adenomatous polyposis
2. colorectal cancer involving at least two generations
3. one or more of the colorectal cancers diagnosed before the age of 50 years.

The criteria were designed to be specific to facilitate research on hereditary non-polyposis colorectal cancer in the days before the mutations responsible for the syndrome had been identified. However, the Amsterdam criteria are overly restrictive, and a large number of individuals who may have hereditary non-polyposis colorectal cancer will be missed if these are the sole criteria used for considering the diagnosis in the clinical setting. In response to this problem, a number of other less stringent diagnostic criteria and guidelines for hereditary non-polyposis colorectal cancer have been promulgated, including the Amsterdam II criteria and the Bethesda guidelines (Table 8.4). At the heart of all of these criteria are certain basic features that are typical of hereditary non-polyposis colorectal cancer

- early age of onset of colorectal or endometrial cancer (less than 50 years of age)
- multiple family members with colorectal, endometrial, or another hereditary non-polyposis colorectal-related cancer
- multiple hereditary non-polyposis colorectal-related cancers in the same individual.

If one or more of these features is identified, the diagnosis of hereditary non-polyposis colorectal cancer should be considered. It should be pointed out, however, that the personal and family cancer history need not be very striking in cases of hereditary non-polyposis colorectal cancer detected in the general population, so vigilance is required.

Genetics The genetic basis of hereditary non-polyposis colorectal cancer is a germline mutation in one of a set of genes responsible for DNA mismatch repair. The growing number of mismatch repair genes include *MSH2*, *MLH1*, *PMS1*, *PMS2*, *MSH3*, *MSH6*, and others. Over 90% of the identified mutations are in two genes, *MSH2* and *MLH1*, located on chromosomes 2 p and 3 p respectively. Upwards of 5% to 10% of mismatch repair hereditary non-polyposis colorectal cancer families will be accounted for by a germline mutation in *MSH6*. Persons with hereditary non-polyposis colorectal cancer have a non-functioning copy of the gene in the germline, usually through an inherited, or occasionally spontaneous, germline mutation. When the remaining working copy of the gene is inactivated by mutation, loss, or other mechanisms, the cell loses the ability to repair the inevitable mismatches of DNA base pairs during DNA replication, as well as short insertion and deletion loops.

Particularly vulnerable to mutation during replication are DNA regions in which nucleotide bases are repeated several or many times. Such DNA repeat sequences are distributed throughout the genome

Table 8.3 Lifetime risk for cancer among hereditary non-polyposis rectal cancer gene carriers.

Cancer type	Lifetime risk
Colorectal	70%–80%
Endometrial	20%–60%
Ovarian	10%–12%
Gastric	5%–13%
Renal pelvis/ureter/kidney	4%–10%
Biliary tract/gallbladder/pancreas	2%–18%
Small bowel	1%–4%
Central nervous system (usually glioblastoma)	1%–4%

Table 8.4	Clinical criteria for hereditary non-polyposis rectal cancer.
Name	Criteria
Amsterdam	There should be at least three relatives with colorectal cancer; all the following criteria should be present: one should be the first-degree relative of the other two; at least two successive generations should be affected; at least one colorectal cancer should be diagnosed before age 50 years; familial adenomatous polyposis should be excluded.
Amsterdam II	There should be at least three relatives with a hereditary non-polyposis rectal cancer-associated cancer (colorectal cancer, cancer of the endometrium, small bowel, ureter, or renal pelvis). All the following criteria should be present: one should be the first-degree relative of the other two; at least two successive generations should be affected; at least one colorectal should be diagnosed before the age of 50 years; familial adenomatous polyposis should be excluded.
Bethesda (modified)	Individuals with cancer in families that fulfill the Amsterdam criteria. Individuals with two hereditary non-polyposis rectal cancer-related cancers, including synchronous or metachronous colorectal cancers or associated extra-colonic cancers. Individuals with colorectal cancer and a first-degree relative with colorectal cancer, and/or hereditary non-polyposis rectal cancer-related extracolonic cancer, and/or colorectal adenoma; one of the cancers diagnosed before the age of 50 years and the adenoma diagnosed before the age of 40 years. Individuals with colorectal cancer or endometrial cancer diagnosed before the age of 50 years. Individuals with right-sided colorectal cancer with an undifferentiated pattern (solid/cribriform) on histopathology diagnosed before the age of 50 years. Individuals with signet-ring-cell-type colorectal cancer diagnosed before the age of 50 years. Individuals with adenomas diagnosed before the age of 40 years.

(most commonly A_n/T_n or CA_n/GT_n), and are called microsatellites. Greater than 90% of colorectal cancers in hereditary non-polyposis colorectal cancer demonstrate multiple change-of-length mutations of these microsatellites, termed microsatellite instability. Microsatellite instability is classified as being absent, low, or high depending on the frequency of microsatellite mutation. The instability of hereditary non-polyposis colorectal cancer tumors is almost always high frequency. Microsatellites are found in the coding regions of genes involved in growth regulation such as the gene for the transforming growth factor β (TGFβ) receptor type II and *BAX*. Mutations of these genes are common in tumors with high frequency microsatellite instability. The binding of TGFβ with its receptor is important in the inhibition of cellular proliferation as is *BAX* in the induction of programed cell death (apoptosis). A simple laboratory assay can detect the presence or absence and degree of microsatellite instability in tumor tissue using a standard set of microsatellite markers (Table 8.5). In addition, tumors that have lost the function of one of the mismatch repair genes show negative staining for the protein product of that gene by immunohistochemistry. Staining tumors for MSH2 or MLH1 may also aide in the diagnosis of hereditary non-polyposis colorectal cancer.

As with *APC*, the specific mutations in the mismatch repair genes (genotype) correlate with the observed phenotype. For example, extracolonic tumors are more common with *MSH2* mutation than *MLH1* mutation. Families with an *MSH6* mutation tend to have a more attenuated phenotype (later age of onset and lower percentage of gene carriers developing cancer) and an abundance of endometrial cancers when compared with *MSH2* or *MLH1* gene-carrying families. As in familial adenomatous polyposis, a better understanding of genotype–phenotype correlation will lead to improved

Table 8.5 International guidelines for evaluation of microsatellite instability (MSI) in colorectal cancer.

Microsatellite markers loci	Microsatellite type
BAT25	mononucleotide
BAT26	mononucleotide
D5S346	dinucleotide
D2S123	dinucleotide
D17S250	dinucleotide
Interpretation	
MSI-high	≥ 2 positive (> 30%–40% if more than 5 loci evaluated)
MSI-low	1 positive, (30%–40% if more than 5 loci evaluated)
Microsatellite stable	0 positive

hereditary non-polyposis colorectal cancer screening, surveillance, and treatment.

Genetic testing for hereditary non-polyposis colorectal cancer, as well as tumor analysis for microsatellite instability and mismatch repair protein immunostaining, is commercially available. Molecular diagnostics for hereditary non-polyposis colorectal cancer is now recommended and, in the correct circumstances, can greatly facilitate the care of individuals and families suspected of having the syndrome (see below).

Screening, surveillance, and treatment

Recommendations for screening and surveillance in individuals with known or suspected hereditary non-polyposis colorectal cancer are summarized in Box 8.5. Colonoscopy is recommended every 1 to 3 years staring at the age of 20 years, or at least 10 years before the earliest age of cancer in the family. Some experts have recommended that the frequency of screening be increased to yearly starting at the age of 40 years. Complete colonoscopy is essential because the preponderance of right-sided tumors in cases of hereditary non-polyposis colorectal cancer. Colonoscopy needs to be repeated frequently because of the accelerated rate at which adenomas transform into invasive cancer in hereditary non-polyposis colorectal cancer. Colonoscopic screening is of demonstrated efficacy in hereditary non-polyposis colorectal cancer. Individuals that undergo regular total colonic screening have a markedly lower incidence of colorectal cancer, colorectal cancer-related mortality and all causes of mortality, than those not undergoing regular screening.

In addition to colorectal cancer screening, screening for endometrial cancer is recommended for individuals at risk for hereditary non-polyposis colorectal cancer. There is no consensus on the optimal method of screening, but choices include yearly endometrial biopsy or yearly transvaginal ultrasound. The latter method of screening may be problematic in premenopausal women, but has the advantage of serving a screening test for ovarian cancer, especially if coupled with a regular (every 6 to 12 months) determination of cancer cell surface antigen 125 levels. Screening for other hereditary non-polyposis colorectal-related cancers is not recommended generally. However, in families in which certain tumors are seen, screening recommendations are often made in the clinical setting. For example, genitourinary cancers may be screened by periodic urine cytology and gastric cancer by upper gastrointestinal endoscopy. All screening in hereditary non-polyposis colorectal cancer, with the exception of that for colorectal cancer, remains unproven in efficacy.

With respect to treatment for hereditary non-polyposis colorectal cancer, many experts advocate total abdominal colectomy with ileorectal anastomosis at the time of the initial cancer resection, because of the high rate of metachronous tumors. However, what appears to be most important is adequate postoperative surveillance, rather than the extent of the initial resection. As with familial adenomatous polyposis, the rate of rectal cancer in hereditary non-polyposis colorectal cancer can exceed 10% over an extended follow-up period, so ongoing surveillance is essential, even if an ileorectal anastomosis is performed. When adenomas are encountered during screening or surveillance colonoscopy, they are removed endoscopically using standard techniques, and in general, colonoscopic surveillance is continued. However, hereditary non-polyposis colorectal cancer-related polyps are often sessile, so adequate endoscopic resection can be difficult to perform. If there is any doubt, one should proceed with operative resection. Because of the high risk of endometrial and ovarian cancer, some experts have advocated prophylactic hysterectomy and oopherectomy for women who have completed

Box 8.5 Options for cancer prevention in hereditary non-polyposis rectal cancer for known or suspected gene mutation carriers

Primary recommendations
 Colonoscopy every 1 to 2 years beginning at age 20 to 25 years (or 10 years before the earliest diagnosis of colorectal cancer in the family, whichever comes first) until age 40 years and then annual colonoscopy.
 Annual transvaginal ultrasound with color Doppler and/or endometrial aspirate beginning at age 25 to 35 years.
Secondary recommendations
 Consider total abdominal colectomy with ileorectal anastomosis at diagnosis of colorectal cancer.
 Consider prophylactic hysterectomy and oopherectomy in known gene carriers at the time of colonic operation, or after child bearing is complete.
 Consider annual measure of cancer cell surface antigen 125 level.
 Consider serial upper endoscopy among families with gastric cancer.
 Consider annual urine cytology among families with urinary tract cancers.

child bearing, especially if they are undergoing a colonic resection for colorectal cancer. A recent panel of experts, however, found insufficient evidence to recommend for or against prophylactic hysterectomy and oophorectomy.

Common familial colorectal cancer

Clinical features The rare hereditary syndromes, such as familial adenomatous polyposis and hereditary non-polyposis colorectal cancer confer the highest risks of colon cancer, however, these entities account for no more than 5% of all colorectal cancers. Nevertheless, familial history is an important risk factor in the development of colorectal cancer, suggesting a critical hereditary component in more than 25% of cases. The magnitude of the risk depends on the number of first-degree relatives affected and the age at diagnosis (Table 8.6). In a recent meta-analysis, individuals with a single first-degree relative with colorectal cancer have a risk about 2.25 times that in the general population. Individuals with more than one first-degree relative with colorectal cancer have a risk about 4.25 times that in the general population, and individuals with a relative diagnosed with colorectal cancer before the age of 45 have a risk about four times higher than the general population. Individuals with a first-degree relative with colorectal adenoma also have a risk of colon cancer about twice that in the general population. Colon cancer in a second- or third-degree relative increases the risk of colon cancer, but it is only about 50% above the average risk. Importantly, individuals with a first-degree relative with a family history of colon cancer have a colon cancer risk at age 40 years which is similar to the general population risk at age 50 years (Figure 8.3). Though family history of colorectal cancer increases an individual's risk for the disease, especially at a younger age than is seen in cases of pure sporadic cancer, there is no convincing evidence yet that the clinical presentation of these common familial colorectal cancers differ in important ways from sporadic colorectal cancer with respect to features such as tumor location or aggressiveness.

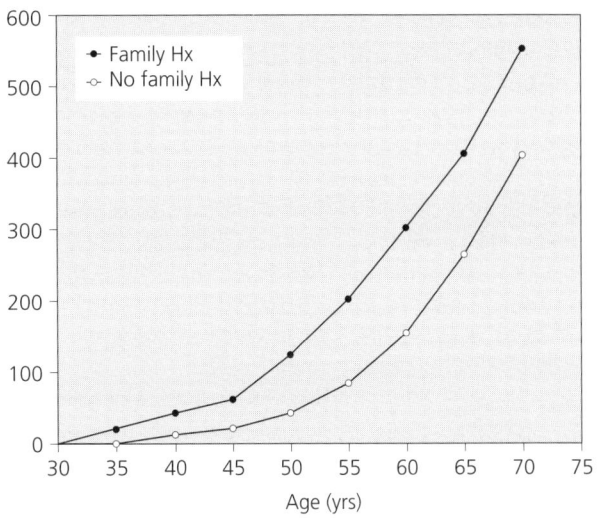

Figure 8.3 Cumulative incidence of colorectal cancer according to age and the presence or absence of a family history of the disease (modified from Fuchs CS, et al: *New Engl J Med* 331: 169–174; 1994, Figure 1, page 1672).

Genetics The gene alterations responsible for common familial colorectal cancer are being discovered in increasingly greater numbers, though for the most part these cancer susceptibility alleles remain unknown. Kindred studies suggest that these genes are dominantly inherited, but unlike in true hereditary colorectal cancer, the altered genes that cause familial colorectal cancer are generally low penetrance. This means that inheriting a disease susceptibility gene increases one's risk for colorectal cancer, but by no means guarantees that the disease will occur. Candidate susceptibility alleles are many and include minor mutations in the same genes that cause hereditary colorectal cancer. An

Table 8.6 Risk for colorectal cancer based on family history.

Family history	Lifetime risk for colorectal cancer
No family history	3%–6%
One first-degree relative with colorectal cancer	2–3 fold increased risk
One first-degree degree relative with colorectal cancer under age 50 years	3–5 fold increased risk
Two first-degree degree relatives with colorectal cancer	3–5 fold increased risk
One second-degree or third-degree degree relative with colorectal cancer	1.5 fold increased risk
Two second-degree or third-degree degree relative with colorectal cancer	2–3 fold increased risk
One first-degree degree relative with adenoma	1.5–2 fold increased risk

example of this is the *I1307K* allele of *APC* found in Ashkenazi Jews. The allele carries an adenine at nucleotide 3920 rather than the normal thymine. This results in a conversion of an A_3TA_4 nucleotide sequence to an A_8 sequence and an isoleucine to lysine difference at amino acid 1307. The protein product of the *APC I1307K* allele is full length and functional. However, owing to the A_8 nucleotide sequence, the allele is over thirty times more likely to mutate than the wild-type allele, most commonly through the insertion of an additional adenine that leads to APC protein truncation. Inheritance of this unstable *APC* allele increases the chance of developing colorectal cancer by approximately one and a half to two-fold, rather than the near 100% risk of colorectal cancer that occurs in classic familial adenomatous polyposis. In the original report I1307K was found in 6.1% of all Ashkenazi Jews tested, in 10.4% of those with colorectal cancer, and 28% with colorectal cancer and a positive family history of the disease. A recent large community-based study of Ashkenazi Jews estimated that by the age of 70 years, 5.1% of allele carriers will develop colorectal cancer compared with 3.1% of non-carriers. It appears that the magnitude of increased risk conferred by carriage of *APC I1307K* is low to modest, and there is no evidence to suggest that colorectal cancer in those with *I1307K* appears at an earlier age or that it differs in presentation or prognosis from sporadic cancer. Nevertheless, even a small increase in colorectal cancer risk conferred by a gene that is common in a particular population will have important implications for that population.

The *I1307K APC* allele is only one example of the minor colorectal cancer susceptibility genes that will be identified with increasing frequency in the future. Other colorectal cancer predisposition alleles are likely to include one of a number of variants of genes involved in carcinogen metabolism, or certain inherited alleles of many of the oncogenes and tumor suppressor genes involved in the molecular progression of sporadic colorectal cancer. Colorectal cancer resistance genes will be described as well. The particular combination of minor susceptibility and resistance genes that a person inherits will prove to be a major determinant of the differing risk of colorectal cancer between individuals.

Screening, surveillance, and treatment

Several different screening recommendations for individuals with familial risk have been published (Table 8.7). A recent task force, comprising several different professional organizations, recommended that colorectal cancer screening in individuals with a family history of colorectal cancer be the same as the screening recommended for the general public, but that this screening start at age 40 years. Screening options for the general population include yearly fecal occult blood testing, or flexible sigmoidoscopy every 5 years, or both, or air-contrast barium enema every 5 to 10 years, or colonoscopy every 10 years. The task force also recommended that special efforts be made to ensure compliance particularly for those in whom the relative had an adenomatous polyp before the age of 60 years or colon cancer before the age of 55 years. In contrast, the American College of Gastroenterology recommends that individuals with a strong family history of colon cancer, for example those with multiple first-degree relatives with colorectal cancer, or a single first-degree relative with cancer diagnosed before the age of 60 years, should undergo screening colonoscopy starting at age 40 years, or 10 years younger than the age at diagnosis of the youngest affected relative. They then recommend that colonoscopy be repeated at 3 to 5 year intervals. The US Preventive Services Task Force does not address familial risk outside the hereditary syndromes.

Genetic testing for hereditary colorectal cancer

Available tests

Genetic tests are commercially available for familial adenomatous polyposis, hereditary non-polyposis

Table 8.7 Screening options for persons with common familial colorectal cancer.

Family history	Recommendation
First-degree relative with colorectal cancer or adenomatous polyps diagnosed before the age of 60 years, or two or more first-degree degree relatives with colorectal cancer or adenomatous polyps regardless of age.	Colonoscopy starting at age 40 years, or 10 years before the youngest case in the family, whichever comes first. Repeat examination every 5 years. OR Perform screening as for persons at average risk but begin at age 40 years.

colorectal cancer (*MSH2* and *MLH1*), and the *I1307K APC* allele. Testing for Peutz–Jeghers syndrome, junvenile polyposis, and Cowden syndrome is also becoming available through commercial laboratories. Genetic testing for common familial colorectal cancer will certainly become common in the near future. The germline genetic tests typically are run on DNA extracted from white blood cells obtained from a blood sample. Rarely DNA for testing can be obtained from another source. The commercial and university-affiliated laboratories that provide these tests, the tests themselves, and their costs are constantly changing. An internet reference to laboratories offering testing for patients with heritable disorders is provided by Helix, a computer-based directory funded by the National Center for Biotechnology Information and the National Library of Medicine. The internet address is (*http://www.genetests.org*). The National Cancer Institute maintains a directory of individuals and institutions providing professional cancer genetics services. Information about cancer genetics education, counseling, and testing can often be obtained by contacting local providers listed in this directory. The Cancer Genetics Services Directory can be accessed on-line at (*http://www.cancer.gov/search/geneticsservices*)

Methods of mutation detection

Commercial laboratories employ various methods of mutation detection. Mutation detection in familial adenomatous polyposis and hereditary non-polyposis colorectal cancer is made difficult because the genes are large and the known mutations are scattered throughout the genes. Further, many families harbor their own unique mutation. Unlike many other genetic disorders, a single or a few very common mutations cannot be easily and rapidly detected. Direct gene sequencing remains the most precise method for mutation detection, but is time consuming and expensive even with robotics. Sequencing is not 100% sensitive as it can miss certain mutations such as large genomic deletions or rearrangements, and high specificity can be difficult to achieve because of the detection of numerous simple amino acid alterations (missense changes) that are often harmless polymorphisms but may be deleterious mutations. Because of insufficient data, these DNA alterations are often labeled variants of uncertain significance.

To circumvent searching for all mutations by sequencing, other techniques for screening mutations are employed and sequencing is then used to confirm positives. Single strand conformational polymorphism and denaturing gradient gel electrophoresis rely on the difference in the movement of mutated DNA compared with normal DNA during gel electrophoresis. The *in vitro* synthesized protein assay, also called the protein truncation test, detects the truncated protein product of a mutated gene. As the majority of *APC* mutations truncate the gene product, *in vitro* synthesized protein assay is currently the main test for familial adenomatous polyposis, and its sensitivity is approximately 80%. However, in the near future more sensitive, complete *APC* sequencing will be commercially available. A variety of mutation detection strategies have been employed for the detection of hereditary non-polyposis colorectal cancer mutations. Most commonly now, complete sequencing of *MSH2* and *MLH1* are undertaken directly. Some laboratories also offer other techniques, such as haploconversion or southern blot analysis, in an effort to detect mutations, such as gene promoter mutations or large deletions, that would be missed by sequencing.

Once a particular mutation has been identified in a family, the search for that mutation in other family members can be accomplished rapidly, accurately, and inexpensively. The most commonly used technique relies on the detection of hybridization between the DNA to be tested and a DNA sequence that carries the known mutation. The *APC I1307K* allele can also be detected in this fashion.

Finally, in large families that appear to have hereditary colorectal cancer, but in whom the deleterious mutation cannot be found by the direct gene detection methods outlined above, linkage analysis can be employed to determine which individuals carry the deleterious allele. Linkage analysis is based on the simple fact that two regions of DNA that are in close proximity will tend to segregate together (stay linked) during meiosis. Linkage analysis is possible in both hereditary non-polyposis colorectal cancer and familial adenomatous polyposis, but rarely undertaken.

Microsatellite instability testing and protein immunohistochemistry in hereditary non-polyposis colorectal cancer

Because the large majority of hereditary non-polyposis colorectal cancer-related tumors (90% to 100%) demonstrate high frequency instability

(MSI-H), microsatellite instability testing of tumors is advocated as a way of screening for hereditary non-polyposis colorectal cancer. The microsatellite instability assay can be performed on tissues that have been formalin-fixed and embedded in paraffin. In unselected colorectal tumors the specificity of MSI-H for hereditary non-polyposis colorectal cancer is low because 10% to 15% of all colorectal cancers will demonstrate MSI-H but only 10% to 15% of these are due to a germline hereditary non-polyposis colorectal cancer mutation. As the sensitivity of MSI-H in hereditary non-polyposis colorectal cancer-related tumors is not 100%, some investigators caution that germline hereditary non-polyposis colorectal cancer testing should not be abandoned if MSI-H is not found when the clinical history is compelling. Immunostaining for the mismatch repair gene proteins in tumors has also been advocated as a method of screening for hereditary non-polyposis colorectal cancer prior to germline genetic testing. As with microsatellite instability testing, the absence of protein staining, especially *MLH1*, does not guarantee hereditary non-polyposis colorectal cancer. This is because the mismatch repair gene proteins may be inactivated solely within the tumor (somatic inactivation) in a minority of sporadic cancers. Furthermore, as with microsatellite instability testing, the sensitivity of protein staining is not 100% because gene inactivation can occur, but protein staining may still be present in the tumor. In fact, protein immunostaining is less sensitive than microsatellite instability testing as a screening test for hereditary non-polyposis colorectal cancer. Both tumor microsatellite instability analysis and tumor *MSH2* and *MLH1* protein immunohistochemistry are commercially available.

Genetic counseling and informed consent

Prior to genetic testing for hereditary colorectal cancer, genetic counseling and informed consent are essential. Genetic counseling for hereditary cancer is often best performed by trained genetic counselors in conjunction with physicians who are experts on the disease, such as gastroenterologists, oncologists, or surgeons. Genetic counselors are health care professionals at masters degree level, who are trained in both the psychosocial and medical aspects of inherited disease, and in adult hereditary cancer syndromes. The role of the counselor can be filled by other trained professionals such as nurses or physicians with a special interest and expertise in hereditary cancer.

The genetic counseling process includes constructing and evaluating a pedigree, eliciting and evaluating the personal and family medical history, and providing information about the genetic risk. For those choosing testing, genetic counseling includes pretest counseling, testing, post-test counseling, and follow-up so that clinical genetic laboratory tests are properly interpreted and patients are educated as to appropriate cancer prevention strategies given their level of risk. The counseling process also includes psychosocial assessment, support, and counseling appropriate to a family's culture and ethnicity. Because genetic risk affects biological relatives, contact with these relatives is often essential to collect an accurate family and medical history. Cancer genetic counseling may involve several family members, some of whom may have had cancer, and others who have not and it often involves multiple visits.

Informed consent is a crucial part of the testing process because of the risks of genetic testing. Risks include psychological harm and genetic discrimination. Positive test results may be accompanied by feelings of anger, anxiety, and depression. Even individuals who have already been diagnosed with cancer may be shocked and saddened to learn that this "trait" may be passed on to their children, or that they are at risk for further cancers. Individuals who test negative may experience relief and joy, they may also experience feelings of guilt and shame (survivor guilt) when dealing with the reality that others in the family carry the deleterious gene. Ambiguous results of tests may, over time, lead to more anxiety and depression than that produced by a positive result.

The gravest negative consequence of genetic testing for hereditary colorectal cancer is the possibility of genetic discrimination. Discrimination may be purely social, for example with respect to dating and marriage. Genetic testing also may lead to the inability to obtain or keep either a job or health, life, or disability insurance. Protections are in place to help prevent genetic discrimination against cancer susceptibility gene carriers, but they are imperfect and largely untested. The federal Health Insurance Portability and Accountability Act of 1996 prohibits employers or insurers from excluding individual employees from group health plans or charging them higher premiums based on genetic information. The Health Insurance Portability and Accountability Act does not bar insurers from excluding coverage, raising rates, or capping benefits for all members of the group as long as individuals are not singled out, nor does this legislation protect individually insured persons. Further the

Health Insurance Portability and Accountability Act permits insurers to demand genetic testing as a condition of coverage. Proposed legislation at the federal level to provide further protection against genetic discrimination has broad bipartisan support but has not yet been passed into law. A large number of states have passed laws to protect individuals against insurance and genetic discrimination, but these vary considerably. The impact of state laws can be limited by the Employee Retirement Income Security Act which preempts self-insured employers from many of the state insurance provisions. Parties interested in genetic testing need to seek updated information about the laws in their state. The National Human Genome Research Institute has a web site that provides updated information about public policy and genetic testing (*http://www.nhgri.nih.gov*). Documented insurance discrimination related to genetic testing for hereditary colorectal cancer is exceedingly rare. Furthermore, the hope is that as genetic predisposition testing becomes more common for a plethora of diseases, genetic discrimination will become increasingly untenable. Fear of genetic discrimination should not prevent patients from obtaining beneficial services, such as cancer predisposition testing, but they need to be made cognizant of these issues.

One of the biggest barriers to the full-scale implementation of genetic testing for hereditary colorectal cancer is cost. The genetic tests are expensive, ranging in price from $750 to $2000 for the germline familial adenomatous polyposis or hereditary non-polyposis colorectal cancer tests depending on the test and the vendor. Once a mutation has been identified, the cost of follow-up testing of other family members is far less expensive, often being in the range of $200 to $300 per test. Health insurance companies are increasingly willing to pay for these tests, though patients often remain reluctant to seek coverage because of fear of discrimination.

Indications and strategy for genetic testing in hereditary colorectal cancer

The American Society of Clinical Oncology recommends that cancer predisposition testing be offered only when

1. the person has a strong family history of cancer or very early age of onset of disease
2. the test can be adequately interpreted
3. the results will influence the medical management of the patient or family member.

The American Society of Clinical Oncology recognizes three general categories of indications for genetic testing. In the first category testing may already be considered part of the standard care, in the second category the value of testing is presumed, but not clearly established, and in the third category the benefit of testing is not yet established. There is no doubt that intensive cancer screening among individuals at risk for familial adenomatous polyposis and hereditary non-polyposis colorectal cancer will save lives and has been found to be cost-effective. Detection of familial adenomatous polyposis and hereditary non-polyposis colorectal cancer gene carriers is beneficial because it will improve the efficiency of cancer prevention in families with these conditions by allowing those who do not carry the predisposition allele to avoid costly and burdensome screening tests, and it has also been found to be cost-effective. Therefore, genetic testing for familial adenomatous polyposis and hereditary non-polyposis colorectal cancer falls under the first American Society of Clinical Oncology category and is now the standard of care for families suspected of having these syndromes. Genetic testing for other rare polyposis syndromes, and for the gene alterations that cause common familial colorectal cancer is becoming commercially available, but the benefits of such testing are not yet clearly established.

Familial adenomatous polyposis

Testing for familial adenomatous polyposis mutations is a standard part of the care of affected individuals and families. The indications and strategy for familial adenomatous polyposis testing are summarized in Figure 8.4. Genetic testing of a family with familial adenomatous polyposis should start with an affected family member. If a mutation is found, then at-risk members of the family can proceed to testing. If the mutation is not found in an affected person, it does not mean that familial adenomatous polyposis is not present, but that the test is non-informative (Table 8.8). Because up to one third of individuals with familial adenomatous polyposis have a spontaneous germline *APC* mutation, testing should not be limited to members of classic familial adenomatous polyposis kindred. Individuals with the familial adenomatous polyposis phenotype, but without a family history, are also eligible for testing. As minors can develop polyposis and therefore require cancer screening, predisposition testing of minors is appropriate, though

Intestinal Polyposis Syndromes and Hereditary Colorectal Cancer

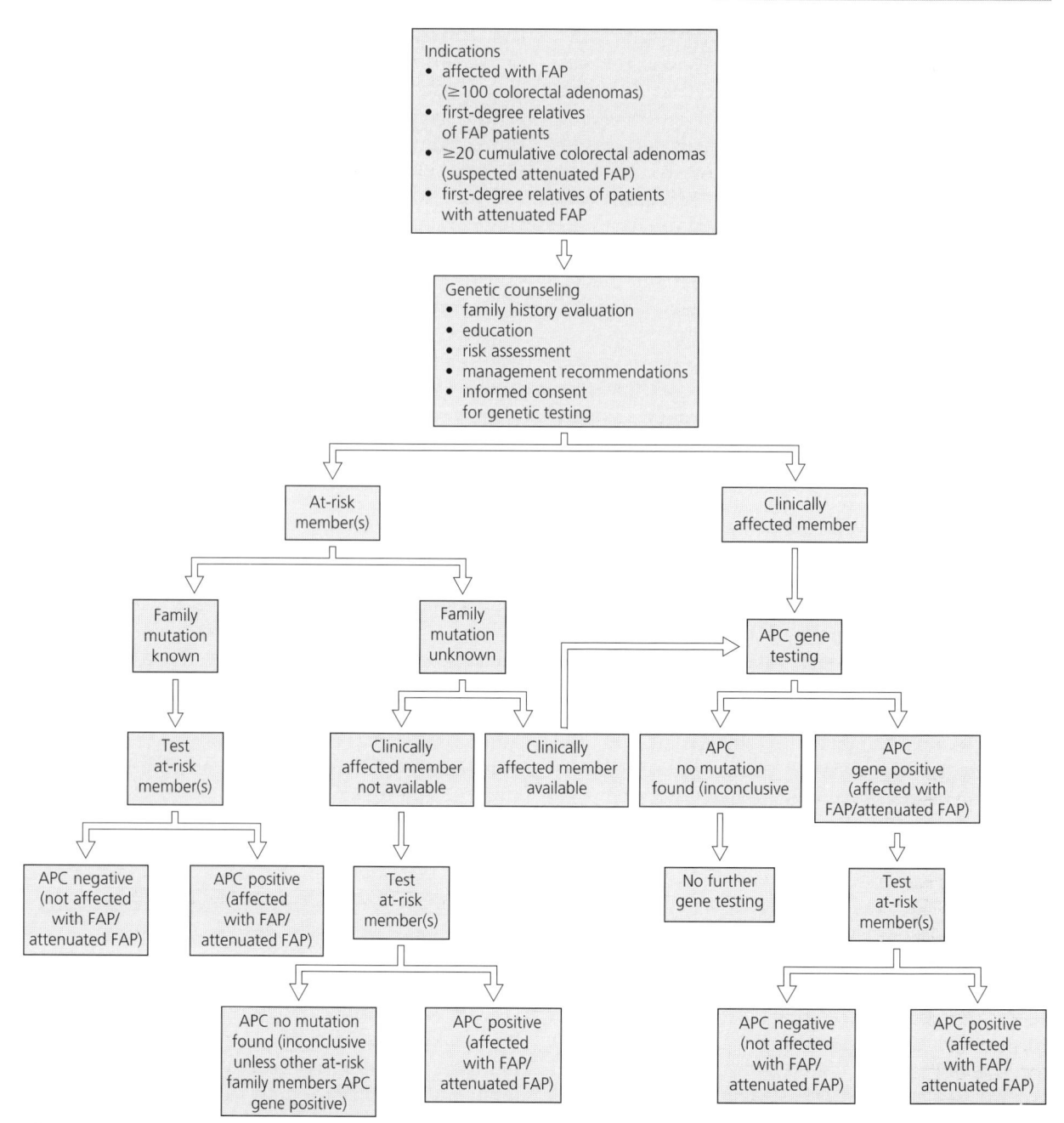

Figure 8.4 Familial adenomatous polyposis (FAP) gene testing recommendations and strategy (reproduced from the American Gastroenterological Association Medical Position Statement: Hereditary colorectal cancer and genetic testing. *Gastroenterology* 121: 195–197; 2001, Figure 1).

this is best deferred until early adolescence. Opthalmological examinations of families with congenital hypertrophy of the retinal pigment epithelium can be used as a surrogate for genetic testing, but the validity of this approach to familial adenomatous polyposis screening has not been conclusively demonstrated. It may be difficult to determine whether an individual has the familial adenomatous polyposis phenotype and therefore merits testing, especially if the diagnosis of attenuated familial adenomatous polyposis is being considered. A finding of multiple polyps in an individual over the age of 45 to 50 years, especially in the absence of a family history, is far more likely to be part of the spectrum of sporadic colonic neoplasms rather than familial adenomatous polyposis, but this remains an area of controversy. Some experts would test patients with twenty or more cumulative colorectal adenomas.

Table 8.8 Appropriate interpretation of genetic test results.

Proband result	Family member result	Interpretation
Positive	Positive	Positive
Positive	Negative	Negative
Negative	Do not test	Not informative*
Ambiguous	Do not test	Not informative*

* Must assume that the family member carries the deleterious gene given the inability to prove otherwise because of the negative test in the proband. Proceed with cancer screening appropriate for a gene carrier in the family member.

Table 8.9 Likelihood of detecting a germline *MSH2* or *MLH1* mutation depending on family history and tumor microsatellite instability (MSI) status.

Clinical criteria met	Likelihood of detecting a mutation
Amsterdam criteria met	35%–65%
Amsterdam criteria met and MSI-H tumor	80%
Near Amsterdam criteria met	15%–45%
Near Amsterdam and MSI-H tumor	50%
Bethesda guidelines met	30%
Bethesda guidelines met and MSI-H tumor	50%
Early onset colorectal cancer w/o family history	0%–30%
Early onset colorectal cancer and MSI-H tumor	30%
Sporadic colorectal cancer	< 1%
Sporadic colorectal cancer with MSI-H tumor	10%

Hereditary non-polyposis colorectal cancer

Determining when genetic testing is indicated for hereditary non-polyposis colorectal cancer is far more difficult than is the case for familial adenomatous polyposis, because individuals with hereditary non-polyposis colorectal cancer do not have a unique phenotype to help establish the clinical diagnosis. Some investigators have suggested direct germline *MSH2* and *MLH1* testing of colorectal cancer patients that meet appropriate and fairly stringent clinical criteria, such as Amsterdam criteria, Amsterdam II criteria, or the first three Bethesda guidelines. The likelihood of detecting a germline *MSH2* or *MLH1* mutation based on clinical criteria being met is summarized in Table 8.9. Other investigators have suggested that tumor microsatellite instability testing or MSH2/ MLH1 protein inmmunohistochemistry should be performed first, and that germline testing be reserved for those found to have MSI-H tumors or those with loss of mismatch repair protein expression. The decision to perform tumor microsatellite instability or immunohistochemistry testing is again based on clinical criteria, though often less stringent criteria than used to decide for germline testing, such as modified Bethesda guidelines. The likelihood of detecting a germline mutation following a positive tumor microsatellite instability test is also summarized in Table 8.9.

Once a germline mutation is detected in the affected proband, germline testing can then be carried out in other family members. In this situation, if family members are found not to carry the family mutation, the result is considered to be a true negative, and their risk for cancer is that of the general population. As with familial adenomatous polyposis, if a mutation is not detected in a family suspected of having hereditary non-polyposis colorectal cancer, the test result is not informative. Failure to detect a mutation in a family without a known mutation does not mean that the family does not have hereditary non-polyposis colorectal cancer (Table 8.8).

The indications and strategy for hereditary non-polyposis colorectal cancer gene testing are summarized in Figure 8.5.

Intestinal Polyposis Syndromes and Hereditary Colorectal Cancer

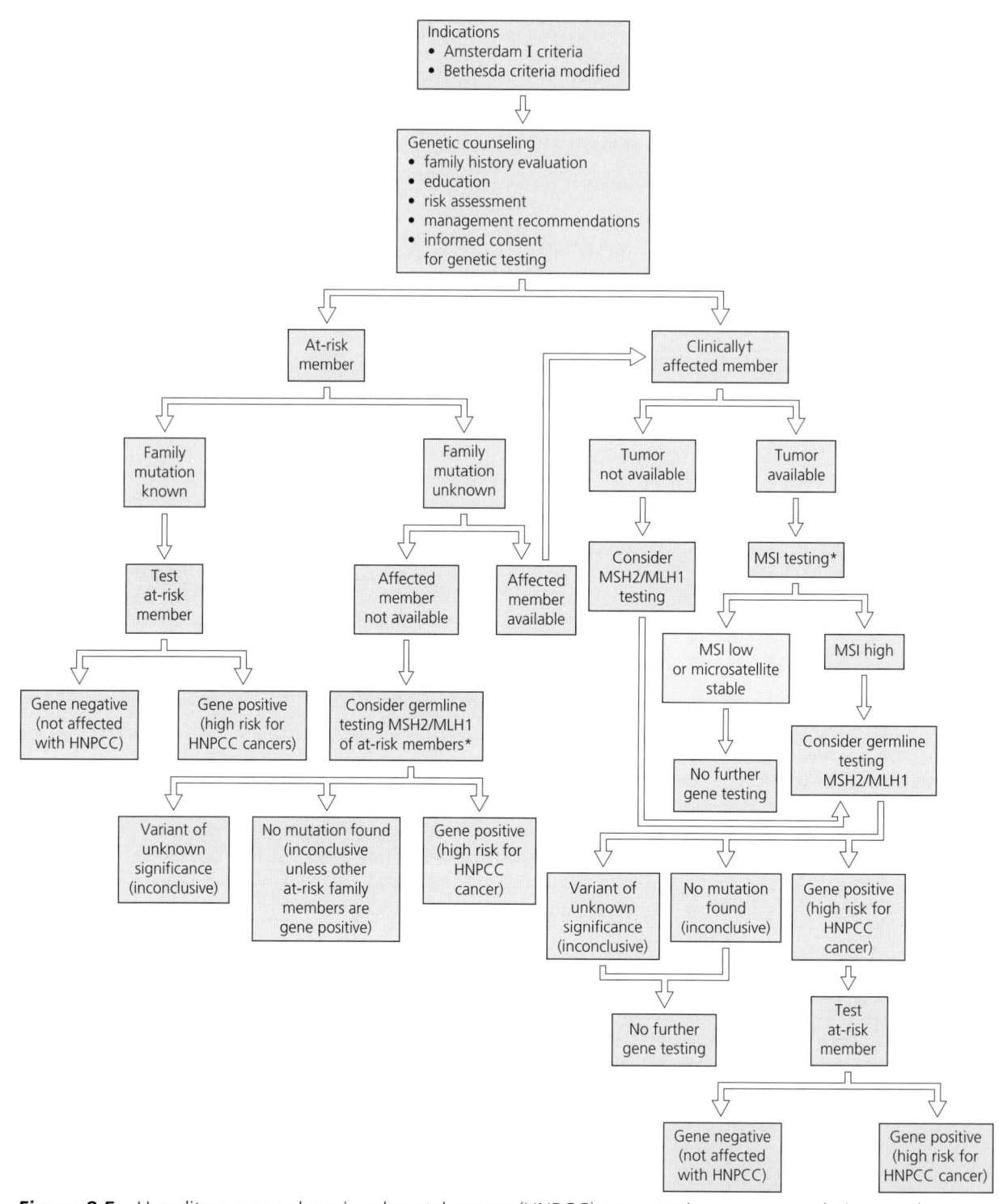

Figure 8.5 Hereditary non-polyposis colorectal cancer (HNPCC) gene testing recommendations and strategy. (reproduced from the American Gastroenterological Association Medical Position Statement: Hereditary colorectal cancer and genetic testing. *Gastroenterology* 121: 195–197; 2001, Figure 2).

Amsterdam I criteria
- 3 relatives with colorectal cancer, 1 of whom is is a first degree relative to other 2
- 2 generations affected
- 1 affected diagnosed < 50 years old

Bethesda criteria modified[1]
- Amsterdam 1 criteria
- Individuals with 2 HNPCC cancers (including synchronous/metachronous colorectal cancers)
- Individuals with colorectal cancer and a first-degree relative with colorectal cancer and/or HNPCC extracolonic cancer and/or colorectal adenoma (cancer < 50 years old and adenoma 40 years old)
- Colorectal or endometrial cancer < 50 years old
- Right sided colorectal cancer with undifferentiated pattern on histology < 50 years old
- Signet cell-type colorectal cancer < 50 years old
- Colorectal adenoma < 40 years old

[1]Bethesda criteria modified with age of cancers changed to < 50 years old vs < 45 years old
* Immunohistochemistry on tumor tissue can be performed prior to germline testing to direct the order of MSH2, MLH1 germline testing
† Initial germline testing without microsatellite instability analysis can be considered in families or individuals meeting the first three Bethesda criteria modified.
MSI = microsatellite instability

Figure 8.5 *continued*

Further reading

American Gastroenterological Association Medical Position Statement: Hereditary colorectal cancer and genetic testing. *Gastroenterology* 2001;121:195–197.

Burt RW. Colon cancer screening. *Gastroenterology* 2000; 119:837–853.

Chung DC, Rustgi AK. The hereditary nonpolyposis colorectal cancer syndrome: genetics and clinical implications. *Ann Int Med* 2003;138:560–70.

Giardiello FM, Brensinger JD, Petersen, GM. AGA technical review on hereditary colorectal cancer and genetic testing. *Gastroenterology* 2001; 121:198–213.

Grady WM. Genetic testing for high-risk colon cancer patients. *Gastroenterology* 2003;124:1574–1594.

Houlston RS, Tomlinson IPM. Polymorphisms and colorectal tumor risk. *Gastroenterology* 2001; 121:282–301.

Johns LE, Houlston RS. A systematic review and meta-analysis of familial colorectal cancer risk. *Am J Gastroenterol* 2001; 96:2992–3003.

King JE, Dozois RR, Lindor NM, Ahlquist, DA. Care of patients and their families with familial adenomatous polyposis. *Mayo Clin Proc* 2000; 75:57–67.

Lindor NM, Greene MH. The concise handbook of family cancer syndromes. *J Natl Cancer Instit* 1998; 90:1039–1071.

McGarrity TJ, Kuline HE, Zaino RJ. Peutz–Jeghers syndrome. *Am J Gastroenterol* 2000; 95:596–604.

Petersen GM, Brensinger JD, Johnson KA, Giardiello FM. Genetic testing and counseling for hereditary forms of colorectal cancer. *Cancer* 1999; 86:1720–1730.

Statement of the American Society of Clinical Oncology: Genetic testing for cancer susceptibility. *J Clin Oncol* 1996; 14:1730–1736.

Terdiman JP, Conrad PG, Sleisenger MH. Genetic testing in hereditary colorectal cancer: indications and procedures. *Am J Gastroenterol* 1999; 94:2344–2356.

Wirtzfeld DA, Petrelli NJ, Rodriguez-Bigas MA. Hamartomatous polyposis syndromes: molecular genetics, neoplastic risk, and surveillance recommendations. *Ann Surg Oncol* 2001; 8:319–327.

Woodford-Richens K, Bevan S, Churchman M, *et al*. Analysis of genetic and phenotypic heterogeneity in juvenile polyposis. *Gut* 2000; 46:656–660.

Chapter 9

Colorectal Neoplasia

Elizabeth E. Half and Robert S. Bresalier

CHAPTER OUTLINE

INTRODUCTION

EPIDEMIOLOGY

ETIOLOGY AND PATHOGENESIS
- *Dietary factors*
- *Chemoprevention*
- *Nutritional agents*
- *Abnormal cellular proliferation.*
- *Genetic alterations*
- *Familial colorectal cancer*
- *Genetic testing*

RISK FACTORS FOR COLORECTAL CANCER
- *Age*
- *Prior colorectal adenoma or carcinoma*
- *Family history*
- *Genetic syndromes*
- *Inflammatory bowel disease*
- *Cholecystectomy*

TUMOR PATHOLOGY AND STAGING
- *Gross appearance*
- *Histology*
- *Tumor configuration*
- *Natural history*
- *Pathological staging*

SYMPTOMS AND CLINICAL SIGNS

PROGNOSTIC FACTORS
- *Pathology*
- *Histology*
- *Molecular markers*
- *Clinical characteristics*

SCREENING AND SURVEILLANCE
- *Screening*
- *Surveillance*

TREATMENT
- *Colon cancer*
- *Rectal cancer*

FURTHER READING

Introduction

The gastrointestinal tract accounts for more neoplastic diseases than any other organ system in the body. Large-bowel neoplasms are common, and appropriate intervention can dramatically modify their morbidity and mortality.

The vast majority of colorectal neoplasias are benign adenomatous polyps which are considered to be pre-neoplastic lesions. The bulk of evidence supports the hypothesis that most colonic cancers arise within previous benign adenomatous polyps. Thus, early intervention and removal of the premalignant polyp interrupts the natural history of the disease.

Epidemiology

Cancer of the colon and rectum represents a major cause of morbidity and mortality in the US and also in countries with similar lifestyles. With an estimated 148 300 new cases and 56 600 deaths in 2002 from colorectal cancer, it is the third most common cancer as well as the second leading cause of cancer-related death among men and women in the US (Table 9.1). Without preventative interventions, about 6% of Americans will develop colorectal cancer at some point during their lives. Similar high rates are found in Canada, the UK, and the white populations of Australia and New Zealand (Figure 9.1). In contrast, in areas of Africa, Asia, and Latin America only about 2% of all reported cancers involve the colorectum. This wide variation in incidence, noted between populations according to geographic region, is not solely the result of genetic factors. Studies of migrant populations demonstrate an increased risk for colorectal cancer in groups that migrate from "low" to "high" risk areas. This was demonstrated in Japanese immigrants to Hawaii and to the US during the 1950s and 1960s. Many of the differences in cancer rates may be due to enviromental factors such as diet. More than 90% of large-bowel cancers arise in individuals who are over 50 years of age. These neoplasms will therefore continue to be a major health problem in western countries with their growing geriatric population. The incidence of colorectal cancer is rising in Japan and other formerly "low risk" areas that have adopted a western lifestyle.

In the US the incidence of colon cancer rose from the 1950s to the 1980s, especially among white men, while the incidence of rectal cancer remained reasonably stable. The incidence of colorectal cancer gradually declined during the 1980s but stabilized thereafter. Currently, both the incidence and mortality rates for colorectal cancer are higher in the black population than in the white population in the US (Table 9.2).

Etiology and pathogenesis

Dietary factors

What accounts for these geographic differences in the incidence of large-bowel cancer? Strong evidence exists for a link between colorectal cancer and environmental factors such as diet (see p. 162). Several types of evidence suggest that diets high in animal fat and low in vegetable fiber predispose individuals to cancer of the large bowel. Mechanisms by which such diets contribute to carcinogenesis in the colon include the enhancement of cholesterol and bile-acid synthesis by the liver, and corresponding elevated amounts of free compounds

Table 9.1 Estimated number of cancer related deaths in the US, 2002.

Both Sexes	Male	Female
Lung and bronchus 154 900	Lung and bronchus 89 200	Lung and bronchus 65 700
Colorectal 56 600	Prostate 30 200	Breast 39 600
Breast 40 000	Colorectal 27 800	Colorectal 28 800
Prostate 30 000	Pancreas 14 500	Pancreas 15 200
Pancreas 29 700	Non-Hodgkin's lymphoma 12 700	Ovary 13 900
Non-Hodgkin's lymphoma 24 400	Leukemia 12 100	Non-Hodgkin's lymphoma 11 700
Leukemia 21 700	Esophagus 9600	Leukemia 9600
Ovary 13 900	Liver 8900	Uterine corpus 6600
Brain 13 100	Urinary Bladder 8600	Brain 5900
Urinary Bladder 12 600	Kidney 7200	Multiple myeloma 5300
All other sites 43 700	All other sites 22 600	All other sites 21 100

Etiology and pathogenesis

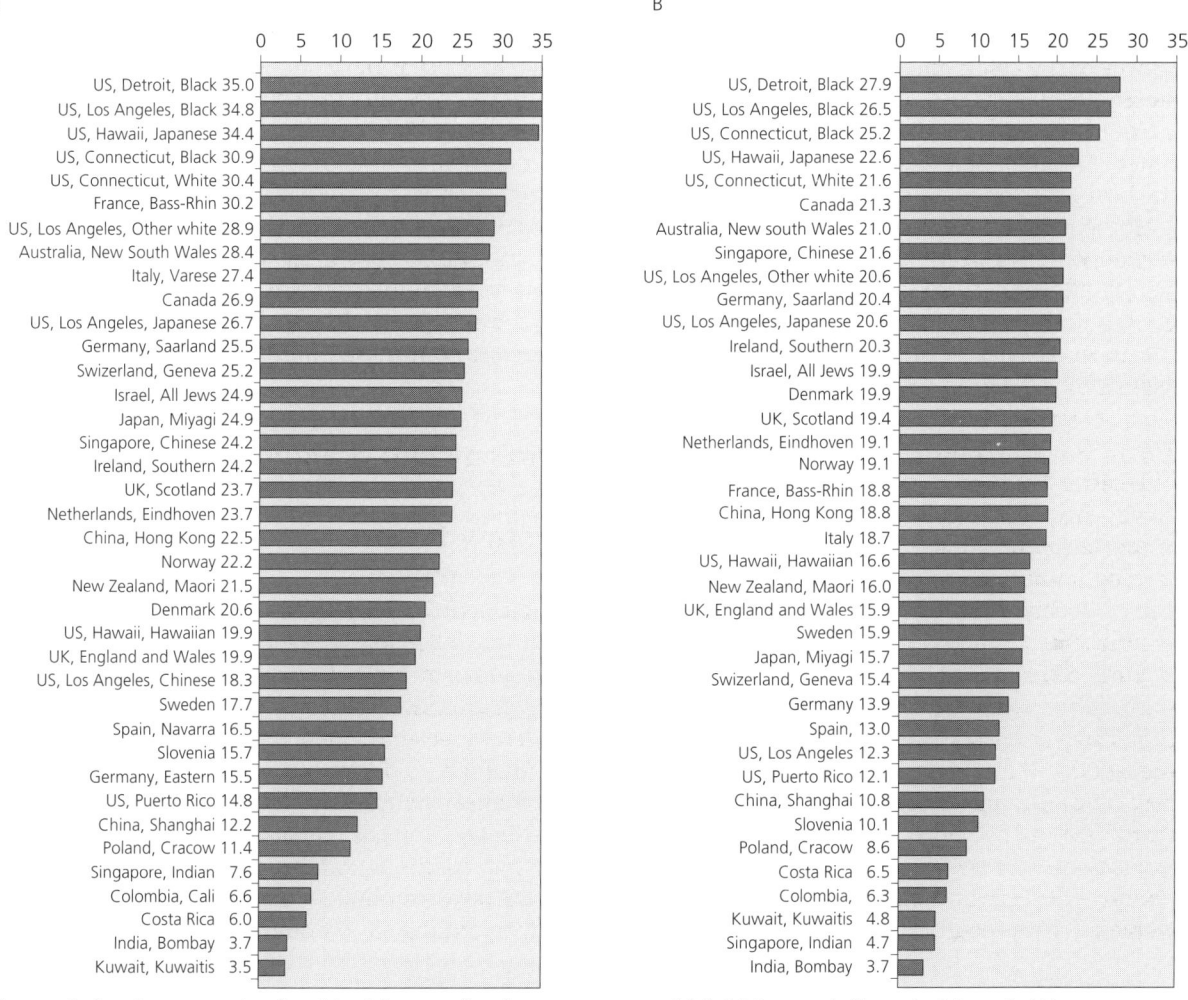

Figure 9.1 Age–standardized incidence of colon cancer per 100 000 population. A. Men. B. Women. Based on data from Parkin DM, Whelen SL, Ferlay J, et al. *Cancer Incidence in Five Continents*. IARC Publication number 143. Lyon Agency for Cancer Research on Cancer, 1997

A. Men

Population	Rate
US, Detroit, Black	35.0
US, Los Angeles, Black	34.8
US, Hawaii, Japanese	34.4
US, Connecticut, Black	30.9
US, Connecticut, White	30.4
France, Bass-Rhin	30.2
US, Los Angeles, Other white	28.9
Australia, New South Wales	28.4
Italy, Varese	27.4
Canada	26.9
US, Los Angeles, Japanese	26.7
Germany, Saarland	25.5
Swizerland, Geneva	25.2
Israel, All Jews	24.9
Japan, Miyagi	24.9
Singapore, Chinese	24.2
Ireland, Southern	24.2
UK, Scotland	23.7
Netherlands, Eindhoven	23.7
China, Hong Kong	22.5
Norway	22.2
New Zealand, Maori	21.5
Denmark	20.6
US, Hawaii, Hawaiian	19.9
UK, England and Wales	19.9
US, Los Angeles, Chinese	18.3
Sweden	17.7
Spain, Navarra	16.5
Slovenia	15.7
Germany, Eastern	15.5
US, Puerto Rico	14.8
China, Shanghai	12.2
Poland, Cracow	11.4
Singapore, Indian	7.6
Colombia, Cali	6.6
Costa Rica	6.0
India, Bombay	3.7
Kuwait, Kuwaitis	3.5

B. Women

Population	Rate
US, Detroit, Black	27.9
US, Los Angeles, Black	26.5
US, Connecticut, Black	25.2
US, Hawaii, Japanese	22.6
US, Connecticut, White	21.6
Canada	21.3
Australia, New south Wales	21.0
Singapore, Chinese	21.6
US, Los Angeles, Other white	20.6
Germany, Saarland	20.4
US, Los Angeles, Japanese	20.6
Ireland, Southern	20.3
Israel, All Jews	19.9
Denmark	19.9
UK, Scotland	19.4
Netherlands, Eindhoven	19.1
Norway	19.1
France, Bass-Rhin	18.8
China, Hong Kong	18.8
Italy	18.7
US, Hawaii, Hawaiian	16.6
New Zealand, Maori	16.0
UK, England and Wales	15.9
Sweden	15.9
Japan, Miyagi	15.7
Swizerland, Geneva	15.4
Germany	13.9
Spain	13.0
US, Los Angeles	12.3
US, Puerto Rico	12.1
China, Shanghai	10.8
Slovenia	10.1
Poland, Cracow	8.6
Costa Rica	6.5
Colombia	6.3
Kuwait, Kuwaitis	4.8
Singapore, Indian	4.7
India, Bombay	3.7

Table 9.2 Average annual incidence and mortality rates for colorectal cancer.[1]

	White population	African-American population
Incidence		
Male	51.4	57.7
Female	36.3	44.7
Total	42.9	50.1
Mortality		
Male	20.6	27.3
Female	13.9	19.6
Total	16.8	22.8

[1] Rates are per 100 000 and are age adjusted to the 1970 US standard population.
[2] CA Cancer J Clin 2002, 52(1) 6–47.

in the colon. Colon bacteria convert these compounds to secondary bile acids (deoxycholic acid, lithocholic acid, 12-ketolithocholic acid), cholesterol metabolites (coprastanol, coprastanone), and other toxic metabolic materials. Bile-acid metabolites are potent promoters of colon cancer in animal models, and higher fecal bile-acid levels have been demonstrated in patients who have large-bowel cancer than in controls. The precise mechanisms by which bile acids and sterols cause colon cancer is not completely understood. Both bile acids and free fatty acids have been shown to damage the colonic mucosa and increase proliferation of the colonic lining cells. Bile acids may also induce the release of arachidonic acid and its conversion to prostaglandins in the colonic mucosa, which can also increase cell proliferation. Preclinical and population-based studies indicate that NSAIDs, which inhibit the enzyme cyclooxygenase (COX) and inhibit prostaglandin synthesis, reduce the incidence of colorectal cancer. Fatty acids may also promote carcinogenesis by altering the fluidity of membranes into which they are incorporated.

High colorectal cancer rates occur in populations with high-fat intakes, and low rates occur in those with low-fat intakes. Total fat comprises approximately 40% to 45% of total caloric intake in western countries, but only 10% to 15% of calories in populations with a low incidence of colorectal cancer. An interesting example is provided by the change in lifestyle of the American black population. In 1940, colorectal cancer was twice as common in American whites as in blacks. By 1980, little difference existed between the two groups. This corresponds to a growing similarity in dietary habits (i.e. diets high in saturated fat and low in fiber) in these populations. Although case control and cohort studies have been less convincing than descriptive epidemiology in demonstrating a link between high-fat diets and colorectal cancer, a prospective study among almost 90 000 US women aged 34 to 59 years supports this relationship. The intake of animal fat and red meat strongly correlated with the risk of colon cancer in this group. Animal studies have provided additional support for the role of dietary fat in the induction of large-bowel cancer. These studies usually involve the injection of carcinogens, such as 1,2-dimethylhydrazine, into rats fed various diets. This carcinogen causes the development of colonic tumors that resemble the human counterpart in histology and, to some extent, distribution within the bowel. Animals fed high-fat diets developed greater numbers of 1,2-dimethylhydrazine-induced colon cancers than did those fed low-fat diets. In fact, increased fat enhanced the induction of colon cancers in animals irrespective of the carcinogen used. The amount and source of dietary fat may, however, influence tumor development. Evidence suggests that fatty acids derived from polyunsaturated fish oils containing omega-3 fatty acids and those from monosaturated oils, such as olive oil, may not promote tumors to the same degree as other polyunsaturated fats.

Similar types of studies favor a protective role for dietary fiber in the development of colon cancer. Dietary fiber is defined as plant material resistant to digestion by the upper gastrointestinal tract. The literature on the subject is sometimes confusing and results may appear contradictory because "fiber" is composed of a heterogeneous mix of carbohydrates, including cellulose, hemicellulose, and pectin, as well as non-carbohydrate substances such as lignin. Nonetheless, numerous epidemiologic studies suggest an inverse relationship between the incidence of large-bowel cancer and the consumption of dietary fiber. In addition, animal studies have demonstrated a decreased incidence of tumors in 1,2-dimethylhydrazine-treated rats fed diets high in fibers, such as wheat bran or cellulose. Dietary fibers, such as cereal bran, may decrease the risk of colon cancer through increasing stool bulk, thereby diluting carcinogens and enhancing their elimination by decreasing intestinal transit time. Contact between these carcinogens and the colon mucosa is therefore decreased. Some fiber components are also converted by fecal flora to short-chain fatty acids, which decrease colonic pH and may therefore inhibit carcinogenesis. Epidemiological, clinical, and laboratory evidence suggest that calcium and vitamin D intake may protect against colon cancer. Calcium has been shown to have an anti-proliferative and differentiating effect on colonic epithelial cells *in vivo*. In a recent prospective randomized trial, Baron and colleagues assigned 930 patients with a recent history of colorectal adenoma to supplemental calcium or placebo treatment and found that calcium supplementation was associated with a significant reduction in the risk of recurrent colorectal adenomas at follow-up colonoscopy. Numerous animal models have demonstrated that the abnormal increase in proliferation in response to diverse carcinogens can be ameliorated in animals receiving supplemental calcium in their diet. It has been suggested that dietary calcium binds to fatty and bile acids in the intestine, converting them to compounds incapable of stimulating proliferation. Furthermore, calcium increases fecal excretion of bile acids decreasing their concentration in the colon. Direct effects of calcium on colonic epithelial cells have also been evaluated by laboratory studies. Epidemiological data indicate that reduced intake of vitamin D is associated with an increased risk of colorectal cancer. Effects of vitamin D have been demonstrated in normal and malignant colonocytes, and several potential mechanisms for colon protection mechanisms have been suggested. The vitamin D receptor is a member of the steroid hormone nuclear receptors, and has been found in normal and transformed cells in many organs including the classic target organs (small intestine, kidney, and bone) and also in the colon. Colon cancer cells not only posses the vitamin D receptor but also are able to synthesize its ligand 1,25-dihydroxyvitamin D3, from its endogenous precursor, 25-(OH)D3. These observations suggest that 1,25-dihydroxyvitamin D3 which is the ligand for the vitamin D receptor may have other biological activities in these cells. This vitamin has been shown to alter the transcription of more than 100 genes involved in important cell processes through binding to the vitamin D receptor and subsequent association of the vitamin D receptor-ligand complex to promotor sequences, termed vitamin D response elements. This receptor complex interacts with the retinoid X receptor, an additional method by which it can effect gene transcription. The major active metabolite, 1,25-dihydroxyvitamin D3, inhibits growth of human colorectal cells *in vitro* and has been shown to induce E-cadherin and modulate β-catenin-TCF-4 target genes in a manner that promotes differentiation of colon carcinoma cells. A recent study detected a significant decrease in intestinal tumor load in Apc(min) mice fed a non-calcemic analog of vitamin D.

Chemoprevention

Chemoprevention is the use of synthetic compounds or nutritional supplements to alter or inhibit the development or recurrence of cancer. The chemoprevention of colorectal cancer has been pursued actively during the last two decades. Because of the long natural history of colorectal cancer, clinical trials have focused on the prevention of its precursor, adenomas. Many clinical trials are now in progress to asses the ability of certain agents to alter either the number of colorectal adenomas or intermediate biomarkers associated with colorectal tumorigenesis. A large number of agents have been evaluated (e.g. folate, calcium, selenium, and hormone replacement therapy), but NSAIDs have had the greatest promise as chemotherapeutic agents.

Epidemiologic studies have demonstrated that long-term use of NSAIDs is associated with a lower risk of colorectal adenomas and a 40% to 50% risk reduction of colorectal cancer compared to controls. The consistency of these findings is striking, despite the diversity of the methods and populations in various trials.

A prospective cohort study among 47 900 male health professionals found that regular users of aspirin (twice or more per week for 4 years) had a lower risk of total colorectal cancer (relative risk 0.68) and advanced (metastatic and fatal, relative risk 0.51) colorectal cancer after adjusting for multiple potentially confounding factors. Data from the Nurses Health Study suggest that this chemopreventive benefit may not be evident until after at least a decade of regular aspirin use. Results of these epidemiologic studies suggest that the duration and consistency of NSAID use may be more important than the daily dose in determining their therapeutic effect. Moreover, the risk of tumor development appears to return to baseline after termination of NSAID treatment.

Colon cancers develop gradually in sequential steps from normal mucosa through adenomatous polyps to overt carcinoma. Therefore, prevention of adenoma development or its recurrence can be used as a surrogate end-point in chemoprevention trials. In familial adenomatous polyposis a germline mutation in the adenomatous polyposis coli (APC) gene results in the development of tens to hundreds of thousands of polyps along the gastrointestinal tract with an associated 100% risk of cancer by the fourth decade. A number of studies have addressed the question of NSAID use in preventing cancer in this high-risk population. Randomized clinical trials have found that two NSAIDs, sulindac and celecoxib, can cause regression of existing polyps in these patients. Treatment with sulindac for 9 months has been shown to decrease both the number of polyps by 56% and their size by 65%. However, 3 months after sulindac treatment was stopped, both polyp number and size increased but remained significantly lower than the value at base line. A prospective randomized placebo control study of 77 patients with familial adenomatous polyposis treated with celecoxib (a selective COX-2 inhibitor) for 6 months demonstrated a significant reduction (28%) in the number of colorectal polyps in patients treated with a high dose of the COX-2 inhibitor, compared to placebo (4.5%). Based on this study, the US Food and Drug Administration approved celecoxib (400 mg twice daily) as an adjunct to the usual care in patients with familial adenomatous polyposis.

The role of NSAIDs in prevention and regression of sporadic adenomas and carcinomas is, at present, unclear. One study, which examined the effect of 150 mg sulindac given twice daily for 4 months versus placebo on polyp size and regression in 22 patients with sporadic adenoma, did not find a significant difference between the treatment or placebo groups. Similar results were associated with another small study of sulindac treatment in only 7 patients during 6 months of treatment. Several ongoing trials are designated to study the effectiveness of NSAIDs and COX-2 specific inhibitors as chemopreventive agents in individuals with a history of sporadic adenoma. Results of one of these trials suggests a significant reduction in adenoma recurrence 3 years after initial polypectomy in patients treated with low dose (80 mg/day) aspirin as compared to controls.

Aberrant crypt foci are abnormally thickened crypts that appear in methylene blue stained colonic mucosa (Figure 9.2). Aberrant crypt foci have been classified as dysplastic (5%) or non-dysplastic. Dysplastic aberrant crypt foci are considered to be precursors of colorectal adenomas and cancers. Aberrant crypt foci are therefore potential markers for use in clinical trials. Limited data exist regarding the effect of NSAIDs on aberrant crypt foci formation. One small study looked at the number of aberrant crypt foci in 20 patients, 11 of whom were then treated with sulindac for 8 to 12 months. After sulindac therapy the number of aberrant crypt foci decreased, disappearing in 7 of 11 subjects, while in the untreated group the number of aberrant crypt foci was unchanged in 8 of 9 patients and increased in 1 patient.

Other potential chemopreventive agents include difluoromethylornithine and HMG-CoA reductase inhibitors. Difluoromethylornithine has been shown in cell culture and animal studies of breast, bladder, and colon cancer to block cell proliferation and inhibit tumor formation by irreversibly inhibiting ornithine decarboxylase, the rate-limiting enzyme in the synthesis of polyamines. In humans, an increased level of polyamines has been documented in colon tumors relative to normal tissue adjacent to the cancer. In addition, data indicate that this enzyme can be transcriptionally activated by c-myc, an oncogene frequently activated early in colonic tumorigenesis. A number of clinical trials are in progress to assess the potential preventive effect of difluoromethylornithine alone and in combination with other drugs on colon cancer development.

The potential benefit of low-fat diets and eliminating bile acids, especially secondary bile acids, from contact with the colonic mucosa is the basis for the use of HMG-CoA reductase inhibitors and ursodeoxycholic acid as potential protective agents. HMG-CoA reductase inhibitors are also known for their antioxidant and anti-inflammatory properties, as well as their effectiveness in suppressing cell proliferation. A reduction in colon cancer incidence was observed in two clinical trials analyzing the effect of HMG-CoA reductase inhibitors in patients with coronary artery disease. Most of these patients were also treated with aspirin. Treatment with pravastatin significantly reduced the incidence of colon cancer in a rat model of colon cancer. The combination of sulindac and lovastatin has also been shown to decrease the total number of aberrant crypt foci per animal in carcinogen-treated rats. Ursodeoxycholic acid is used for the treatment of primary biliary cirrhosis and primary sclerosing cholangitis, and may act as a chemopreventive agent by reducing the concentration of secondary bile-acid deoxycholic acid in the colon. The use of ursodeoxycholic acid as a chemopreventive agent for colon cancer is suggested by preclinical studies and one small clinical study involving 59 patients with ulcerative colitis and primary sclerosing cholangitis. In this study ursodeoxycholic acid was associated with a decreased prevalence of colonic dysplasia ($P = 0.005$), but further randomized placebo controlled studies are necessary to confirm its efficacy in clinical practice.

Nutritional agents

Fiber

The potential protective effect of dietary fiber has been discussed previously (see p. 162). Epidemiological case control studies have frequently reported a risk reduction in colorectal cancer incidence with increasing fiber intake. However several large prospective cohort studies failed to detect such a protective effect. Two recent studies evaluated the effects of high-fiber diets on adenoma recurrence. The Polyp Prevention Trial Study Group assesed the impact of high-fiber and low-fat diets on the recurrence of adenomatous polyps in patients with a history of these polyps. They failed to detect a reduction in adenoma recurrence in the high-fiber low-fat diet group. Further evidence for the lack of association between high-fiber consumption and recurrence of colonic adenomas was provided by the Phoenix Colon Cancer Prevention Physicians Network. They randomly assigned 1429 patients who

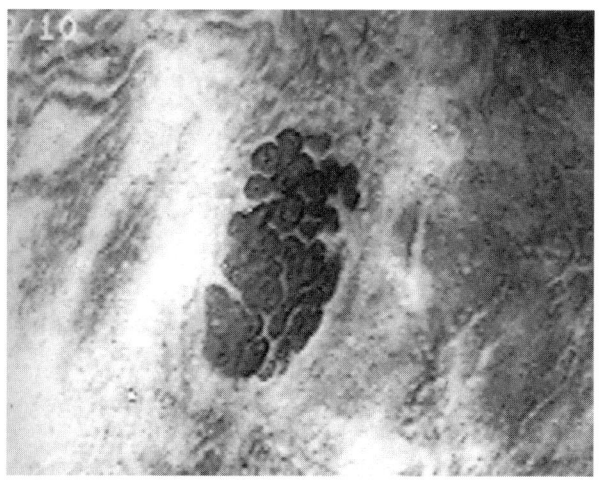

Figure 9.2 Aberrant crypt focus. Colonic mucosa stained with methylene blue and viewed during magnifying colonoscopy.

were 40 to 80 years of age and who had had a prior adenoma removed, to a diet of high (13.5 g/day) or low (2 g/day) wheat bran. After a median follow-up of 35 months, 1303 subjects completed the study and no protective effect of wheat bran on adenoma recurrence was observed.

Calcium

Several studies have found that calcium supplementation or diets rich in calcium is associated with a lower risk of colorectal cancer. However the data is inconsistent and other studies failed to detect this association. The Polyp Prevention Study Group recently reported that subjects treated with calcium carbonate (3 g/day) for 4 years had a significantly lower risk of recurrent adenomas compared to controls. Calcium supplementation was associated with a modest, but not significant, reduction in the risk of adenoma recurrence, however, in a European multicenter, placebo-controlled study.

Folate

Folate plays an important role in deoxyribonucleic acid (DNA) synthesis, repair, and methylation. Folate deficiency may therefore play a role in carcinogenesis. Epidemiological studies have supported the importance of folate in preventing the development of adenomas and colon cancer. Data from the Nurse Health Study indicate that high (over 200 µg/day) folate intake is associated with a lower risk of colorectal adenomas and cancer. The effect of folate on adenoma formation and progression to cancer is the subject of recent clinical trials.

Vitamins C, E, and β-caroten

Studies in animal models and humans have shown that the antioxidant vitamins C, E, and β-caroten reduce epithelial cell proliferation. Some epidemiologic studies suggest that higher intake of these elements might be associated with a reduced risk of colorectal cancer, but the Physician's Health Study found no difference in the incidence of colorectal cancer between individuals with high and low consumption of these vitamins. The only randomized antioxidant vitamin trial, performed by the Polyp Prevention Study Group, failed to detect a protective effect on adenoma recurrence. Furthermore, the Finnish Alpha-Tocopherol, Beta Carotene Cancer Prevention study found that only a modest non-significant decrease in colorectal cancer incidence was associated with vitamin E intake, but not intake of β-carotene. Most studies do not, therefore, support the use of vitamin supplementation in the prevention of colonic adenomas and cancer.

Selenium

Selenium is a trace mineral that, as a constituent of certain selenoproteins, acts as an antioxidant. Results of studies addressing a cancer protective effect of selenium have been controversial. Epidemilogic and animal studies have suggested that dietary selenium reduces the risk of colorectal cancer. In the *min* mouse, heterozygous for a germline mutation of the *APC* gene, a selenium derivate 1,4-phenylenebis(methylene)selenocyanate (p-XSC) was found to decrease the incidence of colon cancer in a dose-dependent manner. The glutathione conjugate of p-XSC (p-Xse-SG) has been found to suppress the multiplicity of azoxymethanol-induced adenocarcinomas and to inhibit COX enzymatic activity. In humans a small, but insignificant, reduction in colon cancer was detected in a phase III randomized placebo-controlled trial using selenized yeast for 4.5 years in patients at risk for skin cancer. These results encouraged the use of these selenium compounds in further trials.

Until now we have talked about environmental factors that may play a role in the development of colorectal cancer. Carcinogens introduced into the bowel lumen act in concert with other luminal factors (e.g. bile-acid metabolites and other tumor promoters) to affect the epithelial cells of the colonic mucosa. It is now recognized that a series of clonal changes in gene expression can be primary or secondary events leading to molecular alterations in the colorectal mucosa resulting in increased proliferation and/or immortalization and uncontrolled cell growth.

Abnormal cellular proliferation

In the normal colon, DNA synthesis takes place and cells divide and proliferate only in the lower and middle regions of the crypts. As cells migrate from lower to upper crypt, the number that continue to proliferate decreases. When these cells reach the upper crypt region they are mature and can no longer divide. Studies have shown that abnormal proliferative activity occurs in the colonic mucosa of families strongly prone to develop colon cancer. Furthermore, in patients with colonic adenomas and cancer, DNA synthesis and cell proliferation may be found throughout the colonic crypt. Increased proliferative activity and distinctive differences in the distribution of tritiated thymidine-labeled cells (i.e. those that actively synthesize DNA) within the crypt have been shown to identify both "at risk" and affected members of families with familial adenomatous polyposis syndrome, as well as non-polyposis inherited colon cancer from groups at lower risk of colon cancer. In addition, proliferative differences have been detected in rectal biopsies from patients with non-familial colonic neoplasia compared to a "normal" proliferation pattern in healthy controls. The proliferation zone and major areas of DNA synthesis are shifted to the intermediate and surface crypt compartments in these individuals. Actively proliferating cells are more sensitive to initiators of carcinogenesis and genetic changes. Conversely, populations at low risk for colon cancer, such as Seventh Day Adventist vegetarians, have relatively low proliferative activity in their colonic mucosa.

Alteration of cell proliferation in the colonic epithelium has been noted after exposure to various carcinogens (e.g. azoxymethane, methylazoxymethanol-acetate) in animal models. Ornithine decarboxylase, an enzymatic marker of rapid cellular proliferation, is increased in the colonic mucosa of family members of familial adenomatous polyposis patients, in rodents exposed to chemical carcinogens, and in colonic adenomas. Bile acids are also known to induce cell proliferation. Activation of protein kinase C may represent an intracellular event by which bile acids stimulate proliferation. Bile acids may also provoke an alteration in mucosal prostaglandin synthesis and release, further increasing cell proliferation. These observations have led investigators to the concept of inhibiting proliferation as a method for preventing colonic neoplasia. Non-steroidal anti-inflammatory drugs, which have been found to block cell proliferation and promote programed cell death or apoptosis, are under active investigation as chemopreventive drugs. Dietary calcium may exert an effect on cellular proliferation in the colon and rectum. Mucosal epithelial proliferation is reduced after the administration of supplemental oral calcium to asymptomatic members of families with hereditary colon cancer. Supplemental calcium also suppresses elevated mucosal ornithine decarboxylase activity in elderly patients with adenomatous polyps.

It is now evident that alterations in multiple proto-oncogenes and tumor suppressor genes lead to disruption of mechanisms that regulate normal cell cycle and proliferation.

Genetic alterations

Major advances in understanding the pathogenesis of colorectal cancer have come from the identification of multiple genetic alterations in colonic mucosal cells that lead to the development of colon cancer (Figure 9.3). Malignant transformation requires several molecular events that disrupt multiple pathways including cell-cycle control, autocrine and paracrine responses to growth factors, motility, and invasion. Three major groups of genetic alterations that lead to the development of colon cancer are recognized

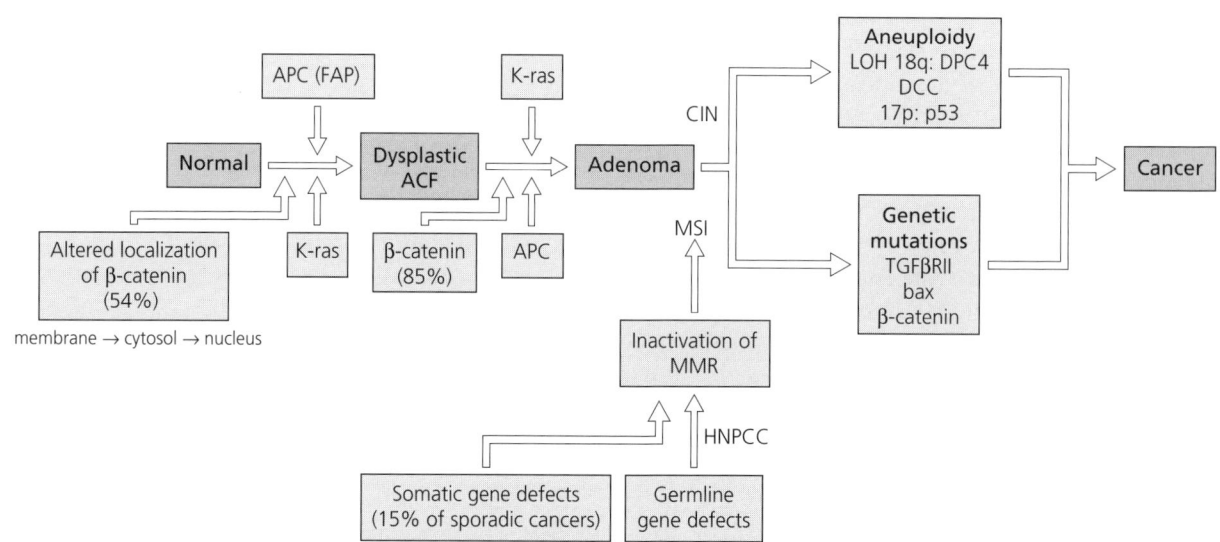

Figure 9.3 Model of colorectal cancer development in which there is an accumulation of molecular genetic alterations during the adenoma to carcinoma sequence.

- changes in proto-oncogenes
- loss of tumor supressor gene activity
- abnormalities in genes involved in DNA mismatch repair.

Cellular proto-oncogenes are human genes thought to play a major role in signal transduction and the regulation of normal cell growth and proliferation. When these genes are mutated (hence, oncogenes), or inappropriately activated, there may be inappropriate transmission of regulatory messages from the cell surface to the nucleus resulting in abnormal growth, uncontrolled proliferation, and neoplastic formation. Several oncogenes have been shown to be amplified or to have altered gene products in colon cancer cell lines and tissues. Elevations in expression of the *ras* oncogene family (*K-ras*, *N-ras*, and *H-ras*) that encode proteins that regulate intracellular signaling pathways have been reported in both pre-neoplastic adenomas and in carcinomas of the colon. *Ras* point mutations are found in 58% of adenomas larger than 1 centimeter in size, in 47% of carcinomas, but in only 10% of smaller adenomas. Thus, *ras* mutations appear to occur during intermediate stages of adenoma growth. *Ras* genes encode membrane proteins involved in signal transduction, abnormalities that may lead to abnormal cell growth and contribute to neoplastic transformation. However, *ras* mutations alone are not sufficient to result in tumor formation.

Tumor suppressor genes were first described in connection with childhood retinoblastoma. The suppressor genes are normal genes whose function is to inhibit the cell cycle and promote apoptosis. Their function is lost when both copies (alleles) of the gene are inactivated. Of the known tumor suppressor genes *p53* is the most commonly mutated in human cancer. Up to 75% of sporadic colorectal cancers display *p53* inactivation. Normal *p53* causes G1 cell cycle arrest to promote DNA repair during replication or to induce cell death. Individuals whose tumors have *p53* mutations have shorter survival rates than those with normal *p53*.

The sequence of genetic changes leading to colorectal cancer usually starts with inactivation of the pathway involving the *APC* tumor suppressor gene and β-catenin. Chromosomal changes have long been reported in colorectal cancer and allelic losses, particularly at chromosome locations 5q, 17p, and 18q, and they appear to contribute significantly to the genesis of colorectal cancer. A deletion of chromosome 5 in a patient with adenomatous polyposis coli (FAP), 5q21, led eventually to the identification and characterization of the *APC* gene. Mutations of the *APC* gene occur in 60% to 80% of sporadic adenomas and the majority of colorectal cancers. Most mutations result in truncation of the APC protein, a finding that has lead to the development of a test for genetic screening of familial adenomatous polyposis families. The adenomatous polyposis coli gene plays an important role in regulating the Wnt signaling pathway (Figure 9.4) which is crucial for colorectal cancer development. Wnt ligands initiate a signaling cascade characterized by movement of cytoplasmic β-catenin to the nucleus. This is achieved by inhibiting the activity of the serine/threonine kinase GSK-3β. Nuclear β-catenin activates a nuclear protein called Tcf-4, which activates a number of target genes (c-myc, cyclin D, PPARδ, TCF-1) that are involved in cell-cycle regulation and cell growth. In the absence of Wnt signals, GSK-3β binds the APC proteins to promote the degradation of β-catenin. Loss of APC function leads to accumulation of β-catenin and continuous stimulation through the Wnt signaling pathway. This leads to absent regulation and increased proliferation as well as inhibition of apoptosis (programed cell death). The *APC* gene is therefore considered to be a tumor suppressor gene. When *APC* is present as a germline mutation it results in familial adenomatous polyposis. Somatic mutation is an early event in the development of sporadic cancer. I1307K mutations in the *APC* gene assist in the development of familial colon cancer in Ashkenazi Jews. Inactivating mutations of both *APC* alleles is the most frequent event that leads to pathological proliferation in colon cancer, however this can also result through dominant mutations of the β-catenin gene. In this case β-catenin-Tcf regulated transcription is insensitive to the regulatory effect of normal wild type *APC*. Abnormalities in the *APC* gene can also cause interference with normal cell to cell adhesion through modified association with E-cadhedrin (a cellular adhesion molecule).

Alleles located at chromosome locus 18q encode additional tumor suppressor genes, the functional loss of which are thought to be important in the transition from pre-neoplastic adenomas to carcinomas. Deletions of these loci are found in over 70% of colorectal cancers. Loss of chromosome 18 is associated with a negative prognosis. At the 18q locus is a gene called *DCC* (deleted in colon cancer). The DCC protein is important in cell adhesion and its loss from Dukes B colon cancers was found in some studies to carry a worse prognosis. Other studies failed to detect this correlation. *DPC4*, belongs to the *SMAD* gene family, is another tumor suppressor gene that is involved in the signal transduction pathways activated through the TGF-β family receptors. Homozygous mutations of

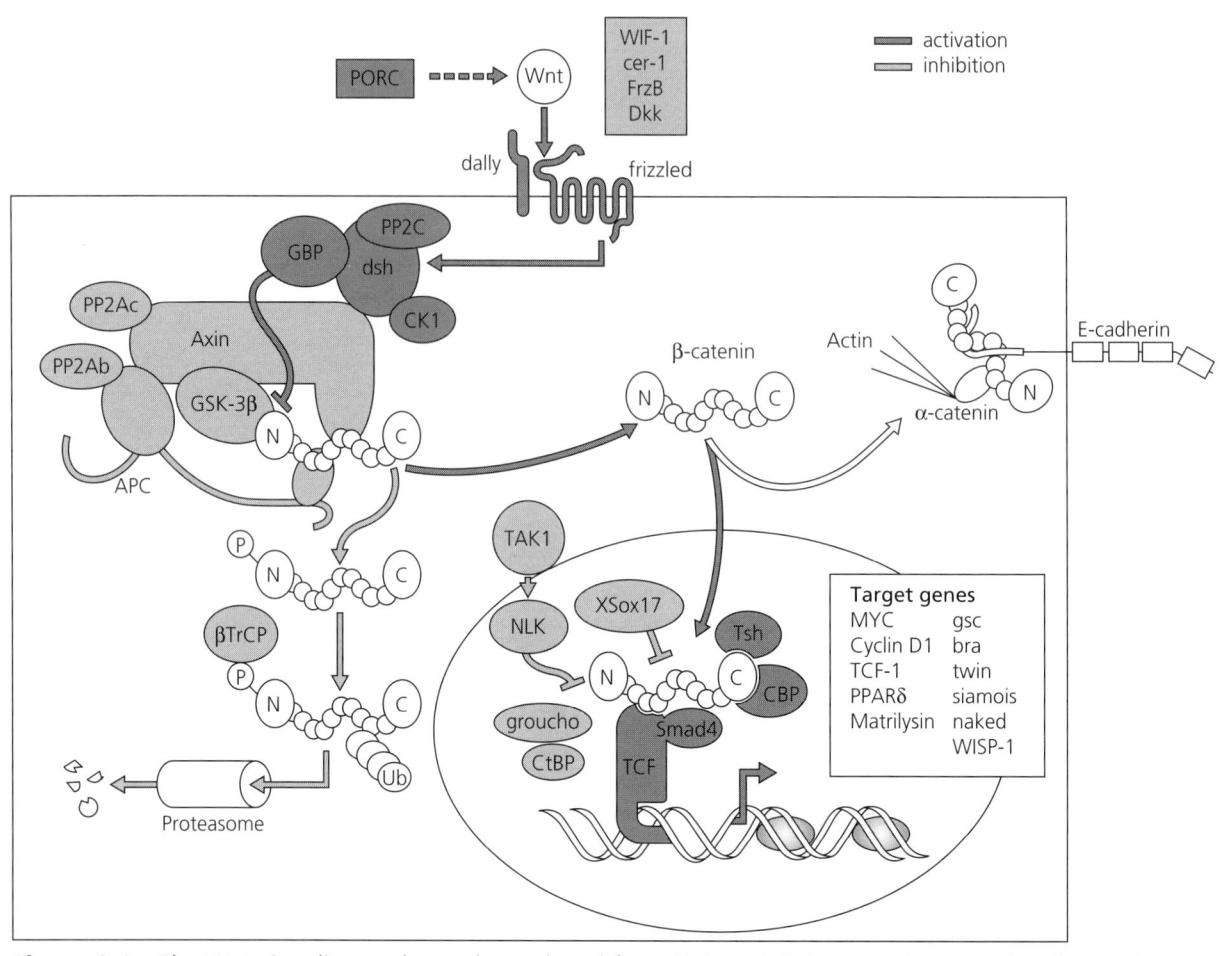

Figure 9.4 The Wnt signaling pathway. (reproduced from Hulsen J, Behens J. The Wnt signaling pathway. J Cell Sci 2000; 113: 3545).

DPC4 are found in 30% of colon cancers. By constructing a knockout mouse model in which its homolog *Dpc4* was inactivated Takaku and colleagues were able to introduce the mutation into the Apc716 knockout mouse (a model for familial adenomatous polyposis). The mice carrying both mutations exhibited a more aggressive disease with extensive cell proliferation, and submucosal invasion. Deletions in chromosome 17p are present in 75% of colorectal cancers and involve the *p53* tumor suppressor gene. The p53 protein prevents cells with damaged DNA from progressing from G1 to the S phase of the cell cycle and its loss enables defective DNA to be synthesized and cells to survive. Inactivation of the *p53* gene mediates the conversion from adenoma to carcinoma. It has been shown that distant colon cancer metastases are associated with high fractional allelic loss and deletions of 17p and 18q.

Genomic instability creates a state in which a potential cancer cell can acquire enough mutations to transform into a cancer cell. Many forms of genomic instability are commonly aquired in colon cancer: microsatellite instability (MSI), i.e. increased rates of genomic mutations in the tandemly repeated DNA sequences known as microsatellites, chromosome instability (CIN), i.e. alterations in the number of chromosomes, and to a lesser extent chromosomal translocations, and gene amplification.

The majority of colon cancers display MSI or CIN at an early stage of cancer development and this indicates that genomic instability is crucial for colon cancer progression. Furthermore, Ried and colleagues used comparative genomic hybridization and detected a gradual increase in the average number of chromosomal copy alterations per case as a polyp progressed from adenoma to low-grade and high-grade dysplasia, and to carcinoma. The early manifestation of MSI and CIN in tumor development provides additional evidence that genomic instability creates a permissive state that results in the accumulation of genetic changes leading to tumor evolution and progression.

Microsatellite instability occurs in most cancers in hereditary non-polyposis colorectal cancer. The loci responsible for hereditary non-polyposis colorectal cancer were linked to chromosome 2p16 and 3p21. Strand and colleagues were the first to suggest that this phenotype might result from defective mismatch repair, i.e a defect in a gene which plays a role in the repair of damaged DNA. Changes in genes that help preserve DNA constancy during replication are characteristic of hereditary non-polyposis colorectal cancer patients. Alterations and inactivation of the mismatch repair system causes genomic instability because of inadequate repair of base pair mismatches resulting from polymerase-generated replication errors. Six genes, *hMLH1, hMSH2, hMSH3, hMSH6, hPMS1,* and *hPMS2* operate in the mismatch repair DNA repair system, and mutations in *hMSH2* and *hMLH1* are the most common causes of MSI tumors. Most patients with sporadic MSI colon cancers, however, do not have mutations in these mismatch repair genes. An alternative method that causes loss of mismatch repair activity is gene silencing by hypermethylation. Kane and others showed that hypermethylation of the *hMLH1* promoter caused bi-allelic silencing of the gene and, hence, loss of mismatch repair function in 70% of sporadic MSI colorectal cancers. The reason for the aberrant methylation is unknown and is under active study.

TGF-βRII and, less frequently, insulin growth factor 2 (IGFRII), Bax, caspases and β-catenin are gene products often affected by defective mismatch repair. Loss of their normal function may contribute to tumor development.

Another form of genetic instability occurs in most malignancies and involves gains and losses of whole chromosomes (CIN) termed aneuploidy. In one study Thiagalingam and colleagues demonstrated that 63% of colorectal cancers exhibit loss of chromosome 18 and 30.6% were associated with complete loss of chromosome 17. Seventy-eight percent of these tumors exhibited partial loss of one chromosome with complete loss of another. Allelic loss has been detected in 90% of colorectal adenomas studied, indicating that it is an early event in colorectal carcinogenesis.

In colorectal cancers a reverse relationship has been found between CIN and MSI. Cancers that manifest mismatch repair deficiency are usually diploid and have normal numbers of chromosomes. On the other hand, mismatch repair-proficient tumors are usually aneuploid with higher rates of chromosomal changes.

Familial colorectal cancer

All cancers have a genetic component which may be inherited or acquired. Approximately 5% to 10% of colorectal cancers have an inherited predisposition. Familial adenomatous polyposis is inherited in an autosomal dominant manner as a result of a mutation in the *APC* gene. Most cases of familial adenomatous polyposis have a family history but one third of the cases arise from a *de novo APC* germline mutation. Classic familial adenomatous polyposis is characterized by the presence of hundreds to thousands of colorectal adenomas (Figure 9.5) and in some instances extracolonic tumors (duodenum, ampulla of vater, jejunum, and ileum) (Table 9.3). The majority of patients with familial adenomatous polyposis eventually develop colorectal cancer by the sixth decade if the colon is left intact. Generally the cancers develop a decade after the appearance of the polyps.

Attenuated familial adenomatous polyposis is characterized by fewer colorectal polyps (less than 100 synchronous or metasynchronous adenomatous polyps), later age of onset of polyps (mean age of polyp diagnosis is 44 years) and cancer (mean age is 56 years), predilection of proximal colon involvement, and infrequent rectal involvement. Patients with attenuated familial adenomatous polyposis are often found in families that also have classic familial adenomatous polyposis. The genetic alteration in attenuated familial adenomatous polyposis is associated with APC mutations most commonly at the 5' or 3' region of the *APC* gene.

Hereditary non-polyposis colorectal cancer accounts for approximately 6% of colorectal cancers. Like familial adenomatous polyposis its mode of inheritance is autosomal dominant. Tumors

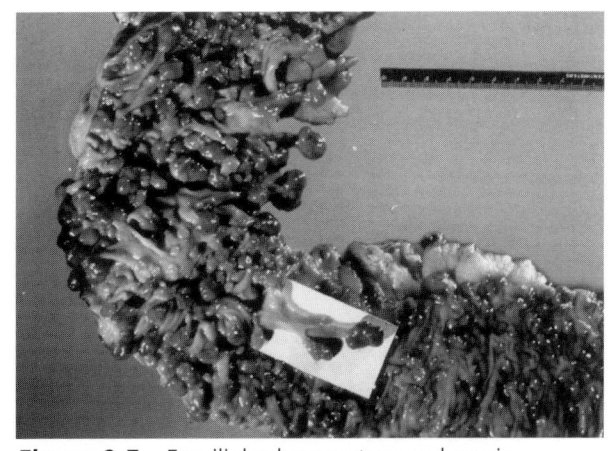

Figure 9.5 Familial adenomatous polyposis. A surgical specimen showing a portion of the colon "carpeted" with multiple adenomatous polyps.

usually arise from a single colorectal adenoma in the absence of polyposis. Hereditary non-polyposis colorectal cancer results from a predisposing germline mutation in genes responsible for the DNA mismatch repair system (see pp. 166–167). Mutations in *hMLH1/MSH2* genes, located on chromosome 3p21 and 2p16 respectively, account for 80% to 90% of all mutations found in hereditary non-polyposis colorectal cancer. However, the prevalence of *hMLH1* and *MSH2* mutations in these families is only approximately 50%. Mutations in a number of other genes, especially *PMS1*, *PMS2*, and *MSH6*, have also been identified in hereditary non-polyposis colorectal cancer families and in some cases of hereditary non-polyposis colorectal cancer no locus has been identified. Individuals with hereditary non-polyposis colorectal cancer gene mutation have about a 70% to 80% life-long chance of developing colorectal cancer. In hereditary non-polyposis colorectal cancer patients colorectal cancer develops at a younger age (average 44 years) relative to sporadic cancers which develop most commonly two decades later. The tumor site is more proximal, with 60% to 80% of the tumors developing proximal to the splenic flexure. In sporadic colon cancers only 23% to 32% are located in this area. Tumors from hereditary non-polyposis colorectal cancer patients tend to have a higher incidence of mucin production. In 45% of the patients metachronous colorectal cancers occur within 10 years of initial resection. In addition to colorectal cancers, hereditary non-polyposis colorectal cancer patients are at increased risk for developing multiple extracolonic tumors (Table 9.3), especially endometrial and ovarian malignancies. Other associated tumors include transitional cell carcinoma of the renal pelvis, as well as carcinomas of the stomach, small bowel, biliary system, pancreas, larynx, breast, and brain tumors. The definition of hereditary non-polyposis colorectal cancer was standardized and defined in 1999 by the International Collaborative Group on Hereditary Non-Polyposis Colorectal Cancer (Box 9.1). In response to concerns that these standards were too strict and did not account for the frequent occurrence of extracolonic malignancies, alternative criteria were developed by the National Cancer Institute-sponsored workshop on hereditary non-polyposis colorectal cancer ("Modified Amsterdam Criteria") (Box 9.1). As mentioned above hereditary non-polyposis colorectal cancer results from a predisposing germline mutation in genes responsible for the DNA mismatch repair system (see pp. 166–167). Mutations of the mismatch repair genes *hMLH1* (on chromosome 3p21) and *hMSH2* (on chromosome 2p16) are the most common mutations found in hereditary non-polyposis colorectal cancer families. However, in some cases of hereditary non-polyposis colorectal cancer no locus has been identified even though "Amsterdam" criteria are fulfilled. Microsatellite instability has been found in more than 90% of hereditary non-polyposis colorectal cancer patients that fulfill the "Amsterdam" criteria.

The Bethesda guidelines (Box 9.2) were developed to identify patients for whom tumor MSI testing was essential. Studies have validated the advantage of these criteria for hereditary non-polyposis colorectal cancer genetic testing.

Twenty percent of colon cancers are considered familial colon cancer in which colon cancer develops more frequently in a specific family compared to the general population, but not in a pattern con-

Table 9.3 Extracolonic features in FAP and HNPCC.[1]

Disorder	Cancers	Other lesions
Familial adenomatous polyposis	Brain (medulloblastoma), thyroid, duodenum, periampullary, pancreas, hepatoblastoma, biliary tree	CHRPE[2] nasopharyngeal angiofibroma osteomas radiopaque jaw lesions supernumerary teeth lipomas, fibromas, epidermoid cysts desmoid tumors gastric adenomas, fundic gland polyps café-au-lait spots sebaceous gland adenomas, carcinomas keratoacanthomas
Hereditary non-polyposis colorectal cancer	brain, glioblastoma[3], stomach, small bowel, biliary tree, ureter and renal pelvis, uterus, ovary	

[1] *Giardiello FM, Brensinger JD, Petersen GM. AGA technical review on hereditary colorectal cancer and genetic testing. Gastroenterology 2001; 121: 198–213.*
[2] *CHRPE Congenital hypertrophy of the retinal pigment epithelium.*
[3] *Turcot's syndrome is characterized by glioblastoma associated with hereditary non-polyposis colorectal cancer.*

Etiology and pathogenesis

> **Box 9.1** Clinical criteria for the diagnosis of hereditary non-polyposis colorectal cancer
>
> **Amsterdam criteria[1]**
> 1. At least three relatives with colorectal cancer; one must be a first degree relative of the other two.
> 2. Colorectal cancer involving at least two generations.
> 3. One or more colorectal cancer case(s) before the age of 50 years.
>
> **Modified Amsterdam criteria[2]**
> 1. At least three relatives diagnosed with hereditary non-polyposis colorectal-related cancers (colorectal, endometrial, small bowel, ureter, or renal pelvis); one must be a first-degree relative of the other two.
> 2. Colorectal cancer involving at least two generations.
> 3. One or more colorectal cancer case(s) before the age of 50 years.

[1]*Criteria defined by The International Collaborative Group on Hereditary Nonpolyposis Colorectal Cancer (ICG-HNPCC) (Amsterdam Criteria) in Vasen HF, Mecklin JP, Khan PM, Lynch HT. Dis Colon Rectum 1991; 34: 424–425.*
[2]*Vasen HF, Watson P, Mecklin JP, Lynch HT. New clinical criteria for hereditary nonpolyposis colorectal cancer (HNPCC, Lynch syndrome) proposed by the International Collaborative group on HNPCC. Gastroenterology 1999;116: 1453–1456.*

> **Box 9.2** Bethesda guidelines for the testing of colorectal tumors for microsatellite instability
>
> 1. Individuals with cancer in families that meet the Amsterdam criteria.
> 2. Individuals with two hereditary non-polyposis colorectal-related cancers, including synchronous and metachronous colorectal cancers or associated extracolonic cancers.[1]
> 3. Individuals with colorectal cancers and a first-degree relative with colorectal cancer, and/or hereditary non-polyposis colorectal-related extracolonic cancer, and/or a colorectal adenoma; one of the cancers diagnosed at age less than 45 years, and the adenoma diagnosed at age less than 40 years.
> 4. Individuals with colorectal cancer or endometrial cancer diagnosed at age less than 45 years.
> 5. Individuals with right-sided colorectal cancer with an undifferentiated pattern (solid/cribriform) on histopathology diagnosed at age less than 45 years.[2]
> 6. Individuals with signet-ring cell-type colorectal cancer diagnosed at age less than 45 years.[3]
> 7. Individuals with adenomas diagnosed at age less than 40 years.

[1]*Endometrial, ovarian, gastric, hepatobiliary, or small-bowel cancer, or transitional cell carcinoma of the renal pelvis or ureter.*
[2]*Solid/cribriform defined as poorly differentiated or undifferentiated carcinoma composed of irregular, solid sheets of large eosinophilic cells and containing small gland-like spaces.*
[3]*Composed of more than 50% signet ring cells (Rodriquez-Bigas MA, Boland CR, Hamilton SR et al. A National Cancer Institute Workshop on hereditary nonpolyposis colorectal cancer syndrome: meeting highlights and Bethesda guidelines. J Natl Cancer Inst 1997; 89: 1758–1762).*

sistent with an inherited syndrome. Recently, the I1307K mutation of the APC gene that occurs in 6% of Ashkenazi Jews was discovered as a cause for an undefined proportion of familial colorectal cancer patients. Patients with this mutation have a 20% life-long risk of colorectal cancer. Further study is indicated to investigate the significance of this family clustering.

Genetic testing

The primary step in evaluating the risk of an individual patient is a detailed family history that allows a determination of whether cancer in a family member is sporadic, familial, or inherited.

When the history indicates the possibility of familial adenomatous polyposis or hereditary non-polyposis colorectal cancer a family pedigree should be performed and the option of genetic testing should be explained to the patient and family.

Genetic testing should be offered only when a person has a strong family history of cancer or early age of onset of the disease, the test can be adequately interpreted, and the results will influence the medical management of the patient or family member.

The indications, accuracy, and cost of commercially available genetic tests are summarized in

Colorectal Neoplasia

Tables 9.4 and 9.5. In brief, familial adenomatous polyposis is caused by a mutation in the *APC* gene and genetic testing for the *APC* gene should be used to screen for this condition. The first test should be performed on the affected family member to establish a detectable mutation in the family, usually by protein truncation testing. If a mutation is detected, then genetic testing of at-risk members (first degree relatives 10 years or older) of the family will provide true positive or negative results. If

Table 9.4 Indications for genetic testing.[1]

Disease	Gene test	Indications
Familial adenomatous polyposis	Adenomatous polyposis coli gene	Patients with more than 100 colorectal adenomas.
		First degree relatives of familial adenomatous polyposis patients.
		Patients with 20 or more colorectal adenomas (suspected attenuated familial adenomatous polyposis).
		First degree relatives of patients with familial adenomatous polyposis.
Hereditary non-polyposis colorectal cancer	Microsatellite instability	Patients that fullfil the "Amsterdam Criteria" or "Modified Amsterdam Criteria".
		Affected person in families meeting the "Amsterdam Criteria" or "Modified Amsterdam Criteria"
		Patients that meet the "Bethesda Criteria".
	Mismatch repair gene	Patients with microsatellite instability-high tumors.
		Affected person in famillies meeting any of the first three criteria of the "Bethesda Criteria", or if tumor tissue was unavailable.
		First degree adult relatives of those with a known mutation.

[1] American Gastroenterological Association medical position statement: hereditary colorectal cancer and genetic testing. *Gastroenterology* 2001; 121: 195–197.

Table 9.5 Summary of commercially available genetic tests for hereditary colorectal cancer.[1]

Disorder mutation	Genetic analysis	Method	Sensitivity/ accuracy	Cost Unknown mutation	Cost Known mutation
Familial adenomatous polyposis	APC[2]	sequencing	> 90%	$800	$200
	APC	linkage	99%	$245–$260 per person $630–$1750 per family	
	APC	protein truncation	70%–90%	$750–$1000	$500
	APC	protein truncation + SSCP + sequencing	80%–90%	$530	
APC I1307K	APC	ASO[3]	99%	$150–$255	
	APC	sequencing	99%	$250	
Hereditary non-polyposis colorectal cancer	hMSH2, hMLH1	sequencing	> 90%	$800–$3000	$200–$500
	hMSH2, hMSH1	CSGE[4] + sequencing	> 90%	$1540	$260
	hMSH2, hMLH1	DOVAM-S[5] (SSCP)	95%–100%	$800	$250
	hMSH2, hMLH1	protein truncation	50%–65%	$750	$500
	MSI testing of tumor	polyacrylamide gel electrophoresis	N/A	$300–$500	

[1] American Gastroenterological Association medical position statement: hereditary colorectal cancer and genetic testing. *Gastroenterology* 2001; 121: 195–197.
[2] APC adenomatous polyposis coli.
[3] ASO allele-specific oligonucleotide.
[4] CSGE conformation strand gel electrophoresis.
[5] DOVAM-S detection of virtually all mutations SSCP.

a mutation is not detected, no advantage has been obtained from testing at-risk relatives (a negative test result may be falsely negative because the assay is incapable of detecting the specific mutation). An allele of *APC* designated I1307K is relatively infrequent in the general population but is found in 6% of Ashkenazi Jews. There is a modest increase in the relative risk for colorectal cancer in individuals with this allele, but the penetrance for colorectal cancer is low compared with carrier frequencies. Genetic testing for APC I1307K gene mutation is commercially available (Table 9.5) for Ashkenazi Jewish people with a personal or family history of colorectal cancer. Extensive research is ongoing to determine the clinical application of this mutation. The results of these studies will allow the establishment of guidelines for this genetic test. To date, genetic testing for I1307K is not recommended.

The genetic testing for hereditary nonpolyposis colorectal cancer (Table 9.5) is more complicated than that for familial adenomatous polyposis because numerous germline mutations of the mismatch repair genes can cause hereditary non-polyposis colorectal cancer. Furthermore, the medical benefit of genetic testing in hereditary non-polyposis colorectal cancer has not been validated. Microsatellite instability testing using a panel of five microsatellite markers: BAT25, BAT26, D2S123, D5S346, and D17S250, known as the "Bethesda panel" should be performed in every patient who meets the Bethesda Guidelines (Box 9.2). If the tumor DNA is MSI-high (evidence for the presence of a germline mutation in a mismatch repair gene) patients should be evaluated for mutations of the hMLH1 and hMSH2 genes (the only two genes that are commercially available for evaluation). If tumors are MSI-low or stable then further genetic evaluation is unnecessary at this stage. If a mutation is detected in an affected family member (i.e. the proband) then genetic testing of at-risk relatives should be performed. If MSI testing is not possible in the proband, or if another family member meets any of the first three conditions of the modified Bethesda criteria, consideration should be given to initial germline testing in that individual. If the germline testing is positive at-risk family members should be tested. If no mutation is detected or the result is inconclusive no further gene testing is indicated. First degree family members remain at risk for developing colorectal cancer and should continue standard screening. The current sensitivity of the tests for hMLH1 and hMSH2 mutations is between 50% and 95% and a family could have a mutation in one of the other hereditary non-polyposis colorectal cancer-associated genes for which genetic testing is not available. If the affected person is not available for testing, then at-risk family members can be tested, however only positive results are conclusive and in most cases the testing would be uninformative.

Altered DNA in stool samples has been demonstrated using a multi-target panel of molecular markers (K-ras, p53, APC, and BAT-26). A recent study evaluated K-ras, p53, and BAT-26 DNA mutations in colorectal tumors and stool samples. The authors were able to identify 71% of total colorectal cancers and 92% of the tumors that harbor a mutation in one of these genes by testing stool DNA samples. Stool testing, unlike other conventional screening approaches is non-invasive and does not require intensive preparation. Further studies are, however, indicated to determine the specificity as well as the sensitivity of these genetic tests for detecting colorectal neoplasia in asymptomatic individuals.

Risk factors for colorectal cancer

The risk of developing colorectal cancer is related to many demographic factors. However, not everyone in high-risk geographic regions develops cancer of the colon or rectum despite similarities in diet. Why one individual develops cancer and another does not is under intensive study at present. Certain groups with an increased risk of developing colorectal cancer have been identified (Box 9.3).

Age

The incidence of colorectal cancer increases with age and is equally distributed between men and woman. The incidence of the disease begins to increase at the age of 40 years, and more than 90% of the cases occur in people older than 50 years of age. The mean age at diagnosis is 70 years. Colorectal cancer does arise in younger patients, especially in the setting of familial syndromes, and it must be considered in younger patients with signs and symptoms of the disease.

Prior colorectal adenoma or carcinoma

The majority of data indicates that subjects with prior adenomas are considered at increased risk for cancer throughout their lifetime. Adenomatous polyps are

> **Box 9.3** Risk factors related to colorectal cancer[1]
>
> **Age over 50 years**
> Probable dietary and lifestyle factors
>   high fat intake (as a percentage of daily calorie intake)
>   low fiber consumption
>   red meat consumption
>   decreased physical activity/ high body mass
> Possible dietary and lifestyle factors
>   reduced intake of vitamin D
>   low dietary selenium
> Hereditary syndromes
>   polyposis syndromes: familial adenomatous polyposis, Turcot's syndrome, Muir–Torre syndrome, Peutz–Jegher's syndrome
>   hereditary non-polyposis colorectal cancer
>   family history of colorectal cancer or adenoma
> Prior colorectal neoplasia
>   colorectal adenoma
>   colorectal carcinoma
> Inflammatory disease[2]
>   ulcerative colitis
>   Crohn's disease
>
> [1]Based on descriptive epidemiology. Data from case-control, cohort, and randomized trials are less convincing.
> [2]Especially with high-grade dysplasia or dysplasia-associated mass lesions.

found in about a quarter of people by the age of 50 years and the prevalence increases with age. The probability that a patient will develop other adenomatous polyps or cancer elsewhere in the colon or rectum, can be estimated from characteristics of the polyp at the time it is first examined. The size of an adenoma is directly related to the probability that 1) it will have high-grade dysplasia, and 2) the patient will develop other adenomatous polyps and cancer elsewhere in the colon or rectum. The National Polyp Study found 1.1% of adenomatous polyps were less than 5 mm in diameter, 4.6% were 5 to 9 mm, and 21% of polyps that were 1 cm or larger in size had high-grade dysplasia. Other studies suggest that less than 1% of small polyps (less than 1 cm in size) are found to be malignant compared to more than 10% of larger polyps. The polyp's histology is another determinant of its potential cancer risk. Atkin and colleagues studied 1618 patients that were followed for a mean of 14 years after the removal of an adenoma. The risk of subsequent colon cancer development depended on the histological type, as well as the size and number of adenomas detected. Individuals whose original polyp was tubulovillous, villous, or larger than 1 cm were more than three times more likely to develop colon cancer when compared to those with small tubular adenomas. Those with multiple tubulovillous or villous adenomas were approximately six times more likely to develop cancer.

Individuals with a personal history of colorectal carcinoma have an increased risk of harboring a synchronous carcinoma (0.7% to 7.5%) or developing a subsequent or metachronous carcinoma (1.1% to 4.7%). Most patients with synchronous cancers have them in different locations, i.e one in the distal and the other in the proximal colon. Fifty percent of metachronous colorectal cancers arise within 5 to 7 years of the primary cancer.

Family history

It has become increasingly clear that genetic predisposition plays a role in a significant number of patients with colorectal cancer (see pp. 166–169). The risk of colorectal cancer increases twofold relative to the general population when one or more first degree relatives have a history of colorectal cancer. The risk increases significantly if the first degree relative had a colorectal cancer or an adenomatous polyp diagnosed before the age of 60 years. Furthermore, the risk is higher if more than one first degree relative is affected at any age. Colorectal cancer, even in second degree relatives (grandparents, aunts, and uncles), or third degree relatives (great grandparents and cousins) was found to increase and individual's risk for this cancer by about 50% compared to the general population.

Genetic syndromes

A number of hereditary forms of colorectal cancer in which the majority of affected people will develop colorectal cancer are well known. These syndromes are inherited in an autosomal-dominant fashion and were widely discussed earlier (pp. 137–158). Briefly, in familial adenomatous polyposis and Gardner's syndrome adenomas develop approximately a decade before the appearance of cancer, and virtually all affected individuals eventually develop large-bowel cancer unless the colon is removed. Cancers often occur between the ages of 30 and 50 years, two decades earlier than sporadic cases in the general population. Molecular diagnosis of familial adenomatous polyposis, now possible in at-risk families, has been discussed (see pp. 170–171). Although perhaps the most dramatic and well-defined, these syndromes account for only a small fraction of hereditary colon cancers.

Turcot's syndrome Turcot's syndrome is a rare variation of familial adenomatous polyposis that consists of a combination of adenomatous polyposis and malignant brain tumors (Table 9.3). Some of these patients have mutations in the *APC* gene or mutation of the mismatch repair genes *hMLH1* or *hPMS2* (typical of hereditary non-polyposis colorectal cancer).

Hereditary non-polyposis colorectal cancer Hereditary non-polyposis colorectal cancer is also inherited in an autosomal dominant fashion. It causes colorectal cancer even though multiple polyps are not present. This disease is caused by mutations in mismatch repair genes located on chromosome 2, 3, or 7. Mutations in the mismatch repair genes *hMLH1* and *hMSH2* account for more than 90% of hereditary non-polyposis colorectal cancer families. However, mutations in *PMS1*, *hPMS2*, and *hMSH2* account for additional cases. Each of these mutations places a person at an approximately 80% risk of developing colorectal cancer at an average age of 44 years.

Muir–Torre syndrome The Muir–Torre syndrome is a rare variant of hereditary non-polyposis colorectal cancer. It is defined as the presence of

1. a sebaceous gland adenoma, epithelioma, or carcinoma, and
2. an internal malignancy such as colorectal cancer, genitourinary tract cancer, uterine cancer, or ovarian cancer.

Microsatellite instability and loss of *hMLH1* and *hMSH2* protein expression indicating a mutation in these genes were noted in 69% of Muir–Torre-associated tumors.

Hamartomatous syndromes Two hamartomatous syndromes are associated with increased risk of colorectal cancer development.

Peutz–Jegher syndrome is an autosomal dominant disease characterized by hamartomatous polyps in the small and large bowel and melanin pigmentation of the skin and mucus membranes. Recently, two groups have identified a new gene that codes a serine threonine kinase STK11 that is responsible for Peutz–Jegher syndrome. Adenomatous changes have been reported in 3% to 6% of these hamartomas and Peutz–Jegher syndrome is associated with an eighteen times greater risk of developing cancer relative to the general population as well as an early age of onset of the disease. The most frequently occurring cancers are colon and breast cancer.

Juvenile polyposis is an autosomal dominant disorder characterized by the development of multiple childhood colonic hamartomas without abnormal pigmentation. Adenomatous features develop in some of these polyps with increased risk of cancer development. Recently, two genes have been connected to this syndrome. Germline mutations in the SMAD4 gene located on chromosome 18q21.1 that encodes an intracellular component in the TGF-β pathway has been reported in certain affected patients. PTEN germline mutations, on chromosome 10, have also been connected with this disease.

Inflammatory bowel disease

Patients with ulcerative colitis and Crohn's disease are at an increased risk for developing colonic adenocarcinomas. The risk associated with both diseases is similar for comparable extent, duration, and age of onset of inflammatory disease. The increased risk begins 8 years after the onset of colorectal symptoms and rises at about 10% per decade, reaching about 30% at 25 years. The strongest predisposing factor for cancer is the extent of inflammation. The highest risk is in patients with pancolitis or in those in whom the disease extends proximally to the splenic flexure, whereas patients with disease limited to the rectum have only a slightly increased risk of cancer over the general population. The cumulative incidence of colorectal cancer in patients with pancolitis is estimated at 30% in 35 years. Difficulties related to study designs, sources of referral, sampling, recognition of disease, follow-up procedures, and methods for detecting the disease account for variations in these numbers. Although once thought to be a risk factor itself, early age at onset of colitis does not appear to exert any independent influence on cancer risk, except that the disease is likely to have a longer duration. In addition, neither the severity of the initial attack nor disease activity have been considered independent risk factors for cancer development. Cancer arising in the setting of ulcerative colitis has traditionally been thought of as a highly malignant lesion with a poor prognosis. Nevertheless, recent studies, using state-matched controls from colon cancer populations without colitis, have failed to demonstrate a significant difference in survival between the two groups.

Both dysplasia and an increased risk of colonic carcinoma also occur in patients with Crohn's disease. The literature on Crohn's disease is not as extensive as that for ulcerative colitis, and the incidence is poorly defined (a four- to twentyfold increased risk compared with the general population has been reported). Again it appears that cancer risk occurs in colonic segments involved by disease and correlates with disease duration. The risk of small-bowel carcinoma in patients with Crohn's disease is also increased. Recently, a large study, that included 259 patients with extensive chronic Crohn's colitis, detected dysplasia or cancer in 16% of the patients and concluded that the rates are very similar to ulcerative colitis.

Cancers in patients with inflammatory bowel disease are generally flat and infiltrating. They do not typically arise from polyps but from areas of dysplasia. Furthermore, patients with moderate or severe dysplasia have been shown to have a high probability of developing colorectal cancer. The term *dysplasia* has already been used in our discussion of colonic adenomas. It is a histologic term that describes abnormalities in both crypt architecture and cytologic detail. As compared with normal epithelium, crypts may be reduced in number, irregularly branched, and crowded together ("back-to-back glands"). Cell nuclei may be enlarged and hyperchromatic (stained deep blue with hematoxylin and eosin stain), demonstrate increased mitoses, and occur at different levels in the cell producing a "picket fence" appearance (pseudostratification). There is good evidence that dysplasia is a precursor to carcinoma in ulcerative colitis, as it is in colonic adenomas. It may be categorized as mild or low-grade, and severe or high-grade. Ninety percent of resected colons from patients with ulcerative colitis and cancer contain dysplastic mucosa somewhere in the colon, and 30% of patients with severe rectal or colonic dysplasia on biopsy have coexistent carcinoma. The risk for cancer appears highest in patients with high-grade dysplasia and patients in whom dysplasia occurs in visible plaques or masses (dysplasia-associated mass lesions).

The most recent surveillance recommendations for patients with both ulcerative colitis and Crohn's disease include colonoscopy with extensive biopsies at every 10 centimeters of the colon every 1 to 2 years beginning after 8 years of disease in patients with pancolitis and similarly in patients with colitis involving only the left colon. The rationale for this frequency is the difficulty in detecting cancer or dysplasia in any single examination. If high-grade dysplasia or dysplasia-associated mass lesions are identified at colonoscopy then a colectomy is advocated.

Cholecystectomy

The question of whether or not cholecystectomy increases the risk of bowel cancer has been debated and results of studies are inconsistent. The removal of the gallbladder results in more continuous flow of bile to the duodenum with less effective physiological pulse release during meals. This results in less dilution of bile with food and gastric juices, and a higher rate of mucosal exposure to bile with increased formation of secondary bile acids. Increased exposure of the bowel mucosa to secondary bile acids has been reported to cause increased proliferation and increased risk of colorectal cancer. An increased frequency of tubular adenomas was demonstrated in patients older than 60 years of age who underwent cholecystectomies more than 10 years earlier. Two large meta-analysis studies failed to establish or refute this relationship. An additional study found an increased risk among women for right-sided colon cancer 15 years or more after the operation. A recent Swedish retrospective population-based cohort study evaluated 278 460 cholecystectomized patients for a mean follow-up of 12.1 years. They found an increased risk of proximal intestinal adenocarcinoma, which gradually declined with increasing distance from the common bile duct. A twofold increase in proximal small bowel cancer and a 16% significantly increased risk was noted for proximal (cecum and ascending colon) colon adenocarcinomas.

Tumor pathology and staging

Gross appearance

The gross appearance of adenocarcinoma in the large bowel depends on the tumor site. Carcinomas of the proximal colon tend to be large bulky tumors that often outgrow their blood supply and undergo extensive necrosis (Figure 9.6A). This polypoid configuration of tumors is more common in the proximal (cecum, ascending, transverse) colon but may also be found in other areas of the large bowel. In

Tumor pathology and staging

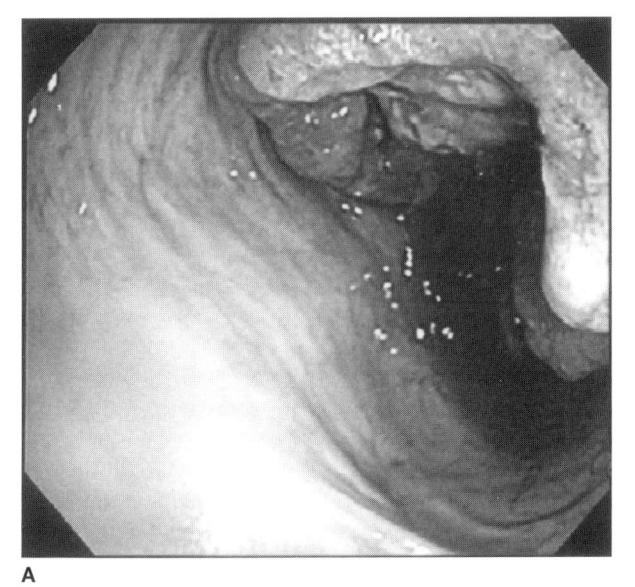

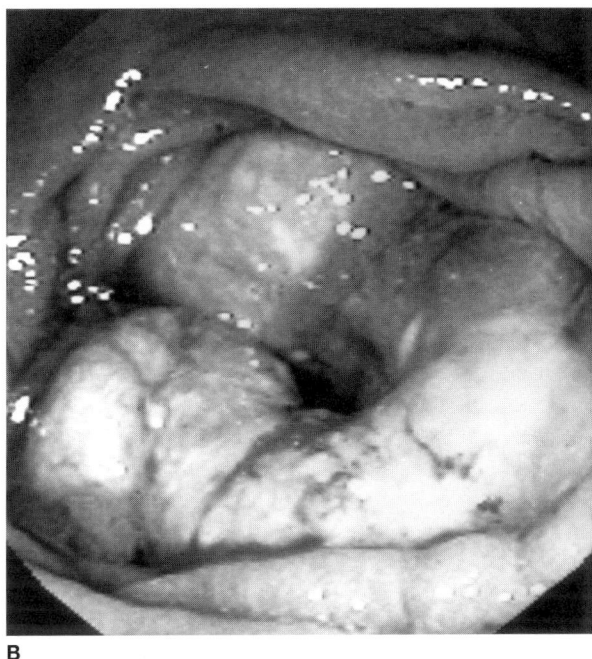

Figure 9.6 Carcinomas of the colon seen at colonoscopy. A) Fungating mass lesion with semi-circumferential involvement of the bowel wall. B) Annular constricting lesion of the sigmoid colon.

the more distal colon and rectum, tumors frequently involve the circumference of the intestine, with an annular constricting or "napkin-ring" appearance (Figure 9.6B). In these tumors, fibrous stroma tissue accounts for constriction and narrowing of the bowel lumen. Occasionally cancers have a flatter appearance with intramural spread, characteristics most frequently seen in cancers arising in the setting of ulcerative colitis. These features have clinical, diagnostic, and prognostic importance.

Many studies have found a change in the distribution of large-bowel tumors over the past several decades, with a proximal shift in colon cancer. Proximal colonic cancers are more common among older individuals (over 65 years) and as the population life expectancy increases, a larger number of proximal cancers may be expected. It has also been hypothesized that there has been a decline in the incidence of left-colon and rectal cancers, while the incidence of right-colon cancers may be unchanged. Currently in the US, the prevalence of colorectal cancer in the white population is higher in the cecum and ascending colon (22% in men, 27% in women) and in the sigmoid colon (average 25% for both sexes) (Figure 9.7). This change in colorectal cancer distribution has important implications for screening methods and it may have a significant effect on the future usefulness of flexible sigmoidoscopy as a screening tool for colorectal cancer as it misses approximately 50% of the colonic cancers.

Synchronous (simultaneous) malignant or benign colorectal lesions are estimated to occur in 1.5% to 9% and 23% to 38% of patients respectively. The lesions may be in the same segment of the colon or in different locations. Total colonoscopy is therefore indicated when a neoplastic lesion is detected in the colon by any other means. This allows the removal of synchronous polyps and permits modification of the surgery if necessary.

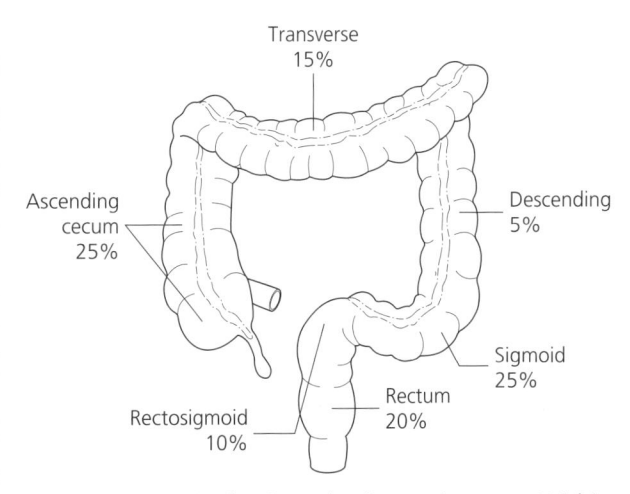

Figure 9.7 Distribution of colorectal cancer. Within the colon approximately 50% of cancers are within the reach of a flexible sigmoidoscope.

Histology

Colorectal cancers can be divided into histological grade and histological type. Histological grade is defined by microscopic features such as degree of gland formation. Most colorectal cancers are moderate or well differentiated (Figure 9.8A). Approximatly 20% of colorectal adenocarcinomas are poorly or undifferentiated tumors (Figure 9.8B) which demonstrate less-defined gland formation and are associated with a worse prognosis. A significant degree of interobserver variability in grading of colorectal cancer has been shown to exist. Histologic grade has repeatedly been shown by multivariate analysis to be a stage-independent prognostic factor with high tumor grade (i.e. less differentiation) conferring a poor prognosis.

Carcinomas of the large bowel are predominantly adenocarcinomas and most represent malignant conversion of a pre-existing adenomatous polyp (Figure 9.9). Adenocarcinomas of the colon form moderately to well-differentiated glands and secrete variable amounts of mucins. Mucins are large-molecular-weight glycoproteins and major secretory products of both normal and neoplastic glands in the colon. Mucins are detected by histochemical stains such as periodic acid-Schiff (Figure 9.10A). "Signet-ring" cells, in which a large vacuole of mucin pushes the nucleus to one side, are a feature of some tumors (Figure 9.10B). In approximately 15% of tumors, large lakes of mucin (more than 50 of tumor) with scattered collections of tumor cells are present. These are the so-called mucinous, or colloid, carcinomas (Figure 9.9A), and are also considered to be associated with poorer 5-year survival relative to non-mucinous tumors. These mucinous tumors more often occur in younger patients, in the proximal part of the colon, and usually present at a more advanced stage. Medullary carcinoma has recently been added as a separate histological type by the World Health Organization. These tumors are associated with high degrees of MSI indicative of loss of normal DNA repair gene function. This cancer type may occur sporadically or in association with hereditary non-polyposis colon cancer. It is characterized by uniform polygonal tumor cells that exhibit solid growth in nested, organoid, or trabecular paterns that only focally produce small amounts of mucin. These tumors are typically infiltrated by lymphocytes and have no immunohistochemical evidence of neuroendocrine differentiation. Small cell carcinoma is a malignant neuroendocrine carcinoma that resembles small cell carcinoma of the lung histologically and biologically.

Histological type *per se* is of limited prognostic value. The exceptions are signet-ring cell carcinoma and small-cell carcinoma, which have an unfavor-

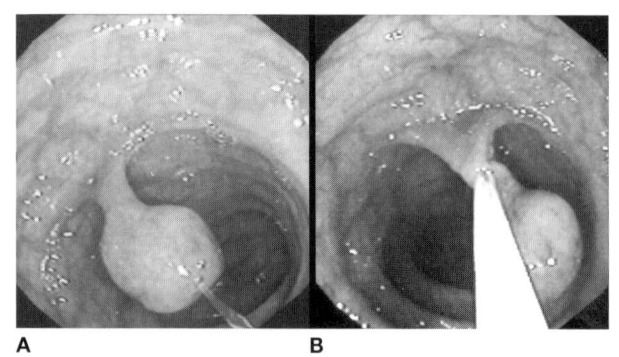

Figure 9.9 Adenomatous polyps of the colon. A) Colonic adenomatous polyp detected at colonoscopy. (see overleaf for figure 9.9, part C & D)

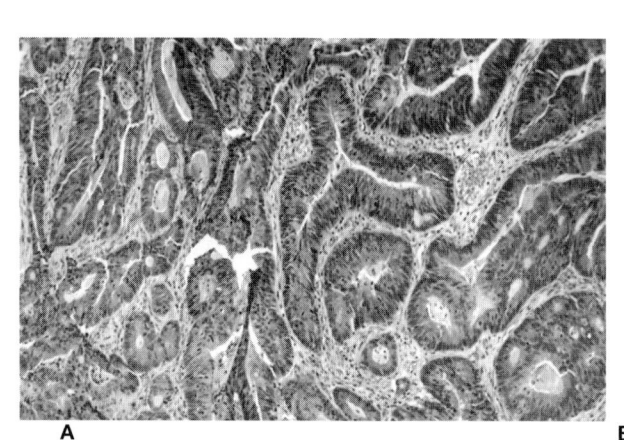

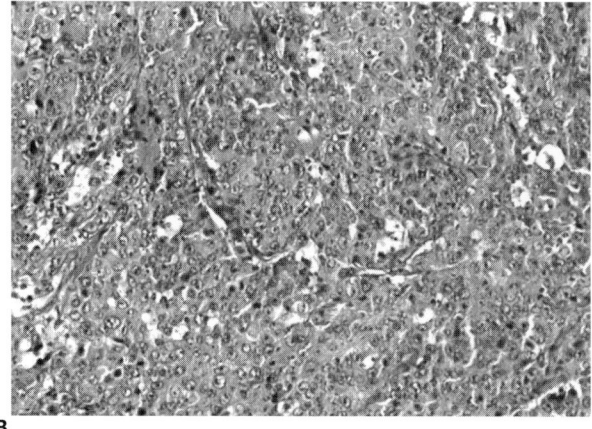

Figure 9.8 Colon cancer histology. A) A well-differentiated adenocarcinoma demonstrating typical gland formation. B) A poorly differentiated adenocarcinoma. Note the lack of gland formation.

Tumor pathology and staging

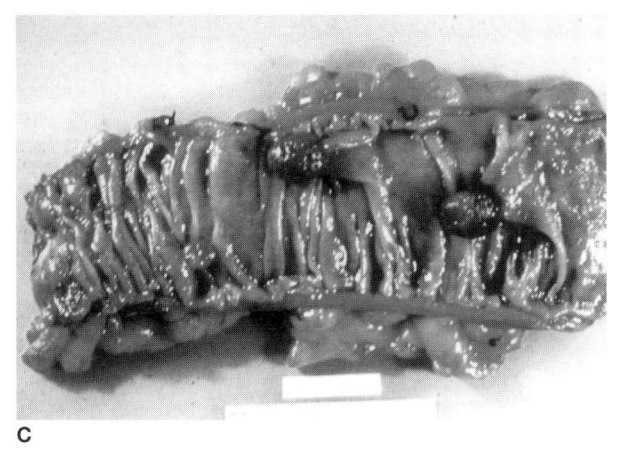

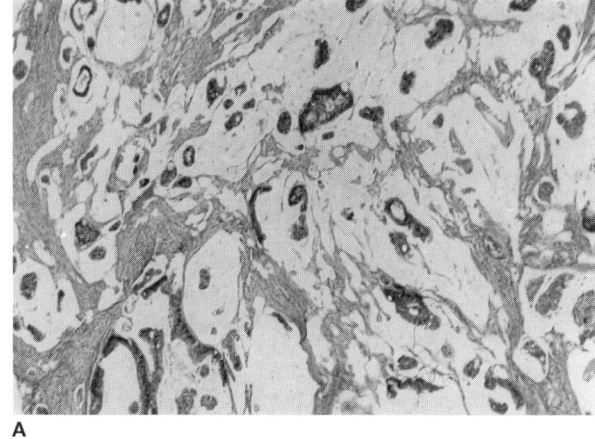

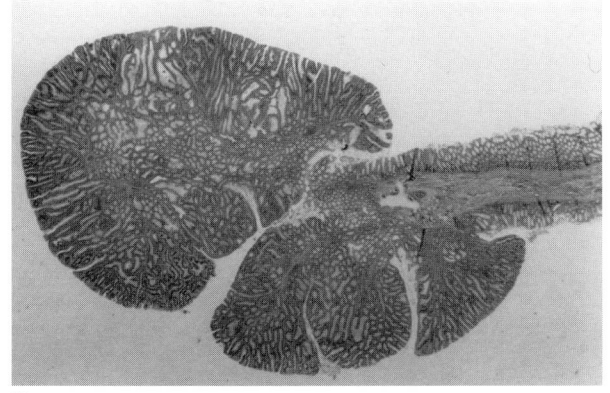

Figure 9.9 (continued) B) Snare polypectomy. C) Surgical specimen containing pedunculated polyps. D) Photomicrograph demonstrating a pedunculated tubular adenoma.

Figure 9.10 A) Mucinous carcinoma of the colon in which tumor cells can be seen floating in lakes of mucin. B) Signet-ring cell carcinoma.

able stage-independent prognosis, and medullary carcinoma, which is prognostically favorable.

Cancers other than adenocarcinomas constitute less than 5% of malignant tumors of the large bowel. Most of these arise at the anorectal junction and include squamous cell carcinomas, cloacogenic carcinomas, and melancarcinomas. Primary lymphomas of the large bowel constitute less than 0.1% of all large-bowel neoplasms. Endocrine tumors such as carcinoids also occur in the colon.

Tumor configuration

The three configurations of colorectal cancers include exophytic (fungating), endophytic (ulcerative), and diffusely infiltrative (linitis plastica) or annular. Overlap between these different types is a common feature of colorectal cancer. Overall configuration has no independent prognostic value with the exception of linitis plastica which is considered to have a worse prognosis.

Natural history

Most colorectal cancers evolve sequentially from intramucosal benign epithelial lesions through accumulation of a series of genetic events. This multi-step pattern of development is known as the adenoma–carcinoma sequence. One of the earliest events is the alteration in the cell proliferative pattern in the colonic crypt.

The initial recognizable histologic lesion is the aberrant crypt focus (Figure 9.2) which may be classified as dysplastic or non-dysplastic. Dysplastic aberrant crypt foci are considered to be microadenomas, they account for approximately 5% of total aberrant crypt foci and have the potential for progression to macroscopic adenomas and carcinomas.

Somatic mutations in the *APC* gene have been reported in up to 40% of dysplastic aberrant crypt foci and infrequent MSI has also been detected. *K-ras* mutations, although more frequently observed in hyperplastic aberrant crypt foci, have also been reported in dysplastic lesions. Dysplastic aberrant crypt foci have been demonstrated to have alterations in the distribution of proliferation markers in colonic crypts and increased expression of carcinoembrionic antigen. In aggregate these data suggest that larger dysplastic aberrant crypt foci progress to more advanced lesions. Only a small fraction of total number aberrant crypt foci ever progress to macroscopic adenomas and cancinomas.

The process of carcinogenesis is usually very long, taking many years, if not decades, to reach the stage of invasive carcinoma. Colon cancers grow at variable rates, the mean doubling time in one study was 620 days. As cancers grow they become invasive, penetrating through muscularis mucosae and beyond. Cells from these tumors eventually invade the lymphatic and vascular systems, metastasizing to local and distant sites (most commonly lymph nodes and liver). Patterns of spread depend on the anatomy of the specific bowel segment that harbors the cancer as well as its lymphatic and blood supply. Colon cancers spread to regional and distant lymph nodes and hepatic artery via the superior and inferior mesenteric vessels to the portal vein and the liver.

Rectal cancers often invade through the bowel wall and extend to nearby local structures. Lymphatic and hematogenous spread is uncommon prior to invasion of the muscularis mucosae except for poorly differentiated tumors which may spread at an earlier stage.

Pathological staging

Surgical resection is still the most effective therapy for colorectal cancer and the best assessment of prognosis is related to the pathological findings obtained from the surgical specimen. In this regard, the anatomical extension i.e the stage of the disease, is the most important independent prognostic factor. In 1929 Dukes proposed a classification for colorectal cancer in effort to increase the prognostic potential (Table 9.6). This classification has been modified many times however, the most commonly used modification was that performed by Astler and Coller in 1954. The Astler-Coller classification designated stage A, as tumors limited to the mucosa; stage B1, tumors extending into, but not through, the muscularis propria; stage B2, tumors invading the mus-

Table 9.6 Classification of colorectal cancer

Stage	Dukes, 1932 (rectum)	Astler-Coller, 1954 (colon and rectum)	Turnbull et al., 1967	Modified Astler-Coller (Gunderson and Sosin, 1974) (colon and rectum)
A	Limited to bowel wall	Limited to mucosa	Limited to mucosa	Limited to mucosa
B	Through bowel wall		Tumor extension into pericolic fat	
B1		Into muscularis propria		Into muscularis propria
B2		Through muscularis propria (and serosa)		Through serosa M = microscopic G = gross
B3				Adherent to or invading structures
C	Regional nodal metastases		Regional nodal metastases	
C1		Same as B1 plus regional nodal metastases		Same as B1 plus regional nodal metastases
C2		Same as B2 plus regional nodal metastases		Same as B2 plus regional nodal metastases
C3				Same as B3 plus regional nodal metastases
D			Distant metastases or adjacent organ invasion	

cularis propria but no lymph node involvement; stage C includes all tumors with lymph node involvement. Stage C is further categorized into C1, which includes tumors that are restricted to the bowel wall and C2 when tumors extend and invade the bowel wall. In 1967, stage D was added by Turnbull *et al.* and included all patients with distant metastasis.

A large number of staging systems for colorectal cancer have been developed over the years in attempt to improve the prognostic value of classification. The College of American Pathologist has recommended the use of the TNM Staging System (tumor invasion, number of nodes, and metastasic status) developed by the AJCC and the International Union Against Cancer (Boxes 9.4 and 9.5). In this classification the letter "T" designates the extent of invasion of the primary tumor, "N" designates the extent of regional lymph node involvement, and "M" indicates distant metastasis. Patients are grouped into 5 stages (0-IV) (Box 9.5). Stage 0 is considered carcinoma *in situ* and includes both malignant cells confined within the glandular basement membrane (intraepithelial carcinoma) and cells that invade the muscularis mucosa but do not penetrate it (intramucosal carcinoma). The 5-year survival rates have been shown to correlate with the TNM stage. The TNM classification system is widely accepted in the US as well as inter-

---

Box 9.5 American Joint Committee on Cancer staging of colorectal cancer

Stage 0
Carcinoma *in situ* (Tis, N0, M0)

Stage I
Tumor invades submucosa (T1, N0, M0)
Tumor invades muscularis propria (T2, N0, M0)

Stage II
T3, N0, M0
T4, N0, M0

Stage III
Any degree of bowel wall perforation with regional lymph node metastasis
Any T, N1, M0
Any T, N2, N3, M0

Stage IV
With evidence of distant metastasis.
Any T, Any N, M1

Based on the American Joint Committee on Cancer Manual for Staging of Cancer 5th edn. Dukes' B (corresponds to stage II) is a composite of better (T3, N0, M0) and worse (T4, N0, M0) prognostic groups as is Dukes' C (corresponds to stage III).

Box 9.4 TNM staging system[1]

Primary tumor (T)
T0 No evidence of primary tumor
Tis Carcinoma *in situ* intraepithelial or invasion of lamina propria[2]
T1 Tumor invades submucosa
T2 Tumor invades muscularis propriae
T3 Tumor invades through muscularis propriae into subserosa, or into non-peritonealized pericolic or perirectal tissue.
T4 Tumor directly invades other organs or structures, and /or perforates the visceral peritoneum[3]

Regional lymph nodes (N)
NX Regional lymph nodes cannot be assessed
N0 No regional lymph node metastases
N1 Metastases in less than four regional lymph nodes
N2 Metastases in more than four regional lymph nodes

Distant metastases (M)
MX Distant metastases cannot be assessed
M0 No distant metastases
M1 Distant metastases

[1]Based on the American Joint Committee on Cancer. Manual for Staging of Cancer, 5th edn, 1997
[2]Tis includes cancer cells confined within the glandular basement membrane (intraepithelial) or lamina propria (intramucosal) with no extension through the muscularis mucosa into the submucosa.
[3]Direct invasion in T4 includes invasion of other segments of the colorectum by way of the serosa, for example invasion of the sigmoid colon by a carcinoma of the cecum.

nationally and has in many cases replaced the Dukes' classification system.

Symptoms and clinical signs

Colorectal adenocarcinomas are slow-growing tumors and may be present for years before symptoms appear. Occult blood can be detected in asymptomatic individuals many years before symptoms emerge, and the bleeding rate increases with tumor size and degree of ulceration.

Symptoms depend on the site of the primary tumor. Cancers of the proximal colon usually grow larger before they produce symptoms. Constitutional symptoms (fatigue, shortness of breath, angina) secondary to microcytic hypochromic anemia are often the principal manner of presentation of right-colon tumors. Less often, blood from right-colon cancers is admixed with stool and appears as "maroon stool". More advanced tumors may produce vague abdominal discomfort or present as palpable masses. Obstruction is uncommon because of the large diameters of the cecum and ascending colon, although cecal cancers may block the ileocecal valve and cause distal small-bowel obstruction.

The left colon has a narrower lumen relative to the proximal colon and cancers of the descending and sigmoid colon often involve the bowel circumferentially and cause obstructive symptoms. Patients may present with colicky abdominal pain, and changes in bowel habits. Constipation may alternate with increased frequency of defecation, as small amounts of retained stool move beyond the obstructing lesion. Hematochezia, i.e the passage of bright-red blood, is present more often with distal colon and rectal lesions than with proximal ones. Rectal cancers also cause obstruction and changes in bowel habits, including constipation, diarrhea, and tenesmus. Rectal cancers may also cause perineal or sacral pain as they invade locally to involve the bladder, vaginal wall, or surrounding nerves. However, this symptom is a late manifestation of rectal cancer.

Prognostic factors

Pathology

The relationship between advanced colorectal cancer stage and patient survival has been consistently observed. The depth of tumor invasion into the bowel wall in addition to the presence or absence of lymph node involvement are by far the most accurate prognostic indicators. The 5-year survival rate for patients with carcinoma *in situ* is approximately 100% while even invasion of the muscularis propria (T2) lowers the 5-year survival to 85%. The degree of tumor invasion is positively correlated with lymph node involvement and the incidence of local recurrence after treatment. Lymph node involvement, however, has been shown to be an important independent risk factor. Lymph node involvement causes a 20% to 25% reduction in patient survival rates for the same degree of tumor invasion.

The importance of involvement of small lymphatic vessels and perineural invasion have been shown by multivariate analysis to be independent risk factors and indicate a worse prognosis. It is not always possible to distinguish lymphatic vessels from small venules. Involvement of extramural veins by tumor and its association with an increased risk of liver metastasis also has prognostic importance.

Histology

The histological grade of the tumor has been shown to correlate with survival. Poor differentiation confers a worse prognosis relative to well- or moderately differentiated tumors. Histological types of colorectal cancer that have been shown to have an adverse prognostic significance independent of stage are signet-ring cell carcinoma and small-cell carcinomas. Paradoxically, signet-ring cell carcinoma may occur in the setting of high MSI, in these cases the prognosis may be determined by the microsatellite status and may therefore be favorable. The correlation between mucinous tumors and prognosis has been less clear. While a poor prognosis has been reported by some studies, other studies failed to detect a correlation with prognosis at all or found a prognostic significance only for some classes of patient such as those with rectal tumors.

Tumor infiltration by lymphocytes is indicative of a host response and has been shown by some workers, but not others to be a positive prognostic factor.

Molecular markers

The DNA content of colorectal cancer has been shown to correlate with prognosis. Survival is better for individuals with diploid tumors, and worse for patients with non-diploid or aneuploid tumors. The value of routine measurements of DNA content in assessing individual prognosis remains to be determined. A wide number of molecular markers have been suggested as potential indicators of prognosis. Deletions in chromosomes 18q and 17p may be independent indicators of prognosis. In addition, alterations in TGF-β1, EGFR, c-erbB-2, VEGF and others are under extensive investigation as potential markers for prognosis after treatment of primary and metastatic colorectal cancer. Patients with tumors demonstrating MSI may have a better prognosis than those with microsatellite stable tumors.

Clinical characteristics

A number of clinical parameters have shown prognostic value. Younger age at presentation has shown to be an adverse progostic factor. Black race has also been shown to be an indicator of worse prognosis. In both these populations the low survival rate may be related, in part, to delayed diagnosis, with late presentation and a higher percentage of more advanced cancers. These patients usually present with symptoms such as rectal bleeding (34%), abdominal pain (30%), or a combination of the two. In addition, a higher percentage of mucinous tumors have been detected in younger patients.

Three of every twenty patients with colon cancer (15%) present with large-bowel obstruction. This presentation confers a worse prognosis with 5-year survival rates ranging from only 12% to 31% relative to non-obstructing tumors with 5-year survival rates of approximately 60%. Bowel perforation is another feature conferring a poor prognosis. In a recent study the 5-year survival in patients presenting with perforation was 46.8% compared to 76.6% in patients without bowel perforation ($P = 0.002$). Most studies have reported a much less favorable outcome for patients presenting with perforation with 5-year disease-free survival rates as low as 14%.

Tumor markers, including carcinoembryonic antigen, are used mainly for tumor follow-up to detect the recurrence of colonic cancer. Preoperative carcinoembrionic antigen levels have been shown to have a prognostic value, with high levels predicting the development of metastases and a poor prognosis. In a retrospective study that followed 318 patients for a minimum of 5 years or until death, the authors found that the incidence of preoperative carcinoembrionic antigen levels were predictive of 5-year survival rates in Dukes' B and C patients. For Dukes' B patients, the 5-year survival was 85% if carcinoembrionic antigen was 5 ng/mL or less, compared to 55% if carcinoembrionic antigen levels were more than 5 ng/mL ($P < 0.05$). Dukes' C patients with carcinoembrionic antigen of 5 ng/mL or less had a 5-year survival rate of 64% compared to patients with carcinoembrionic antigen levels above 5 ng/mL who had a 5-year survival rate of only 37% ($P < 0.05$). In this study, carcinoembrionic antigen was an independent prognostic factor for the recurrence of disease after primary tumor resection.

Expression of tumor-associated carbohydrate antigens such as sialyl Lewis X and the carbohydrate binding protein galectin-3 have been associated with the metastatic potential of tumor cells.

Screening and surveillance

Screening and surveillance are two different entities. Screening (in the context of colorectal cancer) identifies asymptomatic individuals who are at risk for development of colorectal cancer or adenomatous polyps. Surveillance monitors people with previously diagnosed colorectal disease (polyps, colorectal cancer, or inflammatory bowel disease).

Approximately 5.6% of Americans will eventually develop colorectal cancer. When colorectal cancer is diagnosed at an early, localized stage, 5-year survival is 90%, but only 37% of incident cases are diagnosed while still localized. Five-year survival for regional disease is 70%, and 38% of cases are diagnosed at this stage. Five-year survival for metastatic disease is 9%, and unfortunately 22% of patients are diagnosed at this advanced stage.

Screening

The major impact of colorectal cancer screening programs is through the early detection and removal of adenomatous polyps (Figure 9.9A, B), the precursors of colorectal cancers, and through the early detection of localized cancers which may be curable by surgical resection. Screening strategies take into consideration an individual's relative risk for colorectal cancer. High-risk populations include those at increased risk because of a family history of colorectal cancer, genetic syndromes, or a personal history of inflammatory bowel disease.

Individuals with a family history of colorectal cancer, but without any defined genetic syndrome, account for the majority (15% to 20%) of the high-risk population. Those with no predisposing factor are considered to be at average risk and this group constitutes approximately 75% of new cases of colorectal cancers. Screening of asymptomatic individuals at average risk for colorectal cancer should begin at the age of 50 years. Initiation of screening at an earlier age in this group is not indicated. This was supported by a recent study that included 906 consecutive persons 40 to 49 years of age who voluntarily participated in an employer-based screening colonoscopy program. In this age group advanced neoplasms (adenomas of at least 1 centimeter in diameter, a polyp with villous features or severe dysplasia, or a cancer) none of which were cancer, were detected in only 3.5% of individuals. More than half of the adenomas were located distally within the reach of a sigmoidoscope. Although the incidence of invasive cancer at the age of 50 years is relatively low, about 25% of adults at 50 years will have an adenomatous polyp. On the basis of this data the American Cancer Society, the American College of Gastroenterology, the American Gastroenterology Association, The American Society for Gastrointestinal Endoscopy, and the Society of American Gastrointestinal Endoscopic Surgeons have recommended five possible screening strategies for the average risk population (Table 9.7).

Fecal occult blood testing

Three prospective randomized trials have demonstated a 15% to 33% reduction in colorectal cancer-related mortality with fecal occult blood testing. Two case control studies reported a 31% to 57% reduction in mortality with fecal occult blood testing, in agreement with the beneficial effect observed in the prospective studies. The test most commonly utilized is the guaiac-based test for peroxidase activity. The positive reaction with blood results from the pseudo-peroxidase activity of hemoglobin. The most commonly used guaiac-based tests give no indication of the amount of blood lost and are not specific for human hemoglobin. Other substances have peroxidase or pseudoperoxidase activity (red meat, bacteria, and some hyperoxides in fruits and vegetables) and may cause false positive tests. False positive results also occur because other lesions

Table 9.7 Average-risk screening guidelines.

Screening tool	USPSTF[1]	Multidisciplinary Expert Panel[2]	American Cancer Society[3]	American College of Gastrenterology[4]
Fecal occult blood testing	Recommended annually.	Recommended annually.	Recommended annually as an option.	Recommended annually in conjunction with flexible sigmoidoscopy every 5 years.
Flexible sigmoidoscopy	Recommended "periodicity unspecified".	Recommended every 5 years.	Recommended every 5 years as an option.	Recommended every 5 years in conjunction with annual fecal occult blood testing.
Fecal occult blood testing plus flexible sigmoidoscopy	Recommended as an option.	Recommended as an option.	Annual fecal occult blood testing plus flexible sigmoidoscopy every 5 years recommended as an option.	Annual fecal occult blood testing plus flexible sigmoidoscopy every 5 years recommended as an option.
Colonoscopy	Insufficient evidence.	Recommended as an option every 10 years	Recommended as an option every 10 years.	Recommended as preferred strategy every 10 years.
Double-contrast barium enema	Insufficient evidence.	Recommended as an option every 5 to 10 years.	Recommended as an option every 5 years.	Not recommended as a primary screening strategy.

[1] US Preventative Services Task Force.
[2] Winawer SJ, Fletcher RH, Miller L, et al. Colorectal cancer screening clinical guidelines and rationale. Gastroenterology 1997; 112: 594–692. Endorsed by numerous medical and surgical societies. Updated guidelines 2001 provides menu of options rather than recommending any specific option in order to increase compliance with screening. Fecal occult blood testing should use take-home sample method. All positive tests should be followed-up with colonoscopy.
[3] Smith RA, von Eschenbach A, Wender R, et al. American Cancer Society guidelines for the early detection of cancer: update of early detection guidelines for prostate, colorectal, and endometrial cancers. CA Cancer J Clin 2001; 51: 38–75.
[4] American College of Gastroentroogy. Colorectal Cancer Prevention 2000. Colonoscopy is the preferred option for screening. All other options should be utilized when resources, expertise, or reimbursement for screening colonoscopy are not available.

along the gastrointestinal tract may bleed. Prior to the use of guaiac-based tests, individuals should be instructed to avoid non-steroidal anti-inflammatory drugs (in doses greater than 325 mg/day) for 1 week. In addition, vitamin C supplements or citrus fruits (in excess of 250 mg/day), and red meats should be eliminated from the diet for 3 days prior to testing. The positive predictive value for fecal occult blood testing with guaiac-based reagents is approximately 20% for adenomas and 5% to 10% for cancers. Colonic neoplasms bleed intermittently and blood is not present homogeneously throughout the stool. For these reasons the optimal protocol for testing fecal occult blood includes testing two samples from each of three consecutive stools at home. Sampling on one specimen yields a 40% to 50% false negative result. Fecal occult blood testing should be performed annually. The Minnesota fecal occult blood testing trial found a significant 33% reduction in mortality in those screened annually, and a 21% reduction in those screened every other year (biannually) at 18 years' follow-up. Other large prospective trials from Great Britain and Scandinavia have demonstrated a 15% to 18% reduction in mortality with biannual screening. American Cancer Society guidelines recommend annual fecal occult blood testing for men and women aged 50 years and over.

Flexible sigmoidoscopy

Flexible sigmoidoscopy enables visualization of the distal large bowel. Current flexible sigmoidoscopes are 60 to 70 centimeters in length but the amount of bowel visualized will vary depending on individual anatomy, the adequacy of bowel preparation, and the patient's ability to tolerate the procedure. Bowel preparation is performed usually by a saline laxative enema 1 to 2 hours before the procedure. Patients are generally not sedated and about 10% to 15% of patients experience discomfort of at least moderate intensity. Flexible sigmoidoscopy has replaced the rigid sigmoidoscope. A number of case control studies have provided evidence regarding the effectiveness of sigmoidoscopy in reducing mortality from colorectal cancer. In 1992, Selby and colleagues reported a 70% overall reduction in the mortality (adjusted odds ratio 0.41) from distal colorectal cancer in those undergoing rigid sigmoidoscopy compared to age- and sex-matched controls. The investigators tested the validity of their findings by analyzing deaths from cancers proximal to the area reached by the endoscope, and found that the protective effect was not apparent for proximal cancers. In another study, Newcomb and colleagues studied 66 patients who died of large-bowel cancer for history of screening for colorectal cancer and compared them with 196 controls of similar gender and age. While only 10% of case subjects were found to have a history of screening sigmoidoscopy, matched controls (30%) were much more likely to have had the procedure. They reported an 80% reduction in the risk for death from rectosigmoid cancer in patients who had a screening sigmoidoscopy compared with people who had not had this procedure. Since about 50% of colorectal cancers can be detected in the region accessible to the sigmoidoscope, these data suggest that periodic sigmoidoscopy screening could reduce overall colorectal cancer mortality by approximately 30%. In an additional study, Muller and colleagues studied patients with colon ($n = 8722$) and rectal ($n = 7629$) cancer relative to age-, sex-, and race-matched controls for the number of endoscopic procedures of the large bowel that had been performed prior to the diagnosis of colorectal cancer, and which would have allowed polypectomies to be performed. They concluded that endoscopic procedures of the large bowel reduced the risk for developing colon and rectal cancers by 50% and their protective effect lasted for 6 years. On the bases of these trials the American Cancer Society, the American College of Gastroenterology, the American Gastroenterology Association, The American Society for Gastrointestinal Endoscopy, and the Society of American Gastrointestinal Endoscopic Surgeons have recommended flexible sigmoidoscopy every 5 years as a screening option in average-risk individuals (Table 9.7). Sigmoidoscopy, however fails to detect a valuable number of proximal advanced adenomas (at least 1 centimeter in diameter, with villous features or severe dysplasia), and carcinomas. Approximately 50% of patients with advanced proximal lesions do not have distal findings on sigmoidoscopy. Only about 1.5% of patients with no distal adenomas, however, will harbor a proximal advanced neoplasm. It has been assumed that combining flexible sigmoidoscopy and fecal occult blood testing would be preferable to either test alone, but definitive data is lacking.

Double contrast barium enema

Barium enemas have been performed in two ways

1. a single contrast study using barium alone which mainly detects filling defects
2. a double contrast (air contrast) barium enema.

In the latter, after most of the barium has been removed, air is introduced into the rectum and colon and mucosal lesions are outlined by the retained barium. This procedure is capable of detecting mucosal lesions including small polyps that could not be detected by single contrast barium enema. No prospective randomized trial has directly compared the effectiveness of barium enemas with other modalities for colon cancer screening. Individual studies have suggested that the sensitivity and specificity for detection of neoplastic lesions were both approximately 80% to 90%. A Swedish retrospective study compared the yield of double contrast barium enema relative to colonoscopy in 288 people with suspected lower gastrointestinal bleeding and found that the sensitivity of the double contrast barium enema in detecting carcinomas and polyps larger than 1 centimeter was 100% and 98% respectively. However, more recent data are less favorable. Winawer and colleagues evaluated the accuracy of double contrast barium enema relative to colonoscopy in patients 3 to 6 years after a previous polypectomy. They studied 862 paired double contrast barium enema and colonoscopy examinations on 580 patients and found that double contrast barium enema detected only 48% of adenomas larger than 1 centimeter and 39% of smaller adenomas. Although not performed in a screening setting this study proposes that double contrast barium enema may be much less sensitive than previously thought. Complications of double contrast barium enema are minimal and include rare bowel perforation (1 in 25 000), barium impaction which can be prevented by the use of laxatives, and colicky abdominal discomfort after the examination which can be minimized by the use of antispasmodic drugs before the procedure. Furthermore, instilling carbon dioxide instead of air may reduce the incidence of severe pain after the test from 27% to 7%. In practice, approximately 10% of the double contrast barium enemas are unsatisfactory, and necessitate another attempt at double contrast barium enema or colonoscopy in order to image the entire colon. Furthermore, any pathology detected on double contrast barium enema has to be followed by a colonoscopy and potential biopsy of suspected lesions. For these reasons the use of double contrast barium enema for colorectal cancer screening is limited.

Colonoscopy

This is the only technique available that offers the ability to both detect and remove premalignant and small localized malignant lesions throughout the colon and rectum. A growing body of evidence suggests that colonoscopy may be the most effective method for colorectal cancer screening. Rex and colleagues studied 210 asymptomatic average risk people aged 50 to 75 years who had negative fecal occult blood testing and found that 53 (25%) had an adenoma and 2 had cancer. A multi-center trial which evaluated asymptomatic men (96.8%) between the ages of 50 and 75 years reported that a colonoscopic examination demonstrated one or more neoplastic lesions in 37.5%, dysplasia in 1.6%, and invasive cancer in 1% of the patients studied. Moreover, they found that 52% of patients with advanced proximal neoplasia (adenoma larger than 1 centimeter in diameter, villous adenoma, high-grade dysplasia or invasive cancer) had no distal adenomas. Approximately 3% to 15% of colorectal lesions may be missed by colonoscopy depending on the size of the lesion. A prospective study, in which 90 patients underwent two colonoscopies by different experienced examiners, found that adenomas larger than 1 centimeter were rarely missed but smaller lesions were missed in 15% of the cases. The National Polyp Study suggested that 20% of small polyps (less than 1 cm) may be missed by colonoscopy. Other studies have reported that up to 25% of polyps less than 5 millimeters in diameter may be missed by this examination. The direct effect of screening colonoscopy on cancer-related mortality has not been assessed. Since about 45% to 50% of advanced neoplastic lesions are beyond the reach of the sigmoidoscope, and given the proximal shift in colorectal cancer incidence over the past 30 years, the advantage of colonoscopy over sigmoidoscopy has been advocated. Colonoscopy, like sigmoidoscopy, permits the removal of neoplastic polyps with a subsequent lower than expected incidence of colorectal cancer.

The optimal interval at which screening colonoscopy should be performed has not been determined. On the basis of the high accuracy of this test, the time interval between adenoma and carcinoma development (adenoma–carcinoma sequence) and assessments from case control studies utilizing sigmoidoscopes, screening at a 10-year interval seems reasonable and cost effective. Colonoscopy is the gold standard for diagnosis of colonic neoplasia but it is not a perfect test. In one study performed in twenty Indiana hospitals the authors subsequently found 47 cases of colorectal cancer among patients who had a colonoscopy performed within 3 years of cancer diagnosis (sensitivity of 95%). The most frequent reason for not detecting the cancer was failure to reach the specific area. Another study yielded a 5% false negative rate for colonoscopy in a group of colorectal cancer patients who had prior procedures at a mean interval of 23 months (range 4 to 59 months) prior to diagnosis.

Colonoscopy is a relatively safe procedure. The complications can be divided into those attributable to the procedure itself and those caused by the sedation. The current rate of perforation induced by diagnostic colonoscopies is uncertain and ranges from 1 in 1000 to one in several thousand cases. The risk of perforation from the passage of the instrument has decreased over the years. Major hemorrhage is reported in 3 in 1000 colonoscopies and approximately 1 to 3 per 10 000 patients undergoing colonoscopy will die of complications from the procedure. The complication rate is higher if polypectomy if performed. Complications due to the sedation with midazolam plus meperidine mainly occur in older patients and include respiratory depression, hypotension, and bradycardia. Recent data suggest that sedating with propofol may result in fewer complications and increase patient satisfaction.

New screening techniques

Early clinical studies have shown promising results utilizing virtual colonoscopy and DNA stool tests for colorectal cancer screening. Virtual colonoscopy, also known as CT colonography, is a relatively non-invasive imaging method that was first introduced in 1994. Thin-section, helical computed tomography (CT) is used to generate high-resolution, two-dimensional axial images. Three-dimensional images of the colon simulating those obtained with conventional colonoscopy are then reconstructed off-line. This test has many potential advantages over conventional colonoscopy in that it is safe and quick and allows visualization of the whole colorectum in addition to visualization of the depth of the colon wall, lymph node enlargement, and liver metastases. This technique is currently under intensive study as a potential screening tool for detecting colorectal neoplasia. Published studies to date have investigated symptomatic or high-risk patients. The sensitivity of the test is between 83% and 100% and the specificity is 93% to 100% for detection of polyps equal to or larger than 1 centimeter. The sensitivity of the test is only 55% to 80% for detection of polyps 5 millimeters or smaller in size. One study evaluated 42 patients undergoing screening colonoscopy. All patients had CT colonography performed prior to conventional colonoscopy. Their sensitivity rates were similar to those previously reported in high-risk patients (100% for polyps 1 cm or larger, 60% for those between 6 and 9 mm, and 50% for polyps < 5 mm).

The major disadvantages of this test are a relatively low sensitivity for small polyps and the need for high resolution helical CT scanning which at present precludes its wide application for routine colorectal screening. In addition this method does not permit biopsies and removal of adenomatous polyps. High false positive results in early trials are also of concern.

The fecal multi-targeted DNA-based assay panel test is designed to detect DNA shed from colorectal neoplasms. A recent study utilized assay targets which included point mutations at any of 15 sites on *K-ras*, *p53*, and *APC* genes, Bat-26, a MSI marker, and highly amplified DNA. The authors reported a sensitivity rate of 91% for cancer and 82% for adenomas 1 centimeter or larger with a specificity of 93%. A randomized clinical trial is underway to assess the performance of multi-targeted DNA-based assay panel versus fecal occult blood testing or colonoscopy, but more definitive results regarding the potential role for fecal DNA sampling in colorectal screening are not expected for at least 3 to 5 years.

Screening in high risk groups

Approximately 5% to 10% of colorectal cancers occur in individuals at high risk for development of this disease. Those with a family history of colorectal neoplasia make up the majority of the high-risk population. Most cases of familial colorectal cancer are individuals with at least one immediate relative with neoplasia. Familial syndromes such as familial adenomatous polyposis and hereditary non-polyposis colorectal cancer are important because of the extremely high association with colorectal cancer, but they account for only a small portion of colon cancer cases in the US (1% to 2% for familial adenomatous polyposis and 6% for hereditary non-polyposis colorectal cancer). Other high-risk groups also require screening (inflammatory bowel disease) or surveillance (those with a personal history of colorectal cancer or adenomatous polyps).

Familial adenomatous polyposis

Screening of family members of an individual with established familial adenomatous polyposis should begin with genetic testing to determine which family members will eventually need follow-up (Table 9.4). Present methods allow successful recognition of an *APC* mutation in approximately 80% of familial adenomatous polyposis families. Those that carry a mutation should begin annual sigmoidoscopic examinations at 10 to 12 years of age to assess the polyp load and appropriate timing for colectomy. If genetic testing is not feasible or if the specific familial index case is negative for an identified genetic mutation, annual sigmoidoscopic examinations should begin at 10 to 12 years of age, and once polyps appear colectomy should be planned.

Hereditary non-polyposis colorectal cancer

Screening of family members of a patient with hereditary non-polyposis colorectal cancer should begin at the age of 20 to 25 years or 5 years younger than the index case with a full colonoscopy because of the predominance of proximal cancers in these families. Colonoscopy should be repeated every second year until the age of 40 years and annually thereafter. Genetic testing is available and best performed among families that are clinically known to meet the Amsterdam criteria. Unlike familial adenomatous polyposis identifiable mutations are present in only 50% of the index cases of Amsterdam criteria-positive families, and genetic testing is only valuable in these families.

Positive family history

Familial clustering of colorectal cancer cases is common in the absence of evidence for defined syndromes, and confers increased risk. A family history of either colorectal cancer or adenomatous polyps increases an individual's risk of developing colorectal cancer. First degree relatives of those with colon cancer have a two- to threefold increased risk of developing colorectal malignancies, and develop the disease at an earlier age than people without a family history. In a large prospective study Fuchs and colleagues found that in individuals with even a single first degree relative with colon cancer, the incidence of colorectal cancer at the age of 40 years was comparable to that in individuals at the age of 50 years without a family history of cancer. The risk is greatest in those whose relatives develop cancer at a younger age. The findings most predictive of risk severity were the number of immediate relatives with colon cancer and the age at diagnosis. Colon cancer in second and third degree relatives has been reported to increase the risk of colorectal cancer by only 50% above the general population risk. Risk for colorectal cancer is increased even among first degree family relatives of those with adenomatous polyps. In the National Polyp Study, the risk of colorectal cancer in siblings and parents of persons with any size adenomatous polyp was 1.78. If the adenoma was diagnosed before the age of 60 years the risk rose to 2.59 compared to those whose sibling had an adenoma later than 60 years of age.

The American Cancer Society recommends that if colorectal cancer or adenomatous polyps occur in any first degree relative before 60 years of age, or in two or more first degree relatives at any age, then colonoscopy should be performed every 5 to 10 years, beginning at age 40 years, or 10 years before the youngest case in the individual's family. How those with a single first degree relative who developed a neoplasm at a more advanced age should be screened is less clear. The multidisciplinary expert panel recommended that these individuals should be offered the same options as average-risk individuals (Table 9.7) but that screening should begin at 40 years of age. The American College of Gastroenterology has also provided recommendations that stratify screening intervals according to relative risk.

Surveillance

Three groups will be considered.

1. Individuals with a personal history of adenomatous polyps. These individuals should undergo colonoscopy at regular intervals. The National Polyp Study compared colonoscopy to double contrast barium enema in 862 paired procedures and found colonoscopy to be a superior method for surveillance. This study also demonstrated that a similar proportion of adenomatous polyps with advanced pathology (3.3%) was detected in patients who had repeat colonoscopies at 1 and 3 years, as compared to those who had the procedure done at only 3-year intervals. The American Cancer Society suggests that those whose index lesion is a single adenoma less than 1 centimeter in size should have a follow-up colonoscopy 3 to 6 years after the initial polypectomy. If the examination is normal, the patient can be screened according to the average-risk guidelines. In those with a larger (greater than 1 cm) adenoma, multiple adenomas, or adenoma with high-grade dysplasia or villous changes, colonoscopy should be repeated within 3 years of the initial polypectomy. If normal, the examination should be repeated once again in 3 years. If it remains normal, then the patient can thereafter be screened according to the average-risk guidelines. The guidelines for the latter group differ somewhat from previous American Cancer Society

guidelines, and from the procedures that are often practiced (i.e. colonoscopy 3 years after the removal of an adenoma; if it is negative then colonoscopy every 5 years) (Table 9.8).

2. Surveillance after curative-intent resection of colorectal cancer. These patients should have a complete examination of the colon within 1 year after resection. If this is normal, the examination should be repeated in 3 years. If the results are again negative, colonoscopy should then be repeated every 5 years. Serum carcinoembrionic antigen should be monitored at regular intervals since post-operative carcinoembrionic antigen elevation may indicate disease recurrence.

3. Inflammatory bowel disease. This has been extensively covered above (see p. 175). Patients with ulcerative colitis as well as Crohn's colitis develop colorectal cancer at a greater rate and at an earlier age relative to the general population. Risk is proportional to the duration and extent of colonic involvement.

Colonoscopy with frequent mucosal biopsies are effective in detecting pre-neoplastic and neoplastic lesions and is the preferred method for surveillance. The American Cancer Society and the American Gastroenterology Association recommend annual colonoscopies beginning after 8 years of disease duration in patients with extensive colitis, or similarly in those with left-sided colitis. Biopsies should be taken at 10 centimeter intervals with special attention to areas in the mucosa that appear grossly abnormal. In these patients the search is for dysplasia rather than for polyps and random biopsy sampling carries a high false negative rate (because of missing the area with dysplasia). If high-grade dysplasia is detected or macroscopic lesions or masses are found, colectomy is recommended. If low-grade

Table 9.8 Guidelines for surveillance colonoscopy.

Pathology	American College of Gastroenterology[1]	Multidisciplinary expert panel[2]	American Cancer Society[3]
Single adenoma	5 years after initial polypectomy.	No specific recommendation.	3–6 years after initial polypectomy. ↓ If normal as average risk.
Multiple (> 2) non-advanced adenomas	3 years after initial polypectomy. ↓ After one negative colonoscopy at 5-year intervals.	3 years after initial polypectomy.[4] ↓ If normal or single small tubular adenoma at 5-year intervals.	Within 3 years of the initial polypectomy ↓ If normal repeat colonoscopy in 3 years. ↓ If normal as average risk.
Advanced adenomas.	As for multiple non-advanced adenomas.	As for multiple non-advanced adenomas.	As for multiple non-advanced adenomas
Curative-intent resection of colorectal cancer	Not specified.	Preoperative examination within 1 year after cancer resection. ↓ If normal repeat colonoscopy in 3 years. ↓ If normal repeat every 5 years.	Within 1 year after cancer resection. ↓ If normal repeat colonoscopy in 3 years. ↓ If normal repeat every 5 years.
Inflammatory bowel disease	Not specified	Every 1–2 years,[5] Pancolitis: beginning after 8 years of disease. Left-sided colitis: beginning at 15 years.	Every 1–2 years. Pancolitis-beginning after 8 years of disease. Left-sided colitis beginning at 12–15 years.

[1] Bond JH, Polyp guideline: diagnosis, treatment, and surveillance for patients with colorectal polyps. Practice Parameters Committee of the American College of Gastroenterology. Am J Gastroenterol 2000; 95(11): 3053–3063.
[2] Winawer SJ, Fletcher RH, Miller L, et al. Colorectal cancer screening clinical guidelines and rationale. Gastroenterology 1997; 112: 594–692. Endorsed by numerous medical and surgical societies.
[3] Smith RA, von Eschenbach A, Wender R, et al. American Cancer Society Guidelines for the early detection of cancer: update of early detection guidelines for prostate, colorectal, and endometrial cancers. CA Cancer J Clin 2001; 51: 38–75.
[4] If multiple adenomas are detected a shorter than 3-year interval may be necessary, according to the judgment of the clinician.
[5] Looking for dysplasia as a marker of colorectal cancer risk.

dysplasia is detected colonoscopies are recommended at 3 to 6-month intervals. To date, no direct evidence firmly establishes a reduction in colorectal cancer mortality because of surveillance in this group

Treatment

Colon cancer

Surgical resection of the tumor is the treatment of choice for colorectal cancer. Prior to the surgery a full colonoscopic evaluation of the colon and rectum should be performed to rule out synchronous malignancies which occur in about 5% of the patients. If a full colonoscopy is impossible a double contrast barium enema should be performed. Rectal cancer evaluation and treatment differs from colon cancer and will be addressed separately. A preoperative evaluation for metastatic colon cancer should include a thorough physical examination, chest X-ray, liver function tests, and a serum carcinoembrionic antigen level. Computed tomography is not requested as a routine preoperative evaluation tool, it is indicated, however, if clinical or biochemical evaluations indicate a possibility of liver or peritoneal involvement. The aim of surgery is not only resection of a wide area around the involved section (at least a 5 cm margin on each side) of the bowel but also the removal of the segmental lymphatic drainage vessels. The extent of colonic resection is determined by the blood supply and distribution of regional lymph nodes. Segmental resection is preferred when possible. Cancers of the cecum and ascending colon often require right hemicolectomy. The extent of resection in the left colon varies with location. Larger resected areas have not proven to be superior to the segmental resection. The primary tumor should be resected even if distant metastases are present in order to prevent obstruction and bleeding. Surgery is unnecessary for polypoid early colonic tumors that can be resected endoscopically as long as the resection margins (2 mm or more) are negative for tumor cells and the tumor is well or moderately differentiated. Surgery should be performed unless there is a medical contraindication to a surgical procedure. Advanced age should not preclude surgery for colorectal cancer.

Surgical resection of liver metastases

Synchronous liver metastases occur in approximately 20% of patients presenting with colorectal cancer and 25% to 30% develop metachronous liver metastases. Surgical resection for isolated liver metastases results in a 5-year survival of 24% to 38% in selected patients. Only 10% to 15% of patients with liver metastases are appropriate candidates for metastatic resection because of extensive disease, poor general condition, or primary failure to detect occult disease. Accurate staging and the extent of liver involvement is an important factor in selecting patients who will benefit from this surgery. Staging laparoscopy combined with laparoscopic ultrasonography should be a routine for all patients considering resection of hepatic metastases. Up to 45% of patients will be disqualified by this procedure because of unresectable disease. The only absolute contraindications to surgery are an inability to resect all lesions or the presence of extrahepatic spread. A number of factors such as the number of metastases (more than 4), resection margins (less than 1 cm), size of liver metastases (more than 5 cm), and an elevated preoperative carcinoembrionic antigen level are, however, associated with a poor prognosis.

Adjuvant chemotherapy

The prognosis of patients after complete surgical removal of a clinically localized colon cancer depends on the pathological staging of the primary tumor. The 5-year survival for patients with Dukes' A tumors is approximately 90% while patients with locally advanced Dukes' B2 or C tumors have a significantly increased risk of relapse after surgical resection alone, with a 5-year survival rate of only about 40% for patients with Dukes' C tumors. For this reason adjuvant therapies have been targeted at destroying microscopic metastases.

Many studies over the past 40 years have studied different regimens for adjuvant therapy. To date the most common drug in use is fluorouracil (5-FU). This drug is converted into its active metabolite, fluorodeoxyuridine monophosphate (FdUMP), within the cell. Fluorodeoxyuridine monophosphate inhibits the enzyme thymidilate synthase (TS), which catalyzes the conversion of dUMP to dTMP, preventing pyrimidine synthesis and therefore DNA synthesis. Fluorouracil is also falsely incorporated into RNA, interfering with RNA synthesis. A large clinical controlled study evaluated 1296 patients with Dukes' B2 or C colon cancer. Patients were randomly assigned to observation or to treatment for 1 year with 5-FU combined with levamisole. Patients with Dukes' C disease could also enter a levamisole-alone arm. The combination of 5-FU and levamisole in patients with

Dukes' C reduced the relative risk of cancer recurrence by 42% and overall death rate by 33%, while levamisole alone had no detectable effect. The authors concluded that 5-FU and levamisole should be standard therapy for Dukes' C colon cancer. Further studies demonstrated that treatment should be continued for at least 1 year. Similar regimens did not prove superior to surgery alone for Dukes' B colon cancer, and overall survival of these patients was not increased with adjuvant therapy at 7 years (72% in both arms).

Based on these results, in 1990 a consensus development panel convened by the National Cancer Institute decided that patients with Dukes' C colon cancer should be offered adjuvant therapy with 5-FU and levamisole. More recent evidence suggested that the combination of 5-FU and leucovorin was effective in improving overall and disease-free survival when used in the adjuvant setting. A study comparing adjuvent therapies included 2151 patients with Dukes' B and C colon cancer, and found that treatment with 5-FU and leucovorin confers a small disease-free survival advantage (65% versus 60%) and a borderline prolongation in overall survival relative to treatment with 5-FU and levamisole. An additional prospective multi-centre trial studied these two regimens in 680 Dukes' C patients and found that after a median follow-up of 46.5 months, the combination of 5-FU and leucovorin significantly improved disease-free survival ($P = 0.037$) and decreased overall mortality ($P = 0.0089$) in comparison with 5-FU plus levamisole. Recent evidence suggests that treatment with 5-FU and leucovorin for 6 months after curative surgery is as effective, and yet more convenient, than the standard 5-FU and levamisole given for 1 year. Adjuvant treatment with 5-FU and leucovorin for 6 months is therefore considered the best therapeutic regimen for patients with Dukes' C or stage III disease.

Adjuvant chemotherapy for node-negative, stage II, colon cancer remains controversial, and its administration is not routinely recommended except in certain high-risk and selected patients (patients whose tumor invades through muscularis propria into subserosa or into pericoloic tissue (T3) or with tumor invasion into other organs (T4).

Portal vein infusions of chemotherapeutic agents have been extensively studied as a means of delivering adjuvant therapy. This approach is designed to destroy micrometastasis in the liver. A meta-analysis evaluated results from ten randomized studies of portal vein infusion involving approximately 4000 patients. The main cytotoxic drug utilized in these studies was 5-FU, however, mitomycin C was co-administered in two of the trials. Results indicate that portal vein infusion with 5-FU, with or without other cytotoxic drugs for about 1 week after surgery in patients with colorectal cancer, may produce an absolute improvement in 5-year survival of only a few percent. Additional larger randomized studies are necessary before a recommendation for routine portal vein infusion as adjuvant therapy can be made.

Chemotherapy of advanced disease

The approch to patients with advanced colorectal cancer has changed dramatically over the past decade. Until the early 1990s the only effective agent available for the treatment of metastatic disease was 5-FU. During the past decade new cytotoxic agents such as raltitrexed, irinotecan, oxaliplatin, and oral fluoropyrimidines have been evaluated. Three oral fluoropyrimidines have been developed; UFT, eniluracil, and capecitabine. UFT is a combination of uracil and tegafur (prodrug of 5-FU). Recent research has also focused on novel targets and molecular markers. Untreated patients with metastatic colon cancer have a median survival of about 6 months. A meta-analysis comparing the median survival rate of infusional 5-FU with that of bolus 5-FU treatment found that infusion therapy gave a higher response rate (22% versus 14%; $P = 0.0002$) and was also associated with a small but significant survival advantage (12.1 months versus 11.3 months; $P = 0.04$). A major disadvantage of the infusion regimen is the necessity for a central venous catheter for the administration of drugs. Folinic acid increases the intracellular pool of reduced folate and stabilizes the FdUMP/TS complex. Studies have shown that adding folinic acid to bolus 5-FU improves response rates from 11% to 23%. Currently the first line treatment for metastatic colorectal cancer is bolus 5-FU combined with folinic acid. Additional treatment options include CPT-11/irinotecan, and oxaliplatin. The camptothecin analog CPT-11 inhibits DNA topoisomerase I and induces single-strand DNA breaks and replication arrest. This drug has been shown to be of efficiency in patients refractory to 5-FU. A large phase III clinical trial evaluated CPT-11 in a study of 387 patients who had previously not been treated with chemotherapy. The combination of 5-FU and CPT-11 was superior to 5-FU alone, with a response rate of 49% in the combined treatment group compared to 31% in those treated with 5-FU alone ($P < 0.001$). Overall survival was increased from a median of 14.1 months in the 5-FU group to 17.4 months

($P = 0.031$) in the combination group. Oxaliplatin is a third generation platinum analog that induces DNA cross-linkage and apoptotic cell death. This drug, like CPT-11, has been shown to be effective in treating 5-FU refractory advanced colon cancer with response rates of approximately 10% to 20%. It has also shown effectiveness in combination with 5-FU and folinic acid and has been added to the combination of 5-FU and leucovorin in patients resistant to standard 5-FU/leucovorin treatment with a response rate of 27%.

Infusion of chemotherapy directly into the hepatic artery may be utilized to treat hepatic metastases. The rationale for this treatment modality is that metastases travel to the liver via the portal system, however, once they grow beyond 3 millimeters their arterial blood is supplied by branches of the hepatic artery. The liver hepatocytes, on the contrary, gain their blood supply from the portal system. In this way higher concentrations of chemotherapy can be delivered directly to the tumor. The infusion catheter is implanted into the common hepatic artery through the gastroduodenal artery at the time of laparotomy. Fluorinated pyrimidines such as 5-FU and floxuridine (FUDR), have high hepatic excretion which permits a significant concentration of drug within the intrahepatic circulation while minimizing systemic toxicity. Randomized studies of systemic versus intrahepatic infusion of FUDR in patients with liver metastases have shown significantly higher response rates for the latter (54% to 83%) but the influence on survival is unclear as most studies permitted crossover of those patients who progressed.

Complications of the intrahepatic arterial pumps are minimal and include arterial occlusion, infections, and catheter leaks. However, intrahepatic treatment carries a high rate of liver toxicity. Hepatocytic necrosis and cholestasis are observed, and in one autopsy series damage to the biliary tree associated with small vessel necrosis was universal. These changes have been found to be similar to idiopathic sclerosing cholangitis. All patients treated with intra-arterial hepatic chemotherapy should be monitored for changes in liver function tests and if changes develop dose reduction and treatment discontinuation should be considered. Serum bilirubin levels over 3 mg/dL necessitate treatment breaks until normalization to prevent sclerosing complications. While relapse within the liver is reduced, a large percentage (up to 70%) of patients receiving intrahepatic infusion therapy go on to develop extrahepatic metastases. Combination with systemic chemotherapy has been evaluated in a number of trials. This may reduce the rate of extrahepatic disease from 79% to 56%.

Rectal cancer

Approximately 20% of large bowel cancers are located in the rectum. Rectal cancers present a therapeutic challenge because they are located in the pelvis and complete resection of large tumors may be a difficult task, especially if the pelvis is small, necessitating removal of the anal sphincter. Surgical treatment of rectal cancer is also more complicated than for colon cancer because the autonomic innervation lies close to the mesorectum (the fatty tissue surrounding the rectum that contains vessels and lymph nodes) which may be injured in the process of removing the tumor, leading to impotency and neurogenic bladder. The importance of total mesorectal excision has been demonstrated in multiple clinical trials. In a cohort of 381 patients who underwent total mesorectum excision the local recurrence (6% versus 15%) and cancer-related deaths decreased significantly over a period of 2 years. Autonomic nervous system preservation, which includes preservation of the hypogastric nerve, has become the standard care for minimizing bladder and male sexual dysfunction after radical resection of rectal cancer. In view of these results and the potential for fewer surgical complications, total mesorectal excision is the procedure of choice for curative treatment. Preservation of the anal sphincter is dependent on the distance between the lower edge of the tumor and the external sphincter and levator ani muscle. In general, sphincter preservation should be performed as long as a distal margin of 2 centimeters of normal mucosa exists below the tumor.

Adjuvant therapy

Local recurrence of rectal cancer is more common than colon cancer, partially because of the difficulty in obtaining wide surgical margins as discussed previously (see p. 190). Local recurrence for stage II rectal cancer after primary resection approaches 25% to 30%, with a 50% recurrence rate for those with stage III disease. Furthermore, patients with locally invasive rectal cancer are at high risk for systemic relapse. Two major components of adjuvant therapy for rectal cancer include pelvic radiation and fluoropyrimidine-based chemotherapy (5-FU). Radiation therapy (pre- or postoperative) is primarily used to decrease local recurrence and increase the possibility of sphincter preservation, while systemic chemotherapy serves to intensify radiation (radiosensitize) and eliminate distant metastases. Based on two large randomized trials from the Gastrointestinal Tumor Study Group and the Mayo/NCCTG which revealed a significant improvement in local recurrence (Mayo/NCCTG) and survival (both studies) with combined adjuvant therapy, the National Institute of Health Consensus Conference in 1990 recommended adjuvant therapy for patients with stage II to III rectal cancer that includes high-dose pelvic radiation and 5-FU-based chemotherapy. Preoperative adjuvant therapy (neoadjuvant) has been studied intensively during the past decade. This results in tumor regression, facilitating resection of the tumor and sphincter-preserving surgery. Patients diagnosed with rectal cancer should have preoperative staging which includes a thorough physical examination, chest X-rays, CT scan of the abdomen and pelvis, and transrectal ultrasound. Accuracy of transrectal ultrasound in the preoperative setting is as high as 90% to 95% in staging the transmural extent of rectal cancer, and about 80% in the detection of regional lymph node metastasis. It is less accurate following pre-operative radiation. Digital examination of the tumor determines whether the tumor is mobile (T2), tethered (T3), or fixed to the surrounding tissue (T4). Suitable candidates for neoadjuvant chemoradiation are patients with locally advanced rectal tumors (T3 or T4 by digital examination and transrectal ultrasound) without evidence of systemic metastasis. Patients with metastatic rectal cancer may be candidates for neoadjuvant chemoradiation, but evidence for its benefit in this setting is less clear. It is not clear at the present time if there is a difference in outcome in patients treated with preoperative versus postoperative chemoradiation, and several comparative trials are ongoing. Many studies have focused on the addition of intraoperative radiation therapy to preoperative chemoradiation. After tumor resection has been completed, radiation is provided to the tumor bed. Non-randomized studies have found that intraoperative radiation therapy may be superior in reducing local recurrence in patients with microscopically positive tumor margins, however, recurrence rates still remain as high as 60% for these patients.

Further reading

Ahlquist DA, Skoletsky JE, Boynton KA, *et al.* Colorectal cancer screening by detection of altered human DNA in stool: feasibility of a multitarget assay panel. *Gastroenterology* 2000; 119(5): 1219–1227.

Baron JA, Beach M, Mandel JS, *et al.* Calcium supplements for the prevention of colorectal adenomas. Calcium Polyp Prevention Study Group. *N Engl J Med* 1999; 340(2): 101–107.

Cruz-Correa M, Hylind LM, Romans KE, *et al.* Long-term treatment with sulindac in familial adenomatous polyposis: a prospective cohort study. *Gastroenterology* 2002; 122(3): 641–645.

Fuchs CS, Giovannucci EL, Colditz GA, *et al.* A prospective study of family history and the risk of colorectal cancer. *N Engl J Med* 1994; 331(25): 1669–1674.

Gastrointestinal Tumor Study Group. Adjuvant therapy of colon cancer: results of a prospectively randomized trial. *N Engl J Med* 1984; 310: 737–734.

Giardiello FM, Hamilton SR, Krush AJ, *et al.* Treatment of colonic and rectal adenomas with sulindac in familial adenomatous polyposis. *N Engl J Med* 1993; 328(18): 1313–1316.

Hermsen M, Postma C, Baak J, *et al.* Colorectal adenoma to carcinoma progression follows multiple pathways of chromosomal instability. *Gastroenterology* 2002; 123(4): 1109–1119.

Imperiale TF, Wagner DR, Lin CY, *et al.* Risk of advanced proximal neoplasms in asymptomatic adults according to the distal colorectal findings. *N Engl J Med* 2000; 343; 169.

Peltomaki P, Aaltonen LA, Sistonen P, *et al.* Genetic mapping of a locus predisposing to human colorectal cancer. *Science* 1993; 260(5109): 810–812.

Sonneberg A, Delco F. Cost-effectiveness of a single colonoscopy in screening for colorectal cancer. *Arch Intern Med* 2002; 162(2): 163–168.

Steinbach G, Lynch PM, Phillips RK, *et al.* The effect of celecoxib, a cyclooygenase–2 inhibitor, in familial adenomatous polyposis. *N Engl J Med* 2000; 342(26):1946–1952.

Takayama T, Katsuki S, Takahashi Y, *et al.* Aberrant crypt foci of the colon as precursors of adenoma and cancer. *N Engl J Med* 1998; 339(18): 1277–1284.

Vogelstein B. Fearon ER, Hamilton SR, *et al.* Genetic alterations during colorectal tumor development. *New Engl J Med* 1988; 319: 525.

Watanabe T, Wu T-T, Catalano PJ, *et al.* Molecular predictors of survival after adjuvant chemotherapy for colon cancer. *New Engl J Med* 2001; 344: 1196.

Winawer SJ, Stewart ET, Zauber AG, *et al.* A comparison of colonoscopy and double-contrast barium enema for surveillance after polypectomy. National Polyp Study Work Group. *N Engl J Med* 2000; 342(24): 1766–1772.

Chapter 10

Motility Disorders of the Small Bowel and Colon

Henry P. Parkman

CHAPTER OUTLINE

INTRODUCTION

THE SMALL INTESTINE

   Normal small-intestinal motility

   Symptoms related to abnormal small-intestinal motility

   Motility testing of the small intestine

   Disorders of small-intestinal motility

THE COLON

   Normal colonic motility

   Symptoms of colonic motility disorders

   Evaluation of colonic and anorectal motility

   Disorders of colonic motility

SUMMARY

FURTHER READING

Introduction

This chapter will provide an overview of the motility disorders of the small bowel and colon. It will also cover the tests used for the clinical evaluation of patients with these disorders. Small-bowel motility disorders can cause a variety of symptoms from nausea and vomiting to altered bowel habits – either constipation or diarrhea. Similarly, colonic motility disorders may also cause symptoms of constipation, diarrhea, and abdominal pain. Small-bowel and colonic motility disorders can present with varying severity that ranges from mild to severe and incapacitating. Persistent symptoms often lead to a motility evaluation which may include whole-gut scintigraphy, antroduodenojejunal manometry, and/or anorectal manometry. These evaluations can assess the part of the gastrointestinal tract affected and characterize the type of abnormality – either neuropathic or myopathic. Evaluation may guide treatments which target the underlying pathophysiology of the disease.

The small intestine

Normal small-intestinal motility

The small intestine functions mainly to digest and absorb nutrients after the delivery of solid and liquid material from the stomach. The motor function of the small bowel serves two basic purposes, proper mixing of the material with absorption of nutrients and timely propulsion of the bowel contents. These depend on highly coordinated neuromuscular function involving smooth muscle contractility regulated by electrical input from the interstitial cells of Cajal and neural input from both the intrinsic (enteric) and extrinsic nervous systems.

Small-bowel motor function is closely coordinated with that of the stomach with the occurrence of two distinct patterns of motor activity, the interdigestive (fasting) cycle and the digestive (fed) response. The interdigestive (fasting) cycle consists of three phases that recur cyclically. Each sequence begins with a period of motor quiescence (phase I) that is followed by intermittent contractions (phase II), which culminates in a burst of regular rhythmic contractions (phase III, activity front). The appearance of phase III in the duodenum coincides with cyclic increases in biliary and pancreatic secretions. The intense propulsive contractions during phase III are the predominant mechanism by which dietary fiber and indigestible solids leave the stomach and pass into and through the small intestine during the interdigestive period. The term "intestinal housekeeper" has been used to describe the phase III activity front since it sweeps any remaining food in the stomach and small intestine down the gastrointestinal tract into the colon. The cycle then recurs, returning to phase I. Feeding disrupts the characteristic interdigestive migrating motor complex cycles of phase I, phase II, and phase III. The contractile pattern that develops with eating is termed the "fed" or post-prandial pattern and consists of random motor activity with occasional peristaltic traveling over short distances and segmental contractions. This apparent disorganized pattern is, however, responsible for the transport of digestible food out of the stomach and down the small intestine.

Symptoms related to abnormal small-intestinal motility

Symptoms that may arise from slow propagation of small-bowel contents include post-prandial abdominal distension and bloating, nausea and vomiting, abdominal pain and discomfort, constipation, and/or diarrhea (see Box 10.1). Some of these symptoms of small-bowel dysmotility can also be seen in gastroparesis alone (delayed gastric emptying) or in mechanical obstruction. The most important initial clinical question in evaluating a patient with suspected small-bowel motility disorder is whether the symptoms are the result of either a motility disorder or a mechanical obstruction.

Symptoms that may arise from rapid small-bowel transit include post-prandial diarrhea. Rapid intestinal transit also leads to a decreased contact time of the luminal contents with the mucosa preventing proper absorption. Patients may have maldigestion and malabsorption because of poor mixing of the dietary material with the digestive enzymes and bile salts. Accentuated bowel sounds, borborygmi, may also disturb the patient. Diarrhea may also occur with slow transit because of small intestine bacterial overgrowth that arises in part from reduced or absent phase III migrating motor complexes.

Motility testing of the small intestine

Intestinal transit measurements

Barium contrast radiography Radiological studies are important in the diagnosis of structural gastrointestinal lesions that produce symptoms similar to those caused by motility disorders, and can also provide indirect signs of impaired gastrointestinal motility. Upper gastrointestinal series with small-bowel follow-through can give an estimation of transit time to the terminal ileum, but it is not very accurate. In the upper gastrointestinal series with small-bowel follow-through, overview films of the abdomen are obtained at periodic intervals (usually 30 min) after the conventional upper gastrointestinal series with orally administered contrast. When the barium reaches the cecum, spot films are obtained to visualize the terminal ileum; compression of the abdomen is also used to separate the loops of small bowel. The small-bowel follow-through generally provides adequate information in severe obstruction and can usually assess the terminal ileum for Crohn's disease. Conventional small-bowel follow-through examination has limitations that causes it to miss lesser grades of small-bowel obstruction and small focal abnormalities. The barium empties out of the stomach at an uncontrolled rate giving an unreliable and variable passage of the barium through the pylorus with subsequent difficulty in correct timing of serial fluoroscopy. Anatomically, the small-intestinal loops overlap one another preventing adequate visualization. Throughout the test, it is not possible to distend the small intestine for adequate visualization. The test can be made more accurate by more frequent fluoroscopy with manual compression, however, this is seldom done.

In enteroclysis (small-bowel enema), a naso- or oroduodenal tube is used to deliver barium directly into the small bowel. Intubation beyond the

---

Box 10.1 Symptoms of small-bowel motor dysfunction

Abdominal distension or bloating
Nausea and/or vomiting
Postprandial abdominal discomfort or pain
Diarrhea
Constipation

pylorus bypasses gastric emptying and allows careful delivery of contrast material at a controlled rate using gravity or a pump. The radiologist can follow the initial flow of barium through each portion of the small intestine. Infusion of methylcellulose after the barium allows double contrast studies and adequate distension from the ligament of Treitz to the terminal ileum. Intubation with a 10 F tube is a limiting factor in the examination, which occasionally requires sedation using a benzodiazepine. The tip of the nasoduodenal tube is usually advanced to the ligament of Treitz, thus lesions of the duodenum can occasionally be missed. If asked, at the end of the procedure the radiologist can pull the tube back into the mid-duodenum and instill additional barium to visualize this area. Overall, the procedure time for enteroclysis, usually less than 1 hour, is shorter than the time needed for small-bowel follow-through.

At present, enteroclysis is the most accurate technique available for radiologic examination of the small intestine. It is more accurate in detecting small lesions compared to conventional small-bowel follow-through, for mild to intermediate grades of SBO and for detection of small-bowel cancers. For obstructing lesions, the transition site from dilated to non-dilated small bowel is often readily apparent. If an abnormality exists, differentiation between an adhesive band, malignancy, or radiation injury can often be made.

Hydrogen breath test Lactulose, a non-absorbable carbohydrate, is utilized in the hydrogen breath test primarily to assess for bacterial overgrowth, but it can also be used to measure orocecal transit. After oral ingestion, lactulose traverses through the small intestine unaltered and undergoes metabolism by colonic bacteria at the cecum. The hydrogen produced is absorbed into the blood stream and excreted by the lungs. The time from ingestion of lactulose to the onset of a sustained rise in breath hydrogen provides an index of the orocecal transit time (Figure 10.1A). This technique is simple, inexpensive, and non-invasive with no radiation exposure. Lactulose itself, however, may increase orocecal transit. The interpretation of this test in patients is difficult if gastroparesis or small-intestinal bacterial overgrowth is present. In bacterial overgrowth, bacteria in the small intestine metabolize the lactulose giving rise to an early double peak in the breath hydrogen concentration (Figure 10.1B). In some patients, the colonic bacteria metabolize the lactulose to methane rather than hydrogen; often both are measured for clinical evaluation.

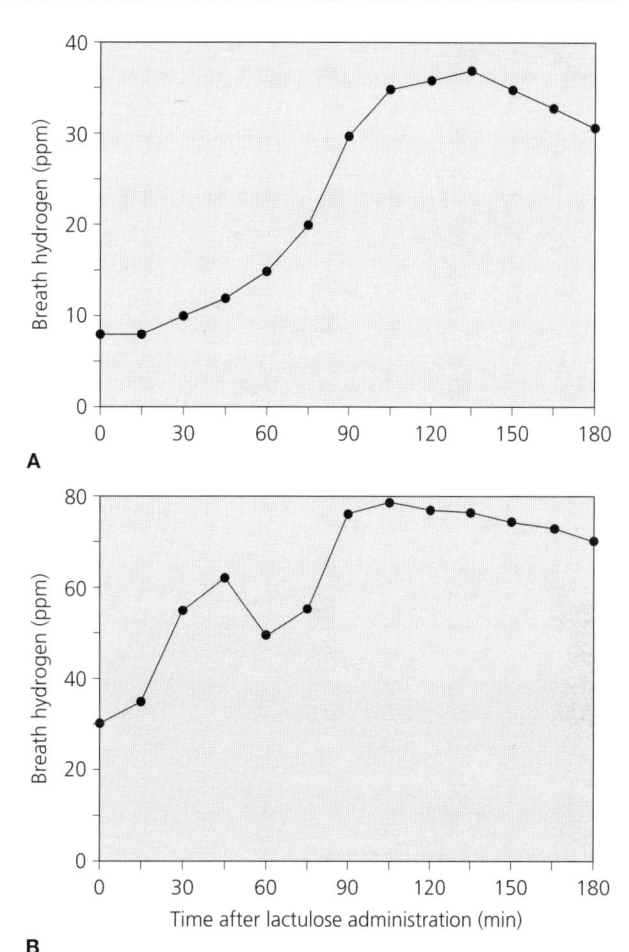

Figure 10.1 Lactulose breath test. A) Normal result. There is a low fasting breath hydrogen concentration less than or equal to 20 ppm. After lactulose administration, there is a single peak of the breath hydrogen. The normal peak breath hydrogen is less than or equal to 64 ppm. In this example, there is an orocecal transit time of 75 min, the time that there is a greater than 10 ppm rise above the baseline breath hydrogen concentration. B) Small-intestinal bacterial overgrowth. There is an elevated baseline hydrogen greater than 20 ppm. After lactulose administration, there is a double peak in breath hydrogen. There is also an elevated peak breath hydrogen of greater than 64 ppm.

Scintigraphic small-intestinal transit Small-intestinal transit can be measured scintigraphically. This is often performed as an addition to the standard solid-phase gastric emptying test using indium-111-DTPA in water to measure liquid gastric emptying and small-bowel transit, as shown in Figure 10.2. Measurement of small-bowel transit requires up to an additional 4 hours of imaging over the usual 2 hours for gastric emptying. There are several methods to measure small-bowel transit

Motility Disorders of the Small Bowel and Colon

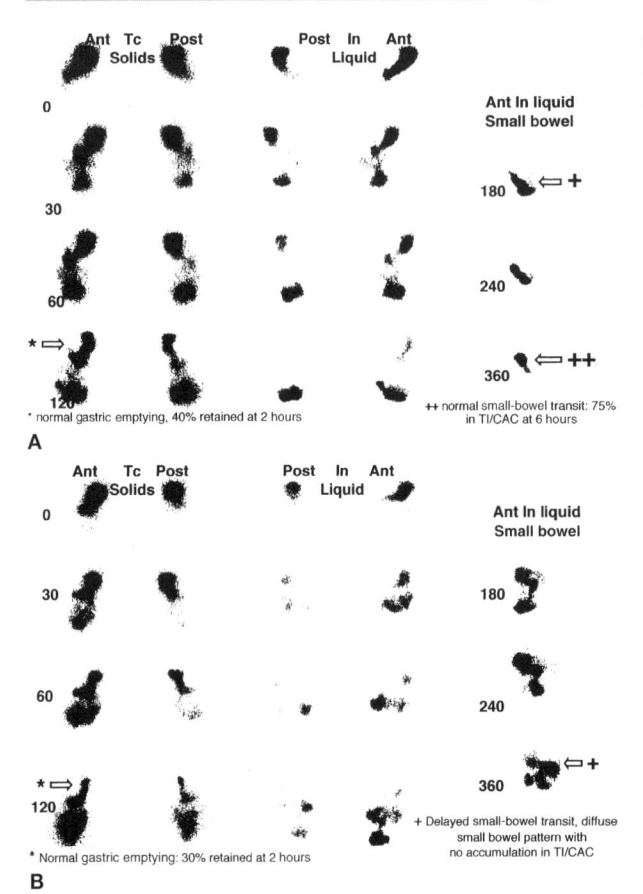

Figure 10.2 Gastric emptying and small-bowel transit scintigraphy. A) Normal gastric emptying and normal small-bowel (SB) transit. On the left are paired anterior and posterior images at 0, 30, 60, and 120 minutes for solids labeled with ^{99m}technetium (Tc), and in the center are similar images for liquids labeled with indium-111 (In). At 2 hours, 40% of the solid activity remains in the stomach (*), consistent with normal gastric emptying. On the right are small-bowel transit images of the liquid indium-111. At 180 minutes there is indium-111 activity spread throughout the small bowel (+), but at 6 hours, 75% of this activity has completed transit through the small bowel and reached the TI/CAC (++). B) Example of normal gastric emptying (*) with delayed small-bowel transit (+) (modified with permission from Bonapace ES, Davidoff S, Krevsky B, Maurer AH, Parkman HP, Fisher RS. Whole gut transit scintigraphy in the clinical evaluation of patients with upper and lower gastrointestinal symptoms. *Am J Gastroenterol* 2000; 95: 2838–2847).

scintigraphically. One approach is to measure the orocecal transit time or initial arrival of an orally administered radiotracer in the cecum. This is analogous to breath hydrogen testing which detects leading edge arrival. Another approach is to measure the total amount of radiotracer that passes into the cecum and/or ascending colon after a defined time, often 6 hours. Often, the orally administered isotope collects in a well-defined region of the pelvis corresponding to the terminal ileum prior to passing into the colon so the terminal ileum is often included with the cecum and/or ascending colon region of interest.

Several centers use small-bowel scintigraphy for clinical evaluation. Small-bowel transit may be useful to detect diffuse gastrointestinal motor dysfunction or isolated small-bowel dysfunction (Figure 10.2). In chronic intestinal pseudo-obstruction caused by either neuropathic or myopathic processes, there is a often delay in both gastric emptying and small-bowel transit. Small-bowel transit may be altered in irritable bowel syndrome, suggesting that this disorder involves the small intestine in addition to the colon. Transit of food through the small intestine and colon is faster than normal in patients with irritable bowel syndrome who have diarrhea, but slower than normal in patients with irritable bowel syndrome who have constipation.

Small-intestinal contractile activity

Antroduodenojejunal (small-bowel) manometry provides information about the coordination of gastric and small-intestinal motor function in both fasting and post-prandial periods (Figure 10.3). Small-bowel manometry helps to identify normal motility features and consequently to identify abnormal motor patterns (Figures 10.4 and 10.5). The procedure is somewhat invasive and lengthy (requiring at least 5 hours of recording), and performed at only select centers. Ambulatory studies can also be performed over 24 hours using solid-state transducers and they allow for correlation of symptoms with abnormal motility. However, catheter migration in the stomach during the ambulatory study prevents quantitation of antral contractility.

Patients who remain undiagnosed after extensive traditional work-up and fail several courses of medical therapy should be referred for small-bowel manometry. The main indications for antroduodenal manometry are to evaluate

1. unexplained nausea and vomiting
2. the cause of gastric or small-bowel stasis (e.g. differentiation of neuropathic or myopathic disorders)
3. suspected chronic intestinal pseudo-obstruction when the diagnosis is unclear.

Antroduodenal manometry may differentiate between a neuropathic or myopathic motility disor-

The small intestine

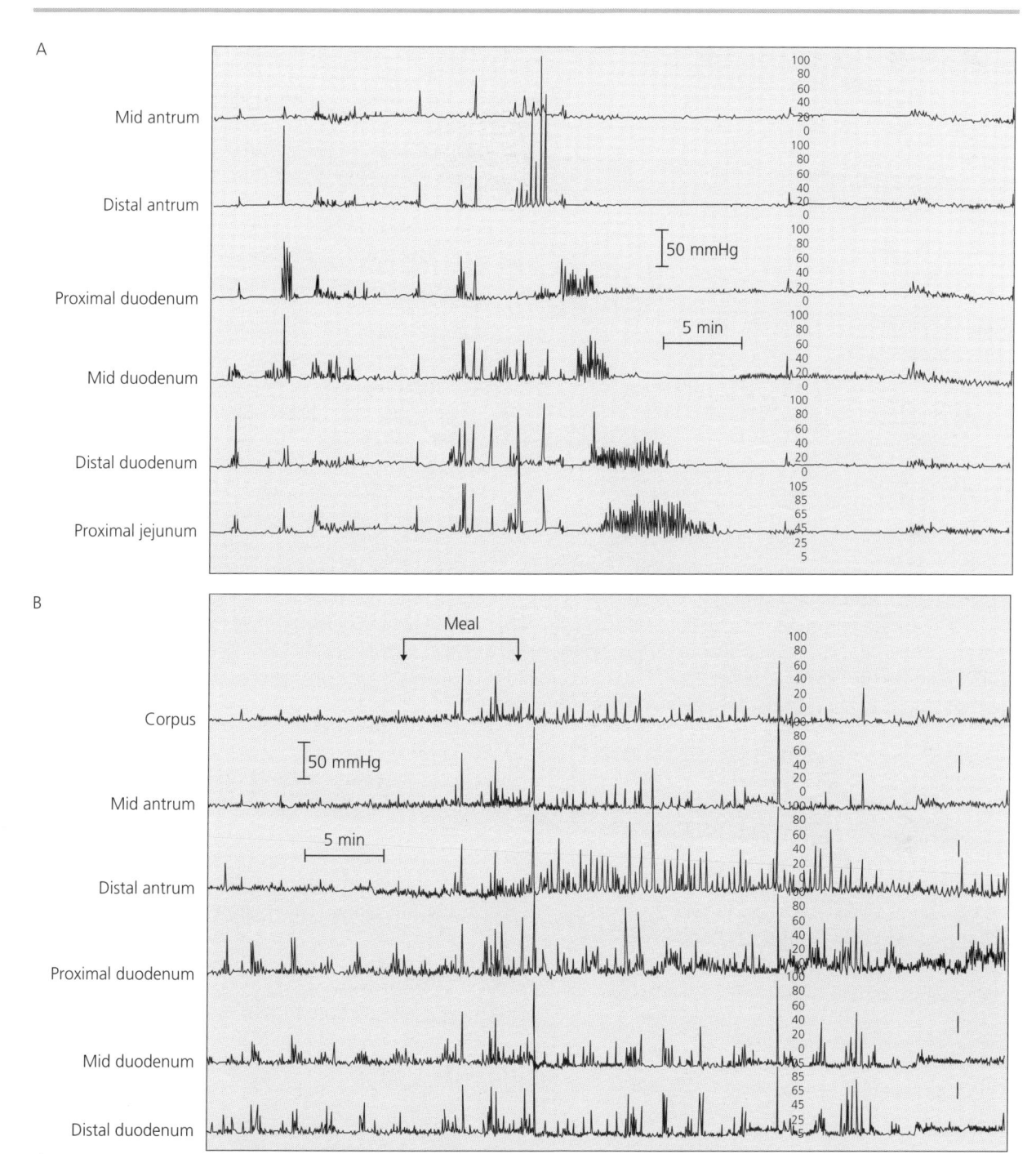

Figure 10.3 Normal antroduodenal manometry. A) depicts the fasting state. In this study, there are recording ports in the stomach, duodenum, and proximal jejunum as depicted. The initial portion of the tracing represents a phase II period which features somewhat irregular contractions. A normal phase III complex starts in the antrum and proceeds in a peristaltic direction down the duodenum into the jejunum. The phase III complex lasts several minutes, followed by relative quiescence (phase 1) for several minutes. B) depicts the conversion from the fasting to the fed state. This manometric recording demonstrates the effect of a meal on antral and duodenal contractility. Ingestion of the meal results in an increase in antral and small-intestinal contractile activity. The cyclical MMC activity is replaced by more random activity in the small intestine (reproduced with permission from Parkman HP, Harris AD, Krevsky B, Urbain J-L, Maurer AH, Fisher RS. Gastroduodenal motility and dysmotility: Update on techniques available for evaluation. *Am J Gastroenterol* 1995; 90: 869–892).

Motility Disorders of the Small Bowel and Colon

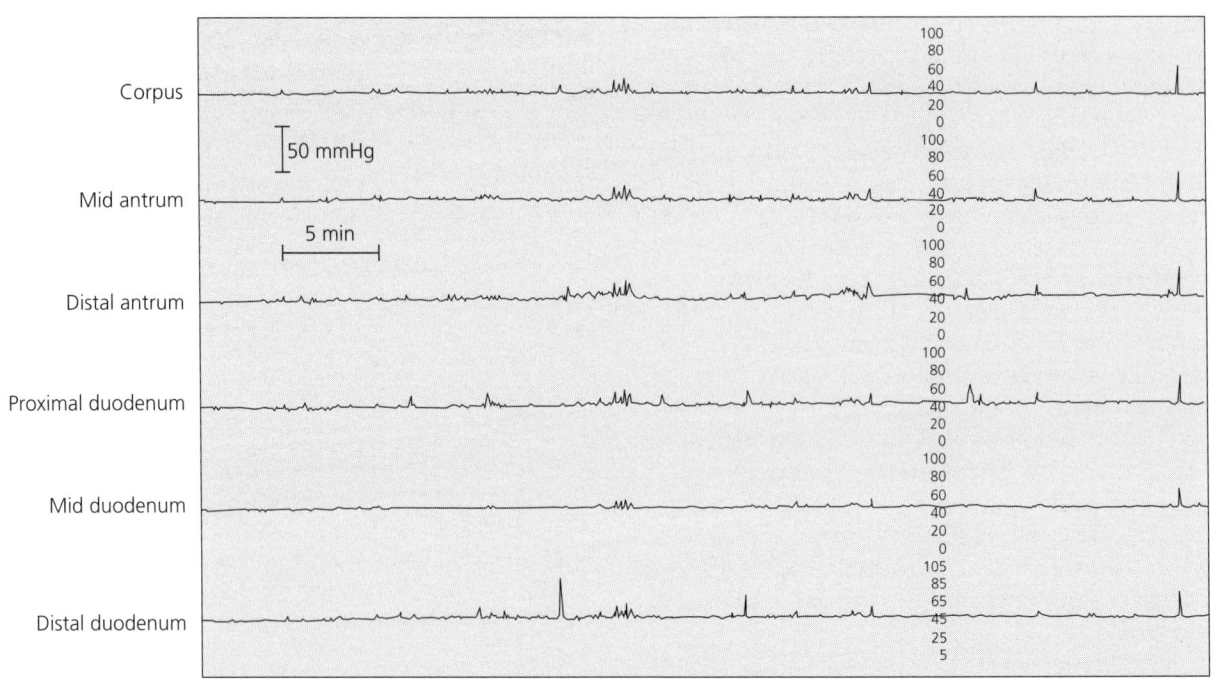

Figure 10.4 Abnormal antroduodenal contractility in a patient with constipation and symptoms suggestive of chronic intestinal pseudoobstruction. Very low amplitude contractile activity (antroduodenal hypomotility) is seen in the antrum and duodenum. This is suggestive of a myopathic process (reproduced with permission from Parkman HP, Harris AD, Krevsky B, Urbain J-L, Maurer AH, Fisher RS. Gastroduodenal motility and dysmotility: Update on techniques available for evaluation. *Am J Gastroenterol* 1995; 90: 869–892).

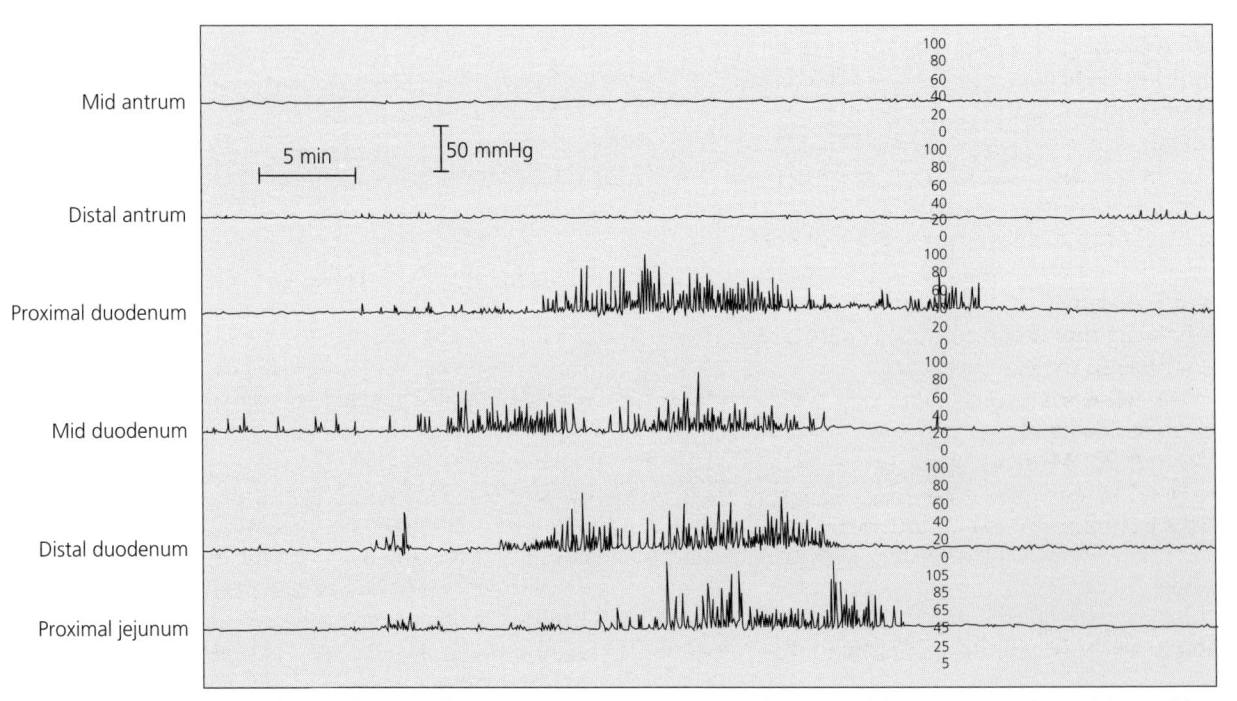

Figure 10.5 Abnormal antroduodenal contractility in a patient with intractable nausea and vomiting with insulin-dependent diabetes mellitus and known gastroparesis. Two abnormalities are seen. First, the phase III activity starts in the duodenum, not the antrum. Second, the phase III contractile activity is irregular with both antegrade and retrograde propagation (reproduced with permission from Parkman HP, Harris AD, Krevsky B, Urbain J-L, Maurer AH, Fisher RS. Gastroduodenal motility and dysmotility: Update on techniques available for evaluation. *Am J Gastroenterol* 1995; 90: 869–892).

der, or it may suggest an unexpected small-bowel obstruction or rumination syndrome. Myopathic disorders, such as scleroderma, amyloidosis, or hollow visceral myopathy have low-amplitude (less than 20 mmHg) contractions with normal propagation. Neuropathic disorders have normal amplitude but abnormal propagative contractions, seen readily in the phase III migrating motor complex, such as bursts and sustained uncoordinated pressure activity, and failure of a meal to induce the fed-type pattern. Occult mechanical obstruction of the small intestine is suggested by non-propagated, prolonged contractions during the post-prandial period. Antroduodenal manometry may demonstrate a characteristic pattern of rumination with an increase in intra-abdominal pressures at all levels of the upper gut (R waves), especially post-prandially. Clustered contractions may suggest irritable bowel syndrome, although these contractions can be seen in other conditions.

Antral contractility is also measured during antroduodenojejunal manometry. Decreased antral contractility and phase III migrating motor complexes originating in the small intestine rather than in the stomach can be seen in gastroparesis. Antroduodenal manometry can help confirm or exclude a gastric motility disorder if the gastric emptying test is normal or borderline. With an accurate stationary recording, a reduced post-prandial distal antral motility index is correlated with impaired gastric emptying of solids. A normal study with a normal transit test strongly suggests that motor dysfunction is not the cause of the symptoms.

Some investigators perform the study with the administration of erythromycin and/or octreotide to predict the patient's response to chronic treatment of these agents. In pediatric studies, the absence of migrating motor complexes is an indicator of a poor response to prokinetic agents.

Medications may have an effect on small-intestinal motility – both transit and contractility (Box 10.2). Most of these medications should be stopped 2 days prior to tests of small-intestinal and/or colonic transit or contractility.

Disorders of small-intestinal motility

Abnormal small-intestinal motility may be caused by decreased, increased, or uncoordinated contractility. Decreased intestinal motility reflects either absent or fewer contractions of phase III of the migrating motor complex during fasting or a minimal increase in post-prandial motility in the differ-

> **Box 10.2** Medications that affect gastrointestinal motility
>
> Medications that delay transit
>   anticholinergics
>   tricyclic antidepressants
>   narcotic analgesics
>   calcium channel blockers
>   adrenergic agents
> Medications that accelerate transit
>   Prokinetic agents
>   metoclopramide
>   cisapride
>   domperidone
>   tegaserod
>   erythromycin

Modified from Camilleri M, Hasler W, Parkman HP, Quigley EMM, Soffer E. Measurement of gastroduodenal motility in the GI laboratory. Gastroenterology 1998; 115: 747–762.

ent regions of the small bowel. Conversely, increased motility is reflected in increased numbers of fasting migrating motor complexes or an augmented contractile response to eating. Uncoordinated intestinal motility can be caused by retrograde migrating motor complexes and clustered contractions.

Small-bowel dysmotility and its associated symptoms may result from diseases affecting the intestinal smooth muscle, enteric nervous system, extrinsic nerves, regulatory hormones, and the intestinal pacemaker cells called the interstitial cells of Cajal.

Chronic intestinal pseudo-obstruction

Chronic intestinal pseudo-obstruction is a syndrome with recurrent clinical symptoms suggestive of intestinal obstruction in the absence of mechanical blockage of the lumen (see Figure 10.6). The symptoms of pseudo-obstruction are caused by ineffective peristalsis and they include nausea, vomiting, and abdominal pain with abdominal distension. Disturbances in bowel habit are common but unpredictable: some patients having constipation, some having diarrhea. Radiologic findings consist of air–fluid levels within the small-intestinal lumen. If the X-ray is normal without air–fluid levels or distension and there is delayed transit, some clinicians refer to this as a diffuse gastrointestinal motility disorder rather than chronic intestinal pseudo-obstruction.

Chronic intestinal pseudo-obstruction is a chronic condition, whereas the syndrome of adynamic ileus

Motility Disorders of the Small Bowel and Colon

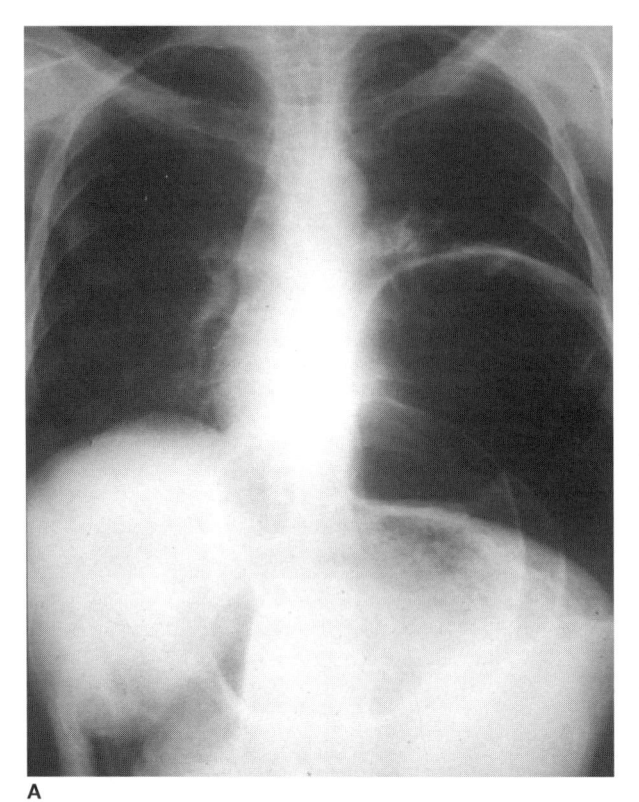

Figure 10.6 Chronic intestinal pseudo-obstruction. A) The chest and B) abdominal radiographs show marked intestinal distension. The chest radiograph by itself might be suggestive of pneumoperitoneum. In this patient the intestinal dilation was primarily the small intestine.

is acute and self-limited. Chronic intestinal pseudo-obstruction was initially a diagnosis applied to small-bowel motor dysfunction. Chronic intestinal pseudo-obstruction may also involve other segments of the gastrointestinal tract besides the small intestine, such as the stomach, colon, and even esophagus, which are also regulated by the autonomic nervous system and contain smooth muscle. The patient's symptoms may reflect this heterogeneity. A consensus working group that included pediatric and adult gastroenterologists defined intestinal pseudo-obstruction as a rare, severe, disabling disorder characterized by repetitive episodes or continuous symptoms and signs of bowel obstruction, including radiographic documentation of dilated bowel with air–fluid levels, in the absence of a fixed, lumen-occluding lesion.

Causes There are many causes of chronic intestinal pseudo-obstruction (Box 10.3). In adults, pseudo-obstruction is more often secondary to a systemic disease. Among the most common causes of adult pseudo-obstruction are scleroderma and other connective tissue disorders, diabetes, use of narcotics or drugs with anticholinergic properties, hypothyroidism, paraneoplastic syndromes, amyloidosis, and radiation enteritis. Recent interest has been paid to viral infections as a cause of pseudo-obstruction, including cytomegalovirus, herpes zoster and Epstein–Barr virus. Mitochondrial disorders have been shown to cause pseudo-obstruction. Severe intestinal dysmotility may be the result of an immune response against an occult neoplasm. Small cell lung carcinoma is the most common tumor among the many that are associated with pseudo-obstruction. Often, however, there is no known cause of the symptoms of pseudo-obstruction and these cases are labelled chronic idiopathic intestinal pseudo-obstruction. An approach to these patients suspected of having CIP is outlined in Box 10.4.

The two main forms of idiopathic pseudo-obstruction are myopathic (involving the intestinal musculature) and neurogenic (involving the nerves and the pacemaker cells – interstitial cells of Cajal) (Box 10.3). Histologically, the bowel wall in patients with the myopathic form (e.g. hollow visceral myopathy) shows thinning and degeneration of the smooth muscle with replacement by fibrous tissue. The neuropathic form (e.g. visceral neuropathy) has abnormalities in neurons and glial cells within the splanchnic ganglia and/or myenteric plexus. The intestinal smooth muscle in the neuropathic form is normal. In patients with intestinal myopathy, manometry typically reveals contrac-

The small intestine

> **Box 10.3** Small-intestinal motility disorders
>
> Myopathic abnormalities (decreased contractility)
>   hollow visceral myopathies (familial, sporadic)
>   collagen vascular disorders (scleroderma, SLE, MCTD, dermatomyositis)
>   amyloidosis
>   muscular dystrophies (myotonic dystrophy, Duchenne's muscular dystrophy)
>   hypothyroidism
>   jejunal diverticulosis
>   jejuno-ileal bypass
> Neuropathic abnormalities (increased and/or uncoordinated contractility)
>   primary visceral neuropathy (familial, sporadic)
>   carcinoma-associated visceral neuropathy (paraneoplastic syndrome)
>   irritable bowel syndrome
>   endocrine abnormalities (diabetes, hyperthyroidism, hypoparathyrodism)
>   carcinoid syndrome
>   Chagas' disease
>   neurofibrimatosis or ganglioneuromatosis of the intestine
>   Parkinson's disease
>   spinal cord injury
> Drug-induced small-intestinal dysmotility
>   anti-Parkinsonian medications
>   phenothiazines
>   clonidine
>   tricyclic antidepressants
>   narcotic analgesics
>   ganglionic blockers

Modified from 1) Anura S, Hodges. Dysmotility of the small intestine. In Yamada T (ed.) Textbook of Gastroenterology. Lippincott, Williams and Wilkins. Philadelphia, PA 1998, and 2) Snape WJ Jr. Cecil Textbook of Medicine (W.B. Saunders Philadelphia, PA 2001.

> **Box 10.4** Evaluation of suspected small-intestinal dysmotility
>
> **Step 1 initial evaluation**
>   history
>   physical examination
>   blood tests: complete blood count with erythrocyte sedimentation rate, complete metabolic panel, TSH, CPK, magnesium, ANA
>   abdominal obstruction series with chest X-ray
> **Step 2 evaluate for mucosal disorders: ulcer, cancer, obstruction**
>   upper endoscopy or enteroscopy
>   upper gastrointestinal series with small-bowel follow-through or enteroclysis
> **Step 3 evaluate for motility disorders**
>   whole gut transit scintigraphy
>   antroduodenojejunal manometry
> **Step 4 evaluate for specific systemic/extraintestinal disorder**
> A evaluate for other specific endocrine/metabolic/autonomic disorders
>   thyroid function tests (free T4, free T3, TSH)
>   adrenocorticotropic hormone stimulation test
>   autonomic nervous system testing
> B evaluate for intracranial disease
>   head computed tomography or magnetic resonance imaging
> **Step 5 therapeutic trial**
>   prokinetic agent
>   5HT4 agonists – cisapride or tegaserod
>   octreotide

tions that propagate normally but with low amplitude (Figure 10.4). In patients with intestinal neuropathy, individual contractions may be of normal amplitude but are disorganized with disruption of the phase III migrating motor complex, bursts of nonpropagating activity during fasting, and failure to convert from the fasting to the fed pattern with a meal (Figure 10.5).

With familial primary intestinal pseudo-obstruction, parts of the urinary system (bladder and renal pelvis) may also be dilated as a result of a generalized disorder of smooth muscle contractility. This may lead to bladder distension and frequent urinary tract infections. Intestinal malrotation is found in 25% of cases of congenital pseudo-obstruction with similar prevalence in myopathic and neuropathic forms. Autonomic nervous system dysfunction, especially vagal dysfunction, is found in most adult chronic intestinal pseudo-obstruction patients with known neurological disorders and in up to 25% of patients without a previously recognized neuropathy. Autonomic nervous system dysfunction may present with postural dizziness and sweating abnormalities.

Treatment The principles of management of patients with chronic intestinal pseudo-obstruction involve

203

1. establishing a correct clinical diagnosis and excluding mechanical obstruction
2. differentiating between idiopathic and secondary forms
3. performing a physiologic assessment of the parts of the gastrointestinal tract involved
4. performing a nutritional assessment of the patient
5. developing a therapeutic plan addressing the patient's symptoms and nutritional status.

The natural history of chronic idiopathic intestinal pseudo-obstruction depends on the underlying cause of the syndrome. Nutritional support and relief of symptoms are the primary management goals of pseudo-obstruction. The management of chronic idiopathic intestinal pseudo-obstruction involves multiple modalities – dietary manipulations, parenteral nutrition, pharmacotherapy, and endoscopic and surgical therapy.

Nutritional support by enteral or parenteral means is an important aspect of management in patients with severe intestinal dysmotility. A low-fat diet, supplemented by liquid formulas, can be tried first. Enteral feedings, particularly jejunal feedings through a jejunostomy tube may be needed, especially if gastroparesis is also present. A trial of several days of naso-jejunal feeding is tried to help ensure that patients can tolerate this form of feeding. Total parenteral nutrition may be needed in select patients. However, total parenteral nutrition is costly and is associated with complications including infection and thrombosis.

Pharmacotherapy consists primarily of prokinetic agents. Unfortunately, these agents are usually less effective in the small intestine than in the stomach. The response to prokinetic agents is less in patients with a myopathic process than in those with a neuropathic process, however, some patients with severe scleroderma may derive symptomatic improvement. They should be tried initially because of their known effect on improving small-bowel transit. Improvement of gastric dysmotility may alleviate the patient's symptoms. The $5-HT_4$ receptor agonists such as cisapride and tegaserod have been shown to increase small-bowel motility and transit. However, cisapride is available only in strict compassionate-use programs. Tegaserod is only currently approved by the FDA for women with constipation-predominate irritable bowel syndrome. Erythromycin and metoclopramide have greater effects on the stomach than on the small intestine. Subcutaneous octreotide may be helpful for small-bowel dysmotility, being particularly helpful in patients with scleroderma. Octreotide exerts its motor effects mainly on the small intestine. Octreotide may, however, delay gastric emptying, so it is often given at night.

Patients with chronic intestinal pseudo-obstruction may develop bacterial overgrowth as a complication of the impaired transit. Antibiotics are used for bacterial overgrowth (see p. 205).

Venting jejunostomy with bowel decompression may be helpful to relieve obstructive symptoms. This simple intervention can substantially reduce the number of hospital admissions and emergency-room visits in selected patients with intermittent obstructive symptoms. Jejunostomies may also provide access to enteral feedings. Parenteral support is reserved for patients in whom trials of tube feedings fail.

Recently, small-bowel transplantation has been used in some centers. Only small series of patients have been reported. The recent success of isolated intestinal grafts, together with the mortality and morbidity associated with total parenteral nutrition therapy, has led to the resurgence of small-intestinal transplantation in select patients.

Acute ileus

Acute ileus, or acute intestinal pseudo-obstruction usually occurs either in the postoperative period or it accompanies severe illness. It may involve either the small intestine and/or the colon. Ileus is generally an acute decrease or absence of small-bowel motility. This often occurs in the postoperative period ("postoperative ileus"), in association with peritonitis, or following spinal cord injury or pelvic fractures. It may occur as the result of severe electrolyte imbalance (potassium, calcium, magnesium). Adynamic ileus tends to be self-limiting, lasting up to 3 days postoperatively after open laparotomy. Sympathetic inhibitory overactivity from the spinal cord, possibly in conjunction with a decrease in parasympathetic activity, may be an important cause in its development. Factors that may prolong postoperative ileus include electrolyte (especially hypokalemia) and metabolic abnormalities, medications (such as opiates), and infections (such as peritonitis). Although ileus is most commonly seen in the postoperative setting, it is being increasingly recognized in non-surgical conditions, usually in the context of severe metabolic or systemic illness. Treatment is largely empirical, based primarily on nothing by mouth, decompression with a nasogastric tube, replacement of fluid volume, correction of electrolyte and acid–base imbalances, and decreasing narcotic analgesics. Recently, peripheral-acting μ-opiate receptor antagonists have been shown to reduce the duration of postoperative ileus.

Small-intestinal bacterial overgrowth

Normally, gastric-acid secretion and intestinal motility play important roles in preventing significant numbers of bacteria in the upper gastrointestinal tract. Common causes of small-intestinal bacterial overgrowth include reduced anti-bacterial defenses due to gastric hypoacidity and small-intestinal stasis from either structural abnormalities or reduced gastrointestinal motility. Intestinal dysmotility is an important factor contributing to the development of clinically significant small-intestinal bacterial overgrowth. Diarrhea, steatorrhea, bloating, gas production, and malabsorption are consequences of bacterial overgrowth. Diagnosis can be made with

1. small-intestinal aspiration of luminal contents with quantitation of bacteria
2. the hydrogen breath test with either lactulose or glucose showing an early hydrogen peak representing metabolism of the lactulose by bacteria in the small intestine, or
3. empiric treatment trial of antibiotics, treatment is with antibiotics, often with metronidazole or ciprofloxicin.

Irritable bowel syndrome

Irritable bowel syndrome is the most commonly diagnosed functional disorder of the gastrointestinal tract (symptoms are believed to originate in the gut but are not associated with any structural or biochemical abnormality). Irritable bowel syndrome affects 10% to 20% of the US population, and patients with this disorder account for up to 25% of the total visits made to gastroenterologists. As generally defined, irritable bowel syndrome is characterized by chronic or recurrent abdominal pain associated with altered bowel function (constipation, diarrhea, or alternating constipation and diarrhea). The diagnosis of irritable bowel syndrome is based on a characteristic history, the absence of significant physical findings, no abnormalities on standard laboratory tests, and normal gross and histologic findings on flexible sigmoidoscopy. The Rome criteria, often used for research studies, defines irritable bowel syndrome as

1. abdominal pain or discomfort which is relieved with defecation and/or associated with a change in the frequency of bowel movements, and
2. disturbed defecation – altered stool frequency, altered stool form, altered stool passage (straining or urgency, feeling of incomplete evacuation), passage of mucus, bloating or a feeling of abdominal distension.

Although irritable bowel syndrome is classically considered to be a disorder of the colon, motility abnormalities can also be detected in the small intestine in a majority of patients with this condition. A number of small-bowel motility abnormalities have been described in irritable bowel syndrome that include clustered contractions, exaggerated post-prandial motor response, and disturbances in intestinal transit. Dysmotility may also reflect autonomic dysfunction, disturbed central nervous system control, and the response to heightened visceral sensation or central perception. Motor abnormalities in the alimentary tract, reported in irritable bowel syndrome, include altered myoelectric activity and prolonged irregular small-bowel and colonic contractions (duodenal and jejunal clustering, ileal high-pressure waves, and a disturbed post-prandial motor response). Abnormal visceral perception, as detected by a lower pain threshold in response to bowel distension, may represent one of the key physiological disturbances.

Symptoms of diarrhea-predominant irritable bowel syndrome may also be caused by bacterial overgrowth, lactose intolerance, and, rarely, celiac sprue disease (gluten sensitive enteropathy). These disorders need to be considered in a patient with abdominal discomfort and diarrhea.

Rapid small-intestinal transit

Rapid gastric emptying with rapid small-bowel transit is responsible for "dumping syndrome" with symptoms that include post-prandial sweating, weakness, orthostasis, tachycardia, and diarrhea. Dumping syndrome, especially of liquids, usually occurs after gastric surgery, especially after gastrectomy (usually antrectomy) and/or truncal vagotomy. Dumping symptoms are often characterized as "early" or "late" relative to their time course after meal ingestion. Early dumping symptoms occur in the first 30 minutes and result from accelerated early gastric emptying of liquids with rapid filling of the intestine with hypertonic fluid leading to bloating, crampy abdominal pain, and explosive diarrhea. Rapid filling of the intestine is associated with osmotic fluid shifts into the gut lumen and reduction of plasma volume resulting in secondary release of vasoactive substances which cause symptoms such as lightheadedness, sweating, flushing, and palpitations with tachycardia. Late dumping symptoms occur 2 to 3 hours after a meal and are associated with reactive hypoglycemia (weakness, palpitations, and diaphoresis); these symptoms are due to the hyperinsulinemic response to an overwhelming carbohydrate load.

The colon

Normal colonic motility

The colon serves three major functions

1. it is a storage and mixing reservoir
2. it absorbs water and electrolytes
3. it slowly propels its contents aborally toward the anus.

There are regional differences in the motor functions of the colon. The ascending colon functions as a reservoir to accommodate ileal chyme, while the descending colon acts as a conduit for ultimate evacuation. The sigmoid colon and rectum serve as a reservoir until evacuation which is ultimately determined by the anal sphincters.

Normal colonic contractile activity is irregular, ranging from quiescence, to isolated contractions, and to bursts of propagated contractions. Segmentation into haustra helps compartmentalize the colon, facilitating mixing, retention of residue, and the formation of solid stool. Colonic transit is associated with propagated contractions over long distances. In contrast to the upper gastrointestinal tract, there is no organized interdigestive, cyclical, migrating motor complex. High-amplitude propagated contractions occur, on average, six times per day, and they originate predominately in the cecum and/or ascending colon and migrate over a variable distance. High-amplitude propagated contractions are responsible for mass movement of colonic contents and they occur with the urge to defecate. Eating is accompanied by a brisk increase in tone and phasic activity throughout the colon. This "gastrocolonic reflex" may last from minutes to several hours and may be responsible for the need to defecate after ingesting a meal.

There are a vast number of neurotransmitters that play a role in normal gastrointestinal motor function. Serotonin is released from enterochromaffin in response to luminal mechanical distension. The released serotonin acts on 5-HT_4 receptors to play a role in initiating the peristaltic reflex with ascending contraction and descending relaxation which helps to propel material through the gastrointestinal tract. The contractile portion is mediated through acetylcholine and substance P; the relaxation portion is mediated through nitric oxide and vasoactive intestinal polypeptide. Other neurotransmitters play a role in mediating the afferent and efferent pathways. These neural and hormonal pathways may be affected by pharmacologic agents. The muscarinic anticholinergic agent atropine, has been shown to reduce tone throughout the colon. The 5-HT_3 receptor antagonists inhibit both colonic tone and the motor response of the colon to feeding. Narcotic analgesics often work at μ-opiate receptors to delay colonic transit. On the muscle level, calcium channel antagonists reduce muscle contractility and can lead to constipation. In a similar analogy, several pharmacological agents alter colonic sensation. Alpha$_2$-adrenergic agents modulate colonic sensation probably via central effects. Octreotide alters colonic and rectal sensory function. The 5-HT_3 receptor antagonists and even 5-HT_4 receptor agonist may also play a role in sensory modulation and may be useful in irritable bowel syndrome.

Defecation is associated with intra-abdominal and rectal contractions associated with relaxation of the internal and external anorectal sphincters. The anal sphincter complex consists primarily of the internal anal sphincter and external anal sphincter. Both the internal and external anal sphincters are essential components for maintenance of continence and for normal defecation. The internal anal sphincter is composed of smooth muscle with autonomic innervation from the sympathetic and parasympathetic nervous systems. The external anal sphincter, a striated muscle receiving pudendal nerve innervation, surrounds the internal sphincter, being separated by a thin band of connective tissue, and extends distally. The normal involuntary brake on stool passage is provided by the tone of the internal anal sphincter. The volitional holding of the stool is provided mainly by the external anal sphincter. Dysfunction of either one may have significant clinical implications.

Symptoms of colonic motility disorders

The common symptoms of colonic dysmotility include constipation, diarrhea, fecal incontinence, and lower abdominal pain (Box 10.5).

Constipation, defined by infrequent bowel movements, occurs in approximately 2% of the general population who seek medical attention, with an

> **Box 10.5** Symptoms of colonic motor dysfunction
>
> Constipation
> Lower abdominal pain
> Diarrhea
> Fecal incontinence

increase in incidence after the age of 65 years to 4% in males and 8% in females (Box 10.6). The actual prevalence of constipation, however, depends on the definition that is used. The most common definition for research studies is less than three spontaneous bowel movements per week. Patients often view constipation differently to physicians. Constipation, as defined by straining at defecation, hard or lumpy stools, and a sensation of incomplete evacuation, is present in 24% of elderly persons.

> **Box 10.6** Secondary causes of delayed colonic transit and constipation
>
> Drug effects
>   see Box 10.2
> Mechanical obstruction
>   intrinsic: colon cancer, diverticular stricture
>   extrinsic: external compression
> Endocrine or metabolic causes
>   diabetes mellitus
>   hypothyroidism
>   hypercalcemia
>   hypokalemia
>   hypomagnesemia
>   uremia
>   pregnancy
> Myopathies
>   amyloidosis
>   scleroderma
>   familial visceral myopathy
> Neuropathies
>   Parkinson's disease
>   spinal cord injury or tumor
>   cerebrovascular disease (cerebrovascular accident, tumor)
>   multiple sclerosis
>   familial autonomic neuropathy
>   Hirschsprung's disease

Modified from Locke GR III, Pemberton JH, Phillips SF. AGA technical review on constipation. Gastroenterology 2000; 119: 1766–1778.

Colonic pain frequently resolves after a bowel movement or the passing of flatus. Although frequently pain of colonic origin is located in the lower quadrants, pain referred from the anatomic location of the colon may occur in any of the abdominal quadrants. Visceral hypersensitivity is an important reason that explains the abdominal pain in patients with irritable bowel syndrome. The pain has also been associated with exacerbated motor response of the colon as well as the small intestine. In addition, colonic contractility, either normal or excessive, may produce symptoms because of coexistent hypersensitivity. The colon has dual innervation by the sympathetic and parasympathetic systems, both of which carry afferent sensory information to the central nervous system. Parasympathetic afferents, comprising the majority of nerve fibers in the vagus and pelvic nerves, convey non-conscious sensory information. Vagal afferents have cell bodies in the nodose ganglion, and signals are relayed to the nucleus of the solitary tract. Sympathetic afferents, which convey painful stimuli, travel to the spinal cord via the dorsal root ganglia. Second-order neurons ascend in the spinothalamic or spinoreticular tracts. Third-order neurons project to the higher sensory centers such as the anterior cingulate cortex.

Chronic diarrhea is also a common gastrointestinal symptom in the general population, with a prevalence of 14% in patients over 65 years of age. The prevalence also depends on the definition used: passing loose, watery stools (12.9%), and/or stool frequency of more than three stools per day (2.5%). For research studies, diarrhea is objectively defined as the daily passage of stools weighing more than 200 grams, and it is defined as chronic diarrhea if it continues for longer than 4 weeks.

Fecal incontinence is an important problem in the elderly, with stool leakage of more than once per week being reported in 3.7% of elderly subjects.

Evaluation of colonic and anorectal motility

Colonic transit

Assessment of colonic transit may be helpful in the evaluation of patients with symptoms of constipation. Colonic transit studies can be conducted using either radiopaque markers (Sitzmarks) or scintigraphy (Figures 10.7, 10.8). These tests can determine if there is an actual delay in colonic transit (confirming patients' subjective complaints of

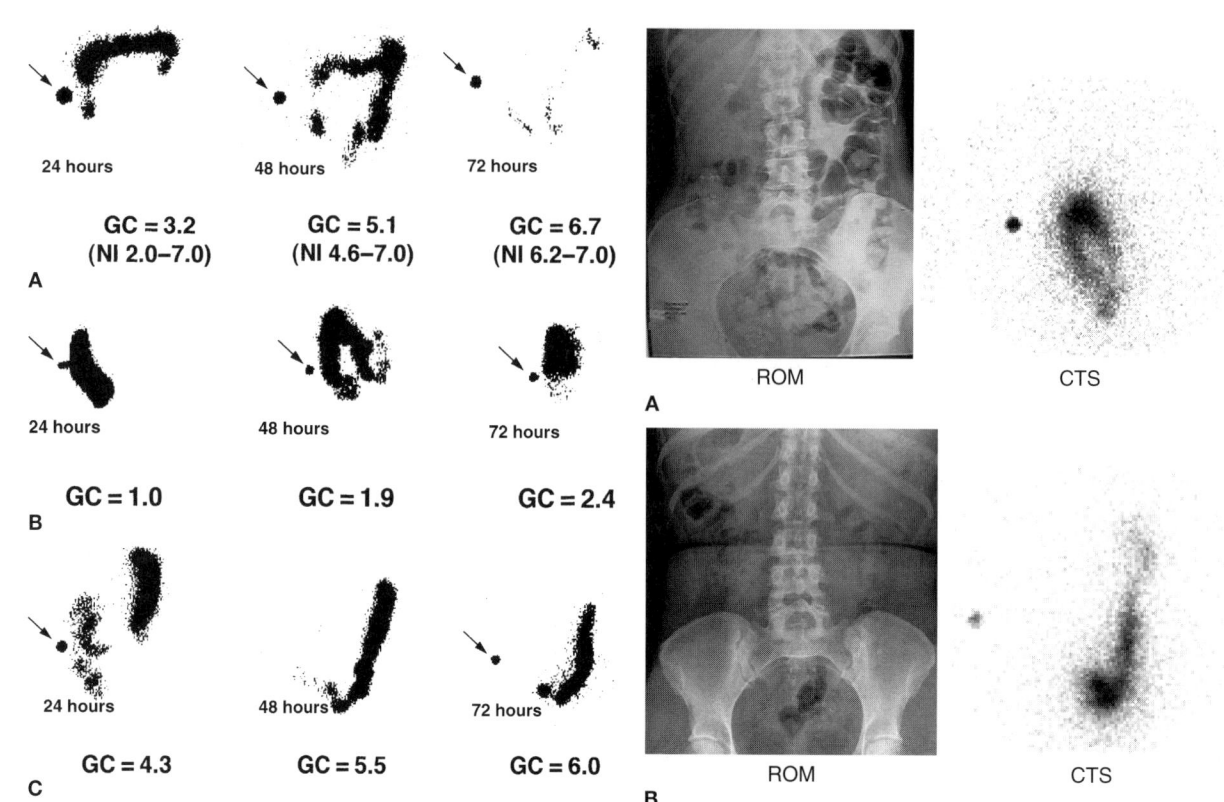

Motility Disorders of the Small Bowel and Colon

Figure 10.7 Colonic transit. A) Normal colonic transit. Images at 24, 48, and 72 hours are shown, along with an iliac crest marker (arrow) for reference. At 24 hours note that the majority of activity is seen in the transverse colon, with a geometric center (GC) of the radioactivity of 3.2, where 1 represents the cecum and 7 represents excreted stool. At 48 hours activity is centered over the descending colon (GC of 5.1). At 72 hours the majority of activity has been evacuated (GC of 6.7). B) Colonic inertia. In this example there is little progression of activity past the hepatic flexure at 48 and 72 hours, with a GC of 1.9 and 2.4 respectively. C) Functional rectosigmoid obstruction. Activity is seen to progress normally at 24 and 48 hours. However, there is little further progression of activity at 72 hours with a GC of 6.0, suggesting obstructed defecation (reproduced with permission from Bonapace ES, Davidoff S, Krevsky B, Maurer AH, Parkman HP, Fisher RS. Whole gut transit scintigraphy in the clinical evaluation of patients with upper and lower gastrointestinal symptoms. *Am J Gastroenterol* 2000; 95: 2838–2847.

Figure 10.8 Colonic transit with Sitzmark radiopaque colonic transit (ROM) and colonic transit scintigraphy (CTS) in two patients with chronic constipation. In these radiographs these techniques were performed simultaneously. A) Colonic inertia. There is accumulation of the radiopaque markers and the radioisotope on the right side of the colon after 72 hours. B) Functional rectosigmoid obstruction. There is accumulation of the radiopaque markers and the radioisotope in the rectosigmoid after 72 hours.

constipation and decreased stool frequency) or if there is normal transit. Furthermore, these tests may help identify the region or site of dysfunction in the colon, i.e., a diffuse delay in colonic transit suggesting colonic inertia or localized delay primarily at the anorectum suggesting functional rectosigmoid obstruction or pelvic floor dyssynergia.

Radiopaque markers For radiopaque marker colonic transit studies, radiographs are taken after ingestion of a capsule containing radiopaque markers (Sitzmark). There are two general ways to measure colonic transit with radiopaque markers.

1. The subject ingests a capsule containing twenty-four radiopaque markers and an X-ray is taken 5 days later. The presence of five or more radiopaque markers on the X-ray suggests delayed colonic transit. If no markers are present, the patient does not have delayed colonic transit. In the constipated patient, localization of the markers to the rectosigmoid region suggests an anorectal-outlet obstruction.

If the markers are distributed throughout the colon, colonic inertia is suggested.

2. Originally this technique involved the subject ingesting a capsule containing twenty-four radiopaque markers each day for 3 consecutive days and an X-ray was taken on the fourth day. This procedure has been modified so that now the subject takes the capsule daily for 4 days with an X-ray being taken on the fifth day. Formulae are available to determine actual colonic transit. Normal mean colonic transit time is 36 hours.

The use of radiopaque markers for assessing colonic transit is simple, inexpensive, and nearly universally available. However, there are some drawbacks to the use of radiopaque markers. It is limited in interpreting regional transit through the colon since only infrequent radiographs are obtained, and localization of the markers in the colon may not be accurate as they are inferred from the intra-abdominal location of the markers relative to bony landmarks, not from the true position in the colon. The solid radiopaque markers are also non-physiologic and may not move through the colon in the same manner as native material (chyme).

Colonic transit scintigraphy Colonic transit scintigraphy is performed with the administration of a radioactive substance with evaluation of the progress of the isotope using gamma camera imaging. Colonic transit scintigraphy is usually performed as part of whole gut scintigraphy (gastroenterocolonic transit scintigraphy) which makes use of the radioactivity as it traverses each section of the gastrointestinal tract, permitting measurement of gastric emptying, small-bowel transit, and colonic transit. This is helpful in patient evaluation as it is important to know if motility disturbances are isolated to the colon, or more diffuse as in intestinal pseudo-obstruction. It is not, however, as widely available and is more expensive than the radiopaque marker technique.

Colonic transit assessment can be used to confirm that delayed colonic transit indeed exists. In addition, scintigraphy can document whether the motor abnormality is diffuse or localized to a specific region of the colon. With scintigraphy, several patterns of colonic transit are seen in constipated patients. Colonic inertia is characterized by delay in transit with failure of progression of activity beyond the splenic flexure. A diffuse slow colon transit can also be recognized which demonstrates generalized retention throughout the colon with no regional abnormality localized in any one segment of the colon. Functional rectosigmoid obstruction is shown with normal transit in the proximal colon, but with accumulation of activity in the descending and rectosigmoid colon. Normal colonic transit can also be seen in some patients complaining of constipation. Differentiation of functional rectosigmoid obstruction from normal colonic transit may be possible scintigraphically only if prolonged imaging to 72 hours is obtained, and is not possible if shorter scanning periods of 24 to 48 hours are used.

Assessment of anorectal function

Anal manometry, anal EMG, balloon expulsion tests, and defecography are useful tests for anorectal anatomy and function.

Anorectal manometry Anorectal manometry uses a thin catheter with either solid state pressure transducers or radially placed water pressure transducers. A balloon is attached to the end of the catheter. The catheter is lubricated and placed in the rectum. Several maneuvers are performed to measure the anal sphincter pressure at rest, during balloon distension, while squeezing, and while simulating a bowel movement (Figure 10.9). Rectal

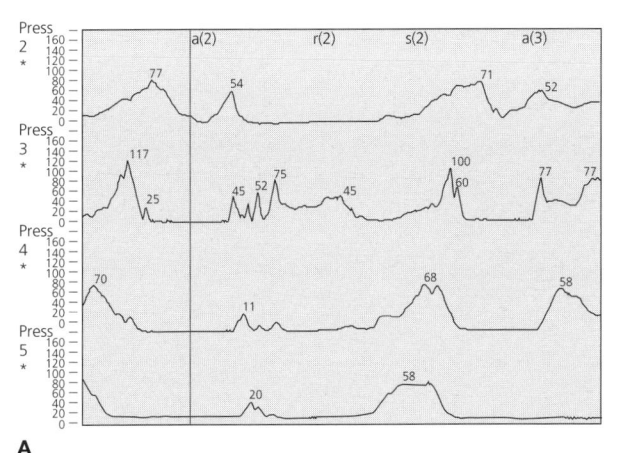

Figure 10.9 Anorectal manometry and anal EMG. A) Basal anal sphincter pressure. This figure depicts the pressure profiles of four perfusion ports radially located at 90 degrees apart and 1 cm apart on the catheter. The catheter is slowly withdrawn and the x axis is time (or distance) of the pull-through procedure. Shown sequentially are the rectal pressure (r), sphincter pressure (s), followed by atmospheric pressure (a). There is a high-pressure zone representing the basal anal sphincter pressure. (see overleaf for figure 10.9, part B & C)

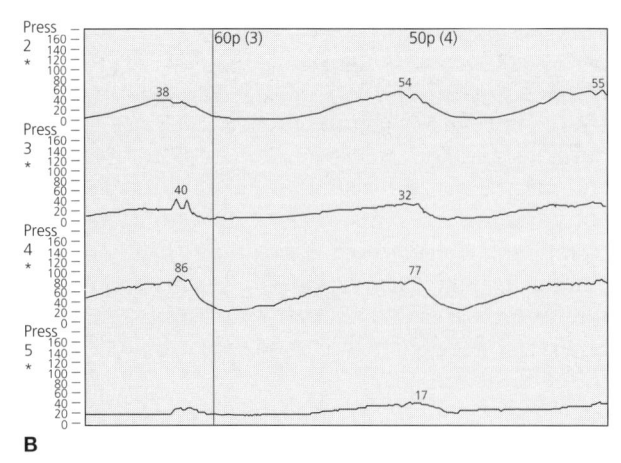

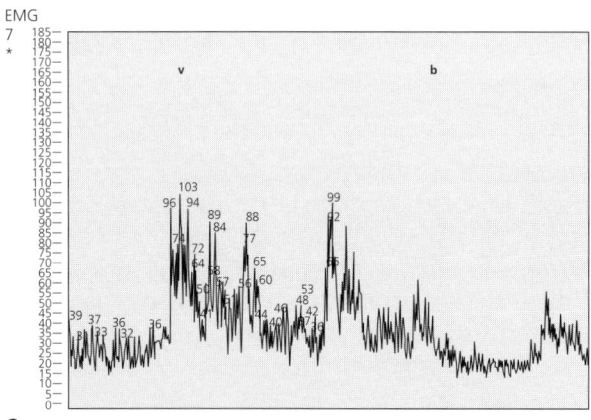

Motility Disorders of the Small Bowel and Colon

Figure 10.9 (continued) B) Normal internal anal sphincter relaxation response to rectal balloon distension. The tracing depicts the high-pressure zone of the internal anal sphincter in the third tracing. Upon rectal balloon distension, first with 60 mL of air and second with 50 mL of air, there is prompt relaxation of the basal anal sphincter pressure. C) Anal EMG with a circumferential anal plug recording electrode. When the patient squeezes volitionally, simulating preventing defecation, there is an abrupt increase in anal EMG activity (v). Upon bearing down towards the end of the tracing, simulating having a bowel movement there is a decrease in anal EMG activity (b). This is a normal tracing.

sensation thresholds and the presence or absence of the rectoanal inhibitory reflex are also determined with inflation of the balloon in the rectum.

Resting anorectal pressures reflect the tonic activities of both the internal and external anal sphincters with most of this pressure derived from the internal anal sphincter. Squeeze pressures primarily reflect the external anal sphincter. Low resting anorectal pressure and squeeze pressures are seen in fecal incontinence and may suggest a good response to biofeedback therapy.

Anal manometry is used to evaluate the anorectal inhibitory reflex; with rectal distension with a balloon there is a decrease in the tonic pressure of the anal sphincters. Impairment of this internal anal sphincter relaxation response to rectal balloon distension suggests a neuropathy with loss of ganglion cells of the myenteric plexus. Absence of this reflex is suggestive of Hirschsprung's disease in the appropriate clinical setting. Occasionally, if the patient has a megarectum, it is necessary to use larger volumes of rectal distension to elicit this reflex. The relaxation reflex can also be partially impaired in functional rectosigmoid obstruction.

Balloon distension is used to detect the threshold for sensation. Three sensations can be tested for – the first detectable sensation (rectal sensory threshold), the sensation of urgency to defecate, and the sensation of pain (maximum tolerable volume). The rectal sensory threshold for the first detectable sensation is the most commonly used measure. This is of value in biofeedback training of patients with fecal incontinence; normalization or reduction of the threshold correlates with success, whereas poor or absent sensation makes a good response to biofeedback unlikely.

Manometry is used to assess anorectal patterns during attempted defecation. During normal defecation, rectal pressures increase while sphincter pressures decrease, allowing expulsion of stool. In functional rectosigmoid obstruction, patients create adequate propulsive forces but a paradoxical increase in sphincter pressure leads to difficulty expelling stools.

Anorectal manometry is performed in patients with constipation and fecal incontinence. In patients with chronic constipation, this test is useful to exclude Hirschsprung's disease and to determine if the patient has functional rectosigmoid obstruction (pelvic floor dyssynergia). Furthermore, biofeedback with anorectal manometry can be performed to treat functional rectosigmoid obstruction. In patients with fecal incontinence, anal manometry can define functional weakness of one or both sphincter muscles, predict patients that may respond to biofeedback therapy, and be used to perform biofeedback therapy.

Anal EMG EMG testing is usually performed together with anorectal manometry. Often a probe is used to monitor anal sphincter muscle electrical activity and assess recruitment during squeezing and simulated defecation (Figure 10.9). Anal EMG is helpful in the evaluation of sphincter function, primarily in the diagnosis of functional rectosigmoid obstruction, where a paradoxical increase in EMG activity is seen when the patient bears down, simulating a bowel movement. Anal EMG is also useful for biofeedback training for functional rectosigmoid obstruction.

Balloon expulsion test The balloon expulsion test is performed by introducing a lubricated balloon attached to a thin catheter into the rectum, filling it with 50 mL of air or water and asking the patient, while sitting on a commode to expel (i.e. defecate) the balloon. Normal expulsion takes less than 60 seconds. This is a test of motor function and coordination, and it has been suggested that it should be used as a screening test for functional rectosigmoid obstruction (pelvic floor dyssynergia).

Defecography Defecography involves imaging the rectum with contrast material and observing the process, rate, and completeness of rectal evacuation using fluoroscopy. In addition to determining rectal diameter and emptying, defecography may detect anatomic abnormalities either at rest or with straining. These include rectoceles, enteroceles, intussusceptions, rectal prolapse, poor relaxation of the puborectalis muscle, and perineal descent.

Defecography is of potential value in patients with constipation in whom the following problems are suspected as being the cause of impaired defecation: inappropriate contraction of the puborectalis muscle (pelvic floor dyssynergia), enterocele, and anterior rectocele. This test is, however, somewhat embarrassing to the patient. The results may detect mild anatomic abnormalities, such as rectoceles, that are not responsible for the patient's symptoms.

Anal ultrasound Anal endosonography allows imaging of the sphincter muscles. It is a simple, reliable, and relatively non-invasive test for the definition of anatomic defects in the internal and external sphincters. It is most useful in evaluating the incontinence that occurs in patients with history of vaginal deliveries, and in patients with prior hemorrhoidal surgery. Abnormalities of the structural integrity involving either the internal or external anal sphincter can be identified. The internal sphincter is seen as a dark homogeneous ring. Anal endosonography also allows delineation of the external sphincter, although interpretation of these images is more difficult. Accurate delineation of structural damage using endosonography allows for correct selection of patients for surgical repair and for postoperative assessment of patients.

Disorders of colonic motility

Hirschsprung's disease

Hirschsprung's disease is the classic congenital colonic disorder characterized by the absence of enteric neurons in the myenteric and submucosal plexus. This occurs because of an arrest of the embryonic caudal migration of the enteric neurons along the gut. The aganglionic segment remains contracted with secondary dilation of the proximal normal bowel. Most cases are recognized in infancy characterized by constipation and obstipation. The severity of symptoms and the age of diagnosis are related to the length of the aganglionic segment. If a short segment of the distal rectum is aganglionic, the patient may present later in life, usually with long-standing symptoms of constipation.

In Hirschsprung's disease, there is a lack of intramuscular nitrergic (nitric oxide containing) nerves leading to an inability to produce nitric oxide, an inhibitory neurotransmitter that normally relaxes the internal anal sphincter. This leads to an absence of the anal sphincter relaxation that occurs to produce a bowel movement. This absence of the internal anal sphincter relaxation is readily apparent on anal manometry. Recent studies also suggest that the distribution of the interstitial cells of Cajal is abnormal in Hirschsprung's disease. Several genetic markers for familial and sporadic forms of Hirschsprung's disease exist. Mutations in the RET proto-oncogene have been associated with long-segment aganglionosis, whereas abnormal endothelin-B receptor genes and endothelin 3 genes have been detected in the shorter forms of the disease. These genetic abnormalities are thought to cause impaired neuronal crest migration and differentiation.

Ogilvie's syndrome

Ogilvie's syndrome (acute colonic pseudo-obstruction, acute megacolon) involves marked colonic dilation with abdominal distension. It is typically seen in older patients who have recently undergone surgery or trauma, or who suffer from a severe systemic illness or infection. It may be associated with or exacerbated by electrolyte disturbances (hypokalemia, hypocalcemia, hypomagnesemia) or medications (anticholinergics, opiate narcotic analgesics, and antidepressants). It may also affect the small intestine, thus there is overlap with acute ileus (see p. 204). In this disorder, there is an abrupt inhibition of colonic neuromuscular function for unclear reasons, possibly representing an imbalance in neural control with an increase in sympathetic inhibitory activity in conjunction with a decrease in the excitatory parasympathetic activity.

With the marked colonic distension, there is a danger of perforation if the cecum distends to larger than 10 cm in diameter. Initial management is conservative with nothing by mouth, intravenous fluids, nasogastric suction, correction of any electrolyte abnormalities, stopping possible offending medications, and, at times, placement of a rectal tube. Changing positions of the patient may help gas movement. If there is a possibility of obstruction, a Gastrografin enema is occasionally performed. If the cecal diameter exceeds 12 cm, colonoscopic decompression may be attempted to reduce the dilation. This will also help rule out an obstruction. However, this "therapeutic" colonoscopy is at an increased risk, being performed without preparation, with minimal sedation, and with minimal air insufflation. Recently, intravenous neostigmine (2 mg) has been used with success and is now often used for treatment prior to colonoscopic or surgical decompression. Surgery with tube cecostomy or right hemicolectomy is needed for marked dilation, or if there is a suspicion of occult or impending perforation with fever or leukocytosis.

Chronic functional constipation

Functional constipation according to the Rome criteria based on symptoms is defined as two or more of the following for at least 3 months

1. two or fewer bowel movements per week
2. straining at defecation at least one fourth of the time
3. lumpy and/or hard stools at least one fourth of the time
4. a sensation of incomplete evacuation at least one fourth of the time.

In general, constipation can result from either delayed transit or outlet obstruction to defecation; other patients may report severe constipation but tests of colonic transit and defecatory function are normal. In patients complaining of intractable constipation, one study found slow transit in 27%, pelvic floor dysfunction in 31%, and irritable bowel syndrome in 23% of these patients.

For constipated patients not responding to simple therapeutic measures (see p. 213), further evaluation is often needed to help determine the cause of symptoms. These procedures include

1. colonoscopy or barium enema to rule out obstructive lesions
2. colonic transit studies to assess for slow colonic transit and regional delay
3. anorectal manometry and anal EMG to evaluate for pelvic floor dysfunction and, rarely, Hirschsprung's disease.

In the evaluation of patients with persistent constipation, symptom diaries are helpful to the history. Diaries allow the patient to record the stool frequency and consistency and the occurrence of other symptoms such as pain. They are helpful aids to the patient's memory and in the documentation of the problem. They are also helpful to monitor the efficacy of treatment and adherence to treatment recommendations.

Physiologic testing, therefore, is an important area in evaluation when management strategies for patients with severe constipation are being planned. Colonic transit tests are often important clinically as regional and generalized motor disturbances cannot be diagnosed solely on the assessment of symptoms. Differentiation between different types of constipation (colonic inertia or functional rectosigmoid obstruction) is also useful therapeutically. For instance, prokinetic agents may be helpful in constipation from colonic inertia, but not from anal sphincter dysfunction or functional rectosigmoid obstruction. Constipation from functional rectosigmoid obstruction may be treated with anal manometry biofeedback. If surgery is contemplated, patients with total colonic inertia will need a colectomy, whereas patients with anorectal dysfunction may need an anorectal myomectomy. Symptoms by themselves do not reliably differentiate these physiologic subgroups of patients with severe idiopathic constipation. A sensation of anal blockage during defecation suggests pelvic floor dysfunction, but this symptom may also be seen in patients with slow transit constipation and those with normal transit.

A normal colorectal transit scan suggests the possibility of irritable bowel syndrome, misrepresentation of bowel habits, misconception of normal frequency of bowel movements, or a psychosocial disturbance. Patients with normal colorectal transit and complaints of constipation appear to suffer more from depression than patients with either slow transit or pelvic floor dysfunction. The documentation of normal colorectal transit enables the physician to re-educate the patient concerning normal bowel function.

Medical therapy for constipation is shown in Table 10.1. Treatment should begin by increasing fluid and fiber intake. Medications should be reviewed for agents that can cause constipation,

Table 10.1 Medical treatment of functional constipation.

Agents	Examples
Bulking and hydrophilic agents	
Fiber	
dietary fiber	bran
psyllium	Metamucil®, Konsyl®, Perdiem Fiber®
methylcellulose	Citrucel®
calcium polycarbophil	FiberCon®
Stool-modifying agents	
ducosate	Colace®
dehydrocholic acid	
mineral oil	
Laxatives	
Osmotic laxatives	
magnesium hydroxide	Milk of magnesia, Haley's M-O®
sodium phosphate	
lactulose	Chronulac®, Enulose®
sorbitol	
polyethylene glycol-electrolytes	MiraLax®, GoLYTELY®, Colyte®, NuLYTELY®
Stimulant laxatives	
bisacodyl	Dulcolax®
ricinoleic acid	castor oil
anthraquinones	senna, cascara, Senokot®, Pericolace®
Prokinetic agents	
5-HT$_4$ receptor agonists	tegaserod, cisapride
prostaglandin analogs	misoprostol (Cytotec®)
Enemas	
water	
sodium phosphate	Fleet®
mineral oil	
Suppositories	
glycerin	
bisacodyl	Dulcolax®

Modified from 1) Schiller LR. Treatment of constipation and diarrhea. Ch. 62 in Wolfe MM (ed.) Therapy of Digestive Disorders. Philadelphia PA, WB Saunders, 2000. 2) Locke GR III, Pemberton JH, Phillips SF. AGA Technical Review on Constipation. Gastroenterology 2000; 119: 1766–1778.

especially narcotic analgesics and calcium channel blockers. Fiber supplementation is the initial treatment of choice. Fiber can be incorporated into the diet or standardized fiber supplements can be used, Metamucil® and Citrucel® are common fiber supplements used. There are a variety of treatments used for patients who do not respond to fiber supplementation. Either hyperosmolar agents or polyethylene glycol-electrolyte solutions can be tried for short-term relief of constipation. Hyperosmolar agents include lactulose and sorbitol. Polyethylene glycol-based purgatives, such as Myralax®, can be helpful in patients not responding to fiber. Stimulant laxatives affect mucosal transport and motility. These include Colace®, Dulcolax®, glycerine. Stimulant (irritant) laxatives may have damaging effects and should not be used chronically. Phenolphthalein was withdrawn form the US market because of carcinogenesis in animal models. Newer prokinetic agents, such as tegaserod, may have a role.

Rarely, for selected patients with chronic intractable constipation, surgery may ultimately be needed. For patients with slow colonic transit or colonic inertia, subtotal colectomy with ileorectal anastomosis is the procedure of choice. Limited colonic resection is often unsatisfactory. For patients with functional rectosigmoid obstruction with an impaired rectoanal inhibitory reflex not responding to biofeedback, a limited posterior anal myomectomy with interruption of the internal sphincter may be tried. For patients with both colonic inertia and impaired rectoanal inhibitory reflex, ileostomy is occasionally needed.

Irritable bowel syndrome

Usually, constipation is self-limiting or it responds to diet alteration and/or the addition of fiber. The condition most commonly diagnosed in patients with mild constipation is irritable bowel syndrome. This condition is described in detail in Chapter 00. Although irritable bowel syndrome has a variety of definitions, it generally refers to a symptom complex characterized by abdominal pain and altered bowel habit (constipation and/or diarrhea) that occurs in the absence of identifiable structural disease. In the evaluation of patients with constipation, careful review of underlying illnesses, medications, diet, activity, and other potential contributors to constipation is important. Initial diagnostic testing is to exclude underlying causes of constipation, such as malignancy, intestinal obstruction, or hypothyroidism. On occasion, constipation may be the presenting sign for colon cancer, especially if the change of bowel habits is of recent onset. Most often, however, the barium enema or colonoscopy do not reveal organic lesions.

Functional diarrhea

Normal stool frequency is up to two bowel movements per day; three or more stools per day is considered abnormal. Stool weights above 200 g/day also fulfill the criteria for abnormality. Evaluation of patients with chronic diarrhea generally entails studies to evaluate for infectious etiologies, inflammatory bowel disease, malabsorption disorders, and surreptitious laxative abuse. After careful evaluation, however, 10% to 25% of patients with chronic diarrhea remain without a diagnosis and are often labelled with "functional" or "idiopathic" diarrhea. This is discussed in detail in Chapter 5 on Chronic Diarrhea.

Rapid colonic transit can be seen with functional diarrhea, irritable bowel syndrome, bile-salt diarrhea, surreptitious abuse of laxatives, and carcinoid syndrome. Although rare, carcinoid syndrome can present with incapacitating diarrhea. In this disorder there is increased jejunal secretion combined with increased small-intestinal and colonic motor activity, but a reduction in proximal colonic capacitance. Treatments for diarrhea aimed at reducing colonic transit are shown in Table 10.2.

Fecal incontinence

Fecal incontinence, often underreported to physicians, is not uncommon. Next to dementia, it is a major reason for placing elderly people in nursing homes. Some degree of fecal incontinence develops in 3% of women who give birth by vaginal delivery. Fecal incontinence is traditionally divided into two categories – partial and major incontinence. Partial incontinence is defined as loss of control to flatus and minor soiling of the underwear. Major incontinence is the frequent and regular inability to control stools of normal consistency. Evaluation of fecal incontinence consists initially with several simple procedures. Diagnostic procedures of value for the evaluation of fecal incontinence include

1. symptom diaries for diagnostic evaluation
2. digital rectal examination allowing a simple qualitative assessment of resting and squeeze pressures
3. flexible sigmoidoscopy to evaluate for inflammation, melanosis coli, tumors, and even fecal impaction which may result in overflow incontinence
4. anorectal manometry with sensory and compliance testing to define functional sphincter weakness and to perform and predict response to biofeedback training
5. anal ultrasound examination for structural damage to the anal sphincter.

Initial treatments include bulking or antidiarrheal agents. Anorectal manometry not only assesses anal sphincter pressure and rectal sensation, but may be used for treatment using biofeedback techniques. Further treatments include biofeedback training. This can increase sensation and sphincter muscle strength. For patients who meet the criteria (motivation, ability to comprehend directions, and some degree of rectal sensation), success has been achieved with anal manometry biofeedback in up to 70% of cases, including patients with incontinence caused

Table 10.2 Treatments for diarrhea aimed at reducing colonic transit.

Class	Examples
Opiates	
loperamide	Imodium®
diphenoxylate with atropine	Lomotil®
Alpha$_2$-adrenergic agonists	
clonidine	
Somatostatin analogs	octreotide
Calcium channel blockers	

Modified from Schiller LR. Treatment of constipation and diarrhea. Ch. 62 in Wolfe MM (ed.) Therapy of Digestive Disorders. Philadelphia PA, WB Saunders, 2000.

by prior sphincter surgery or anorectal disease, idiopathic incontinence, and diabetes mellitus.

Surgical therapy is reserved for situations with marked incapacity from fecal incontinence. Surgical procedures involve direct sphincter repair of injured sphincters, posterior sphincter plication for weak sphincters, and, at times, a colostomy where stool diversion is needed. New treatments that are being tried include applying electric radiofrequency to the anal sphincters or injecting collagen into the anal sphincters.

Summary

This chapter has provided an overview of the motility disorders of the small bowel and colon. It has discussed the tests for patient evaluation and discussed several classic conditions that affect small-bowel and colonic motility. Management of these patients requires an understanding of the pathophysiology, clinical tests, and treatment options for these conditions.

Further reading

Anura S, Hodges. Dysmotility of the small intestine. *Textbook of Gastroenterology*. Yamada T (ed) 1998.

Bonapace ES, Davidoff S, Krevsky B, *et al*. Whole gut transit scintigraphy in the clinical evaluation of patients with upper and lower gastrointestinal symptoms. *Am J Gastroenterol* 2000; 95: 2838–2847.

Camilleri M, Hasler W, Parkman HP, *et al*. Measurement of gastroduodenal motility in the GI laboratory. *Gastroenterology* 1998; 115: 747–762.

Di Lorenzo C. Pseudo-obstruction: Current approaches. *Gastroenterology* 1999; 116: 980–987.

Diamant NE, Kamm MA, Wald A, Whitehead WE. AGA Technical review on anorectal testing techniques. *Gastroenterology* 1999; 116: 735–760.

Donowitz M, Kokke FT, Saidi R. Evaluation of patients with chronic diarrhea. *New Eng J Med* 1995; 332: 725–729.

Herlinger H. Guide to imaging of the small bowel. *Gastroenterol Clinics NA* 1995; 24: 309–329.

Locke GR III, Pemberton JH, Phillips SF. AGA Technical Review on Constipation. *Gastroenterology* 2000; 119: 1766–1778.

Parkman HP, Harris AD, Krevsky B, *et al*. Gastroduodenal motility and dysmotility: Update on techniques available for evaluation. *Am J Gastroenterology* 1995; 90: 869–892.

Quigley EM. Acute intestinal pseudo-obstruction. *Curr Treat Options Gastroenterol* 2000; 3: 273–286.

Quigley EM. Chronic intestinal pseudo-obstruction. *Curr Treat Options Gastroenterol* 1999; 2: 239–250.

Quigley EM. Disturbances in small bowel motility. *Baillieres Best Pract Res Clin Gastroenterol* 1999; 13: 385–395.

Quigley EMM, Hasler WL, Parkman HP. AGA Technical Review on Nausea and Vomiting. *Gastroenterology* 2001; 120: 263–286.

Soffer EE. Small bowel dysmotility. *Curr Treat Options Gastroenterol* 1998; 1: 8–14.

Wald A. Constipation and fecal incontinence in the elderly. *Gastroenterology Clinics North America* 1990; 19: 405–418.

Chapter 11

Mesenteric Ischemia and Intestinal Vascular Disorders

Ross Milner and Omaida C. Velazquez

CHAPTER OUTLINE

CHRONIC INTESTINAL ISCHEMIA
- *Pathophysiology*
- *Presentation and differential diagnosis*
- *Imaging studies*
- *Treatment options*
- *Postoperative management and complications*
- *Patency rates for chronic intestinal ischemia revascularization*

ACUTE MESENTERIC ISCHEMIA
- *Pathophysiology and diagnosis*
- *Diagnosis and imaging studies and percutaneous treatment modalities*
- *Operative treatment*
- *Postoperative care*

NON-OCCLUSIVE MESENTERIC ISCHEMIA
- *Pathophysiology and presentation*
- *Diagnosis and imaging studies*
- *Treatment*
- *Outcome*

MESENTERIC VENOUS THROMBOSIS
- *Pathophysiology*
- *Presentation*
- *Diagnosis and imaging studies*
- *Treatment*
- *Outcome*

FURTHER READING

Chronic intestinal ischemia

Pathophysiology

Chronic intestinal ischemia may result from diseases of either the small or large arteries of the mesenteric circulation. The most common cause of chronic intestinal ischemia is arteriosclerosis of the mesenteric arteries. This results in either severe stenosis or occlusion of the proximal segments of two or three of the three main axial splanchnic arteries (Figure 11.1). The most common normal anatomy of these vessels is depicted in Figures 11.1 to 11.5. These arteries are the celiac axis (Figure 11.2) (that gives rise to the common hepatic artery, the left gastric artery, and the splenic artery), the superior mesenteric artery (Figure 11.3) that supplies circulation to the small bowel from the distal duodenum to the mid-transverse colon, and the inferior mesenteric artery (Figure 11.4) that provides inflow to the colon from the mid-transverse colon to the rectum. Extensive collateral channels connect the branches of these main mesenteric vessels (Figure 11.5). Most commonly, chronic intestinal ischemia results from occlusive or stenotic disease that is limited to the ostium of the axial splanchnic vessels (Figure 11.6) and many normally occurring collateral vessels enlarge in caliber and become much more prominent and hemodynamically

Mesenteric Ischemia and Intestinal Vascular Disorders

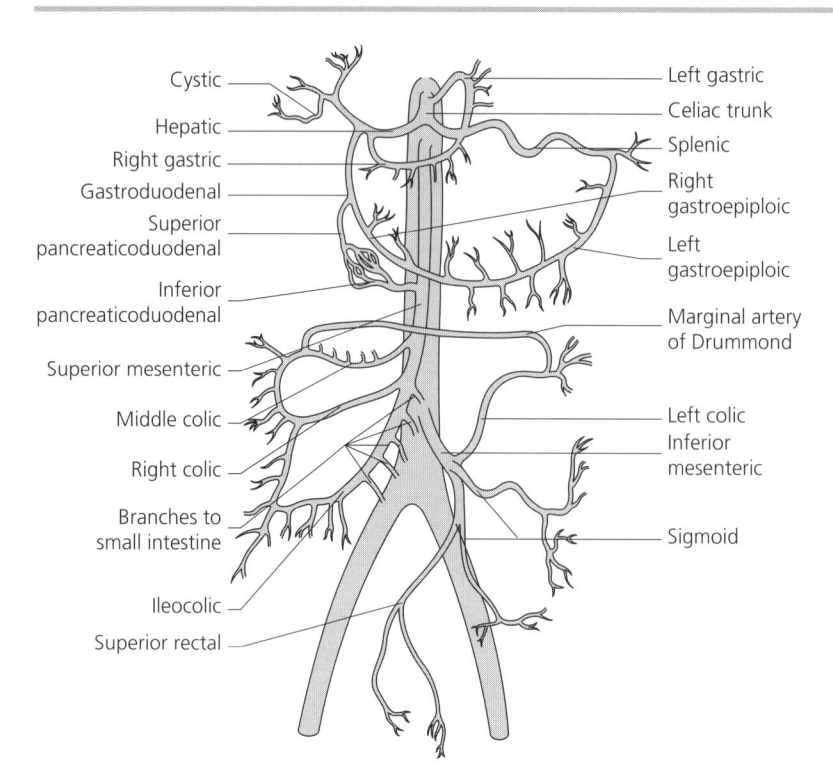

Figure 11.1 Schematic of the mesenteric circulation (reproduced from: Schwartz LB, Davis RD Jr, Heinle JS, *et al*: The vascular system. In Lyerly HK, Gaynor JW Jr (eds) *The Handbook of Surgical Intensive Care* 3rd edn, St Louis, Mosby Year Book, 1192, p. 287, 1992).

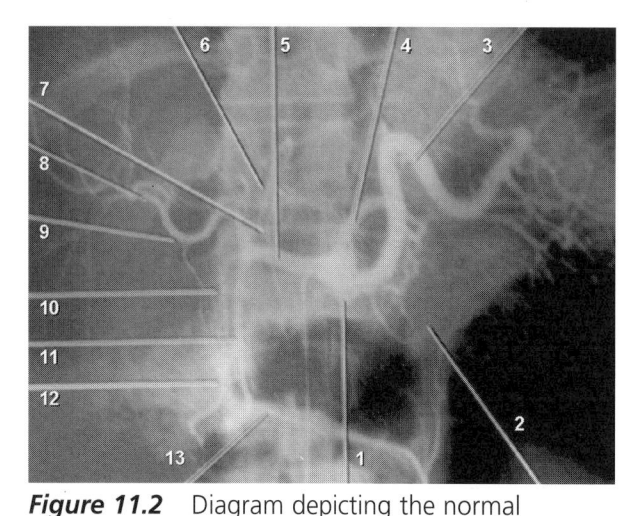

Figure 11.2 Diagram depicting the normal anatomy of the celiac axis. 1 = celiac trunk; 2 = left gastroepiploic; 3 = splenic artery; 4 = left gastric artery; 5 = proper hepatic artery; 6 = right gastric artery; 7 = cystic artery; 8 = right hepatic artery; 9 = common hepatic artery; 10 = superior pancreaticoduodenal artery; 11 = gastroduodenal artery; 12 = inferior pancreaticoduodenal artery (from the superior mesenteric artery); 13 = right gastroepiploic artery.

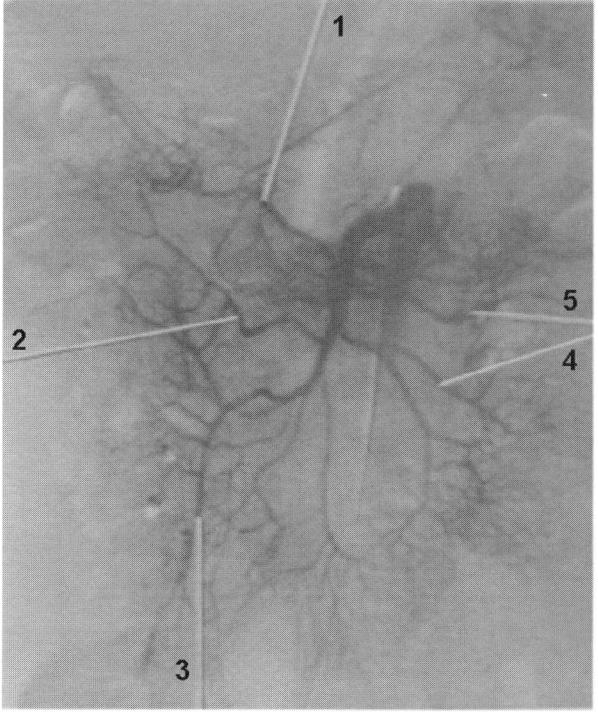

Figure 11.3 Selective superior mesenteric arteriogram depicting the normal superior mesenteric artery and its branches. 1 = middle colic branch; 2 = right colic branch; 3 = iliocolic branch; 4 and 5 = multiple branching arcades to the small intestine.

218

Chronic intestinal ischemia

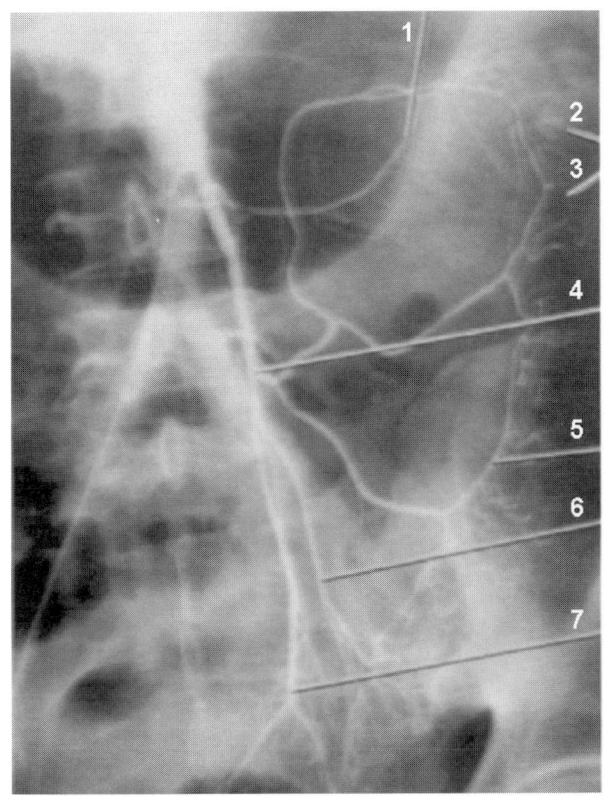

Figure 11.4 Selective inferior mesenteric arteriogram depicting the normal inferior mesenteric artery anatomy. 1 = left colic branch; 2, 3, and 5 = multiple communications of the marginal artery of Drummond; 4 and 6 = sigmoid branches; 7 = superior rectal branch.

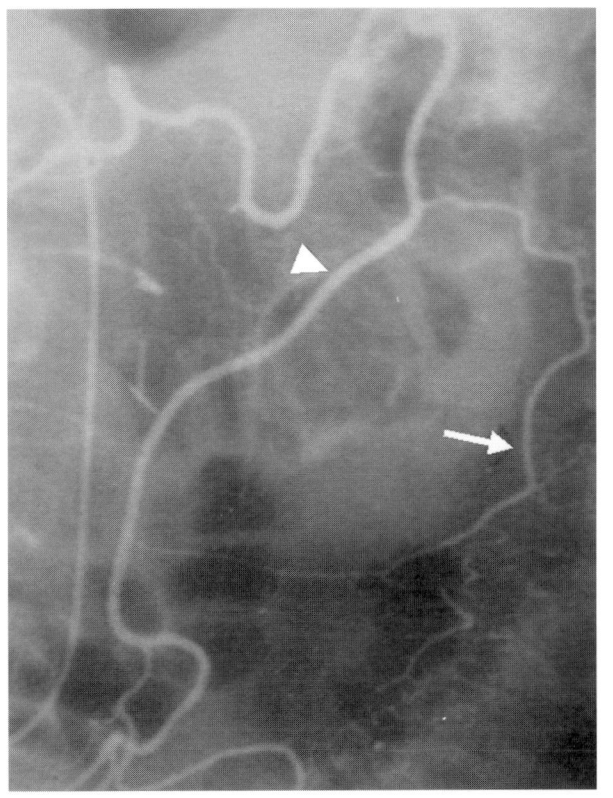

Figure 11.5 Branches of the superior mesenteric artery communicate with branches of the inferior mesenteric artery at the periphery of the colon via multiple collateral connections of the marginal artery of Drummond (long arrow). The superior mesenteric artery and inferior mesenteric artery also communicate via a more centrally located vessel known as the arc of Riolan (short arrow), also referred to as the meandering mesenteric artery.

important to the bowel inflow circulation (Figure 11.7). Under physiologic conditions, the mesenteric vessels vasodilate after a meal leading to significant post-prandial hyperemic intestinal arterial flow. A failure in the normal physiologic effect is seen with atherosclerotic disease of the mesenteric arteries. This is the basic pathophysiologic mechanism for the clinical entity of chronic intestinal ischemia. However, there are many other known clinical entities that are associated with chronic, acute, or subacute mesenteric ischemia. These less common diseases are listed in Box 11.1. Visceral artery dissection is commonly associated with aortic dissection and may present as chronic, subacute, or acute mesenteric ischemia (Figure 11.8). Even less common causes include visceral artery aneurysms with acute or chronic distal embolization (Figure 11.9) and median arcuate ligament syndrome.

Box 11.1 Conditions associated with mesenteric ischemia

Visceral artery atherosclerosis
Neurofibromatosis
Visceral artery dissection
Fibromuscular hyperplasia
Buerger's disease
Radiation injury
Rheumatoid arthritis
Systemic lupus erythematosis
Polyarteritis nodosa
Cogan's syndrome
Coarctation repair
Ergor poisoning
Cocaine abuse

219

Mesenteric Ischemia and Intestinal Vascular Disorders

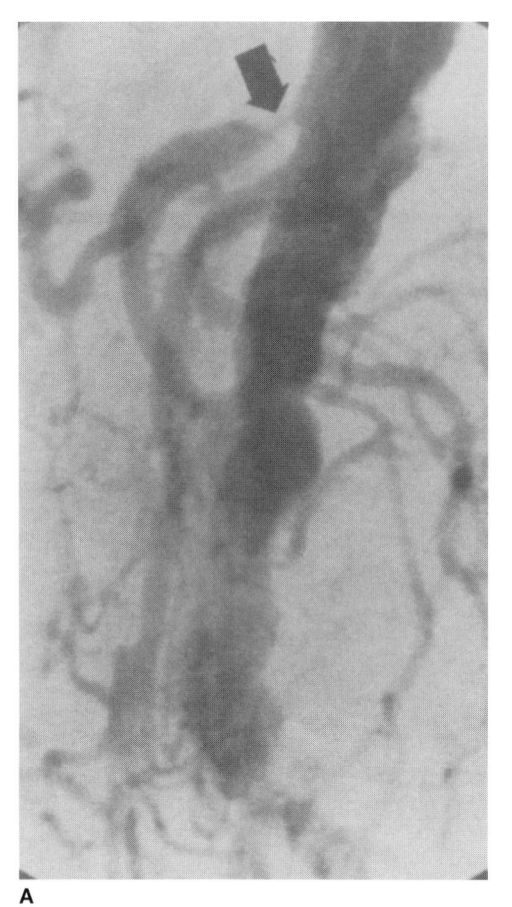

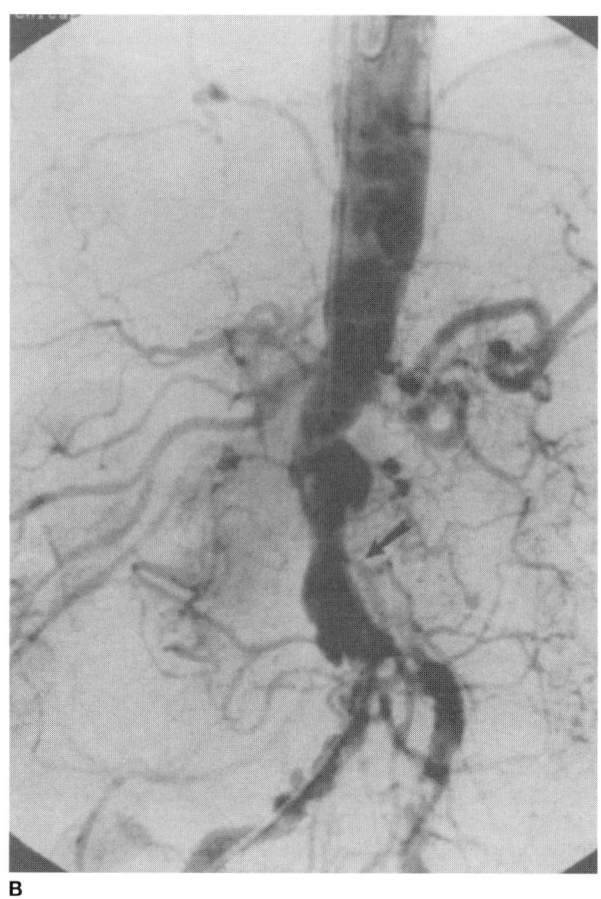

A **B**

Figure 11.6 Chronic mesenteric ischemia in a 78-year-old woman who had undergone coronary artery bypass and carotid endarterectomy and who presented with claudication, 30-pound weight loss, and postprandial pain. A) Lateral aortogram showing critical celiac axis stenosis (arrow). B) Anteroposterior aortogram showing severe infrarenal aortic disease and critical inferior mesenteric artery stenosis (arrow) (reproduced from: Schwartz LB, Gewertz BL: Intestinal ischemia disorders. In Yao JST, Pearce WH (eds) *Modern Trends in Vascular Surgery*. Norwalk, CT Appleton & Lange, 1999, pp. 347–367).

Presentation and differential diagnosis

Atherosclerotic disease causes stenosis of the proximal mesenteric arteries and is frequently asymptomatic. Collateral circulation develops that effectively compensates for these stenotic lesions (Figures 11.5, 11.7). Autopsy studies have demonstrated that as many as 10% of unselected patients have evidence of 50% or greater stenosis in at least one of the three main mesenteric arteries. The prevalence of this disease appears to increase with age.

Chronic mesenteric ischemia is also associated with other forms of systemic atherosclerosis. Approximately one third of patients undergoing diagnostic aortography as part of the work-up for peripheral vascular disease have been found to have evidence of chronic stenotic disease of the mesenteric vessels. These patients are generally asymptomatic from the classic symptoms of chronic mesenteric ischemia (Figure 11.10).

Anatomic routes for compensation via collateral circulation include the pancreaticoduodenal arteries, the arc of Riolan (ascending branch of the left colic artery), and the internal iliac arteries (Figures 11.2–11.5, 11.7). In the presence of a hemodynamically significant stenosis of the superior mesenteric artery, collateral routes can allow for inflow from the hepatic artery to the gastroduodenal artery and into the superior mesenteric artery branches through the superior and inferior pancreaticoduodenal arteries. Similarly, a hemodynamically significant lesion of the celiac axis can lead to collateral flow in the opposite direction through these same routes with filling of the celiac branches retrograde from the superior mesenteric artery flow. In the clinical situation where both the celiac axis and

Chronic intestinal ischemia

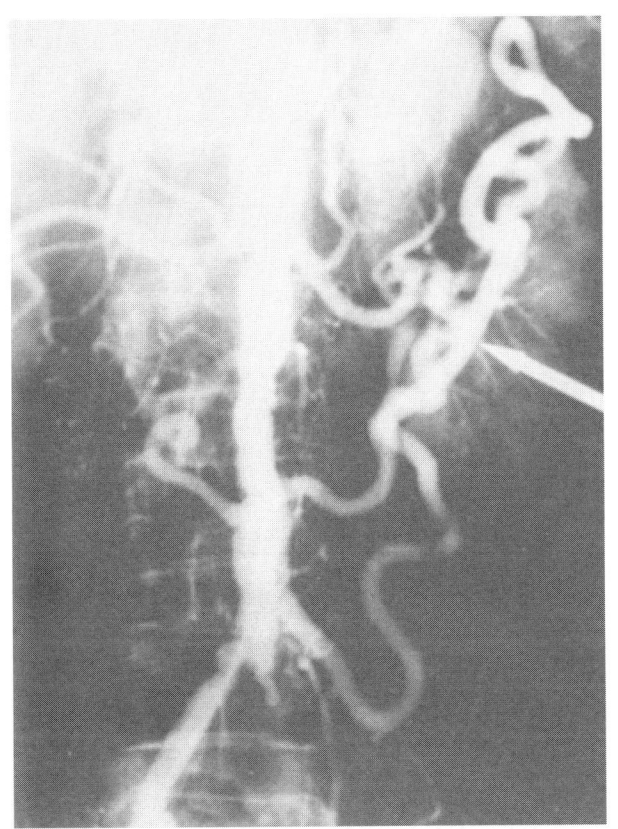

Figure 11.7 Angiogram from an asymptomatic patient with proximal occlusion of the celiac and superior mesenteric arteries. The arterial supply to the foregut and midgut is via a large collateral vessel of the inferior mesenteric artery, the arch of Riolan (arrow) (reproduced from Lloyd M. Taylor. Management of visceral ischemic syndromes. In Rutherford RB *et al.* (eds) *Vascular Surgery* 5th edn. Philadelphia PA, WB Saunders, 2000, p. 1503).

interrupted the normally occurring collateral circulation. When clinical symptoms are present, most commonly they include pain in the mid-abdominal and epigastric area after meals. The pain is usually described as a deep, dull, or colicky intense ache. There is occasional radiation of this discomfort toward the back. The individual usually comes to associate eating with this pain and develops a fear of food and there is an associated significant weight loss. Malabsorption is not a significant component of the weight loss associated with chronic intestinal ischemia. Rather, the significant decrease in nutritional intake appears to be the most important etiology for the weight loss. Occasionally, patients may present with a constant, mild, generalized abdominal pain that is not necessarily associated with food intake. This syndrome will completely disappear after surgical revascularization of the mesenteric circulation.

In general, physical examination is unremarkable except for the significant weight loss that is often seen. In addition, there might be evidence of diffuse atherosclerotic occlusive disease. Arthrosclerotic and/or calcified plaque within the aorta and its branches may result in abdominal bruits that are noted on physical examination. Bruits are not specific for mesenteric ischemia. There is also no specific pattern of bowel habits associated with chronic mesenteric ischemia. The differential diagnosis includes abdominal malignancies, ulcer diathesis, and symptomatic cholelithiasis.

superior mesenteric artery have hemodynamically significant stenoses, the inferior mesenteric artery can provide retrograde flow to the branches of these two mesenteric vessels. This occurs via the arch of Riolan through the marginal anastomotic arteries and then to the middle colic and pancreaticoduodenal arteries. The internal iliac arteries, which have many collateral branches to the inferior mesenteric artery, can also provide significant collateral flow when both the superior mesenteric artery and celiac axis are involved with significant disease.

The symptoms of chronic intestinal ischemia are usually present when at least two of the three major splanchnic vessels are severely stenotic or completely occluded. Infrequently, severe disease of the superior mesenteric artery only may result in clinical symptoms. This is particularly true with a history of prior abdominal operations that have

Imaging studies

Digital subtraction arteriography is the diagnostic study of choice for the detection of chronic and/or acute intestinal ischemia (Figures 11.6, 11.11). It is important that both anteroposterior and lateral views of the abdominal aorta and its branches are obtained. Unless a therapeutic percutaneous intervention is planned, the selective catheterization of the main visceral vessels, as depicted in Figures 11.11C, 11.11D, is not required or advised. This is because most lesions are ostial (Figures 11.6, 11.10), and therefore are best imaged with standard aortogram techniques. In addition to demonstrating any significant stenoses of the visceral branches of the abdominal aorta, the arteriogram can demonstrate evidence of well-developed collateral circulation (Figure, 11.11D 11.6–11.7). These latter findings may suggest that the stenoses visualized in the visceral vessels are in fact hemodynamically significant. However, the presence of a pronounced

Mesenteric Ischemia and Intestinal Vascular Disorders

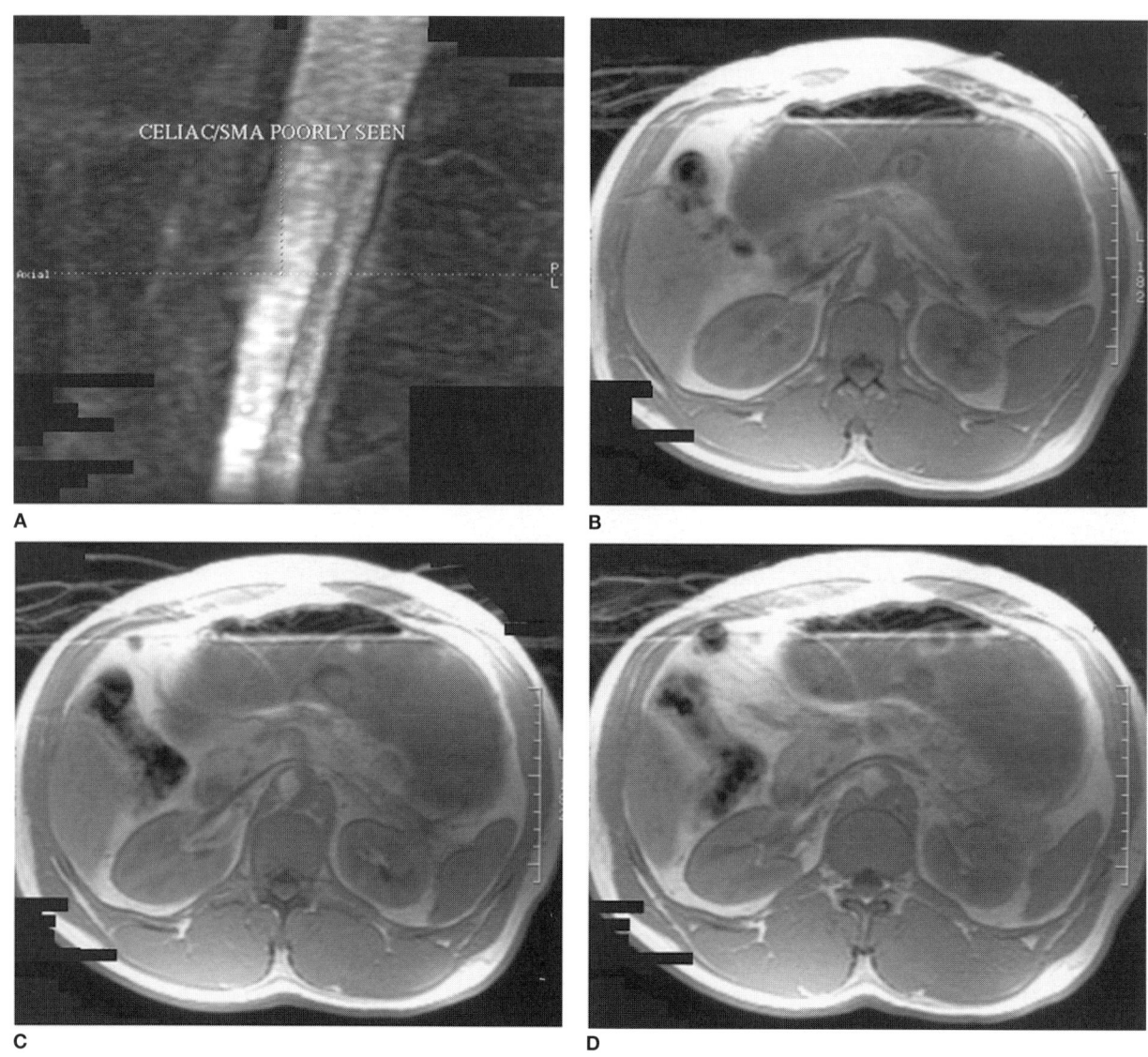

Figure 11.8 Gadolinium-enhanced magnetic resonance angiography in a 39-year-old patient presenting with acute onset of abdominal pain and uncontrolled hypertension with a history of cocaine abuse. A) The abdominal aorta is dissected and the celiac axis and superior mesenteric artery are poorly visualized on lateral projection. B, C and D) On cross-sectional views there is an abrupt cut-off noted in the flow to the proximal superior mesenteric artery and there is no visualized enhancement in the distal superior mesenteric artery.

collateral circulation does not necessarily correlate with symptoms since many patients are well compensated by these same well-developed collaterals.

Magnetic resonance angiography (MRA) is a very useful non-invasive imaging technique for evaluating patients who are suspected as having chronic mesenteric ischemia (Figures 11.8, 11.10). Magnetic resonance angiography can also clearly demonstrate any associated stenoses or abnormalities of the renal arteries and the pelvic circulation. The MRA technique requires institutional validation and comparison with standard arteriographic methods. It is a useful technique that avoids an arterial puncture as well as contrast dye nephrotoxicity that has been reported with conventional arteriography. In addition, magnetic resonance techniques provide useful images of the intra-abdominal organs and retroperitoneum. Moreover, the venous anatomy can be easily visualized by magnetic resonance techniques. Post-prandial hyperemia can be documented in the superior mesenteric vein by phase contrast cine magnetic resonance imaging. Computed tomography scanning can visualize the proximal mesenteric circulation (Figure

Chronic intestinal ischemia

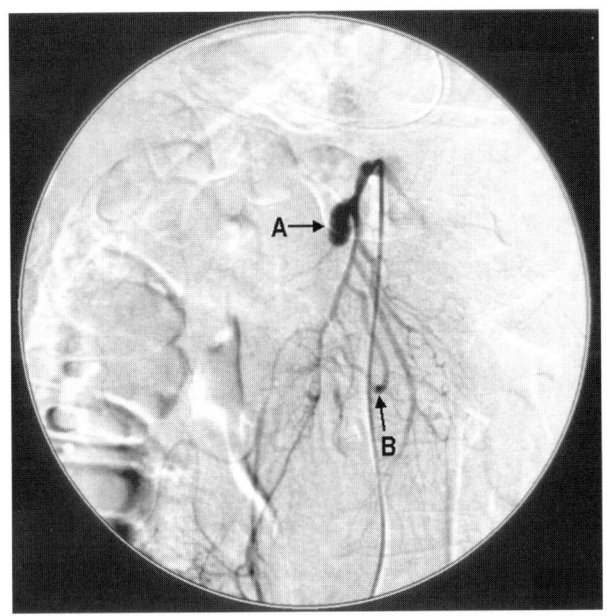

Figure 11.9 Selective arteriogram of the superior mesenteric artery demonstrates a sacular aneurysm of the proximal superior mesenteric artery (A) with abrupt cut-off of flow in some of the small-bowel branches of the superior mesenteric artery (B), in a 48-year-old man presenting with an acute abdomen and segmental small-bowel necrosis secondary to distal embolization of an aneurysm-derived thrombus.

11.12) and may demonstrate advanced findings of bowel necrosis but is not considered ideal for the early diagnosis of mesenteric ischemia. Improvements in CT scanning may increase its utility in evaluating the mesenteric circulation.

Duplex ultrasonography is another non-invasive modality that can be utilized in the diagnosis of chronic mesenteric ischemia. It has significant limitations related to the skill of the operator, bowel gas, postoperative changes, and body habitus. Studies have demonstrated that superior mesenteric artery peak systolic velocity of greater than 275 cm/s is highly predictive of a 70% or greater stenosis within this vessel. The sensitivity, specificity, and predictive value of ultrasound in identifying stenoses within the superior mesenteric artery is slightly higher than for the same modality when studying the celiac axis. Similar duplex scanning criteria have been developed for diastolic velocities. In interpreting duplex scanning velocities, one must keep in mind that the Doppler angle needs to be approximately 60 degrees. Doppler angles larger than 70 degrees may result in falsely elevated peak systolic velocities. The degree of respiratory motion and the depth of the vessels that are being studied

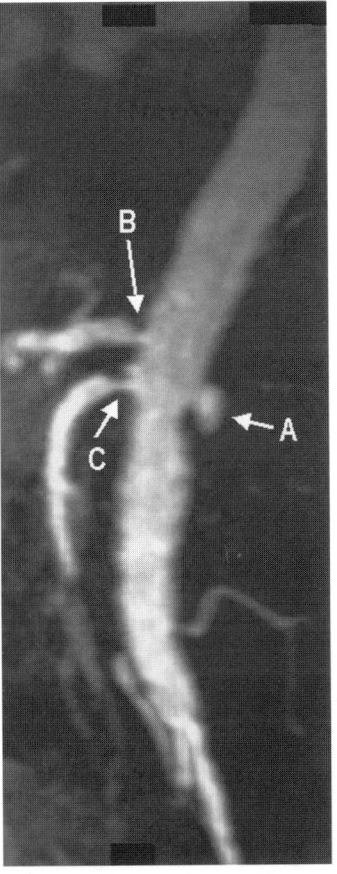

Figure 11.10 Gadolinium-enhanced magnetic resonance angiography of the abdominal aorta in lateral projection in a 79-year-old woman presenting with embolization to the toes bilaterally. The aorta demonstrates a penetrating ulcer (A) (this was likely to be the source of a distal embolus) and the incidental finding of moderate celiac axis (B) and superior mesenteric artery (C) proximal stenosis. The inferior mesenteric artery was widely patent and there were no clinical signs or symptoms of chronic mesenteric artery ischemia.

may significantly influence the results obtained with the duplex scanner. There are some proponents of replacing diagnostic arteriography with duplex, however, because of the above-mentioned limitations we believe the diagnosis of chronic mesenteric ischemia needs to be confirmed by either standard arteriography or MRA.

Treatment options

Intestinal infarction can occur in chronic intestinal ischemia weeks, months, or years after the history of chronic recurrent abdominal pain has

Mesenteric Ischemia and Intestinal Vascular Disorders

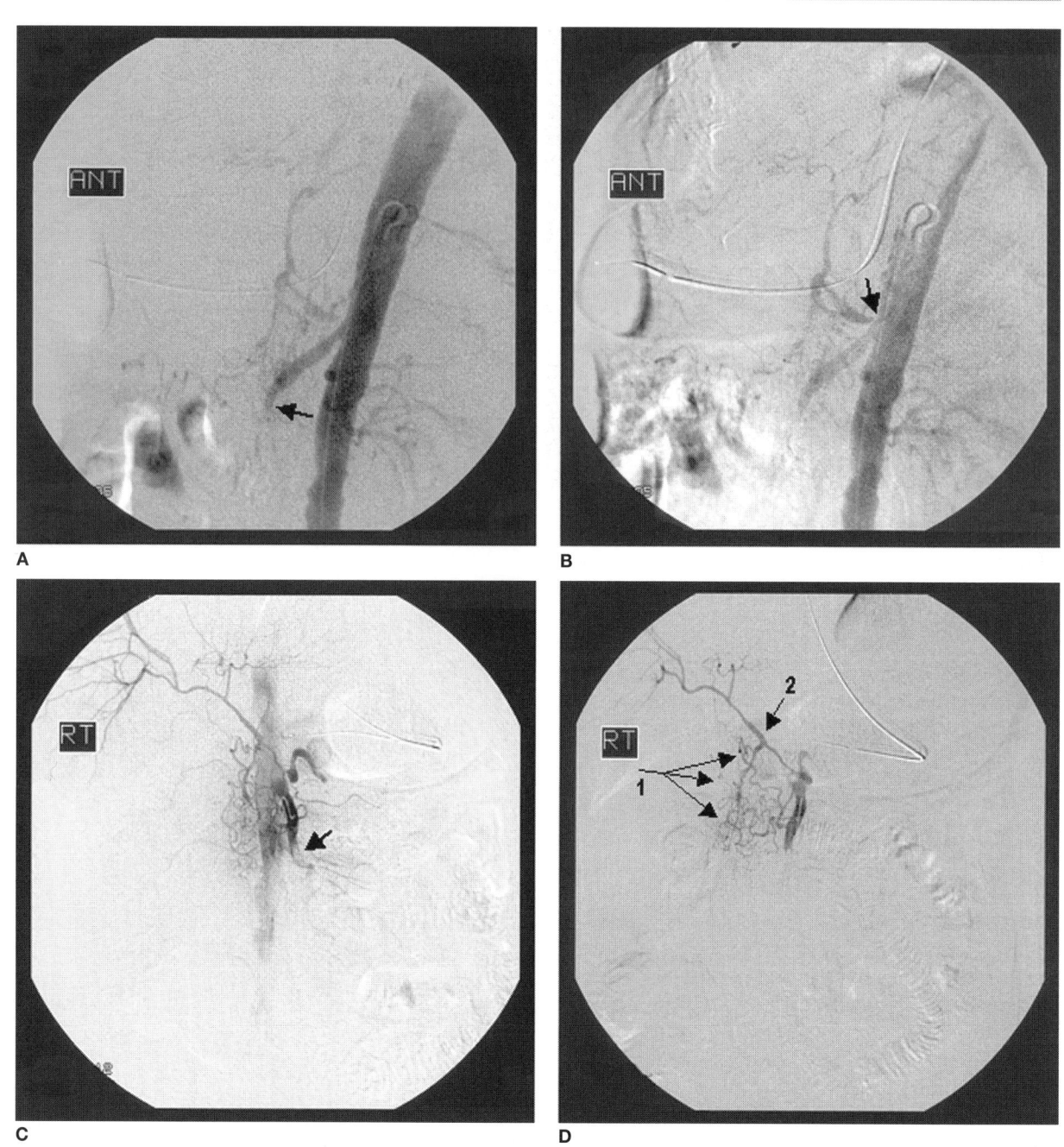

Figure 11.11 Aortogram in lateral (A and B) and anteroposterior (C and D) projections in a 63-year-old man presenting with a history of atrial fibrillation and long-term smoking that presented with sudden onset of severe abdominal pain out of proportion with physical examination findings. The study demonstrates evidence of an acute cut-off of flow in the superior mesenteric artery (arrow in A) suggestive of an embolus. However there is also evidence of moderate proximal stenosis of the celiac axis (arrow in B) and well-formed pancreaticoduodenal collaterals channels (arrows 1 and 2 in D), which suggests the concurrent diagnosis of chronic asymptomatic mesenteric stenosis. The absence of ostial disease in the superior mesenteric artery and the characteristic flow void produced by intraluminal clot (arrow in C) confirms the diagnosis of an acute embolus to the superior mesenteric artery.

been documented. Mikkelson first proposed the possibility that surgery may alter the natural history of this disease in 1957. Shaw and Maynard performed the first surgical reconstruction for mesenteric ischemia. Since that time, it has been well accepted and well documented that the symptoms of chronic intestinal ischemia can be successfully eliminated by surgical revascularization. One

Chronic intestinal ischemia

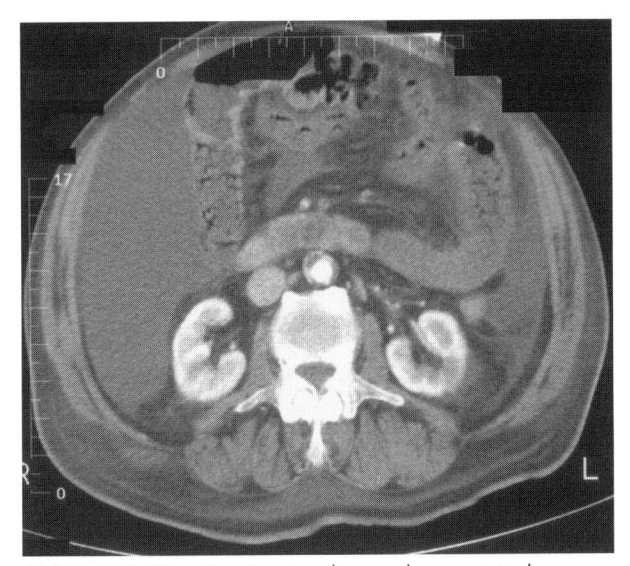

Figure 11.12 Contrast-enhanced computed tomography scan showing lack of visualization of contrast in the distal superior mesenteric artery as it emerges inferior to the pancreas, in a 47-year-old patient with abdominal pain and tenderness.

case report suggested that the use of octreotide could improve the symptoms of chronic mesenteric ischemia. This was done in an extremely high-risk patient.

Surgical intervention for chronic intestinal ischemia

Indications There is no data to suggest that asymptomatic lesions need to be treated. However, patients with significant stenosis or occlusion of the superior mesenteric artery who must undergo other aortic or renal artery reconstruction, may undergo simultaneous reconstruction of the superior mesenteric artery. This may be performed in the absence of pre-existing clinical symptoms. However, the additional intervention may add risk to the procedure with increased mortality as previously published by the Mayo Clinic and Cleveland Clinic. Clearly, it has been documented that intestinal ischemia may occur after such aortic or renal reconstructions if the superior mesenteric artery is not also revascularized. Asymptomatic lesions of the celiac axis, however, do not require any surgical intervention.

For symptomatic patients, it is important to rule out the possibility of commonly occurring malignancies that may also present with abdominal pain and weight loss. This possibility may be ruled out with cross-sectional imaging of the abdomen by CT or MRI. Symptomatic patients may benefit from a short period of preoperative cessation of oral intake and support with total parenteral nutrition. The rationale for a short-term course of total parenteral nutrition preoperatively relates to potentially decreasing complications associated with severe pre-existing malnutrition.

Techniques Revascularization of the mesenteric vessels can be accomplished by a variety of techniques. These techniques include re-implantation of the vessels beyond the stenoses, endarterectomy of the obstructing plaque, and bypass grafting. Inflow for bypass grafting with either prosthetic or autologous veins (Figure 11.13) has been described as arising from either the supraceliac (Figure 11.14)

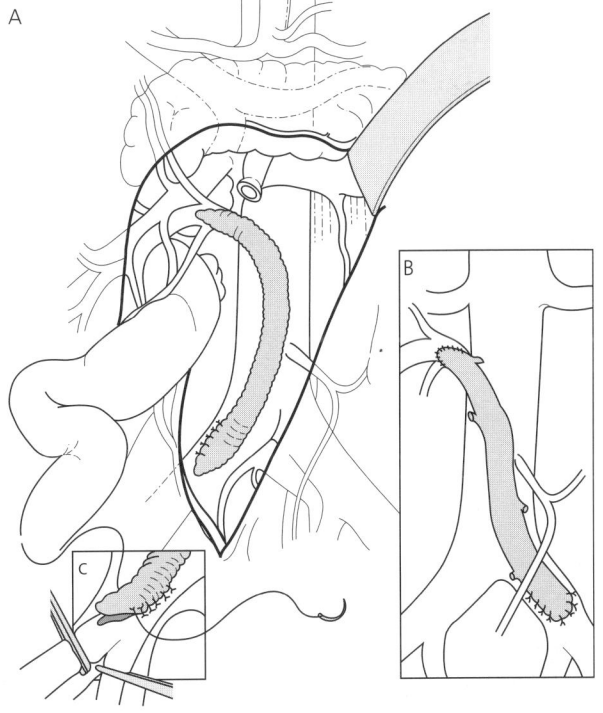

Figure 11.13 (A) Iliac to superior mesenteric artery bypass using a prosthetic for cases in which superior mesenteric artery thrombosis produces ischemic but salvageable bowel. (B) Iliac to superior mesenteric artery bypass using saphenous vein for cases in which some segments of necrotic or perforated bowel must be resected. (C) Detail of distal anastomosis (from Kazmers A: Operative management of acute mesenteric ischemia. *Ann Vasc Surg* 12: 127–197; 1998. Reproduced with permission from Lloyd M Taylor Jr, Gregory L Moneta, John M. Porter. Treatment of acute intestinal ischemia caused by arterial occlusions. In Rutherford RB *et al.* (eds) *Vascular Surgery* 5th edn. Philadelphia PA, WB Saunders, 2000, p. 1517.)

Mesenteric Ischemia and Intestinal Vascular Disorders

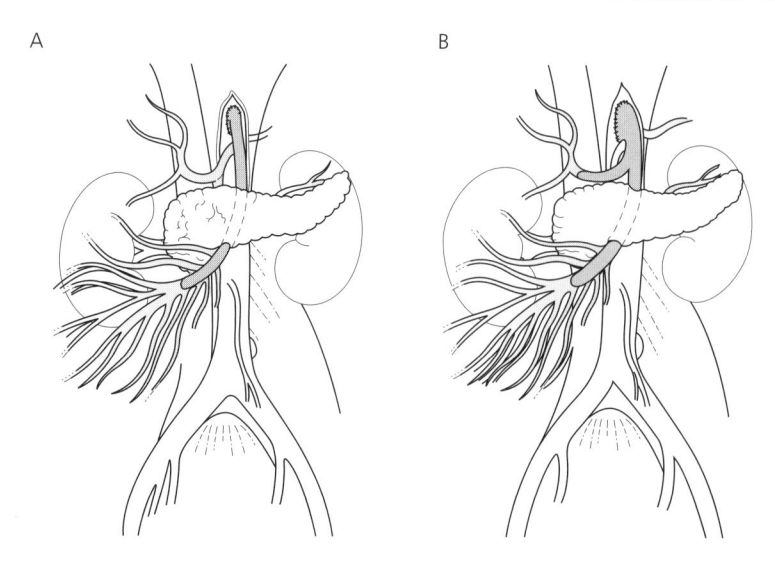

Figure 11.14 (A) Supraceliac aorta–superior mesenteric artery bypass. The graft origin is best cut from a bifurcation graft, as illustrated in Figure 11.14B. (B) Supraceliac aorta–superior mesenteric and hepatic bypass. (from Taylor LM Jr, Porter JM: Treatment of chronic intestinal ischemia. *Semin Vasc Surg* 3: 195; 1990. Reproduced with permission from Lloyd M, Taylor Jr, Gregory L. Moneta, John M. Porter. Treatment of chronic visceral ischemia. In Rutherford RB *et al.* (eds) *Vascular Surgery* 5th edn, Philadelphia PA, WB Saunders, 2000, p. 1538.)

or infrarenal aorta (Figure 11.15). Alternatively, the iliac arteries may serve as adequate inflow (Figure 11.13). In addition, several abdominal vessels have been described as a potential source for inflow.

Endarterectomy Exposure to the celiac axis and superior mesenteric artery can be obtained via a midline transabdominal incision utilizing a medial visceral rotation technique. Alternatively, a thoracoabdominal exposure may be utilized for exposure of the proximal part of the visceral arteries.

Utilizing a transabdominal approach, the distal mesenteric artery can be exposed. A distal arteriotomy is created through which a blind retrograde endarterectomy can be performed. This operation, however, offers little control of the desired endarterectomy endpoint and for this reason has been essentially abandoned. Obtaining vascular control of the suprarenal aorta and performing the arteriotomy across the origin of the superior mesenteric artery allows an endarterectomy with direct visualization of the endpoint. Again, this exposure

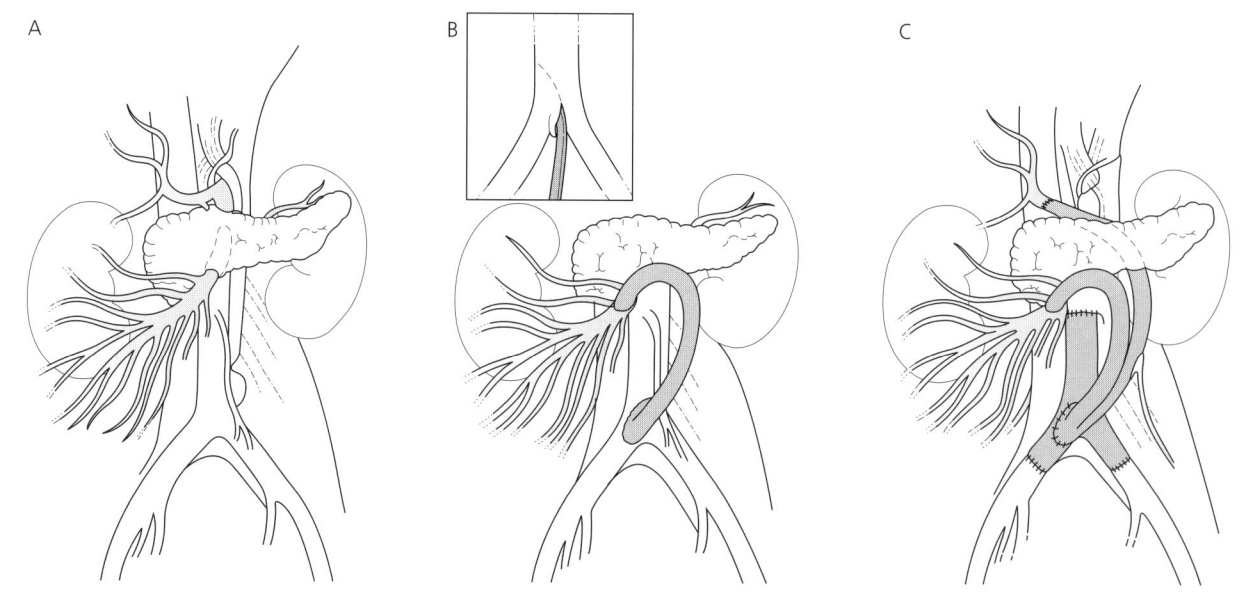

Figure 11.15 (A) Exposure of the infrarenal aorta and the superior mesenteric and celiac arteries. (B) Method of infrarenal aorta–superior mesenteric artery bypass; inset, method of forming the graft origin. (C) Method of infrarenal aortic graft placement with bypass to the superior mesenteric and hepatic arteries. Note the reimplantation of the inferior mesenteric artery (from Taylor LM Jr, Porter JM: Treatment of chronic intestinal ischemia. *Semin Vasc Surg* 3: 195; 1990. Reproduced with permission from Lloyd M, Taylor Jr, Gregory L. Moneta, John M. Porter. Treatment of chronic visceral ischemia. In Rutherford RB *et al.* (eds) *Vascular Surgery* 5th edn, Philadelphia PA, WB Saunders, 2000, p. 1536.)

may be obtained transabdominally, using a medial visceral rotation. Alternatively, the aorta may be exposed through a retroperitoneal incision that exposes the posterior-lateral aspect of the aorta. A transaortic endarterectomy can be performed with this approach such that the aorta is opened in a "trap-door" fashion. The origin of the visceral arteries can then be visualized directly and a direct endarterectomy can be performed with full control of the endpoint. In addition, this method allows for simultaneous endarterectomy of the renal arteries and the celiac axis.

Bypass grafting to the mesenteric vessels

Although endarterectomy is a well-accepted approach to the treatment of stenosis of the visceral arteries, the surgical exposure to accomplish this operation is very technically demanding. In addition, the vascular control for this operation requires clamping both the visceral and renal circulation and carries a significant risk of ischemia to the kidneys with resulting renal failure, embolization to the lower extremities, the viscera, or the spinal cord resulting in paraplegia. In addition, there is a significantly increased risk of cardiac and pulmonary complications. For these reasons, a more popular approach to the revascularization of the mesenteric vessels is bypass grafting from either the suprarenal or infrarenal abdominal aorta (Figures 11.13–11.15). The level of the aorta preferred for the source of inflow in these revascularizations is highly dependent on whether or not the aorta is diseased at these levels.

When the infrarenal aorta is amenable for inflow, a short reversed saphenous vein graft can be utilized from the infrarenal aorta to the superior mesenteric artery as it emerges from the inferior border of the pancreas (Figure 11.16). Acute angulation may pose significant technical difficulties with this particular graft configuration. These short grafts are at particular risk for kinking and extrinsic compression. Prosthetic grafts made from double-velour Dacron are often preferred as the source of conduit. This is not true in the setting of active intra-abdominal infection and bowel ischemia at the time of operation. When the infrarenal aorta is severely diseased as a result of either occlusive or aneurysmal disease, the inflow can be obtained from a prosthetic utilized to replace the diseased segment of the aorta. Alternatively, the common iliac arteries may be utilized as a source of inflow as long as there is no evidence of occlusive disease.

As a general rule, the procedure of choice for revascularizing the mesenteric vessels depends on the extent of disease along the length of the aorta

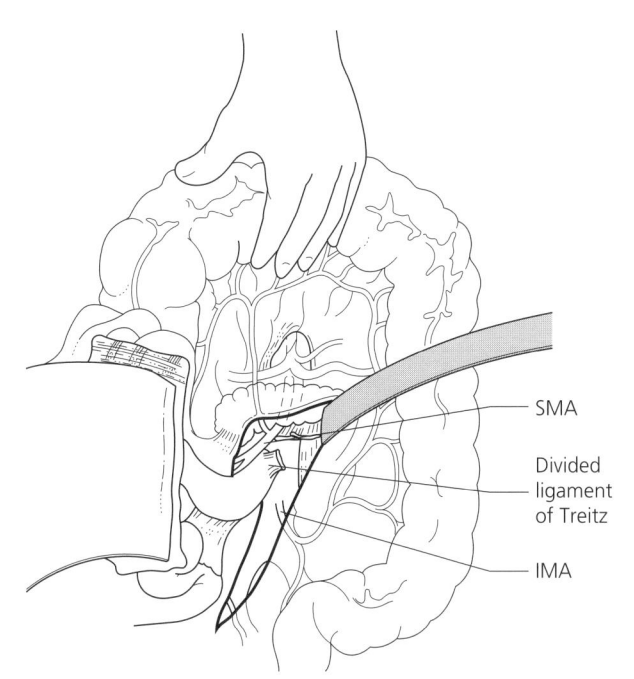

Figure 11.16 Exposure of the infrarenal aorta, proximal right common iliac artery, and proximal superior mesenteric artery (SMA) achieved by intestinal retraction and division of the posterior peritoneum, ligament of Treitz, and base of small-bowel mesentery. IMA = inferior mesenteric artery (from Kazmirs A. Operative management of acute mesenteric ischemia. *Ann Vasc Surg* 12: 187–197; 1998. Reproduced with permission from Lloyd M, Taylor Jr, Gregory L. Moneta, John M. Porter. Treatment of chronic visceral ischemia. In Rutherford RB *et al.* (eds) *Vascular Surgery* 5th edn, Philadelphia PA, WB Saunders, 2000, p. 1515.)

and whether or not infrarenal aortic grafting has been required. Choosing the infrarenal aorta as the source of inflow significantly lessens the associated risks. The infrarenal aorta avoids a long ischemic period to the kidneys and minimizes the extent of the surgical dissection. However, special attention to the configuration of the graft is required in order to minimize the risk of graft kinking.

A bifurcated Dacron graft originating from the junction of the aorta and the right common iliac artery going to the base of the superior mesenteric and celiac arteries accomplishes revascularization from the infrarenal aorta with a geometry that avoids kinking. The celiac artery is revascularized by tunneling the graft in the retropancreatic plane. The distal anastomosis is usually performed to the hepatic artery, although it can also be performed to the splenic artery. This effectively revascularizes the distribution of the celiac axis. The limb to the superior mesenteric artery terminates in an antegrade fashion with an end-to-side anastomosis at the level of the inferior border of the pancreas. If only the superior mesenteric artery needs to be revascularized, a single lumen Dacron graft is used as the conduit. In fact, some authors feel adequate results can be achieved with revascularization of the superior mesenteric artery alone. A unusual variant of single-vessel revascularization is grafting to the inferior mesenteric artery alone. This reconstruction is dependent on a patent collateral circulation.

The supraceliac aorta has also been advocated as a good choice of inflow with the thought that it may improve long-term patency rates. However, given that most studies have utilized only historical controls, it is difficult to conclude that greater technical success with revascularization from either the supraceliac or infrarenal aorta may occur. Clearly, success in revascularization from infrarenal aorta inflow (or any other inflow) is dependent upon the fact that the infrarenal aorta is not severely diseased. When utilizing the supraceliac aorta as the origin of the revascularization, a partially occluding clamp may avoid prolonged ischemia to the liver, bowel, and kidneys. This may not necessarily decrease the risk of distal embolization. However, when the operation is reserved for patients that have a segment of supraceliac abdominal aorta that is angiographically normal, the risk of embolization is minimized.

The approach for revascularization from the supraceliac aorta is through a midline laparotomy incision. The crus of the diaphragm are incised after dividing the gastrohepatic ligament. The anterior and lateral surfaces of the supraceliac aorta are carefully dissected. A bifurcated (usually a 12 × 6 mm or 10 × 5 mm) Dacron graft is anastomosed in an end-to-side fashion to the anterior surface of the supraceliac aorta. One limb is anastomosed in an end-to-side fashion to the common hepatic artery. The other limb is tunneled behind the pancreas and anastomosed in an end-to-side fashion to the anterior surface of the superior mesenteric artery as it emerges from the inferior border of the pancreas.

In a recent report from the Mayo Clinic, it is suggested that antegrade reconstruction is the preferred location for reconstruction. The authors retrospectively reviewed their data and concluded that this reconstruction decreased turbulent flow, decreased the likelihood of graft kinking, and the supraceliac aorta was less likely to be diseased than the infrarenal aorta. However, an individualized approach to each patient was clearly recommended.

In fact, patients may be revascularized by an isolated graft to the hepatic artery in instances when the standard techniques are not possible. An iliac artery-to-hepatic artery bypass was successfully performed in two patients in this report, once again supporting the use of an individualized approach to each patient.

Percutaneous treatment Percutaneous treatment is becoming more common in the management of chronic mesenteric ischemia. Older patients and patients with significant co-morbid disease appear to have good results without the risk of operative intervention. Femoral or brachial access can be used for angioplasty and stenting. The celiac axis or superior mesenteric artery (Figure 11.17) can be treated with percutaneous techniques.

Even with initially successful angioplasty and stenting, additional procedures may be needed. Hallisey *et al.* report a 25% repeat angioplasty rate in their report. Each additional intervention was successful. The initial intervention may require thrombolytic therapy in order to achieve a successful result. Salvage of a failed angioplasty and stenting may require an operative approach.

The role of operative management in comparison to percutaneous treatment continues to be debated. Due to the recurrent stenoses that occur with percutaneous management as mentioned above, some authors prefer an operative approach. This is especially true in good risk patients.

Percutaneous treatments have also been employed to salvage bypass grafts that appear to be failing. Phipp *et al.* report a case in which a Palmaz stent was used to salvage a vein graft used for a mesenteric revascularization.

Postoperative management and complications

Postoperatively, it is frequently observed that patients do not easily resume adequate oral intake. Total parenteral nutrition can be continued postoperatively and is a very useful adjunct to the surgical treatment of chronic mesenteric ischemia. A post-revascularization syndrome has been reported that includes abdominal pain and tachycardia as well as leukocytosis and intestinal edema. This syndrome can eventually lead to multi-system organ failure

Chronic intestinal ischemia

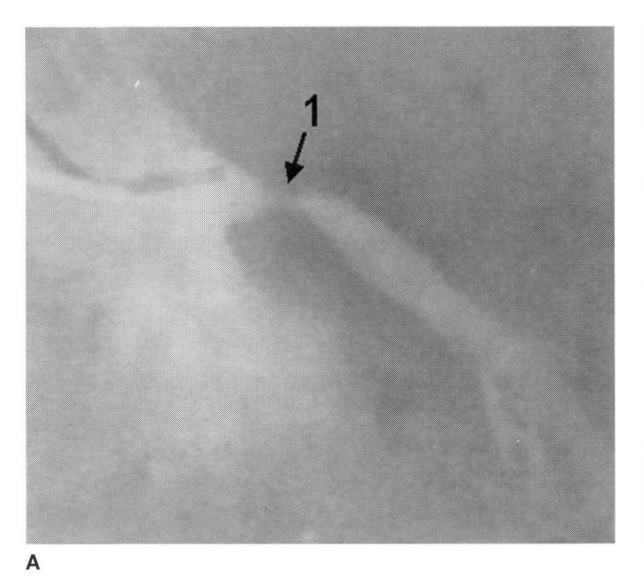

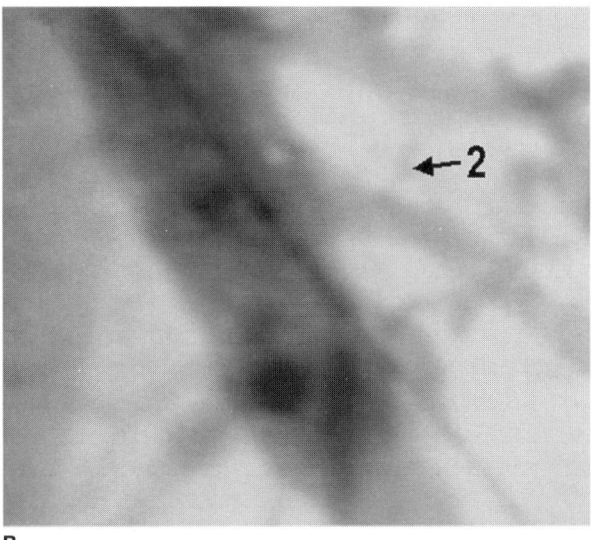

Figure 11.17 (A) Lateral view of aortogram demonstrating a proximal superior mesenteric artery stenosis (1) prior to percutaneous transluminal angioplasty (B) and stent (arrow 2 points to an area of superior mesenteric artery with wall stent). This patient is a 77-year-old woman with post-prandial pain and 15-pound weight loss. The patient is a long-term smoker with significant coronary artery disease and chronic obstructive pulmonary disease, deemed to be a poor candidate for open mesenteric revascularization.

and death. If the patient has abdominal pain, it is mandatory to investigate the etiology further.

Postoperative graft occlusion is a potentially fatal complication. Any delay in diagnosing such an event may result in extensive bowel ischemia and necrosis. This is easily a lethal event. For this reason, one must keep a high index of suspicion in these patients postoperatively. Any concerns may require early diagnostic arteriography. Even with an uncomplicated recovery, some groups advocate angiography before discharge from the hospital.

Other acute complications include myocardial infarction, hemorrhage, stroke, asymptomatic graft limb thromboses, or abdominal compartment syndrome. Late graft occlusions may occur in one or more of the limbs utilized to revascularize the mesenteric vessels. These events can occur as late as ten years after the initial operation.

Patency rates for chronic intestinal ischemia revascularization

Multiple series indicate the outcome achieved for various operative methods and the expected success rates are in the 80% to 90% patency at 5-year follow-up (Table 11.1). The operative mortality ranges from 0% to 12%. Most centers would feel that a mortality rate less than 5% is to be expected with the current operative techniques and postoperative care.

Table 11.1 Results of revascularization for chronic intestinal ischemia.

Study	No. of patients (%)	Operative mortality (%)	Female (years)	Follow-up	Late success (%)
McAfee et al. 1992	58	10	79	5*	90
Cunningham et al. 1991	74	12	82	5*	85
Rheudasil et al. 1988	41	5	51	3.5	84
Current series	84	11	67	11	95
Moawad et al. 1997	24	4	76	2.4*	78
Johnston et al. 1995	21	0	48	NA	86

* Life table follow-up.
NA = not available.

Acute mesenteric ischemia

Pathophysiology and diagnosis

Acute mesenteric ischemia is frequently a life-threatening event because of the difficulty in accurate and efficient diagnosis. Many patients have a history of untreated chronic mesenteric ischemia that is acutely worsened by an occlusive event. But, it is important to recognize that previously unaffected patients may present with an acute mesenteric ischemic episode from embolic phenomenon. A large percentage of affected patients are women over seventy years of age.

Most patients present with significant abdominal pain not associated with abdominal tenderness. Commonly, patients will also complain of vomiting and diarrhea. Unless the initial evaluation prompts concern for acute mesenteric ischemia, then a delay in diagnosis easily occurs. Laboratory values are commonly unremarkable at initial presentation as well. Plain films may show dilated loops of bowel, but not routinely. Significant physical findings will only begin to develop as the process worsens. Tachycardia, hypotension, and marked abdominal tenderness arise in the setting of newly detected acidosis. This constellation of findings leads to an emergency laparotomy that is likely too late. Necrotic bowel is commonly found and resection with an attempt at revascularization is required. Second-look laparotomies to assess the viability of the remaining bowel are usually necessary.

Unfortunately, the outcome of patients treated still remains poor. Mortality remains high despite advances in operative technique and postoperative care. Early recognition is clearly the most important aspect in a patient's survival. Even if patients survive, it is not uncommon for them to be dependent on parenteral nutrition in a temporary or possibly permanent way. In an elderly population of patients, this is a physically and financially demanding situation.

Acute mesenteric ischemia occurs as the result of the abrupt reduction in blood supply to the either the small or large intestine. The most likely situation is an embolic event to the superior mesenteric artery (Figure 11.18). Embolic events can arise from a cardiac source or from an atherosclerotic plaque within another artery. Cardiac sources are less common now with the prevalent use of anticoagulation in the setting of cardiac arrhythmias and valvular heart disease. Unlikely causes include thrombotic emboli to the celiac axis, tumor emboli, or iatrogenic cholesterol emboli. Iatrogenic emboli are becoming more common as percutaneous interventions have increased. This possibility exists even with intra-aortic balloon pump insertion. Any patient who complains of abdominal pain after an arterial intervention needs to be evaluated carefully.

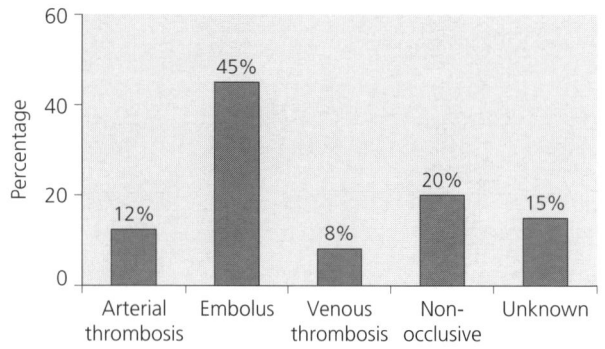

Figure 11.18 Etiology of mesenteric ischemia 1980–1990 (reproduced from Rivers S. Acute nonocclusive mesenteric ischemia. *Semin Vasc Surg* 3: 172; 1990).

Superior mesenteric artery embolism appears to have a better prognosis than an occlusion. The reason for this is that emboli tend to travel distally, sparing some patent branches of the superior mesenteric artery (Figure 11.19). An occlusion of the superior mesenteric artery usually causes a loss of its entire distribution. In patients with chronic mesenteric ischemia and an acute thrombosis, the collateral vessels via the celiac axis and inferior mesenteric artery are also heavily diseased. This leads to a catastrophic event.

Unusual causes of acute ischemia are spontaneous dissections of the celiac axis or superior mesenteric artery. Another unusual cause of acute mesenteric ischemia is chemotherapy treatment. It is important to recognize this as a possibility in patients receiving chemotherapeutic agents so an early diagnosis can be made. Patients with anticardiolipin antibodies also appear to be at risk for acute mesenteric ischemia secondary to thrombosis. These patients can present with acute gastrointestinal hemorrhage secondary to ischemia. They can also present with abdominal pain.

Hyperhomocystinemia has been associated with acute arterial thrombosis. This hypercoagulable state can lead to an acute mesenteric thrombosis. Small bowel volvulus (Figure 11.20) can lead to strangulation of the segmental mesenteric circulation with ischemia of the involved bowel seen as a late finding.

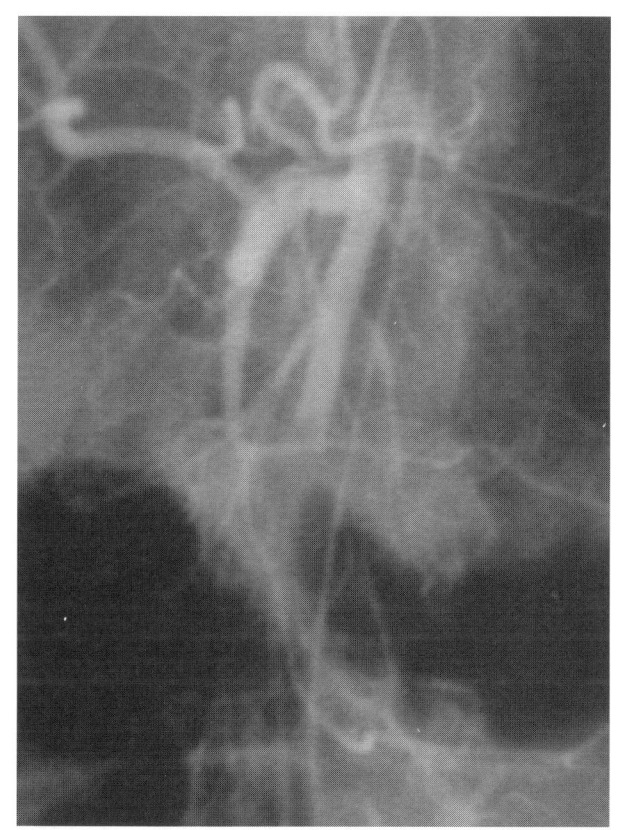

Figure 11.19 Lateral aortogram demonstrating an abrupt cut-off of flow in the distal superior mesenteric artery with spearing of some proximal superior mesenteric artery branches. This patient presented with sudden onset of abdominal pain out of proportion with the physical examination. The findings are typical of superior mesenteric artery embolus.

Diagnosis and imaging studies and percutaneous treatment modalities

There is no specific laboratory value that is diagnostic for acute mesenteric ischemia. An elevated lactate level is indicative of bowel infarction. There is recent evidence that D-dimer measurements may confirm the diagnosis of acute mesenteric ischemia. Further work needs to be done to validate this finding.

It has been shown that Duplex can be diagnostic for acute mesenteric ischemia. CT scan may also be useful. However, significant findings on CT scan such as distended bowel, free air, pneumatosis of the bowel wall (Figure 11.21) or air within the biliary tree (Figure 11.22) clearly represent a very advanced stage of mesenteric ischemia with full-thickness necrosis of the bowel wall that often resulted from a delay in the diagnosis. Conventional arteriography remains the gold standard in imaging for acute mesenteric ischemia. This radiographic method can lead to the diagnosis early in the course of the disease before full-thickness death of the bowel. However, this also raises a dilemma in the management of the disease. Hours taken to perform arteriography will delay the diagnosis and potentially compromise outcome. The corollary alternative consideration is that an error in diagnosis leading to an unnecessary laparotomy can significantly increase morbidity and mortality. In patients with pain alone and without other physical or laboratory findings, an arteriogram is likely worthwhile when mesenteric ischemia is suspected. In general, when the diagnosis of acute mesenteric ischemia is clinically suspected, one must proceed to expeditiously rule it out by a diagnostic arteriogram, as long as the patient does not have clear peritoneal signs that indicate bowel necrosis. The arteriography must be obtained immediately without delay and with concurrent fluid resuscitation and broad spectrum antibiotic coverage since the ischemic bowel mucosa can allow bacterial translocation into the blood stream from the enteric lumen. If patients have already developed peritoneal findings on exam or systemic acidosis, then arteriogram should be avoided and emergent laparotomy recommended concurrent with fluid resuscitation and systemic antibiotics.

The additional benefit of arteriography is the potential for percutaneous treatment. Catheter-based interventions include thrombolytic therapy, mechanical thrombectomy, balloon angioplasty, or the combination of all these techniques. Proponents of percutaneous treatment point to the poor outcomes seen with traditional operative management. Even with successful percutaneous treatment, most patients will still require an exploratory laparotomy. Some authors advocate using laparoscopy after thrombolytic therapy to assess the bowel viability. The majority of patients with a thrombotic event will have some necrotic bowel. The only appropriate management of this is operative resection. In fact, if patients develop a worsening physical exam or acidosis during the course of thrombolytic treatment, then an emergent laparotomy and cessation of thrombolytic therapy is indicated. If percutaneous revascularization is successful and abdominal complaints persist, then laparotomy is once again indicated. Further work is being to done evaluate and improve the percutaneous techniques for acute mesenteric ischemia.

Mesenteric Ischemia and Intestinal Vascular Disorders

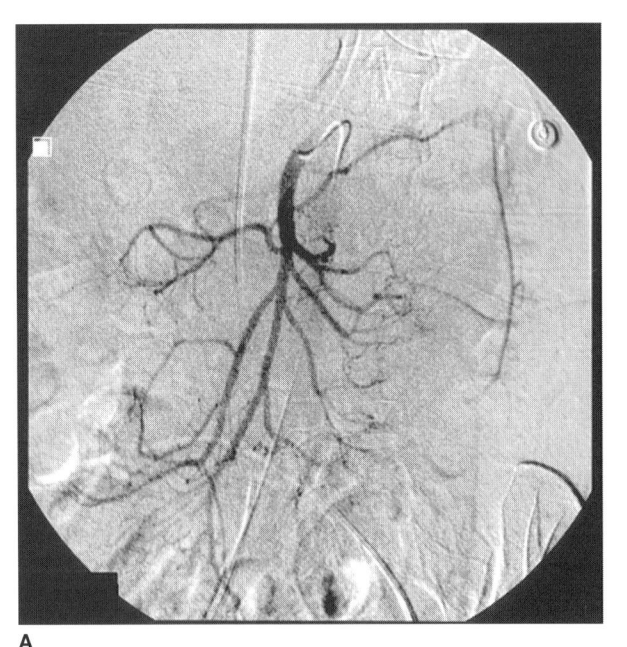

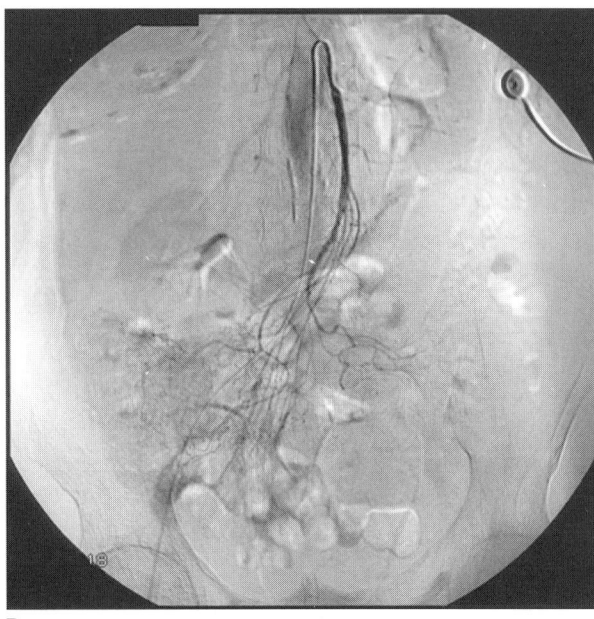

Figure 11.20 Anteroposterior views of an abdominal aortogram showing (A) normal superior mesenteric artery flow and (B) 'bunching' of the superior mesenteric artery small-bowel arcades toward the right lower quadrant, suggestive of mechanical twisting of the small-bowel mesentery. On exploratory laparotomy, the patient in (B) was found to have a jejunum volvulus.

Operative treatment

The initial steps in the operative management of acute mesenteric ischemia are the inspection of the bowel for viability and palpation of mesenteric pulses. The presence of foul-smelling fluid at initial inspection is worrisome for bowel perforation. The inspection of the bowel is important to determine the extent of necrotic bowel and its distribution. The distribution of the necrosis is important in

Figure 11.21 Computed tomography demonstrating (A) small-bowel distension and (B) air within the small-bowel wall in a patient found to have segmental small-bowel necrosis on exploratory laparotomy.

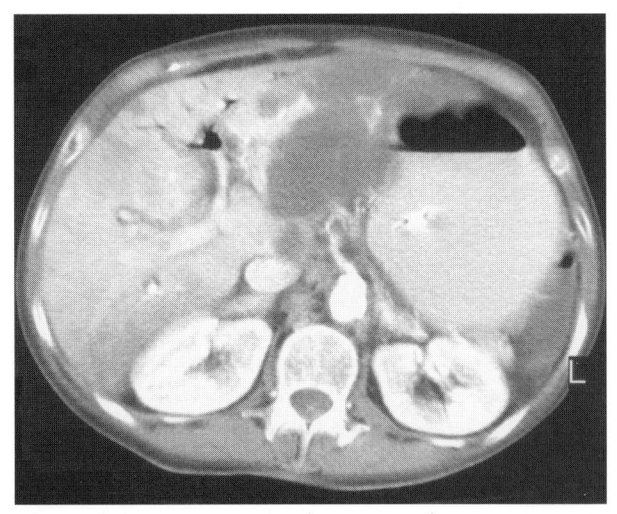

Figure 11.22 Computed tomography demonstrating air within the biliary tree suggestive of advanced bowel ischemia. Peritoneal fluid and a small amount of free air are also noted, again indicative of a late diagnosis of ischemic bowel with full-thickness bowel necrosis, ascites, and perforation. The findings are not specific and may be present with intra-abdominal catastrophes of other etiologies.

defining whether or not a thrombosis or embolism caused the event. The palpation of the mesenteric pulses is further confirmation of the etiology and extent of the ischemic event. In a thrombotic occlusion, the superior mesenteric artery pulse is usually non-palpable. In the setting of an embolic event, the superior mesenteric artery pulse is usually palpable and some of its branches lack pulsations. Doppler evaluation is an additional adjunct to evaluate the blood supply and viability of questionable intestine.

Revascularization

Revascularization is usually performed in the setting of viable bowel. If the extent of necrosis is so widespread that the patient will likely not survive, then a revascularization procedure is usually not performed. If a revascularization is to be performed, it is important to perform the revascularization prior to resecting the bowel, except for the obviously necrotic segments. Successful revascularization will likely salvage some of the involved intestine. Therefore, the intestine should be carefully inspected again and further necessary resections performed when the revascularization is complete.

Superior mesenteric artery embolectomy

The surgical approach to the superior mesenteric artery for the performance of an embolectomy is different than previously described in the section of operative techniques for chronic mesenteric ischemia. The artery is identified at the base of the mesenteries of the small bowel and transverse colon. The artery is exposed for sufficient length to obtain proximal and distal arterial control. Silastic vessel loops are used to control the artery in the proximal and distal locations. Vessel loops are also used to control any side-branches.

A transverse arteriotomy is performed after systemic heparin (5000 units) is administered and arterial control obtained (Figure 11.23). Proximal embolectomy is performed first with a 3 or 4 French Fogarty embolectomy catheter. If brisk flow is obtained after passage of the embolectomy catheter, then attention is turned to the distal blood supply. If brisk flow is not reinstituted, then concern is raised for a thrombotic occlusion and not an embolic event. If this scenario occurs, preparation should be made to perform a surgical bypass procedure.

Distal embolectomy can be very challenging. A small (2 French) embolectomy catheter is used. The vessels are small, tortuous, and friable. At our

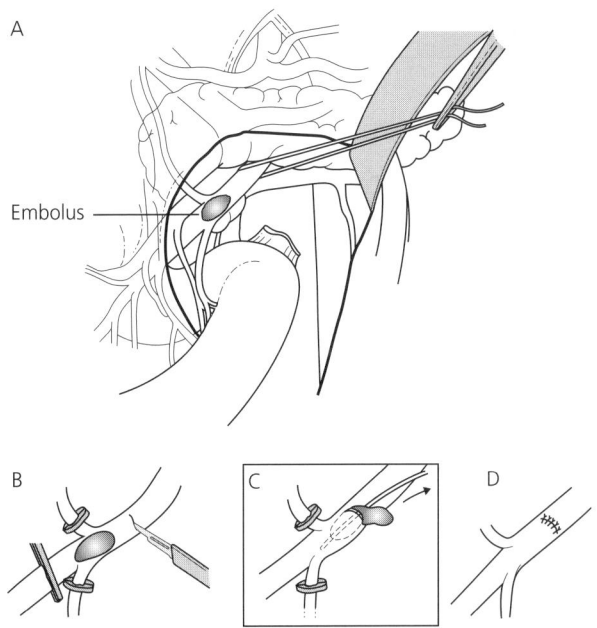

Figure 11.23 (A) Superior mesenteric artery embolectomy. (B) Transverse or longitudinal arteriotomy is followed by (C) balloon catheter embolus extraction and (D) arteriotomy closure. Primary closure suffices for a transverse arteriotomy, whereas a vein patch is usually required to close a longitudinal arteriotomy (from Kazmers A. Operative management of acute mesenteric ischemia. *Ann Vasc Surg* 12: 187–197; 1998. Reproduced with permission from Lloyd M, Taylor Jr, Gregory L. Moneta, John M. Porter. Treatment of chronic visceral ischemia. In Rutherford RB *et al.* (eds) *Vascular Surgery* 5th edn, Philadelphia PA, WB Saunders, 2000, p. 1516)

institution, after catheter embolectomy has yielded as much clearance of the embolus as possible, we prefer to complete the treatment of the distal superior mesenteric artery distribution using intra-operative thrombolytic therapy. This is done by slowly infusing 6–10 mg of tissue plasminogen activator (tPA) through the arteriotomy. The tPA is flushed with heparinized saline. We have found that bleeding complications are very rare and that there is significant improvement in distal perfusion with this technique. The arteriotomy is closed in a transverse fashion as previously described. This prevents a stenosis at the site of the repair. Attention can then be turned to resecting any residual non-viable intestine.

Superior mesenteric artery bypass We previously described the specific techniques for bypass grafting of the superior mesenteric artery in the section on chronic mesenteric ischemia. The significant difference in the setting of acute mesenteric ischemia is the choice of conduit. As mentioned earlier, either prosthetic or autologous vein can be used for reconstruction. If the entire bowel is viable and there is no evidence of intra-abdominal infection, then a prosthetic can potentially be used. At our institution, we tend to perform bypass grafting with reversed saphenous vein when dealing with acute mesenteric ischemia. We believe that the infectious risks and complications associated with it are too great to perform a prosthetic repair.

The bypass graft can once again arise from the suprarenal aorta, infrarenal aorta, or iliac vessels. The location is determined by the quality of the aorta or iliac vessel. It is also important to place the vein graft in a position that kinking will not occur. When inspecting that the graft is appropriately placed, it is important to allow the bowel to return to its normal position within the abdomen.

Intestinal viability

Intestinal viability is reassessed after revascularization has been completed. In certain circumstances, restoration of normal blood supply will be sufficient to reverse the viability of the affected intestine. The bowel will either be viable, necrotic, or be questionable in terms of its viability. There are several methods to assist in assessing the bowel that appears questionable. Visual inspection, palpation of pulses, Doppler examination, intravenous fluorescein, infrared plethysmography, surface oximetry, and laser Doppler velocimetry are the reported techniques.

Inspection of the bowel for viability includes coloration, presence of peristalsis, palpation and visualization of pulsatile flow, and bleeding from cut edges. Although none of these techniques are definitive, experienced surgeons are accurate in using these criteria to assess bowel viability.

Doppler examination of the bowel is performed by placing the probe within the mesentery and on the anti-mesenteric border of the bowel. Pulsatile signal in both of these locations allows a decision to be made that the bowel has sufficient blood flow to remain viable. Lack of signal raises the concern that bowel is not perfused. The doppler is usually available in any operating room and is one of the advantages of this technique.

Intravenous fluorescein is injected systemically and then the bowel is inspected for viability. A Wood's lamp is required for this technique. Approximately 10–15 mg/kg of the fluorescein is injected. It is allowed to circulate and then the bowel is inspected. A Wood's lamp will demonstrate the bowel that fluoresces. Any part of the intestine that does not fluoresce is not perfused. The intra-operative findings are not usually this obvious, though, and clinical judgment needs to be employed.

Surface oximetry detects PO_2 levels on the surface of the bowel. Previous work has demonstrated that abnormal values can detect non-viable bowel. Infrared plethysmography and laser Doppler velocimetry have both been experimentally proven but are infrequently used. Infrared plethysmography relies on detecting differences in reflected infrared light.

No method is 100% accurate and false negatives can be lethal to the patient if non-viable bowel is not resected. A combination of the techniques appears to the most accurate. Most surgeons will combine the techniques of visual inspection, palpation of pulses, and Doppler examination. As previously mentioned, the Doppler is easily available in the operating room and there is little time wasted in making a sound decision. Minimizing operative time for these critically ill patients is as essential as performing a technically appropriate operation.

Second look laparotomy

The decision to operate a second time should always be made at the initial operation. If there is concern for the viability of a portion of the remaining intestine, then a second look laparotomy is recommended. The rationale for making this decision at the initial operation is that a significant percentage of patients will be improved in the first 12 to 24 hours after the initial procedure with removal of the source of sepsis. It is easy to be dissuaded from re-operating with the clinical improvement seen. This is inappropriate management and when a second look is felt necessary at the initial operation, then it should always be performed.

The usual time frame for a second operation is approximately 24–36 hours after the first operation. This amount of time in the intensive care unit allows for aggressive resuscitation as needed and optimization of the patient's physiologic parameters. A safe return trip to the operating room is possible. This time will also allow the bowel to be re-assessed for its true viability. Further intestinal resection can be performed as needed. If needed, a third look laparotomy can be planned at this operation.

Second-look laparoscopy is feasible and some authors feel that is the safest possibility. This is true even in obese patients. Laparoscopy, however, is not our preferred approach for second look exploratory laparotomies.

The decision as to whether or not to construct intestinal anastomoses at the initial operation is controversial, and remains mostly the surgeon's preference. Some feel that the creation of an anastomosis that may need to be resected at the second look laparotomy is wasted operative time. Others feel that is worthwhile to accomplish this at the initial operation to minimize the work needed at the second operation. There is no proof that one technique is superior. We will make this decision based on the extent of bowel necrosis and the physiologic state of the patient. A critically ill patient in the operating room is better served by not wasting time performing anastomoses. In a stable patient with limited bowel necrosis, we will perform the necessary anastomoses at the initial operation.

Postoperative care

Patients suffering from acute mesenteric ischemia tend to be older patients with significant co-morbidities. These patients require aggressive post-operative monitoring. All patients will require intensive care unit admission. Swan-Ganz catheters are usually inserted to monitor appropriate fluid resuscitation in this patient population with significant incidence of concurrent underlying cardiac disease. If not inserted in the operating room, a Swan-Ganz catheter should be inserted promptly after admission to the intensive care unit.

Broad-spectrum antibiotics are usually administered. The compromised integrity of the intestine allows for bacterial translocation. The optimal duration of this antibiotic therapy has not been clearly defined. Untreated bacteremia will accelerate a poor outcome in an already compromised patient.

As mentioned earlier, acute mesenteric ischemia has a high mortality rate. This is a result of a delay in diagnosis and the pre-operative fragility of these patients. If patients survive the initial insult, total parenteral nutrition is a key to their further recovery. They are usually unable to sustain themselves with oral intake for one to four weeks after the initial insult. The bowel needs to recover its ability for peristalsis and absorption. As long as a few feet of small intestine remain, patients will not usually require permanent parenteral nutrition.

Nonocclusive mesenteric ischemia

Pathophysiology and presentation

Mechanical obstruction of the arterial or venous mesenteric systems is not the sole cause of mesenteric ischemia. Nonocclusive mesenteric ischemia occurs in patients suffering from compromised end-organ perfusion. This occurs when severe systemic illness leads to vascular compromise. Cardiogenic or septic sources are common etiologies.

Mesenteric vasoconstriction (Figure 11.24) can occur in the setting of normovolemic or hypovolemic shock. After the shock state is reversed, the mesenteric blood supply usually takes several hours to correct itself. In most circumstances, the local situation allows for dilation of the smaller blood

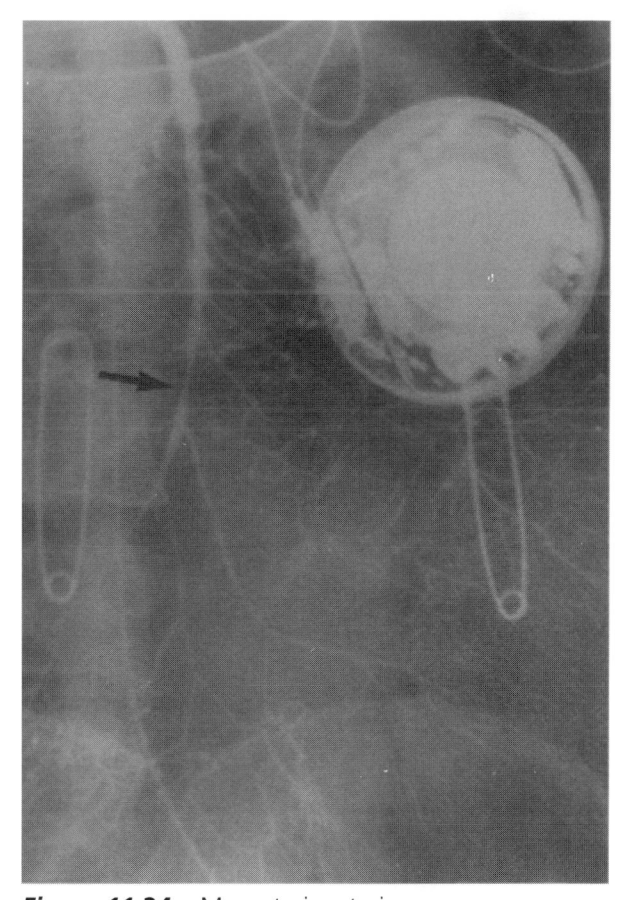

Figure 11.24 Mesenteric arteriogram demonstrating areas of vasoconstriction or 'spasm' (arrow) within the superior mesenteric artery, typically seen in non-occlusive mesenteric ischemia. The patient is a 74-year-old critically ill woman in cardiogenic shock and presenting with abdominal pain and distension.

vessels and preservation of bowel integrity. Nonocclusive mesenteric ischemia develops when the normal adaptation does not occur properly.

The renin-angiotensin axis appears to play a role in the development of nonocclusive mesenteric ischemia. In experimental models where a bilateral nephrectomy or ACE inhibitor is administered, the ischemic response to the mesenteric circulation is blunted. The true etiology of the disruption in the normal physiologic response remains unclear. It is a multifactorial abnormal response that occurs in a certain subset of patients. Our current level of expertise does not allow us to identify those patients that appear most at risk. Patients with congestive heart failure are the most likely to be affected. Sepsis, dehydration, or renal and hepatic dysfunction appears to lead to nonocclusive ischemia in some patients. Drug administration, including the use of cocaine, may also lead to vasoconstriction and ischemia.

Patients affected by nonocclusive mesenteric ischemia present in a similar fashion to patients with acute embolic or thrombotic mesenteric ischemia. Abdominal pain is the most common presenting complaint. Unfortunately, a number of these patients are critically ill and unable to phonate to describe the abdominal pain. As with acute mesenteric ischemia, a high index of suspicion needs to remain in place with these patients. Early detection and correction of the underlying problem are the best treatment plan.

There is a subset of patients with nonocclusive mesenteric ischemia that resolves without operative intervention. These patients have intermittent episodes of abdominal pain or distension that occur when local perfusion is compromised. The extent of malperfusion never leads to necrosis in this setting and the intermittent ischemia resolves without further complications.

Three of the more common scenarios for the development of nonocclusive mesenteric ischemia will be discussed further. These are postcoarctectomy syndrome, drug-induced ischemia, and vasospasm following revascularization. Postcoarctecomy syndrome can occur in approximately 4% of the patients undergoing repair of an aortic coarctation. The mechanism is felt to be a result of the increased flow to the mesenteric vasculature after correction of the coarctation. This change in flow dynamics leads to a necrotizing vasculitis. This abnormal response seems to occur more frequently in the younger population. This is part of the reason a delay until three to five years of age is reached prior to repair. There have also been reports of nonocclusive mesenteric ischemia occurring after cardiopulmonary bypass. This event occurs more frequently in the setting of emergency operations.

Drug-induced mesenteric ischemia can be a result of self-administered or hospital-administered agents. Cocaine and ergot chemicals have been implicated in nonocclusive mesenteric ischemia. Both of these agents are vasoconstrictors that predispose to mesenteric vasospasm and the potential for ischemia.

Vasoactive agents used to treat patients with septic physiology and hypotension also predispose to mesenteric vasospasm. In the usual physiologic administration of these medications, they should not produce nonocclusive ischemia. In patients who are already critically ill and experiencing a low-flow state, there is likely a predisposition to develop ischemia from the administration of vasoactive medications.

Vasospasm after mesenteric revascularization may also occur. As described in the section on chronic mesenteric ischemia, patients tend to have a tenuous postoperative course in the first twenty-four to forty-eight hours. Vasospasm can severely complicate this difficult clinical situation. It is thought to be secondary to reperfusion edema, or possibly celiac neural plexus injury. Other operative procedures also seem to induce vasospastic events in certain patients. This is also a problem with a high mortality rate.

Hemodialysis patients also appear to be affected by nonocclusive mesenteric ischemia. It has been reported that nine percent of the deaths in the hemodialysis population are secondary to nonocclusive mesenteric ischemia. It is important to recognize that an acute abdomen in these patients may be a manifestation of ischemic bowel. This syndrome of nonocclusive mesenteric ischemia associated with hemodialysis can also occur in patients undergoing peritoneal dialysis.

Diagnosis and imaging studies

It is important to recognize that prompt diagnosis is the critical issue in successfully managing patients with nonocclusive ischemia. This is obviously the same caveat given for the management of acute mesenteric ischemia. Patients with abdominal pain should be evaluated with plain abdominal radiographs. If there is evidence of pneumoperitoneum, then an emergent laparotomy is required. Unremarkable plain films do not eliminate the possibility of nonocclusive mesenteric ischemia.

When the clinical suspicion of nonocclusive mesenteric ischemia arises in a hemodynamically stable patient, a conventional arteriogram is obtained. The findings consistent with nonocclusive ischemia include: narrowed origins of the major branches of the superior mesenteric artery; beading, tapering, or segmental narrowing of intestinal branches; spasm of intestinal arcades; and reduced or absent filling of mural vessels (Figure 11.24). This diagnostic study also allows for a potential intervention with the infusion of papaverine. This is performed by selectively cannulating the orifice of the superior mesenteric artery and placing an infusion catheter. Papaverine can then be infused as a therapeutic maneuver in some patients. These patients will resolve their vasospasm and never require an operation. Their signs and symptoms improve throughout the course of the infusion. They remain asymptomatic afterwards when a good result is obtained.

Other patients will worsen during the initial stages of non-operative therapy and will require an emergent laparotomy. In those patients, the catheter can be left positioned within the orifice of the superior mesenteric artery for infusion postoperatively. This will help eliminate the severe complication of further spasm after operative intervention.

Several other imaging modalities can be used to evaluate for nonocclusive mesenteric ischemia. Duplex imaging, phosphorous magnetic resonance imaging, radiolabeled leukocyte scintigraphy, and intraperitoneal xenon injection have been attempted. None are as effective as diagnostic arteriography in confirming the diagnosis of nonocclusive ischemia. Also, they do not allow the option of potential percutaneous intervention with the selective infusion of papaverine.

Treatment

The mainstay of treatment of nonocclusive mesenteric ischemia is reversal of the vasospasm. This includes appropriate fluid resuscitation, elimination of vasopressor agents, and treatment of heart failure. All of these maneuvers are designed to improve perfusion to compromised intestine. Nasogastric tubes are inserted to decompress dilated and fluid-filled intestine. The decompression also improves perfusion to affected intestine.

The effectiveness of direct papaverine infusion has not been well documented, but it clearly reverses the vasospasm. The correction of the factors listed above is usually performed at the same time an intra-arterial infusion of papaverine is being performed. Therefore, it is difficult to assess the role of the intra-arterial papaverine alone. The infusion of papaverine is performed at a rate of 30–60 mg/hour. The infusion is usually continued for twenty-four hours. Arteriography is performed at selected times during the infusion to confirm the reversal of the vasospasm. As mentioned above, even if a patient's physical exam findings or laboratory evaluation deteriorates and a laparotomy is needed, the infusion catheter can remain in place for postoperative infusion.

The decision to operate on a patient with nonocclusive mesenteric ischemia can be very difficult. If a patient develops peritoneal findings, the decision is not difficult and a laparotomy needs to be done. Arteriography should not be considered as a diagnostic or therapeutic maneuver in those patients with peritoneal signs. For patients with a waxing and waning physical examination, but no evidence of peritoneal signs, the best approach is non-operative management. Arteriography can be both diagnostic and therapeutic in this subset of patients, especially if their physical findings or laboratory values worsen. If the patient worsens, the operative approach to nonocclusive mesenteric ischemia is to resect only the obviously affected bowel. Resection of gangrenous bowel is performed as with acute mesenteric ischemia. The decision to perform anastomoses and a second look operation are surgeon dependent as previously described. The intention of this operative approach is to remove affected bowel only. There is no effective surgical approach to correct the underlying vasospasm. Postoperative care is directed at appropriate fluid resuscitation and hemodynamic management plus the potential intraarterial infusion of papaverine. The care is very similar to the patients described above with acute mesenteric ischemia.

Outcome

The survival of patients with nonocclusive mesenteric ischemia has been reported to be as low as 0–29%. The cause of death is usually an irreversible shock state with progressive intestinal infarction. As with acute mesenteric ischemia, the high mortality rate is a reflection of the difficulty of early diagnosis and successful treatment. As mentioned above, the key is to diagnose early and intervene aggressively. The use of vasodilator therapy appears to have improved the mortality rates quoted above.

Mesenteric venous thrombosis

Pathophysiology

Mesenteric venous thrombosis is a relatively uncommon cause of acute mesenteric ischemia. It was well characterized by Warren and Eberhard in the 1930's. It is thought to occur in 5–15% of patients that are diagnosed with acute mesenteric ischemia. Patients with a prior history of mesenteric venous thrombosis or lower extremity venous thrombosis are the most likely candidates to develop this problem. Mesenteric venous thrombosis occurs in an equal distribution between the sexes. It more commonly affects patients older than fifty.

The normal venous anatomy closely mimics the arterial blood supply of the bowel. A venous arcade drains the small bowel and right colon through the ileocolic, middle colic and right colic veins. These veins converge to form the superior mesenteric vein. The confluence of the superior mesenteric vein and splenic forms the portal vein.

Mesenteric thromboses are defined as primary or secondary. Primary mesenteric venous thrombosis is unknown in its etiology. Secondary mesenteric venous thrombosis occurs in the setting of liver disease, splanchnic venous injury, or a hypercoagulable state. Liver disease, such as cirrhosis, leads to portal venous stasis. The portal venous stasis is a nidus for mesenteric venous thrombosis. Splanchnic venous injury can occur during routine operative procedures such as a splenectomy. The resulting venous injury can be a nidus for venous thrombosis. Splenectomy is commonly performed to correct the complications of hematologic diseases. This underlying problem can lead to a hypercoagulable state and increase the chances of developing a postoperative venous thrombosis.

Hypercoagulable states are most commonly thought of as the underlying etiology for mesenteric venous thrombosis. The hypercoagulable states associated with mesenteric venous thrombosis are: protein C and S deficiency, protein C resistance, antithrombin III deficiency, anticardiolipin antibody, polythycemia vera, and certain malignancies. Malignancies can lead to venous thrombosis by mechanical compression of the portal venous system or due to their hypercoagulable state. Oral contraceptive use is the underlying etiology in young women. This hypercoagulability secondary to oral contraceptives accounts for 9–18% of cases in young women. It is currently thought that approximately one-half of the diagnosed mesenteric venous thromboses are secondary to a hypercoagulable state. In fact, it is likely that a number of primary mesenteric venous thromboses are actually undetected hypercoagulable states.

Intra-abdominal infections can also predispose to mesenteric venous thrombosis. This is especially true in the pediatric population. Children with a delayed diagnosis of appendicitis can develop a venous thrombosis.

Mesenteric venous thrombosis causes acute ischemia by obstruction of venous outflow. This can lead to hemorrhagic infarction of the small intestine. It is extremely unusual for the large intestine to be involved. Venous thrombosis, when symptomatic, presents with ascites, variceal hemorrhage, or intestinal infarction. Some patients, though, may develop a venous thrombosis and remain asymptomatic.

The mechanism of intestinal infarction can be better described in this fashion. Acute obstructive venous thrombosis leads to intestinal fluid sequestration with resultant hypovolemia and hemoconcentration. Arteriolar vasoconstriction results from the portal venous pressure. Reduction of intestinal blood flow also occurs as a result of the obstruction to venous outflow. All of these factors combined lead to impairment of the arterial inflow. The end result is the development of hemorrhagic infarction of the small intestine. The ischemia may be limited to the intestinal mucosa, leading to abdominal pain and diarrhea. More severe ischemia leads to transmural necrosis with gastrointestinal bleeding, perforation, and peritonitis. As the integrity of the bowel becomes compromised, bacterial translocation can occur. This leads to a severe septic response. The intestinal ischemia and bacteremia are the first step to the development of multi-system organ failure.

An unusual variant of mesenteric venous thrombosis is mesenteric inflammatory veno-occlusive disease. This disorder occurs more commonly in men and does not affect a specific age group. The affected patients do not have a known connective tissue disorder or vasculitis. The diagnosis is made after careful histologic analysis of resected intestine. The histology reveals a lack of arterial involvement, but transmural phlebitis is seen within the bowel. It is possible that this small venous process has been underdiagnosed, as histologic analysis is the only modality that can confirm the diagnosis.

Presentation

Mesenteric venous thrombosis can present as an acute, subacute, or chronic problem. Acute mesenteric venous thrombosis is characterized by sudden onset of abdominal pain whereas subacute presents with days or weeks worth of abdominal pain. It is unusual for this subset of patients with subacute symptoms to develop intestinal infarction or variceal hemorrhage. Chronic obstruction of mesenteric venous flow usually presents with complications of the venous thrombosis such as variceal hemorrhage.

Similar to mesenteric arterial occlusion, patients with venous ischemia present with abdominal pain that is out of proportion to the physical examination. Nausea, vomiting, anorexia, and diarrhea are other common presenting complaints. Less commonly, patients present with hematemesis, hematochezia, or melena. Occult blood is detectable in 50% of patients on initial presentation. As described earlier with mesenteric ischemia of arterial etiology, the nonspecific complaints with minimal physical findings often lead to delay in diagnosis. The development of physical findings is worrisome for full thickness bowel necrosis. Fever and peritoneal signs develop once intestinal infarction has occurred.

Other diagnoses that are commonly entertained are peptic ulcer disease, gastrointestinal infection, inflammatory bowel disease, and pancreatitis.

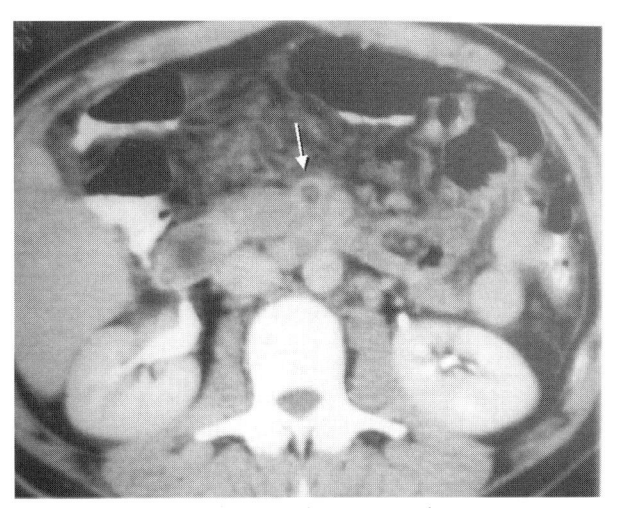

Figure 11.25 Computed tomography demonstrating the typical appearance of a thrombus within the superior mesenteric vein.

Diagnosis and imaging studies

Routine laboratory values are not helpful in making the diagnosis of mesenteric venous thrombosis. Findings on physical examination such as peritoneal signs of inflammation, tachycardia, hypotension, and an elevated lactate level are indicative of intestinal infarction and a delay in diagnosis. Abdominal plain radiographs are abnormal in 50–75% of patients, but it is infrequent to have findings specific for ischemia. Thumbprinting, pneumatosis intestinalis (Figure 11.21), portal venous air (Figure 11.22), or pneumoperitoneum are non-specific late findings for bowel ischemia with necrosis that occur in five percent of patients.

Duplex examination has been used as an attempt to confirm the diagnosis, but computed tomography remains the gold standard for venous thrombosis. CT is able to make the diagnosis in 90 percent of patients. An acute thrombus is detected by a central lucency in the mesenteric vein (Figure 11.25). Other findings include enlargement of the superior mesenteric vein and a sharply defined vein wall with a rim of increased density. Acute mesenteric venous thrombosis is occasionally an incidental finding on CT scan when performed for other reasons, including postoperative scans. Chronic mesenteric venous thrombosis is defined on CT by a well-developed collateral circulation in the mesentery and retroperitoneum venous channels.

Magnetic resonance venography is also a sensitive study to diagnose mesenteric venous thrombosis. At our institution, MRV is readily available and commonly used to evaluate the venous anatomy. This is not uniformly the case and MRV is still limited in its utility. As MRV becomes widely available, it will likely replace CT as the diagnostic study of choice. However, currently CT provides better imaging of diseased bowel and it is also better at defining other etiologies of abdominal pain.

Selective mesenteric angiography is not commonly performed to diagnose mesenteric venous thrombosis. Delayed venous images are obtained from an arterial injection. Findings consistent with venous thrombosis are: thrombus in the larger veins, late visualization of the superior mesenteric vein, impaired filling of mesenteric veins, arterial spasm, and prolonged opacification of the arterial arcades. One of the difficulties in interpreting this study is that the superior mesenteric vein is not routinely seen with the required arterial injection of contrast. Therapeutic interventions are limited to systemic lysis as opposed to selective catheterization of an affected arterial branch as mentioned earlier. In light of the sensitivity of CT and MRV, the need for mesenteric venous angiography is limited.

Other proposed techniques include paracentesis, laparoscopy, gastroduodenoscopy, and colonoscopy. These techniques are limited in their utility and carry inherent risks. CT remains the gold standard for diagnosis.

Once the diagnosis of mesenteric venous thrombosis is confirmed, a hematologic evaluation is needed. An appropriate workup for hypercoagulable states should rule out protein C and S deficiency, factor V Leiden, hyperhomocystinemia, and paroxysmal nocturnal hemoglobinuria. Prothrombin 20210G/A is an unusual cause of hypercoagulability leading to mesenteric venous thrombosis.

Treatment

The treatment of mesenteric venous thrombosis involves a combination of anticoagulation and operative therapy. It is appropriate to manage venous thrombosis without surgical intervention as long as there is no evidence of bowel ischemia. This is at times a difficult determination to make. There is not a clear role for antibiotic therapy unless there is a perforation. It is clear that early introduction of heparin is beneficial. Heparin therapy increases the chances of survival for the acute event and reduces the risk of recurrent episodes. Heparin is administered as an intravenous bolus (5000 units) and then infused continuously. The goal therapeutic value is to maintain the partial-thromboplastin time at twice normal. Other supportive measures include nasogastric decompression, NPO, and the initiation of parenteral nutrition. Oral anticoagulation is started as soon as a diet is safely initiated which may not be possible for up to four to six weeks in some patients with severe symptoms. The duration of anticoagulation therapy is determined by the hypercoagulable workup.

Operative intervention is limited to patients with peritoneal findings on examination. As soon as the diagnosis of a venous thrombosis is confirmed, intravenous heparin therapy should be initiated. As with the previous discussions, surgical therapy is directed at removing infarcted bowel. Mesenteric venous thrombosis presents a similar challenge as nonocclusive ischemia in that surgery is limited to resecting bowel and is not able to treat the underlying etiology. A second look laparotomy is almost uniformly required for mesenteric venous thrombosis to accurately determine the extent of bowel involvement. As arterial spasm is often a component of the problem, intra-arterial papaverine therapy may improve the outcome. The main goal of operative intervention is to preserve as much small intestine as possible.

Some authors have advocated the use of laparoscopy in patients with mesenteric venous thrombosis. This technique allows inspection of the bowel without the potential complications of a laparotomy but has not yet been popularized in many centers.

Lytic therapy has been of limited value in the management of mesenteric venous thrombosis. It requires either systemic infusion or transhepatic portography. Both procedures have high complication rates, especially hemorrhage.

Outcome

The current mortality rate for mesenteric venous thrombosis ranges from 20 to 50 percent. Patients who require an operative intervention tend to be sicker, have longer hospital stays, and thus a more complicated course. The extent of bowel resection will determine the need for postoperative parenteral nutrition.

Long-term survival is dependent on the underlying cause. Malignancy is associated with a worse prognosis. Mesenteric venous thrombosis tends to have a high recurrence rate. The recurrence most commonly occurs within thirty days of the initial presentation. Appropriate anticoagulation is beneficial in preventing recurrence.

It is possible that patients with recurrent abdominal pain may have developed an intestinal stenosis secondary to chronic ischemia. Gastrointestinal contrast studies can confirm the diagnosis of bowel strictures. Bowel resection is needed to correct stenosis secondary to ischemic strictures and carries with a good long-term functional outcome.

Further reading

Baden JG, Racy DJ, Grist TM. Contrast-enhanced three-dimensional magnetic resonance angiography of the mesenteric vasculature. *J Magn Reson Imaging* 1999; 10(3): 369–375.

Bech FR. Celiac artery compression syndromes. *Surg Clin North Am* 1997; 77(2): 409–424.

Bonariol L, Virgilio C, Tiso E, *et al*. Spontaneous superior mesenteric vein thrombosis (Smvt) in primary protein S deficiency. A case report and review of the literature. *Chir Ital* 2000; 52(2): 183–190.

Brountzos EN, Critselis A, Magoulas D, Kagianni E, Kelekio DA. Emergency endovascular treatment of a superior mesenteric artery occlusion. *Cardiovasc Intervent Radiol* 2001; 24(1): 57–60.

Further reading

Choudhary AM, Grayer D, Nelson A, Roberts I. Mesenteric venous thrombosis: a diagnosis not to be missed! *J Clin Gastroenterol* 2000; 31(2): 179–182.

Danse EM, Laterre PF, Van Beers BE, *et al*. Early diagnosis of acute intestinal ischaemia: contribution of colour doppler sonography. *Acta Chir Belg* 1997; 97(4): 173–176.

Donnelly WJ. Management of acute mesenteric ischemia. *N Engl J Med* 1996; 335(8): 595–596; discussion 96.

Hassan HA, Raufman JP. Mesenteric venous thrombosis. *South Med J* 1991; 92(6):558–562.

Jarvinen O, Laurikka J, Salenius JP, Lepantalo M. Mesenteric infarction after aortoiliac surgery on the basis of 1752 operations from the National Vascular Registry. *World J Surg* 1999; 23(3): 243–247.

Kasirajan K, O'Hara PJ, Gray BH, *et al*. Chronic mesenteric ischemia: open surgery versus percutaneous angioplasty and stenting. *J Vasc Surg* 2001; 33(1): 63–71.

Matsumoto AH, Angle JF, Spinosa DJ, *et al*. Percutaneous transluminal angioplasty and stenting in the treatment of chronic mesenteric ischemia: results and longterm followup. *J Am Coll Surg* 2002; 194(1): Suppl S22–31.

Moawad J, McKinsey JF, Wyble CW, *et al*. Current results of surgical therapy for chronic mesenteric ischemia. *Arch Surg* 1997; 132(6): 613–618; discussion 18–19.

Park WM, Cherry KJ Jr, Chua HK, *et al*. Current results of open revascularization for chronic mesenteric ischemia: a standard for comparison. *J Vasc Surg* 2002; 35(5): 853–859.

Schwartz LB, McKinsey JF, Gewertz, BL. Visceral ischemic syndromes. In: Moore WS (ed.) *Vascular Surgery: A Comprehensive Review* 2002; 571–584.

Trompeter M, Brazda T, Remy CT, Vestring T, Reimer P. Nonocclusive mesenteric ischemia: etiology, diagnosis, and interventional therapy. *Eur Radiol* 2002; 12(5): 1179–1187.

Chapter 12

Irritable Bowel Syndrome

Kevin W. Olden

CHAPTER OUTLINE

DEFINITION

DIAGNOSTIC CRITERIA FOR IRRITABLE BOWEL SYNDROME

Rome II criteria for the diagnosis of irritable bowel syndrome

Are the Rome criteria for irritable bowel syndrome valid?

EPIDEMIOLOGY

ECONOMIC IMPACT

PATHOPHYSIOLOGY

Motility abnormalities

Visceral hypersensitivity

Inflammatory factors in irritable bowel syndrome

Psychosocial factors

Psychiatric comorbidity in irritable bowel syndrome

Abuse history

Brain–gut axis

Other factors

THE BIOPSYCHOSOCIAL APPROACH TO IRRITABLE BOWEL SYNDROME

Diagnosis

TREATMENT

The physician–patient relationship

Stratification of treatment

The patient with mild symptoms

The patient with moderate symptoms

The patient with severe symptoms

Drug treatment of irritable bowel syndrome

Behavioral treatment of irritable bowel syndrome

PROGNOSIS

SUMMARY

FURTHER READING

Definition

Irritable bowel syndrome is a chronic functional gastrointestinal disorder characterized by abdominal pain or discomfort *in combination with* changes in stool frequency and/or stool form.

Diagnostic criteria for irritable bowel syndrome

A symptom-based approach to the diagnosis of irritable bowel syndrome is essential in that there are no pathophysiologic markers to discriminate irritable bowel syndrome from other disorders. All of the symptom-based criteria for irritable bowel syndrome assume an absence of structural or biochemical abnormalities that could explain the patients' symptoms. The first symptom-based criteria for the diagnosis of irritable bowel syndrome were put forth by Manning in 1978. The Manning criteria have been shown to be a sensitive and specific tool to correctly diagnose irritable bowel syndrome.

In an attempt to improve on this process, multinational working teams have been convened to develop contemporary diagnostic criteria for the functional gastrointestinal disorders. These teams have been meeting in Rome, Italy, since 1988. The "Rome" committees are comprised of experts from a variety of disciplines around the world. These committees have developed symptom-based diagnostic criteria that have become known as the "Rome criteria" for the diagnosis of irritable bowel syndrome as well as for the other functional gastrointestinal disorders. The Rome Committees have classified the functional gastrointestinal disorders by anatomic regions that include esophageal, gastroduodenal, bowel, and anorectal disorders. In addition, the Rome committees have addressed special topics such as the basic science and psychosocial aspects of the functional gastrointestinal disorders. The Rome Committees have also developed recommendations for the design of clinical treatment trials. Finally, diagnostic criteria have been developed for the pediatric functional gastrointestinal disorders. The original Rome I diagnostic criteria were published in 1992, and the revised Rome II criteria followed in 1999.

Rome II criteria for the diagnosis of irritable bowel syndrome

The current Rome II diagnostic criteria for irritable bowel syndrome are given in Box 12.1.

Irritable bowel syndrome is often classified as diarrhea-predominant or constipationpredominant, although many patients will have alternating diarrhea and constipation if observed over long periods of time. The Rome II criteria presume the absence of anatomic, metabolic, or infectious causes for the patient's symptoms. The most effective approach to diagnosis is discussed below.

Are the Rome criteria for irritable bowel syndrome valid?

A number of studies have shown the predictive value of the Rome I criteria to be good. One study

> **Box 12.1** Rome II criteria for irritable bowel syndrome
>
> At least 12 weeks, which need not be consecutive, in the preceding 12 months, of abdominal discomfort or pain that has two of the following three features:
> - it is relieved with defecation; and/or
> - the onset is associated with a change in frequency of stool; and/or
> - the onset is associated with a change in form (appearance) of stool.

showed a positive predictive value of 100%, a negative predictive value of 76%, a sensitivity of 65%, and a specificity of 100%. Preliminary validation data on the Rome II criteria are encouraging. In one study, Talley and colleagues surveyed a rural county population with the presence of irritable bowel syndrome. The study found that the Manning criteria discriminated irritable bowel syndrome and all non-irritable bowel syndrome gastrointestinal disease with a sensitivity of 58% and 42%, and a specificity of 74% and 85% respectively. They concluded that the symptom-based approach to the diagnosis of irritable bowel syndrome was reasonable, but that the Manning criteria were not highly sensitive. Saito and colleagues evaluated the sensitivity and specificity of the Manning criteria versus the Rome I criteria for the diagnosis of irritable bowel syndrome, again using a population-based survey. Using a threshold of two symptoms as defined by the Manning criteria, a prevalence of 2.4% for irritable bowel syndrome was found. Using the Rome I criteria, a prevalence of 8.5% was found. The difference in the prevalence of irritable bowel syndrome using the two different diagnostic criteria was quite significant. This study concluded that the diagnostic criteria used to detect irritable bowel syndrome was less important than evaluating symptoms within the criteria. The positive predictive value of the Rome I criteria for irritable bowel syndrome was tested in a novel way by Vanner and colleagues. In this study 98 patients, who met the Rome criteria for irritable bowel syndrome but who lacked "red flags" such as rectal bleeding, weight loss, a family history of inflammatory bowel disease, or colorectal cancer, were evaluated. The investigators found that the Rome I criteria, and absent "red flags", had a sensitivity of 65%, specificity of 100%, and a positive predictive value of 100%. Over a 2-year follow-up period, none of the patients required revision of their initial irritable bowel syndrome diagnosis upon review of their medical charts. In a second part of the same study, the investigators prospectively followed 95 patients referred to the gastrointestinal clinic over a 9-month period. Patients diagnosed with irritable bowel syndrome by the gastrointestinal consultant at the initial visit were then followed for 1 year. In this series, the positive predictive value of the Rome criteria was 98%. The investigators concluded that the Rome criteria combined with an absence of "red flags" have a very high predictive value for diagnosing irritable bowel syndrome.

In a more recent study of a community-based sample of irritable bowel syndrome patients, it was found that while the Rome I criteria were more specific, the overall sensitivity of the Rome II criteria was good. In this study, a national community-based sample was surveyed, specifically investigating the lifetime prevalence of irritable bowel syndrome. Using the Rome I criteria, the investigators found that 5.4% of the population met diagnostic criteria for irritable bowel syndrome. When the subjects with irritable bowel syndrome were specifically identified, the Rome I and Rome II criteria were then applied. The results showed that the Rome I criteria was significantly more sensitive than the Rome II criteria (84% versus 49%, $P < 0.001$). However, there was 40% agreement between Rome I and Rome II criteria. Of the 58% of patients who met irritable bowel syndrome by the Rome I criteria, these same subjects also met the diagnostic criteria for irritable bowel syndrome using the Rome II criteria. The investigators concluded that the Rome I criteria tended to be more sensitive when surveying a large community-based sample of female irritable bowel syndrome patients. These and other studies suggest that the Rome I and Rome II criteria are reasonable diagnostic tools for detecting and diagnosing irritable bowel syndrome. It is clear they will undoubtedly undergo further revision as our understanding of this disorder continues to improve. However, it is safe to say at this point, that the use of the Rome criteria in combination with an absence of so-called "alarm" or "red flag" signs is a safe strategy for accurately diagnosing irritable bowel syndrome.

Epidemiology

The prevalence of irritable bowel syndrome has been shown to be between 15% and 25% worldwide. One large community-based epidemiologic survey reported an 11.2% prevalence of irritable bowel syndrome in the US. Similar prevalence rates have been shown in Japan, the Netherlands, Denmark, and Singapore. These and other studies have not demonstrated any strong cultural differences that would influence the prevalence of irritable bowel syndrome. In fact, the prevalence of irritable bowel syndrome worldwide seems to remain amazingly stable, at between 10% and 20%. However, it is clear that only a certain percentage of people with irritable bowel syndrome ultimately seek treatment. One study of a community-based sample in England found the prevalence of irritable bowel syndrome to be 13% in women and 5% in men. However, only half of the subjects ultimately sought medical care. Moreover, people with multiple bowel symptoms, occurring simultaneously, were much more likely to consult a physician. The dichotomy between patients who meet the diagnostic criteria for irritable bowel syndrome in the community versus those who actually seek medical care for their irritable bowel syndrome was further demonstrated in a study by Drossman and colleagues. In this study, subjects were recruited from three populations, as follows

1. patients from a university-based functional gastrointestinal clinic that consisted of individuals who chose to seek medical care for irritable bowel syndrome
2. subjects recruited from the same university's undergraduate student population who met the diagnostic criteria for irritable bowel syndrome but chose not to seek care (positive controls)
3. undergraduate students who had no symptoms suggestive of irritable bowel syndrome (negative controls).

All subjects were administered the McGill pain questionnaire as well as other psychological instruments to measure levels of pain, psychological distress and coping abilities. This study was dramatic in that subjects with irritable bowel syndrome who chose to seek medical care were significantly different psychologically from both the positive control group and subjects who had no symptoms suggestive of irritable bowel syndrome. This study suggested that irritable bowel syndrome care seekers represent a unique subset of individuals who are more physically and emotionally distressed than people who have identical symptoms but who chose not to seek care.

These findings were replicated by Whitehead and colleagues who studied a group of urban churchgoers who met the diagnostic criteria for irritable bowel syndrome (study population) as well as subjects with documented lactose intolerance (positive controls) and individuals with no bowel symptoms (negative controls). In this study, as in the study by Drossman described above, the irritable bowel syndrome patients, although they had symptoms quite similar to individuals with lactose intolerance, were more likely to seek health care and also more likely to be emotionally distressed and in more pain than either the lactose-intolerant individuals or the normal controls. Patients who seek care for irritable bowel syndrome tend to be a special subgroup of the universe of individuals with irritable bowel syndrome. They appear to benefit from treatment delivered from a psychosocial perspective as opposed to a purely medical approach.

Economic impact

Health care costs associated with irritable bowel syndrome are comprised of

- direct costs – costs stemming directly from the diagnosis and treatment of irritable bowel syndrome, such as radiologic testing, doctor visits, and hospitalizations
- indirect costs – lost productivity because of the presence of illness causing absence from work or school
- intangible costs – the pain and suffering experienced by irritable bowel syndrome patients.

Accurately measuring and calculating these various "costs of illness" can be difficult and isn't an exact science. However, a number of studies have suggested that there is not an insignificant economic cost related to the presence of irritable bowel syndrome. One recent study estimated that functional bowel disorders (including irritable bowel syndrome) account for 0.5% to 1% of national health care budgets annually.

Pathophysiology

The pathophysiology of irritable bowel syndrome is incompletely understood. Multiple pathophysiological mechanisms have been proposed to explain the genesis of irritable bowel syndrome. These mechanisms include altered motility, inflammatory factors, visceral hypersensitivity, psychological factors, and alterations in brain function. However, no single pathophysiologic mechanism has been shown to explain the multiple symptoms of irritable bowel syndrome.

Motility abnormalities

Between the late 1940s and the early 1990s, the majority of research within the field of irritable bowel syndrome was focused on disturbances of gastrointestinal motility. At first glance, this approach seems to be reasonable. The symptoms of irritable bowel syndrome, such as diarrhea, constipation, and bloating, are all suggestive of abnormal gastrointestinal motility. Indeed, altered motor function has been identified in patients with irritable bowel syndrome. However, symptom correlation with motility abnormalities has been poor. A number of studies have demonstrated that patients can experience significant symptoms of irritable bowel syndrome while showing no abnormalities in motility. Likewise, patients found to have significant abnormalities in motility of the colon or small bowel often have no symptoms of irritable bowel syndrome suggesting that factors other than abnormal motility play a role in the generation of irritable bowel syndrome symptoms.

Visceral hypersensitivity

In the last 20 years, a number of studies have demonstrated abnormalities in visceral sensation in patients with irritable bowel syndrome. Studies of balloon distension in the sigmoid colon, ileum, and rectum as well as studies using electrical stimulation of the rectum all have demonstrated lower pain thresholds in patients with irritable bowel syndrome when compared with non-irritable bowel syndrome controls. In addition, studies have demonstrated abnormal somatic pain thresholds in patients with irritable bowel syndrome, suggesting that the hyperalgesia is not localized to the viscera. Studies have also shown that patients with irritable bowel syndrome can have an increased awareness of normal gastrointestinal motility function. Abnormal central nervous system processing of pain may also play a role in generating symptoms in irritable bowel syndrome patients. Studies have demonstrated abnormal activation of the anterior cingulate gyrus and the pre-frontal cortex in the brains of patients with irritable bowel syndrome compared to non-irritable bowel syndrome controls.

Inflammatory factors in irritable bowel syndrome

One third of patients with irritable bowel syndrome report the initial onset of symptoms following an episode of gastrointestinal infection. This finding has led to the idea that there may be an infectious and/or inflammatory etiology for irritable bowel syndrome. However, one study showed that the presence of psychosocial difficulties was a more powerful predictor of which patients with these physiological abnormalities would go on to develop symptoms of irritable bowel syndrome.

Psychosocial factors

During the past 10 years, research efforts at the interface of psychiatry and gastroenterology have led to a greater understanding of the psychosocial factors associated with irritable bowel syndrome. Although the diagnostic criteria for irritable bowel syndrome do not require the presence of psychosocial factors, these factors can have a significant impact on patients' perceptions of their symptoms, on a patient's decision to seek care, and on the clinical outcome. These findings led to an increased emphasis in understanding the role of psychological disturbance, social stress, and the significance of having a history of physical and sexual abuse in patients with irritable bowel syndrome.

Psychiatric comorbidity in irritable bowel syndrome

Irritable bowel syndrome is one of several gastrointestinal disorders that can be associated with psychiatric disturbance. Patients with irritable bowel syndrome can suffer from a wide spectrum of psychiatric disorders. These include anxiety disorders such as panic disorder, generalized anxiety disorder, and post-traumatic stress disorder; mood disorders including major depression and dysthymic disorder; and the somatoform disorders such as somatization and pain disorder. The implications of psychiatric diagnoses in patients with irritable bowel syndrome are incompletely understood. It has been demonstrated that the presence of psychiatric disorders can impact on prognosis as well as on health care seeking behavior in patients with irritable bowel syndrome.

One obvious question that arises from this line of investigation is the following. Are psychiatric disorders etiologic to a functional bowel disorder? The answer to this question seems to be unequivocally "No." Although there is a high prevalence of comorbidity in irritable bowel syndrome patients of various psychiatric disorders as outlined above, there does not seem to be any predisposing psychiatric state that places an individual at particular risk for irritable bowel syndrome. Although there is a lack of causality between psychiatric disturbance and irritable bowel syndrome, the presence of psychiatric disturbance can influence care seeking considerably. In a study of a large community-based population in Germany, Herschback and colleagues surveyed 2201 individuals for the presence of gastrointestinal symptoms and psychological disturbance. The workers found that individuals with functional gastrointestinal disorders who consulted a physician for their gastrointestinal symptoms differed significantly on psychological measures from individuals who met the diagnostic criteria for a functional gastrointestinal disorder but who chose not to seek medical care. The health care seekers were more likely to have more severe depressive symptoms, as well as greater concerns about the cause of their illness. This difference was even more pronounced when the care seekers with a functional bowel disorder were compared to normal controls. These findings are similar to the findings in studies of non-gastrointestinal illness where individuals who tend to be more anxious and concerned about disease are more likely in general to seek medical care in response to acute life stressors, as opposed to individuals without psychiatric disturbance. These findings are consistent with a classic work by Drossman and colleagues who found that individuals with irritable bowel syndrome who chose to seek health care were more likely to have a pattern of abnormal personality structure, greater illness behaviors, and lower stressful life-event scores than either irritable bowel syndrome non-patients or normal controls.

What are the implications of these findings for the clinician? It would seem that the patient with irritable bowel syndrome is more likely to be emotionally distressed and have more difficulty coping with life stressors. Investigating these issues more carefully has implications not only for improving the patient's bowel symptoms, but also for improving the overall quality of their life by addressing untreated anxiety, depressive, and other psychiatric disorders.

Abuse history

In 1990, Drossman and colleagues made the unique observation that 44% of the patients who presented at a university gastroenterology clinic had suffered a history of physical or sexual abuse in childhood or in later life. They further discovered that in this sample, patients with functional gastrointestinal disorders, as opposed to structural gastrointestinal disorders, were essentially twice as likely to have suffered physical or sexual abuse. When patients with positive abuse histories were studied in more detail, it was found that they were more likely to suffer pelvic pain, multiple somatic symptoms, and more lifetime surgeries compared to the controls with organic gastrointestinal disorders. These findings were replicated by Walker and colleagues who studied 71 patients with irritable bowel syndrome and compared them to 40 patients with inflammatory bowel disease. The investigators found that patients with irritable bowel syndrome had significantly higher numbers of medically unexplained physical symptoms and higher levels of disability compared to inflammatory bowel disease patients. Delvaux and colleagues further explored this area in a study of 196 irritable bowel syndrome patients seen in eight university hospitals compared to healthy controls, as well as patients consulting gastroenterologists for non-neoplastic organic digestive diseases. A 31.6% prevalence of sexual abuse in the irritable bowel syndrome patients compared to only 14% in the subjects with organic digestive diseases was found ($P = 0.0005$). The prevalence of an abuse history was even lower in ophthalmology patients (12.5%) and lower still in healthy controls (7.6%).

To evaluate whether this finding was true outside the gastrointestinal clinic setting, Talley and colleagues surveyed 909 individuals in a community-based sample. They found an age-adjusted prevalence of abuse of 41% in women and 11% in men resulting in an overall age- and sex-adjusted prevalence of 26%. They further found a significant association between irritable bowel syndrome and sexual abuse, emotional abuse, or verbal abuse both in childhood and in adult life. Finally, they found that the odds of visiting a physician for gastrointestinal complaints were highest in those individuals reporting a positive history of abuse. Similar to the presence of a psychiatric disorder, it is unlikely that abuse *per se* is etiologic of irritable bowel syndrome. Moreover, the overwhelming majority of patients with functional bowel disorders have had no history of physical or sexual abuse. The major implication for the presence of abuse, as with a psychiatric disorder, is in health care seeking behavior and the disability–health status. Lesserman and colleagues studied 239 patients attending a university gastroenterology clinic. They found an overall prevalence of abuse in this population of 66.5%. As the severity of abuse increased, from minor physical abuse through to rape, the severity of the patients' gastrointestinal symptoms, as well as their levels of disability, also increased. These findings certainly suggest that in patients with irritable bowel syndrome, particularly those with more severe symptoms, a history of abuse could influence the perception, expression, and burden of their symptoms. Investigating for the possibility of a history of abuse seems to be reasonable and can constitute an important part of formulating the patient's care plan.

Brain–gut axis

The "brain–gut axis" refers to the juxtaposition of the enteric nervous system and the central nervous system. It links visceral afferent sensation and intestinal motor function with higher cortical centers that modulate and modify their activity. A variety of neurotransmitters including the enkephalins, substance P, calcitonin gene-related polypeptide, nitric oxide, serotonin (5-hydroxytryptamine), and cholecystokinin participate in the regulation of gut function. Deregulation of brain–gut function induced by abnormalities in gut neurotransmitter function has been proposed as a major contributing factor in the etiology of irritable bowel syndrome.

Better understanding of the role of serotonin in visceral perception and the regulation of gastrointestinal motility has led to a number of new agents developed specifically for the treatment of irritable bowel syndrome symptoms. The first of these agents, alosetron, was approved for use in the US in 1999. This agent which is a 5-HT_3 antagonist has been shown to decrease visceral sensitivity and reduce irritable bowel syndrome-associated pain, slow colonic transit, and reduce rectal urgency in patients with diarrhea-predominant irritable bowel syndrome. This drug, unfortunately, has been associated with ischemic colitis. The exact mechanism for the development of ischemic colitis in patients taking alosetron remains unclear. After being removed from the market for a short period, the drug has now been re-introduced under controlled prescribing and aggressive surveillance of patients receiving the drug. It is clear that alosetron is an effective drug for the treatment of diarrhea-predominant irritable bowel syndrome in women. Its efficacy and full safety have not been demonstrated in men, and the drug is not approved for use in men. However, alosetron represents a cutting edge treatment for patients with diarrhea-predominant irritable bowel syndrome.

Alosetron was followed by a second agent, tegaserod. This drug, an aminoguanidine indole, is a 5-HT$_4$ partial agonist. Tegaserod has been shown to be effective for the treatment of constipation-predominant irritable bowel syndrome in women. The drug has not been associated with ischemic colitis or any serious complications to date. Tegaserod has been shown to be effective in relieving the pain, bloating, and constipation associated with irritable bowel syndrome. These agents are revolutionary in that they are the first agents designed specifically to treat the entire spectrum of irritable bowel syndrome symptoms, as opposed to individual symptoms such as abdominal pain or changes in bowel habits. Newer agents following this line of investigation are currently in development. Cilansetron, a 5-HT$_3$ antagonist, is currently in clinical trials, as is dexoxyglutamide, a CCK$_1$A antagonist. The former is being developed for irritable bowel syndrome with diarrhea and the latter for irritable bowel syndrome with constipation.

Other factors

A variety of other mechanisms of altered intestinal function have been proposed, including malabsorption of lactose bile acids and short chain fatty acids. Food allergens have also been suspected of contributing to symptoms of irritable bowel syndrome. None of these factors has been definitively shown to be etiologic for irritable bowel syndrome but they can contribute to irritable bowel syndrome-like symptoms

The biopsychosocial approach to irritable bowel syndrome

Current models for the diagnosis and treatment of irritable bowel syndrome utilize a biopsychosocial approach. In this model, the symptoms of irritable bowel syndrome are believed to be the result of multiple interacting factors. These factors include the physiological mechanisms of pain modulation, neuroendocrine regulation of motility, environmental stressors, psychological and psychiatric comorbidity, and cognitive factors such as illness behavior and individual coping styles.

Diagnosis

Irritable bowel syndrome has traditionally been perceived as a "diagnosis of exclusion." By this is meant that in a patient presenting with symptoms suggesting irritable bowel syndrome, other "more likely" organic diagnoses should be considered first with a diagnosis of irritable bowel syndrome being made only after other diagnostic possibilities have been ruled out. There are a number of problems associated with this approach. First, irritable bowel syndrome is the most common disorder seen in gastroenterologic practice. Therefore, the pre-test probability of a diagnosis of irritable bowel syndrome being made correctly is much greater than for other gastrointestinal illnesses. Clearly, at first glance the prudent gastroenterologist would disagree with this assumption. However, this schema can be made more workable by using the concept of "red flags." This means that the approach to the patient with irritable bowel syndrome should be made first on epidemiologic grounds, i.e. is this a patient who is likely to have irritable bowel syndrome (e.g. a patient who is 50 years old or younger, or female) and does the patient have any findings suggesting other diagnostic possibilities based on history, physical examination, and screening laboratory studies? Certainly the patient who reports weight loss, rectal bleeding, or a family history of inflammatory bowel disease or colon cancer would be viewed differently from the patient without these factors. This approach is supported by a number of studies that have been conducted over the last 8 years. Tolliver and colleagues evaluated 196 patients presenting to a gastrointestinal clinic who ultimately were diagnosed with irritable bowel syndrome. Attending clinicians were allowed to order *ad libitum* diagnostic studies they felt were appropriate. In this study, thyroid function testing, sedimentation rate, examination of the stool for ova and parasites, as well as the structural evaluation of the colon via endoscopy or barium X-rays had very low yields. The investigators concluded that erythrocyte sedimentation rate, thyroid testing, and examination for parasites should not routinely be performed in patients presenting with irritable bowel syndrome-like symptoms. They recommended that colon cancer screening should be performed in accordance with the recommendations of the American Cancer Society.

Hamm and colleagues evaluated 1452 patients entering a clinical trial for a proposed irritable bowel syndrome medication. All patients met Rome I criteria for the diagnosis of irritable bowel syndrome. All underwent imaging of the colon, either endoscopically or via barium X-ray. In addition, all subjects underwent thyroid function testing, fecal ova and parasite examination, as well as lactose breath testing. Investigators found a 23% prevalence of lactose malabsorption and a 6% prevalence of thyroid abnormalities. They noted that both of these prevalence rates were consistent with the background prevalence of thyroid disorders and lactose malabsorption in the population at large. They concluded that for subjects fulfilling the workers own criteria for irritable bowel syndrome, additional investigations were not likely to alter the diagnosis of irritable bowel syndrome, and additional diagnostic testing was probably not indicated. These two studies suggest that the "positive" diagnosis of irritable bowel syndrome is a reasonable strategy. However, once a diagnosis of irritable bowel syndrome is made and treatment is initiated, it is the responsibility of the clinician to continue to follow the patient. Patients who fail to respond to reasonable treatment for irritable bowel syndrome, or who deteriorate during a period of observation of 1 to 2 months should have their diagnosis re-evaluated. Given this practice, the initial step in diagnosis should be based upon both the patient's epidemiologic profile and their meeting the Rome II criteria for irritable bowel syndrome. Limited laboratory studies, including a complete blood count and routine chemistry studies, should be performed. Colon screening in the form of colonoscopy should be undertaken only in patients over the age of 50 years, in individuals with a family history of colon cancer, or in patients with alarm symptoms such as occult blood positive stools or with a frank history of hematochezia. Routine abdominal ultrasound is considered unnecessary in diagnosing irritable bowel syndrome and can even be counterproductive because of the detection of minor, unrelated abnormalities that could lead to further unnecessary testing. Testing for lactose intolerance should be limited to patients from high-risk populations. This diagnostic approach is outlined in Figure 12.1.

In taking a history, the importance of alarm symptoms cannot be underemphasized. Weight loss, nocturnal symptoms, blood mixed in the stools, recent antibiotic use, family history of colon cancer or inflammatory bowel disease, or recent travel history to areas endemic for infectious causes of diarrhea need to be inquired about and, if present, further evaluated. Likewise, any abnormalities found on physical examination, such as an abdominal mass, should prompt more extensive evaluation. Once a tentative diagnosis of irritable bowel syndrome is made and a treatment regimen is begun the patient needs to be followed over time. A change in the clinical picture or failure of the patient's symptom pattern to improve over time may also be an indication for re-evaluation of the irritable bowel syndrome diagnosis.

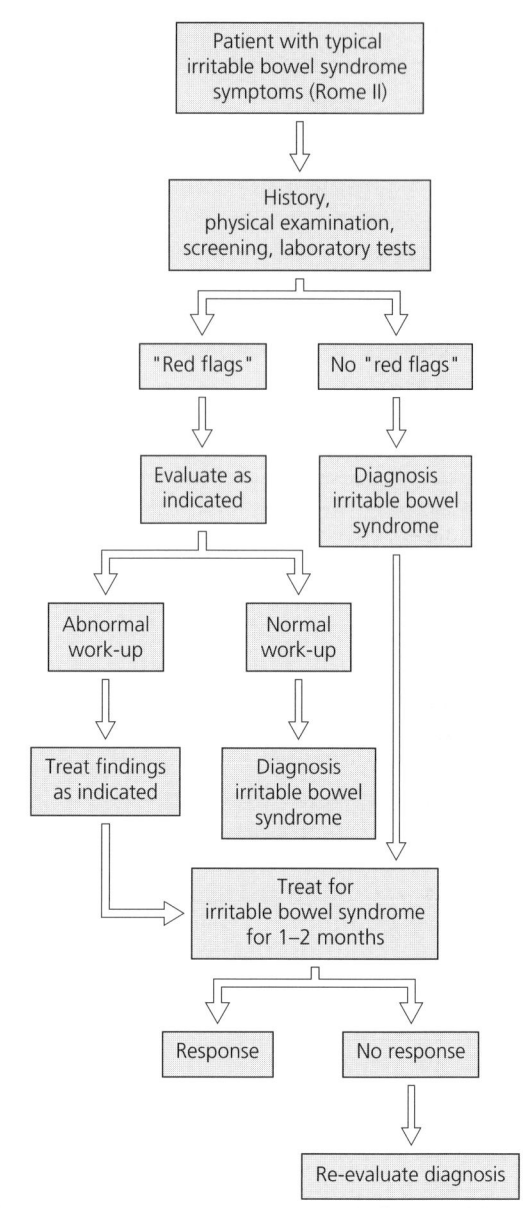

Figure 12.1 Diagnostic approach for irritable bowel syndrome.

Treatment

The physician–patient relationship

An effective physician–patient relationship is an integral aspect of the treatment of irritable bowel syndrome. This is supported by the fact that patients with irritable bowel syndrome have up to a 90% placebo response rate. It is important to obtain a thorough history, including a psychosocial and abuse history using a non-judgmental, patient-centered approach. The physician should provide a thorough explanation of the diagnosis and reassure the patient using terminology that the patient can understand. The physician should give the patient realistic expectations regarding prognosis. It is important for patients with irritable bowel syndrome to have an ongoing relationship with their physician. Allowing patients to ask questions and offering reassurance has been shown to improve prognosis in irritable bowel syndrome. Together, these measures can have a significant impact upon patient anxiety and can help patients participate fully in their care. An effective physician–patient relationship can also decrease the need for additional testing in patients concerned about a "missed" diagnosis.

Stratification of treatment

Treatment recommendations for patients with irritable bowel syndrome have been categorized into subgroups based on symptom severity. Although these subgroups were originally created to assist with the stratification of patients enrolled in clinical trials, categorization of patients based on symptom severity is also useful in clinical practice.

The patient with mild symptoms

Approximately 70% of patients with irritable bowel syndrome have "mild" symptoms that can be managed with measures such as patient education, reassurance, and lifestyle modification. Dietary modification to reduce the intake of lactose and other non-absorbable sugars such as sorbitol and fructose, as well as fat, alcohol, and caffeine may be recommended in these patients. Patients in this subgroup with constipation-predominant symptoms may benefit from a high fiber diet or fiber supplementation. One key element of the treatment of irritable bowel syndrome patients is education. It has been shown that patients with irritable bowel syndrome report a need for more and better information regarding their illness.

The patient with moderate symptoms

Approximately 25% of patients with irritable bowel syndrome have "moderate" symptoms. Although these patients may have increased levels of psychological distress, they do not tend to have severe psychosocial or psychiatric disturbances. Pharmacotherapy in these patients should be symptom-focused. In addition to bowel-directed medical treatment, such as fiber supplementation, anticholinergics, and smooth muscle relaxants, the use of antidepressants may also be helpful in these patients (see p. 252). It has been suggested that these patients may benefit from a more multi-dimensional approach to treatment including behavioral treatments such as hypnosis and relaxation training in addition to medication. Patient education also plays a key role in helping these patients fully understand and cope with their illness.

The patient with severe symptoms

Five percent of patients with irritable bowel syndrome are classified as having "severe" symptoms. These patients describe constant pain and have high levels of disability. They often have significant functional impairment and lower overall quality of life. These patients are quite likely to have comorbid psychiatric diagnoses including anxiety disorders, major depressive disorder, and somatoform disorders as a part of their clinical picture. These patients also have high rates of major social trauma in their lives such as the death of a parent or spouse. Finally, these patients are much more likely to have high rates of physical and/or sexual abuse. Multi-modal approaches combining medical management and education seem to be particularly promising for the patient with moderate-to-severe irritable bowel syndrome. Likewise, psychotherapeutic approaches have also been demonstrated to be particularly helpful in patients with severe refractory irritable bowel syndrome.

Drug treatment of irritable bowel syndrome

The selection of medications for use in patients with irritable bowel syndrome is based on the patient's predominant symptom pattern and the severity of the symptoms.

Irritable bowel syndrome with constipation

Fiber may be useful in patients with constipation-predominant irritable bowel syndrome. However, the literature on the efficacy of fiber for the treatment of irritable bowel syndrome is equivocal. Fiber supplementation certainly can reduce constipation associated with irritable bowel syndrome, however, it can also be associated with bloating and abdominal cramping which makes its use in the treatment of irritable bowel syndrome less than optimal. The recommended fiber intake for these patients is 20 to 30 g/day. In addition to fiber, polyethylene glycol solution has been shown to be useful in alleviating the constipation associated with irritable bowel syndrome.

Irritable bowel syndrome with diarrhea

Loperamide, a non-absorbable opioid, has been shown to slow intestinal transit, increase water and ion absorption, and increase rectal sphincter tone leading to improvement of diarrhea and rectal urgency in patients with diarrhea-predominant irritable bowel syndrome. Because loperamide does not cross the blood–brain barrier, it is preferred over other narcotic medications. Cholestyramine has also demonstrated benefit in diarrhea-predominant irritable bowel syndrome. It has been suggested that the mechanism of action may relate to bile-acid sequestration in patients with idiopathic bile-acid malabsorption contributing to symptoms of irritable bowel syndrome. However, patients may have difficulty tolerating cholestyramine.

Antidepressants

Antidepressants have been used for many years in the treatment of irritable bowel syndrome. The initial rationale for using these medications was their proven efficacy for the treatment of peripheral neuropathy and other neuropathic pain syndromes. However, the rationale for the use of antidepressants in irritable bowel syndrome is more complex. Tricyclic antidepressants have been shown in numerous studies to relieve diarrhea, constipation, abdominal pain, and bloating in patients with irritable bowel syndrome. This effect is independent of their antidepressant effect. Likewise, tricyclic antidepressants seem to have an effect independent of their anticholinergic effect. They seem to be helpful in treating both the constipation- and diarrhea-predominant forms of irritable bowel syndrome. However, their usefulness is limited by the fact that many patients find adverse side effects associated with antidepressant use.

In addition, antidepressants have been shown to be useful in irritable bowel syndrome patients with concomitant psychiatric disorders, as well as in irritable bowel syndrome patients who show no signs of psychiatric disturbance. Psychiatric disorders that are most commonly associated with irritable bowel syndrome are panic disorder, major depressive disorder, and phobias. All of these conditions have been shown to be responsive both to tricyclic antidepressants as well as the selective serotonin reuptake inhibitors. The importance of screening for psychiatric disorders in patients with irritable bowel syndrome, particularly those who are refractory to standard medical management, can help identify individuals who will benefit particularly well from the addition of antidepressant agents to their regimen. For patients who do not have a concomitant psychiatric disorder, tricyclic antidepressants, in doses far lower than usually used for the treatment of depression and anxiety, can be employed. In patients who have a concomitant psychiatric disorder, standard antidepressant doses are usually needed (Table 12.1).

Serotonergic agents

It has been known for many years that 90% of the serotonin receptors present in the body are located in the gut. Research over the last 10 years has shown multiple roles for various serotonin receptor subtypes in both visceral perception and motor

Table 12.1 Antidepressant dosing guidelines.

Antidepressant	GI dosage (mg)	Range (mg/day)
Amitriptyline	10–200	50–300
Imipramine	10–200	75–300
Clomipramine	25–250	25–250
Doxepin	10–200	75–300
Fluoxetine	10–20	20–80
Paroxetine	10–20	20–50
Sertraline	25–50	50–200
Trazodone	25–300	150–600

function of the gut. There has been aggressive research to develop serotonergically active agents that could influence the disturbances of bowel sensation and function seen in irritable bowel syndrome. This line of investigation has led to the development of a number of new agents, some of which are currently available and others which are still in development. A list of newly available and emerging agents is given in Table 12.2. The first of these is alosetron, a 5-HT$_3$ antagonist. Alosetron has been shown to decrease visceral sensation, thereby reducing pain and rectal urgency in irritable bowel syndrome associated with constipation. Alosetron has been associated with high degrees of patient satisfaction and significant improvement in the patient's overall well-being. The major issue confronting alosetron is the fact that it has been associated, for reasons which remain unclear, with ischemic colitis that led to the drug being transiently withdrawn from the market. However, because of its high efficacy and high degree of patient satisfaction, regulatory authorities in the US have re-approved the drug under controlled prescribing circumstances. Alosetron is currently approved for the treatment of *severe* irritable bowel syndrome in women. Another new agent is tegaserod which has been developed as a 5-HT$_4$ partial agonist. Tegaserod is currently available in the US for the treatment of irritable bowel syndrome with associated constipation in women. To date, no significant safety issues have been seen with this drug. Likewise, patient satisfaction, improvements in global well-being, and improvement in the specific irritable bowel syndrome symptoms of pain, bloating, and constipation have all been documented with this drug.

In addition to the two agents discussed above, there are additional serotonergically active agents that are in development. One is prucalopride a 5-HT$_4$ *full* antagonist. This drug currently remains in development and has not yet entered clinical trials, therefore no clinical data are available. Cilansetron is a 5-HT$_3$ antagonist that has also been designed to treat irritable bowel syndrome with associated diarrhea. It is currently in clinical trials and, as yet, no definitive data are available for it.

Novel agents

In addition to antidepressants and serotonergically acting agents, a number of new compounds aimed at other receptor sites in the gut are being investigated for the treatment of irritable bowel syndrome. For some time the kappa opiate antagonist, fedotozine, has been studied in the treatment of irritable bowel syndrome, specifically for the treatment of pain and bloating. Kappa opiate receptors are found only in the gut. The theoretical advantage of fedotozine is that it does not interact with the mu opiate receptor that is responsible for the euphoria and extraintestinal pain relief seen with traditional narcotic analgesics. The results have been mixed. To date, clinical trials using fedotozine have been inconclusive, and it remains unclear whether this agent offers significant therapeutic benefit to patients with irritable bowel syndrome.

In addition to the kappa opiate agonists, antagonists to the inflammatory mediator neurokinin (NK1 antagonists) are currently being investigated to treat a presumed inflammatory response in irritable bowel syndrome. It has been postulated that this inflammatory response may lead to stimulation of visceral afferent nerve endings causing pain, discomfort, and altered motility. One new agent that is currently in clinical trials is dexoxyglutamide which is a CCK$_1$A antagonist. This drug has shown preliminary evidence suggesting that it is efficacious for the treatment of irritable bowel syndrome with constipation. It is currently in phase III trials, and preliminary data are encouraging. We will need to await the completion of the phase III trials of this agent to make any definitive comments on its efficacy for the treatment of irritable bowel syndrome. However, it certainly represents another innovative approach to the treatment of this common disorder. These agents are outlined in Table 12.2.

Table 12.2 New drugs for irritable bowel syndrome.

Name	Action	Indication	Status
Alosetron	5-HT$_3$ antagonist	Women IBS-C	Available
Tegaserod	5-HT$_4$ partial agonist	Women IBS-C	Available
Cilanseron	5-HT$_3$ antagonist	In trial	In trials
Prucalopride	5-HT$_4$ full agonist	In development	In development
Dexoxyglutamide	CCK$_{1A}$ antagonist	In trial	In trials

Behavioral treatment of irritable bowel syndrome

The biopsychosocial nature of irritable bowel syndrome suggests that its effective treatment does not depend only on medical management. This typically seems to be the case. An emerging body of literature is appearing to support the efficacy of a variety of behavioral interventions for the treatment of irritable bowel syndrome. Psychotherapy, particularly cognitive behavioral therapy, hypnosis, and psychodynamic psychotherapy have all been used with great effectiveness in the treatment of patients with irritable bowel syndrome. A number of studies have now demonstrated that the use of psychotherapy can decrease gastrointestinal symptoms and the use of health care services, as well as increase the patient's overall sense of well-being. In one study by Guthrie and colleagues, 101 patients with severe refractory irritable bowel syndrome, which had not responded to traditional medical management, were referred for psychotherapeutic intervention. Patients were randomized either to standard medical treatment in combination with "supportive listening". This latter modality consisted of the psychiatrist investigator spending time with the control subjects to correct for the therapeutic effect of her presence. However, during these sessions the investigator did not engage in delivering psychotherapy but rather engaged in noncommittal supportive listening to the patient's concerns. The active treatment group was randomized to twelve sessions of psychodynamic interpersonal psychotherapy. Outcomes were rated by gastroenterologists, blinded to the patient's treatment status, who assessed the patient's gastrointestinal symptoms. In addition, health care utilization was measured. The investigators found that patients who received psychotherapy had significant improvements in their gastrointestinal symptoms both as measured by standardized rating scales and ratings by the treating gastroenterologist who was blinded to the study. Emotional well-being also significantly improved in the treatment group compared to controls. Finally, the treatment group had a 75% reduction in health care utilization during the 1-year follow-up period after the study was completed. This study demonstrates that psychotherapy, when properly delivered by a therapist experienced in irritable bowel syndrome, can produce improvements not only in gastrointestinal symptoms but also in overall emotional well-being, and can significantly decrease health care utilization.

Prognosis

Although irritable bowel syndrome tends to be a chronic disorder, there is a tendency toward symptomatic improvement. Approximately 30% of patients will have resolution of symptoms over time. Studies have shown that the level of chronic life stress is a powerful predictor of clinical outcome in patients with irritable bowel syndrome. One retrospective study of 136 patients diagnosed with irritable bowel syndrome at the Mayo Clinic in Rochester, Minnesota and then followed via their medical records for an average of 30 years, showed that overall survival of patients with irritable bowel syndrome was as good as, or better than, non-irritable bowel syndrome medical controls. In addition, this study showed that the presence of a positive doctor–patient relationship could have a positive impact on prognosis by reducing patients' concerns, the number of doctor visits, and the number of hospitalizations for irritable bowel syndrome-related complaints. It is clear that irritable bowel syndrome is a chronic disease. However, its overall prognosis seems to be quite good with a general tendency for patients to improve. More importantly, the presence of a positive doctor–patient relationship has major implications for relieving long-term suffering.

Summary

Irritable bowel syndrome is a common, chronic gastrointestinal disorder that is commonly seen both in primary care and in gastrointestinal specialty practice. It is a disorder of gastrointestinal motility, which is influenced by, but not caused by, stress and psychosocial dysfunction. The evaluation of the patient with irritable bowel syndrome-like symptoms needs to be prudent. The use of symptom-based criteria as typified by the Rome II diagnostic criteria to make a "positive," as opposed to an exclusionary approach to diagnosis, has been shown to be a safe and rational approach to diagnosing irritable bowel syndrome. When evaluating the patient with suspected irritable bowel syndrome, it is important to evaluate the psychosocial dimensions of the patient's life. Specifically, inquiring about the presence of physical or sexual abuse and about social losses, such as the death of a parent while in childhood, is critical to fully evaluating patients with irritable bowel syndrome. In addition, screening for *selected* psychiatric disorders is also of great importance. It is only by exploring all of these dimensions, physical, social, and psychological, that an appropriate treatment plan for patients with irritable bowel syndrome can be formulated.

The treatment of patients with irritable bowel syndrome depends not only on effective medical management, such as dietary manipulation and the use of medications directed at gut function, but also may include the judicious use of antidepressants and even newer agents that act on the various neurotransmitter systems in the gut. Behavioral interventions such as hypnotherapy and psychotherapy increasingly play an important role in the treatment of irritable bowel syndrome. Adopting a multi-modal approach to the treatment of irritable bowel syndrome seems to be the most effective approach for these patients. It allows the physician to bring a perspective that is both reassuring and empowering for the patient. Most importantly, it provides the foundation for an effective physician–patient partnership to maximize the combined energy of both parties to ameliorate the symptoms of the patient with irritable bowel syndrome.

Further reading

Bardhan KD, Bodemar G, Geldof H, *et al*. A double-blind, randomized, placebo-controlled dose-ranging study to evaluate the efficacy of alosetron in the treatment of irritable bowel syndrome. *Aliment Pharmacol Ther* 2000; 14:23–34.

Chey WD, Olden KW, Carter E, *et al*. Utility of the Rome I and Rome II criteria for irritable bowel syndrome. *Am J Gastroenterol* 2002; 97:2803–2811.

Drossman DA, McKee D, Sandler R, *et al*. Psychosocial factors in the irritable bowel syndrome. A multivariate study of patients and nonpatients with irritable bowel syndrome. *Gastroenterology* 1988; 95:701–708.

Friedel D, Thomas R, Fisher RS. Ischemic colitis during treatment with alosetron. *Gastroenterology* 2001; 120:557–560.

Guthrie EA, Creed FH, Dawson D, *et al*. A randomised controlled trial of psychotherapy in patients with refractory irritable bowel syndrome. *Br J Psychiatry* 1993; 163:315–321.

Heaton KW, O'Donnell LJD, Braddon FEM, *et al*. Symptoms of irritable bowel syndrome in a British urban community: consulters and nonconsulters. *Gastroenterology* 1992; 102:1962–1967.

Jackson JL, O'Malley PG, Tomkins G, *et al*. Treatment of functional gastrointestinal disorders with antidepressant medications: a meta-analysis. *Am J Med* 2000; 108:65–72.

Olden KW, Drossman DA. Psychological and psychiatric aspects of gastrointestinal disease. *Med Clin North Am* 2000; 84(5):1313–1327.

Silverman DHS, Munakata J, Ennes H, *et al*. Regional cerebral activity in normal and pathological perception of visceral pain. *Gastroenterology* 1997; 112:64–72.

Whitehead WE, Bosmajian L, Zonderman AB, *et al*. Symptoms of psychologic distress associated with irritable bowel syndrome: comparison of community and medical clinic samples. *Gastroenterology* 1988; 95:709–714.

Whitehead WE, Holtkotter B, Enck P, *et al*. Tolerance for rectosigmoid distention in irritable bowel syndrome. *Gastroenterology* 1990; 98:1187–1192.

Zar S, Kumar D, Benson MJ. Review article: food hypersensitivity and irritable bowel syndrome. *Aliment Pharmacol Ther* 2001; 15:439–449.

Chapter 13

Anorectal Diseases
Samantha K. Hendren and John L. Rombeau

CHAPTER OUTLINE

ANATOMY

PHYSIOLOGY

EVALUATION

HEMORRHOIDS
    Internal hemorrhoids
    External hemorrhoids

ANAL FISSURE

ANORECTAL ABSCESS

FISTULA IN ANO

PILONIDAL DISEASE

HIDRADENITIS SUPPURATIVA

ANAL PRURITIS

FECAL INCONTINENCE

RECTOVAGINAL FISTULAS

RECTAL PROLAPSE

ANORECTAL STENOSIS
    High rectal strictures
    Anastomotic strictures

SEXUALLY TRANSMITTED DISEASES OF THE ANUS
    Anal condylomata
    Herpes simplex virus
    Syphilis
    Gonorrhea
    Chlamydia
    Human immunodeficiency virus
    Anal ulcers

ANAL NEOPLASMS
    Cancers of the anal canal
    Cancers of the anal margin

FURTHER READING

Anatomy

The rectum extends from the sacral promontory to the levator ani muscles, and has a length of 12 to 15 cm. Histologically, the rectum is comprised of mucosa, submucosa, inner circular, and outer longitudinal muscle. The rectum has a continuous outer, longitudinal muscle layer, unlike the colon. The anterior and lateral proximal rectum is covered by peritoneum (serosa), however the posterior and distal rectum is devoid of peritoneum.

The anal canal is about 4 cm long, and extends from the levator ani muscles to the anal verge. The internal anal sphincter is a thickening of the circular muscle layer, which is tonically contracted and provides the resting anal tone. In addition there are three muscular slings around the anus. Proximally is the puborectalis muscle, arising from the pubis and forming a sling around the anus. This muscle is contracted at rest and can be felt as the anorectal ring on digital examination. Next is the superficial external sphincter muscle which arises from the coccyx where it is called the anococcygeal ligament.

Anorectal Diseases

Finally, the subcutaneous external sphincter muscle is the most superficial of the three.

The mucosa of the anal canal is divided histologically by the dentate or pectinate line, about 2 cm proximal to the anal verge. Distal to this line, the mucosa is squamous epithelium, called anoderm; proximal to it for approximately 1 cm is the transitional or cloacogenic zone that may have transitional, columnar, or squamous epithelium. Proximal to this is columnar epithelium. A variable number of anal glands (four to ten glands) are lined with columnar epithelium and mucus-secreting goblet cells. They open directly into the anal crypts at the dentate line (Figure 13.1).

The pelvic floor muscles support the viscera in the upright position and are important to rectal function, continence, and the prevention of prolapse of the pelvic organs. The levator ani is a group of thin muscles that form the pelvic cavity floor. Traditionally, it was considered to be comprised of the iliococcygeal, pubococcygeal, and puborectal muscles. However, the puborectalis muscle is probably better classified as a part of the external anal sphincter. The pubococcygeus muscle arises from the pubis and the obturator fascia, extending ventrally around the anus and to the coccyx and sacrum. The ileococcygeus muscle arises from the ischial spine and obturator fascia, passing ventrally and medially to insert on the sacrum and anococcygeal raphe. Contraction of the levator ani widens the hiatus and elevates the anorectum for defecation.

There are several potential spaces surrounding the anus and rectum that are clinically important because abscesses can form in these spaces. The spaces are filled with areolar or fatty tissue in the normal condition and include the following

- the perianal space surrounds the anus and is continuous with the fat of the buttocks laterally
- the ischioanal space lies under the levator ani muscles and above the transverse septum of the ischiorectal fossa, it contains the inferior rectal vessels and lymphatics
- the deep postanal space connects the ischioanal spaces posteriorly, between the levator ani and the anococcygeal ligament
- the intersphincteric space is the route of spread of intersphincteric abscesses
- finally, the supralevator spaces, overlying the levator ani, may allow infection to spread into the retroperitoneum.

Arterial supply of the rectum and upper anal canal is from the superior rectal (hemorrhoidal) artery, the continuation of the inferior mesenteric artery. The middle rectal (hemorrhoidal) arteries arise from the internal iliac vessels bilaterally, and enter the rectum at about the level of the levator ani. The inferior rectal (hemorrhoidal) arteries arise from the internal pudendal arteries bilaterally (from the internal iliacs) and travel through the ischioanal space to the sphincter muscles.

The venous drainage of the rectum and anus follows the arterial supply and results in a systemic and portal drainage. The superior rectal vein drains the rectum and upper anus by way of the inferior

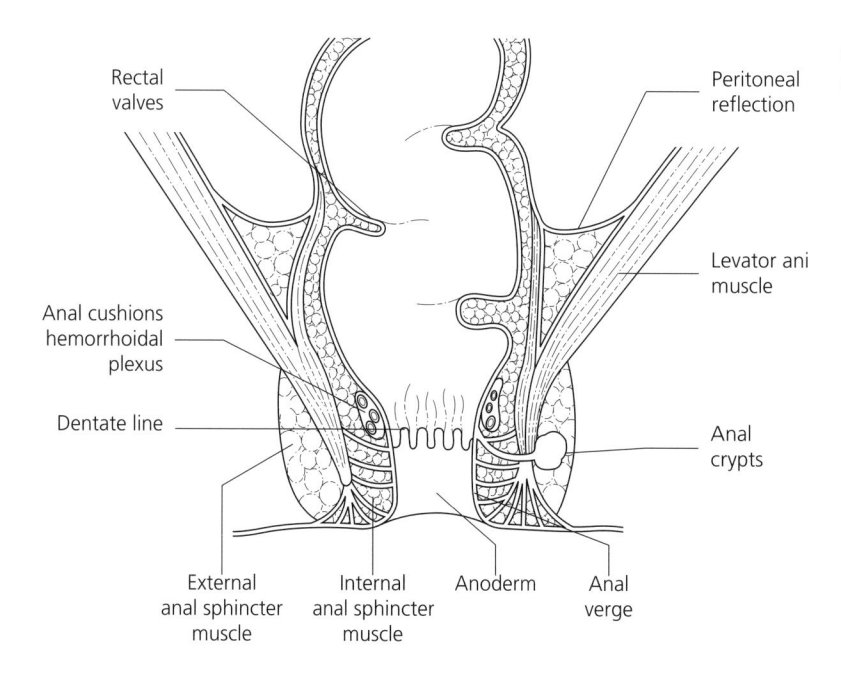

Figure 13.1 Anatomy of the rectum and anus.

mesenteric vein. The middle and inferior rectal veins drain into the internal iliac veins, leading to the systemic venous system.

The lymphatic drainage is clinically significant for the spread of malignancies from the anus and rectum. The upper and middle rectum drain into the inferior mesenteric lymph nodes. The lower rectum drains in two directions: via superior rectal lymphatics to the inferior mesenteric lymph nodes and via middle rectal lymphatics to the internal iliac lymph nodes. Similarly, the anal canal above the dentate line drains to both the inferior mesenteric and internal iliac nodal basins. The anal canal below the dentate line usually drains into the inguinal lymph nodes, unless this drainage is obstructed, in which case internal iliac or inferior mesenteric drainage can occur.

Sympathetic nerve fibers to the rectum arise from the first three lumbar segments of the spinal cord. The parasympathetic nerve supply arises from the second, third, and fourth sacral nerve roots. The internal anal sphincter is an involuntary muscle normally contracted at rest, supplied by inhibitory sympathetic and parasympathetic fibers. The external sphincter, voluntary striated muscle, is supplied by the inferior rectal branch of the internal pudendal nerve and the perineal branch of the fourth sacral nerve. The levator ani is supplied by pudendal and sacral nerves. Anal sensory innervation comes from the inferior rectal nerve branch of the pudendal nerve. Pain sensation may be felt up to 1.5 cm proximal to the dentate line.

Physiology

Fecal continence is an important physiologic function of the anorectum. Several anatomic features promote this function. Maintenance of the anorectal angle by tonic contraction of the puborectalis muscle is essential for continence, this muscle pulls the anus forward to an 80- to 90-degree angle with the rectum. This angle is straightened by assuming the sitting or squatting position. Also, the anal cushions contribute to higher pressure in the anal canal, preventing rectal contents from descending.

The involuntary internal anal sphincter is contracted at rest, creating the high-pressure zone of the anal canal. Via the rectoanal reflex, the internal sphincter relaxes when the rectum is distended, and a bolus of stool can move down into the anal canal. The external anal sphincter reflexively contracts when the rectum is distended to provide voluntary continence, and this "squeeze pressure" is entirely a function of the external anal sphincter. The external sphincter is the most important contributor to voluntary continence. Anorectal sensation is also essential for normal functioning, including the ability to sense rectal fullness and to discriminate between solid and gaseous contents of the rectum. This sensation is probably mediated through the levator ani muscles and the anorectal mucosal nerve fibers.

Defecation is a complex process involving voluntary and involuntary features. When stool enters the rectum stretch receptors mediate the urge to defecate. The internal sphincter relaxes and the external contracts. The solid or gaseous character of the contents is sensed by the anal mucosa. Defecation proceeds when the sitting position is assumed, the rectal muscles contract, and the patient "pushes". After defecation the sphincters contract and resting tone is resumed.

Evaluation

Evaluation of anorectal complaints begins with a complete history and physical examination. Examination of the anorectum has four components: inspection, palpation, anoscopy, and flexible or rigid proctosigmoidoscopy. Examination may be performed in the prone jackknife or left lateral decubitus position. Inspection may reveal skin tags, fissures, various lesions, and prolapsed hemorrhoids. Gentle internal examination with a well-lubricated finger reveals sphincter tone, and the presence of masses, fluctuance, and tenderness. If a painful condition such as a perirectal abscess or fissure exists, internal examination is performed under anesthesia. Anoscopy is an essential portion of the examination, providing a complete examination of the anal canal. Finally, rigid or flexible proctosigmoidoscopy should then be performed after one or two saline or phospho-soda enemas.

Hemorrhoids

Hemorrhoids are cushions of vascular tissue found within the anal canal. They are classified as either internal or external, depending on their position relative to the dentate line. Pathologic conditions of hemorrhoids are common problems that prompt medical attention.

Internal hemorrhoids

In the submucosa of the anal canal are three cushions containing arterioles and venules in a connective tissue matrix. These cushions are located in left lateral, right anterior, and right posterior positions. The normal function of these cushions is the maintenance of continence by filling the space within the anus and in cushioning the anus during defecation, during which the vessels fill with blood. The pathologic condition know as "internal hemorrhoids" arises from prolapse and consequent engorgement of these cushions, due to the breakdown of the connective tissue matrix.

Etiology

The pathophysiology of internal hemorrhoids is incompletely understood. Chronic straining during defecation may result in dilated cushion venules and eventual prolapse. However, there is no clear correlation between constipation and hemorrhoids. Alternatively, increased resting pressures in the anal canal may lead to decreased venous return and vascular engorgement with eventual disruption of the cushion connective tissue. Hemorrhoids are not varices and are not related to portal hypertension as commonly thought.

Clinical presentation and evaluation

The most common presentation of internal hemorrhoids is painless, bright-red blood per rectum associated with bowel movements, often described as "blood dripping into the toilet bowl." The sensation of incomplete rectal emptying is also common, but pain is an uncommon symptom and suggests a thrombosed external hemorrhoid or other pathology. Chronic prolapse of hemorrhoids can cause staining on the underwear or present as a mass. Internal hemorrhoids are classified on the basis of the extent of prolapse

- first degree – the hemorrhoids descend beyond the dentate line on straining
- second degree – the anal cushions prolapse through the anus but reduce spontaneously
- third degree – the hemorrhoids require manual reduction
- fourth degree – the prolapse is not reducible.

Examination of a patient suspected as having hemorrhoids is facilitated by giving the patient an enema prior to the examination. The examination may take place in the prone jackknife or left lateral decubitus position. Perianal examination will reveal associated "sentinel" skin tags, fissures, and fistulas if present. Chronic hemorrhoid prolapse may result in maceration or edema of the perianal area. An incarcerated fourth degree hemorrhoid may be identified. Digital examination should be performed to evaluate tone and rule out a stricture or distal mass, but internal hemorrhoids generally can not be discerned by digital examination.

Anoscopy is usually diagnostic of hemorrhoids. With anoscopy, the anal canal can be examined completely, and the patient can be asked to strain to allow for an estimation of the degree of prolapse. Proctoscopy should also be used to rule out rectal disease that can mimic hemorrhoids. Of note, in young patients the finding of hemorrhoids is sufficient to explain typical bleeding symptoms, but in an older patient (greater than 50 years of age) or a patient with a family history of colon cancer, a colonoscopy must be performed in addition to the hemorrhoid examination and treatment. Any patient presenting with anemia should be worked-up with a colonoscopy, regardless of age.

Treatment

A variety of treatment options exist. Initial therapy is generally conservative, consisting of a high-fiber diet and bulk-forming laxative therapy. Most first- and second-degree hemorrhoids respond to these measures. Hemorrhoids that fail to respond may be treated with elastic-band ligation, sclerotherapy, photocoagulation, cryosurgery, excisional hemorrhoidectomy or other therapies that induce scarring of the prolapsing cushion to the underlying tissues. Several of these procedures will be discussed in more detail.

Rubber-band ligation is one of the most common techniques for treatment of first- and second-degree hemorrhoids. It has the benefit of being a relatively painless office procedure. Technically, the procedure involves grasping hemorrhoidal tissue 1 to 2 cm above the dentate line, pulling the tissue into an elastic-band applicator device and applying two bands to the base of the tissue. In approximately 10 days the banded tissue sloughs, removing part of the prolapsing tissue and causing a scar which prevents further prolapse. Banded tissue must be above the transitional zone above the dentate line, because this mucosa is highly innervated, and rubber-band placement will cause severe pain. Rare cases of sepsis following rubber-band ligation have been reported, especially in patients with bands applied to an unrecognized rectal prolapse or in immunosuppressed patients. Patients must abstain from any therapies that impair blood clotting for at least 10 days after banding, or bleeding may occur.

Injection sclerotherapy is used for first- or second-degree hemorrhoids with persistent bleeding. One to two milliliters of sclerosing agent is injected into the submucosal loose connective tissue above the hemorrhoid, causing scarring. A trial injection should be performed to ensure the placement of the sclerosing agent in the submucosa. The depth of injection is important because transmural injections may result in a prostatic abscess or impotence if the nerves are involved. Superficial injections may result in musocal necrosis and ulceration. The effectiveness of the procedure is probably because of the induction of fibrosis which "fixes" the cushion, preventing prolapse.

Surgical hemorrhoidectomy, the so-called Milligan–Morgan procedure, is usually reserved for third- and fourth-degree hemorrhoids, incarcerated hemorrhoids, or mixed internal and external hemorroids. This procedure is accepted to be the most effective treatment for third- and fourth-degree hemorrhoids, and is the treatment against which newer procedures are compared. This procedure is usually performed in the operating room under spinal or general anesthesia. The vascular pedicle of the hemorrhoid is coagulated or suture ligated, and the redundant mucosa is excised to the level of the anal verge. The defect can be left open or closed. Complications of the procedure include severe pain, urinary retention, bleeding, and fecal impaction. Long-term complications include anal stenosis, if inadequate anoderm is left between excised hemorrhoids or, rarely, incontinence. Postoperatively, stool bulk-forming agents, stool softeners, and adequate pain medication are essential.

Because of the severe pain that often accompanies open hemorrhoidectomy, surgeons have sought a less painful alternative therapy. Technical alterations in the open hemorrhoidectomy such as diathermy dissection and preoperative metronidazole and lactulose have yielded some improvement in pain relief, but not sufficient to create great enthusiasm for the open hemorrhoidectomy.

Several new techniques may address the pain issue. The harmonic scalpel® device divides tissue using high-frequency ultrasonic energy. It coagulates blood vessels at a relatively low temperature, and therefore causes less thermal injury compared to other electrocautery methods. A randomized trial compared standard hemorrhoidectomy using electrocautery versus hemorrhoidectomy using the harmonic scalpel®. Postoperative pain was statistically and clinically significantly less in the harmonic scalpel® group. This device appears to hold promise for decreased pain with open hemorrhoidectomy.

The circular stapler rectopexy, or "stapled hemorrhoidectomy", has been used to treat tens of thousands of patients in Europe with third- and fourth-degree internal hemorrhoids; it is currently under clinical trial in the US. Rather than excising the hemorrhoids, the stapler excises mucosa and submucosa at or above the level of the hemorrhoids, eliminating prolapse and interrupting the blood supply to the hemorrhoids.

Several randomized trials comparing standard excisional hemorrhoidectomy with stapled hemorrhoidectomy have shown early treatment success and significantly reduced postoperative pain with the stapled procedure. In addition, preoperative and 6-month postoperative anorectal function, endoanal ultrasonography, and continence scores were prospectively studied in twenty patients undergoing stapled hemorrhoidectomy. No long-term functional problems were identified, but transient fecal urgency was experienced by several patients, as well as a single case of transient incontinence. This small study supports the safety of the procedure with regard to continence.

Reports of significant complications of circular stapler rectopexy have dampened enthusiasm for the procedure in the US. While precautions are taken to avoid incorporation of muscle into the excised tissue, histologic examination has shown that this phenomenon occurs in many patients. Muscular incorporation places patients at theoretical risk for anal stenosis, incontinence, and rectovaginal fistulas. At least one case of rectovaginal fistula has been reported. Furthermore, in a single series 5 of 22 patients were found to have a syndrome of persistent pain and fecal urgency of unclear etiology.

Most worrying are three cases of pelvic sepsis occurring after stapling procedures, at least one of which was life threatening. Sepsis is rare after elastic-band ligation, and is extremely uncommon after open hemorrhoidectomy. Patients must also be cautioned not to engage in anoreceptive sexual activity until examination has confirmed the absence of sharp staple points. One patient reported pain and bleeding after engaging in anoreceptive intercourse after stapled hemorrhoidectomy. Finally, the cost of the stapler device is relatively high ($350 US), but a faster return to normal activity and possible decreased overall medical costs probably balance this factor.

In summary, additional controlled safety and efficacy data are needed before there will be a wide acceptance of the circular stapler rectopexy procedure in the US. Studies are underway to assess perioperative pain and complications, especially sepsis, short-term and long-term anorectal function, and long-term complications such as anal stenosis and recurrence of hemorrhoid symptoms.

External hemorrhoids

External hemorrhoids arise from the inferior hemorrhoidal plexus below the dentate line and produce significant pain if thrombosed. They can also become congested and swollen causing discomfort. Treatment of external hemorrhoids is usually that used for an acute thrombosis that is treated urgently, given the debilitating pain. The treatment is surgical, with complete excision of the thrombosed vein. Simple incision and clot removal is a less adequate treatment, because the recurrence rate is high. If a patient presents more than 48 hours after the thrombosis, non-operative treatment with warm sitz baths, stool softeners, and stool bulk-forming agents is recommended because the hemorrhoid is more difficult to excise, and decreased pain may not be achieved with surgery.

Anal fissure

Anal fissure or fissure in ano is a painful linear tear in the anoderm at the anal verge (Figure 13.2). This condition affects all age groups, but is commonly seen in young, healthy men and women. The pathophysiology of anal fissures is usually related to initial trauma due to the passage of hard stool. This area is controversial since a majority of patients report no history of constipation. It has been established, however, that a majority of patients with chronic fissures have elevated resting internal anal sphincter pressures. This pressure persists after healing, implying that it may be a cause, not an effect, of the fissure. Modern treatments for fissures use surgical or pharmacologic means to decrease the internal sphincter pressure.

Local ischemia may play a role in fissure formation or chronicity, because of the relatively low baseline blood flow to the posterior anal verge, and/or compression of blood vessels by the hypertonic sphincter muscle. Multiple therapies that decrease sphincter pressure have been shown to increase local tissue perfusion. Postpartum patients have a higher incidence of anterior fissures and may have an alternate pathophysiology related to birth trauma, although this is unproven.

Classic symptoms are anal pain, often severe, during and after defecation, followed by scant bright-red blood. Pruritis is also present in about 50% of cases. On examination, the fissure is seen as a split in the anoderm at, or near, the anal verge, often with spasm of the anal sphincters. Examination may be limited by severe pain with retraction of the buttocks, and digital examination is frequently impossible because of the pain. Early fissures may be subtle with a small mucosal split. Granulation tissue may be present at the base.

Chronic fissures are identified by their indurated edges and the fibers of the internal sphincter visible at the base of the fissure. Skin tags, or other findings of chronic inflammation, sometimes develop, and help distinguish chronic from acute fissures. Fissures are usually solitary and found in the posterior midline or, much less commonly, in the anterior midline (10% of women, 1% of men). Multiple fissures or lateral fissures raise suspicion for an underlying disease such as inflammatory bowel disease, syphilis, or immunosuppression. Fissures failing to heal after sphincterotomy should be biopsied to rule out other lesions.

Initial therapy for acute anal fissures is conservative. A high fiber diet, increased oral fluid intake, sitz baths, and stool-softening laxatives are recommended therapies. Approximately 90% of acute fissures will heal either spontaneously or with these treatments. While preparations of local anesthetics and/or hydrocortisone have also been used, they have the theoretical disadvantage of sensitizing the anoderm to pain or precipitating flares of anogenital viral pathogens. Fissures failing to heal after 6 weeks to 2 months are considered chronic, and require further treatment because they are unlikely to heal spontaneously.

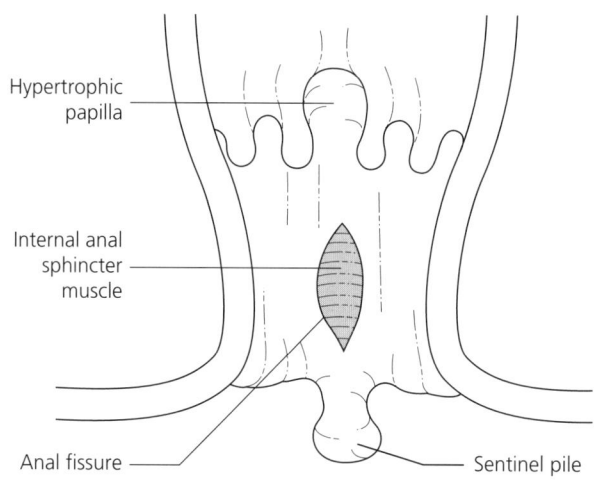

Figure 13.2 Anal fissure.

Treatment of chronic anal fissures failing to heal within 6 weeks is directed at the hypertonic internal anal sphincter. The definitive treatment is surgical lateral internal sphincterotomy. This minor surgical procedure results in healing in 98% of patients, with a very low rate of recurrence (less than 3%). An "open" or "subcutaneous" technique can be used to divide the internal anal sphincter over the length of the fissure. While some authors advise dividing the internal sphincter to the level of the dentate line, this may increase risk of incontinence, especially in women; therefore, a more conservative sphincter division is more commonly used. The procedure is performed as outpatient surgery.

The argument against the use of this procedure is the morbidity of gas or fecal incontinence, with a reported incidence of 0% to 30%. The frequency of this complication varies widely depending on the surgical group. For example, in a recent randomized trial in which 38 patients underwent internal sphincterotomy, no patients developed a change in continence, as formally analyzed by the Jorge and Wexner continence index. In contrast, an older, large, retrospective analysis of patients returning surveys after sphincterotomy showed an alarming rate of 5.3% for "accidental bowel movements", and 35% for incontinence of flatus. Certainly, this study was biased toward reporting complications, and technical improvements have since occurred. None the less, such data led to caution in the application of sphincterotomy in some settings. Certain patients are at increased risk for postoperative incontinence and in these cases this procedure should be considered cautiously. These patients include individuals who have undergone previous anal surgery, previous episiotomy, or a third degree vaginal tear during childbirth. Others at risk are patients with inflammatory bowel disease, irritable bowel syndrome, chronic diarrhea, diabetes, and the very elderly. In these patients, anorectal physiology studies and endoanal ultrasound should be performed to confirm the presence of increased internal sphincter tone prior to surgery. Occasionally at the time of surgery no fissure is discovered. In these cases it is best to abort the planned sphincterotomy.

Other invasive procedures have been tried but are not commonly in use today. Anal dilation procedures have been used in the past, and were effective in many patients. However, high recurrence rates and relatively high rates of incontinence – probably caused by the uncontrolled nature of the sphincter disruption – have led to this technique being abandoned. Similarly, midline internal sphincterotomy has been used but poor wound healing and incontinence problems were more pronounced than in lateral internal sphincterotomy. Anal mucosal advancement flap therapy still has a place in the surgical armamentarium. This procedure, which involves resection of the involved mucosa and advancement of normal proximal mucosa into the defect, is useful for patients with persistent or recurrent fissures and low or normal sphincter tone.

Pharmacological sphincter tone-lowering therapies have gained prominence in the last several years because, while less effective than surgery, they avoid the potential morbidity of gas or fecal incontinence. The most prominent of the recent pharmacological therapies is topical nitrate therapy. The biological basis for this therapy is the recognition that nitric oxide is the neurotransmitter responsible for muscular relaxation in the internal anal sphincter. In several studies topical glyceryl trinitrate ointment (0.2% twice daily for 8 weeks) and isosorbide dinitrate (2.5 mg three times daily for 4 to 8 weeks) have resulted in fissure healing in approximately 60% to 80% of patients. However, one relatively large randomized trial including 132 patients showed no difference between glyceryl trinitrate and placebo in fissure healing, both resulting in healing in about 50% of patients. In the same trial, 34% of the patients experienced headaches with the nitrate therapy, and 6% experienced orthostatic hypotension. It is worth noting that some of these patients received therapy for as little as 4 weeks, rather than the full 8 weeks of therapy utilized in other trials.

Several trials have randomized patients to lateral internal sphincterotomy versus topical nitrate therapy for chronic fissures. In one trial 0.5% or 0.25% nitroglycerin applied three times per day was compared to lateral internal sphincterotomy. Of patients in the internal sphincterotomy group, 89.5% had healed by 6 weeks, while 29.5% of the patients in the nitroglycerin group had healed. This was highly statistically significant. There were no cases of incontinence in either group and patients were significantly more satisfied with their treatment in the sphincterotomy group. Another trial compared lateral internal sphincterotomy with 0.2% glyceryl trinitrate paste applied three times per day. In the sphincterotomy group 97% of patients had healed in 8 weeks, while 60.6% of patients in the glyceryl trinitrate group had healed; this result was statistically significant. The patients who had not healed were crossed over into the sphincterotomy group and the fissures subsequently healed in 12 of 13 patients. Compliance was found to be poor in the glyceryl trinitrate group, because of side effects and perceived lack of effect. Presumably the intensive nature of the therapy, with three times per day dosing contributed to this problem. Minor incontinence to flatus was transiently experienced by two (6.9 %) patients, but resolved within 2 months.

Botulinum A toxin injection (20 units injected into the internal anal sphincter bilaterally) has been shown to heal anal fissures, although the mechanism is unclear. This potent neurotoxin binds to presynaptic cholinergic nerve terminals and inhibits the release of acetylcholine at the neuromusclular junction. The effect remains for 3 to 4 months, until new nerve terminals are regenerated. The site of action of the botulinum toxin is unclear, however, because the smooth muscle of the internal sphincter would not be expected to be relaxed with acetylcholine receptor blockade. A published randomized trial of 50 patients showed healing in 96% of patients treated with botulinum toxin compared to healing in 60% of patients treated with topical nitrate therapy, there were no adverse effects from the botulinum toxin treatment. The healing was durable, with no recurrences in 15 months of follow-up. Advantages of botulinum toxin therapy include its apparent efficacy, its ease of administration and its reversibility. None the less, it is not in common usage at the time of writing, perhaps because of rare cases of serious morbidity that have been reported.

Other pharmacologic therapies have been proposed, based on the neuromuscular blockade of internal anal sphincter contraction. These therapies include calcium channel blockers, alpha-adrenergic receptor agonists, beta-adrenergic receptor agonists and parasympathomimetics. None of these therapies is well established to date.

In summary, while lateral internal sphincterotomy is the definitive treatment for chronic anal fissures, medical therapy with nitrates or other agents avoids the rare possibility of fecal incontinence. Some authors feel these medical therapies are labor intensive, relatively ineffectual, and significantly morbid and, therefore, lateral internal sphincterotomy should be the first line therapy for chronic fissures. Other authors argue that a trial of 8 weeks of pharmacologic therapy is warranted, those patients failing nitrates or other medical therapy then being offered surgery. Botulinum toxin shows promise as an alternative therapy.

Anorectal abscesses

Anorectal abscess is a common condition seen in emergency departments, primary care offices, and surgical clinics. While the evaluation and treatment of this condition is usually straightforward, complex and recurrent cases challenge even the most experienced colorectal specialist.

Etiology

The most accepted theory as to the etiology of anorectal abscess is the "cryptoglandular theory". The anal crypts open into the anus at the dentate line and extend into the underlying sphincter muscle. Presumably, anorectal abscesses start with infection or inflammation of the anal glands at the base of the anal crypts. Initially a small, intersphincteric abscess is formed. This can enlarge and extend laterally, superiorly, or inferiorly into surrounding tissues, resulting in the several anatomic types of abscess and fistula.

Crohn's disease and HIV infection are associated with anorectal abscesses and fistulas, although the vast majority of patients with anorectal sepsis have no such predisposing condition. Other uncommon causes include carcinoma, tuberculosis, actinomycosis, radiation, trauma, and foreign bodies. Abscesses are classified according to the space occupied by the abscess cavity, and the types include perianal, ischiorectal, intersphincteric, deep postanal space, and supralevator abscess.

Clinical presentation and evaluation

Similar to abscesses elsewhere in the body, pain, erythema, soft-tissue swelling, and occasional fever are the presenting symptoms and signs of an anorectal abscess. The presentation will vary depending on the location of the abscess. For perianal and ischiorectal abscesses (Figure 13.3), patients complain of progressive pain in the perianal region or buttocks. Fever may or may not be present. An exquisitely tender, erythematous mass is usually obvious on physical examination, with or without surrounding cellulitis. Postanal-space abscesses are a variation of the ischiorectal abscess, but they are more difficult to diagnose because this space is surrounded by muscle inferiorly and superiorly. The patient complains of symptoms suggestive of an anorectal abscess, but the physical examination may show no external signs of an abscess. A careful digital rectal examination or an examination under anesthesia may reveal a tender posterior mass. A deep postanal-space abscess can spread laterally into the ischiorectal spaces leading to a "horseshoe" abscess.

The symptoms of intersphincteric abscesses are the same as those above, but the physical examina-

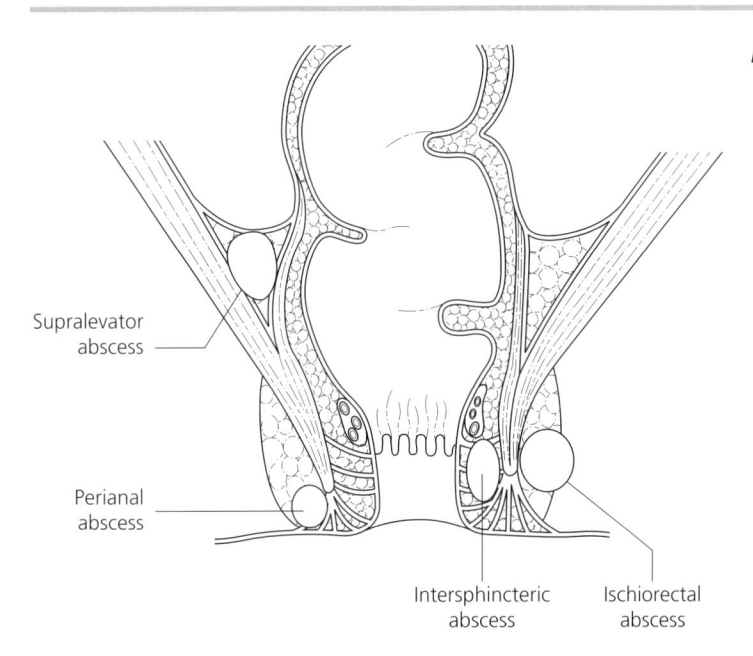

Figure 13.3 Types of anorectal abscesses.

tion is subtle. External signs are generally absent but digital rectal examination reveals swelling, tenderness, and sometimes fluctuance. The patient may be unable to tolerate the examination because of pain, in which case an examination under anesthesia is required. Finally, supralevator abscesses are rare and extremely difficult to diagnose. They may originate from diverticular or pelvic inflammatory diseases in addition to the usual cryptoglandular source. The presentation is of progressive pain with or without fever. Digital rectal examination can reveal a tender mass within the rectum.

Imaging studies are occcasionally used to detect an anorectal abscess, particularly a supralevator abscess. In these conditions it is important to identify associated diverticulitis, pelvic inflammatory disease, or Crohn's disease as the underlying etiology. The optimal treatment will depend on the results of imaging studies; CT scanning, gastrointestinal contrast imaging, and endorectal MRI or ultrasound have been used, depending on the clinical course. In some centers ultrasound is routinely used in the drainage of perianal infections to help localize the collections. As already mentioned, anorectal sepsis can occasionally be the initial presentation of inflammatory bowel disease, and an index of suspicion must be maintained for this etiology.

Treatment

Treatment of an acute anorectal abscess is urgent incision and drainage. A delay in the drainage of an abscess, even with antibiotic treatment, will result in further tissue destruction and increase the possibility of a severe or necrotizing soft-tissue infection. The technique of the drainage procedure varies depending on the location of the abscess. For the most part, infected spaces are left open to heal by secondary intention. However, some groups advocate "primary suture" closure of the debrided cavity under antibiotic coverage as an alternative technique.

Perianal and ischiorectal abscesses are the most common type and are treated similarly. They can often be drained in the outpatient setting. With the patient in the left lateral or prone jackknife position, the skin overlying the mass is prepared and local anesthesia is infiltrated. Note that the effectiveness of local anesthesia in the acidic tissues of an abscess may be diminished, and general or regional anesthesia may be needed. A cruciate incision over the most fluctuant area is usually made and the loculations inside the cavity are "broken up" using a finger or instrument, to ensure that all pus is drained. Incisions nearer to the sphincter muscles are preferable, as this creates a shorter fistula tract if a fistula eventually develops. Some surgeons remove the corners of the "cross" to increase the size of the opening. Usually, gauze packing is placed inside the cavity and removed on the first postoperative day. Sitz baths are prescribed at least twice per day. Antibiotics are used only when significant cellulitis is present or if the patient is immunocompromised. An alternative method for drainage is to use a smaller incision with placement of a 10 to 16 French "mushroom" catheter into the cavity. Patients are discharged with the catheter in place and instructions for sitz baths. The catheter is removed once the suppuration has resolved.

Postanal-space abscesses are usually treated in the operating room under general or spinal anesthesia. An anal retractor is inserted and the posterior anus is examined. The postanal space may be entered via an internal sphincterotomy in the posterior midline. If a horseshoe abscess has developed the lateral extensions should be drained by counter-incisions into the ischiorectal fossae.

Similarly, an intersphincteric abscess is usually treated in the operating room under general or spinal anesthesia. An anal retractor is inserted, and the point of maximal fluctuance is identified within the anus. Often, a crypt internal opening can be identified at this site. An incision is made over this area and the internal sphincter muscle fibers are spread for wide drainage of the purulence into the anus. The edges are sometimes marsupialized for hemostasis.

The optimal treatment of supralevator abscesses depends on the underlying cause of the disease. As mentioned, it is important to obtain preoperative imaging to define the etiology. In draining a supralevator abscess, one should avoid the creation of an extrasphincteric fistula. Therefore, an abscess arising from ascending cryptoglandular disease should be drained into the rectum. An abscess arising from pelvic diseases may be drained either into the rectum or via the ischiorectal fossa, depending on where the fluctuance is greatest. In addition, transabdominal drainage is sometimes most appropriate for a pelvic abscess, and bowel resection may be required depending on the source.

In general it is not recommended that fistula tracts be addressed at the time of drainage of an abscess, even if the internal opening is clearly identified. The majority of abscesses will heal without a persistent fistula. This area is somewhat controversial with some authors advocating immediate fistulotomy if a low fistula is identified.

Perianal sepsis in the immunosuppressed patient deserves special consideration. Patients with AIDS, solid organ transplantation, malignancies, steroid therapy, and insulin-dependent diabetes mellitus may be expected to have increased susceptibility to severe infections, as well as poor wound healing after surgical interventions. A retrospective review of 83 such patients treated with early abscess drainage and fistulotomy reported similar outcomes when compared to immunocompetent patients. None the less, the potential for life-threatening infection, such as necrotizing soft-tissue infection is increased in immunocompromised patients, and they should be treated promptly with surgical drainage and antibiotics and closely observed.

Perianal abscesses in Crohn's disease are usually a manifestation of fistula disease, and are discussed below.

Fistula in ano

An anorectal fistula is an abnormal communication between the anal or rectal lumen and the perianal skin. These fistulas are classified according to their relationship to the anal sphincter muscles. Fistulas may be intersphincteric (the most common), transsphincteric, suprasphincteric, or extrasphincteric.

Etiology

Anorectal fistulas are sequellae of anorectal abscesses. Occasionally, a patient with a fistula will have no antecedent episode of abscess, and the etiology is presumed to be a subclinical episode of perianal suppuration. Trauma, Crohn's disease, tuberculosis, and hidradenitis suppurativa are rarer etiologies for perianal fistulas.

Clinical presentation and evaluation

The clinical hallmark of an anorectal fistula is the persistent drainage of purulent material from an opening in the perianal skin. Symptoms may be intermittent, with temporary closure of the opening followed by recurrent drainage. Physical examination and proctoscopy are usually diagnostic, revealing a perianal site draining purulent material spontaneously or at the time of digital rectal examination. Evaluation in the outpatient setting may be difficult because of patient discomfort, and in these cases an examination under anesthesia is required. Blunt-tipped probes, hydrogen peroxide injected via an angiocatheter, or dilute blue dye may be used to define the fistula tract in the operating room.

Radiologic testing is occasionally useful, especially in the complex patient with multiple fistulas, recurrent fistulas, and/or Crohn's disease. The most commonly used studies are an endoanal ultrasound or MRI with endoanal coil. Fistulogram, the injection of contrast dye into the fistula, is also used to define the size and direction of the tract.

Treatment

The treatment of fistula in ano is primarily surgical. The type of surgical treatment depends on the anatomy of the fistula tract with respect to the sphincter muscles. In many instances, the exact location of the fistula tract will not be identified until the time of surgery. None the less, the path of the fistula tract can often be predicted on the basis of Goodsall's rule, which states that fistulas draining to the skin anterior to the anus will open via a radial tract into the anus or rectum, while fistulas with posterior external openings will drain into the posterior midline via a curved tract. Exceptions to this rule will be encountered, especially with very long tracts.

Superficial, intersphincteric and low transsphincteric fistulas are treated with a similar surgical approach (Figure 13.4). Simple fistulotomy may be performed safely when it involves division of the internal sphincter only or a very small portion of the external sphincter. The entire tract should be identified if possible, using a probe or an injection, although vigorous probing must be avoided to avoid the creation of false fistula tracts. The tract is opened along the probe, and the granulation tissue at the base is cauterized or curetted to destroy it. Marsupialization of the edges is optional. The wound is left open, and postoperative sitz baths, stool softeners, and analgesics are used.

Fistulotomy has the disadvantage of the risk of postoperative incontinence, particularly in patients with preoperative sphincter dysfunction. Situations in which there is an increased risk for postoperative incontinence include multiparous females, fistulas traversing the anterior sphincters, and patients who have undergone previous anorectal surgical procedures. Alternative treatments for low fistulas include advancement flaps, fibrin glue injection, or the use of a seton. In our institution, definitive treatment of a fistula not amenable to fistulotomy involves an advancement flap procedure, while non-cutting setons are used as a temporizing measure to bring perianal sepsis and inflammation under control, in preparation for a definitive fistulotomy or advancement flap. While reports of the successful use of fibrin glue for anorectal fistulas exist, we have had little success with this technique at our institution.

Suprasphincteric and extrasphincteric fistulas are rare fistulas extending above the level of the anorectal ring, where the levator ani muscles insert. These fistulas cannot be treated with fistulotomy, because of ensuing incontinence. Non-cutting setons, advancement flaps, and fibrin glue injection are treatment options. Similar to supralevator abscesses, a pelvic source of sepsis may be present. If an obvious cryptoglandular connection is not found, a thorough search for another source is indicated.

In patients with Crohn's disease or tuberculosis, medical therapy is the dominant mode of treatment. In Crohn's disease, perianal fistulas may be

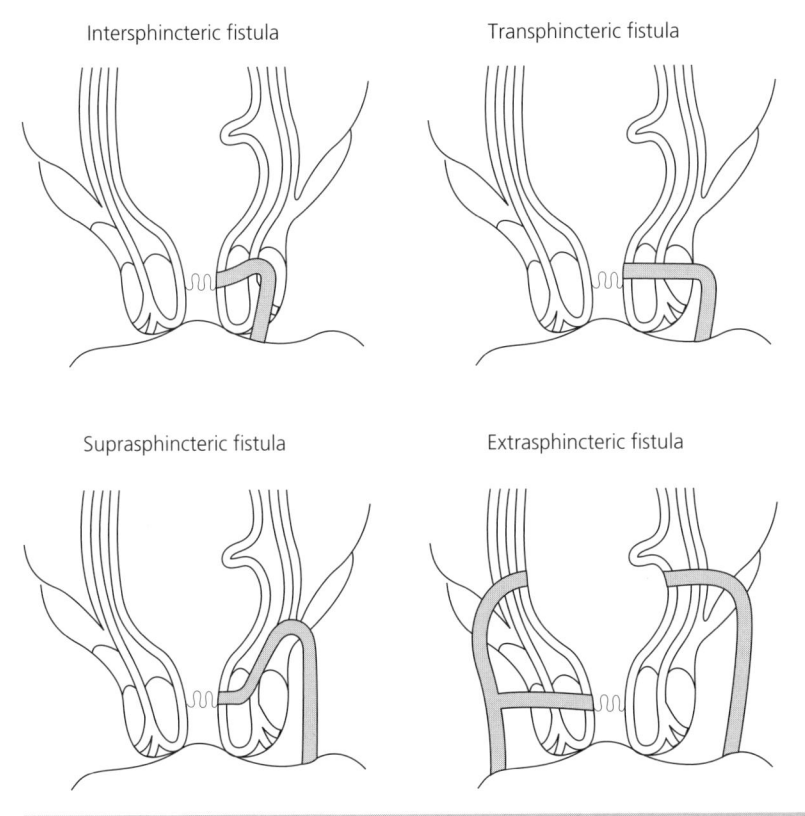

Figure 13.4 Types of anorectal fistulas.

Intersphincteric fistula

Transphincteric fistula

Suprasphincteric fistula

Extrasphincteric fistula

multiple and recurrent, and the management may be complicated by ongoing proctitis, inflammatory scarring, and fecal incontinence. Medical treatments include metronidazole, other antibiotics, azathioprine, other immunosuppressive agents, and infliximab, a monoclonal antibody directed against tumor necrosis factor. Success rates of approximately 60% have been reported with the use of these agents, although fistulas often recur once medical therapy is stopped.

Perianal abscesses in Crohn's disease are usually associated with fistulas. They should be surgically drained, using a non-cutting seton through the fistula tract or via a surgical incision, sometimes with the insertion of a drainage catheter. Standard surgical therapies, such as the fistulotomy and advancement flap procedures, are contraindicated in Crohn's patients with active anorectal inflammation. One exception is the non-cutting seton, which can be used as definitive therapy to control perianal sepsis, even where active inflammation is present. In Crohn's patients without active anorectal inflammation, patients may be treated with fistulotomy or advancement flap; some authors recommend the use of perioperative antibiotics in this setting. Fecal diversion or proctectomy is occasionally required in severe perianal Crohn's disease.

Pilonidal disease

A pilonidal sinus is generally an asymptomatic tract from the skin into the subcutaneous tissues overlying the sacrococcygeal region. The tract opening is usually 3.5 to 5 cm posterior to the anus, and it may have hairs protruding from the opening. The lesion usually comes to medical attention when the sinus or cyst becomes infected forming a pilonidal abscess. Pilonidal sinuses, cysts, and abscesses occur predominantly in young Caucasian men.

Etiology

The etiology of pilonidal disease was previously an area of controversy. The predominant early theory was that the sinus was congenital. It has been proposed that the sinus is a vestige of the medullary canal or neural tube, a dimple remaining after disappearance of the embryologic "human tail", a dermoid remnant buried during folding of the neural canal or the equivalent of an avian "preen gland". In fact, congenital sinuses do occur and are likely to be due to the etiologies proposed above. However, most routine pilonidal sinuses presenting in adults are acquired and are discussed further below. It is, none the less, important to remember that a sinus may be of the congenital type, although these are usually lumbar rather than sacral, communicate with the spinal canal and contain no hair.

The theory that pilonidal sinuses are acquired lesions is supported by the observation of recurrences after complete sinus removal, suggesting de novo formation of another sinus. Furthermore, there are no follicles or glands in the wall of the cyst to explain the formation of the hairs found inside. The proposed mechanism of sinus formation is by penetration of external hairs into enlarged midline hair follicles, leading to a foreign body–granuloma reaction and chronic, low-grade infection with subsequent enlargement of the sinus and/or cyst. Discomfort or discharge from chronic infection or frank abscess formation within the sinus are frequent presentations.

Clinical presentation

The clinical and pathological features of pilonidal disease are well established. Patients present with a small opening or openings in the presacral region, often with hairs protruding. The hairs are usually not attached to the inside of the cavity. A midline sinus is felt to be the entry point for the offending hairs, but lateral openings may also be present and probably represent secondary drainage sites for the chronic infection. An infected cyst will have symptoms of pain and tenderness, usually with a mucoid or purulent discharge. A frank abscess is a tender mass with erythema and induration. Grossly, the sinus leads to a tract or cyst containing granulation tissue, debris, and hairs. Histologically, the sinus and cyst are lined by squamous epithelium. No skin appendages are present within. Acute and chronic inflammation are marked by inflammatory cells, including foreign-body giant cells.

Treatment

Treatment options are primarily surgical, although simply shaving the lumbosacral area may help to ameliorate the course of the disease. Antibiotics are used only when significant cellulitis is present, or in the immunocompromised patient. Many different surgical procedures have been used in the treatment of pilonidal disease, and a definitive procedure of choice has yet to be established. Several general points may be made. First, acute abscesses must be treated by urgent incision and debridement, with the wound usually left open to heal by secondary intention. It is possible that this will provide definitive treatment; a second procedure may, however, be required. Second, it was traditionally felt that the entire cyst or sinus should be surgically removed, leaving a large tissue defect that would heal secondarily or be under excessive tension when closed. However, complete en bloc excision is not always necessary, as evidenced by the success of several procedures that leave the cyst wall in place. Currently, most recommended surgical treatments consist of incision, debridement, and destruction of the tracts, sometimes combined with special maneuvers to prevent recurrence.

A number of authors have reported decreased rates of recurrence by "lateralizing" their surgical incisions away from the midline where sinuses form. Abscess drainage and debridement through a lateral incision that is left open with simple excision and closure of the midline pits is recommended by a number of authors. Procedures with reportedly excellent results are the asymetric excision and primary closure techniques popularized by Karydakis and Bascom. With these procedures, incisions extending lateral to the natal cleft are used to excise the sinus tract. Mobilization of a medial flap and closure result in lateralization of the natal cleft skin and flattening of the cleft. It is proposed that the anatomic alterations decrease recurrence by moving the "at risk" skin laterally, placing the incision lateral to the midline and decreasing the depth of the cleft. In some severe cases formal flap closure may be required, often with the help of a plastic surgeon.

In conclusion, pilonidal disease is a common surgical problem affecting predominantly young men. When it presents as a frank abscess, emergent surgical drainage is essential. Several elective surgical procedures may be used successfully in the definitive treatment of this disease.

Hidradenitis suppurativa

Hidradenitis suppurativa is a chronic inflammatory skin disease that may involve the perianal region, axilla, groin, nipple areola, and other sites. The etiology is a chronic infection of apocrine glands leading to sinus and abscess formation, fibrosis, and scarring. While the disease is generally chronic and indolent, it can result in death from cancer or sepsis, especially in the perianal area. Epidemiologically, young adults are most commonly affected, and there is a male predominance.

Etiology

The pathophysiology of the disease is obstruction of the apocrine glands, with bacterial overgrowth, abscess formation and rupture into the surrounding tissues. Staphylococci and streptococci are the most common organisms, but in the perianal region enteric organisms are also often present.

Clinical presentation and evaluation

The clinical presentation of the acute disease is of a painful abscess requiring urgent drainage, or of the chronic disease is multiple draining sinus tracts and nodules. The perineum or buttocks may be extensively involved with sinuses, abscesses, cellulitis, or disfiguring fibrosis. Chronic disease with pain and drainage may result in social isolation and unemployment. The differential diagnosis of perianal hidradenitis suppurativa includes pilonidal disease, extensive perianal fistula disease, and suppurative dermatologic disorders, although these can usually be differentiated on clinical grounds. If there is any question as to the diagnosis, the apocrine gland involvement of hidradenitis suppurativa is distinct histopathologically.

Treatment

The treatment of hidradenitis suppurativa depends on the presentation. Acute abscesses require urgent drainage, usually accompanied by sitz baths and antibiotic treatment. After healing of any acute abscess, the definitive treatment is complete excision of the involved skin and all sinus tracts, with primary closure if possible. Chronic disease is unlikely to heal without surgical excision and may progress to involve a wider area of skin, making primary closure impossible. Larger wounds can be covered with a split-thickness skin graft, although ocasionally these wounds are left open to heal by scarring. Fecal diversion is rarely needed. It should be emphasized that medical therapies for hidradenitis suppurativa result in a high rate of recurrence, especially in the perianal area, and surgical excision should be considered the standard of care.

In summary, hidradenitis suppurativa should be treated by early surgical excision to prevent the complications of wide extension with debilitation and disfiguring scarring, squamous cell cancer, and sepsis.

Anal pruritis

Pruritis ani is the symptom of perianal itching that may be idiopathic or caused by underlying inflammatory or neoplastic disease. One to five percent of the population experiences this symptom which may be debilitating. Either gender may be affected but there is a male predominance.

The idiopathic form of pruritis ani may be associated with anal seepage, dietary factors, poor hygiene, underlying anorectal or systemic disease, radiation, and psychologic factors. The American Society of Colon and Rectal Surgeons lists the following drinks and foods that may exacerbate pruritis ani: caffeinated beverages, beer, milk, citrus fruit juice, chocolate, fruits, tomatoes, nuts, and popcorn. Some authors have proposed that an association between an excessive intake of caffeinated beverages and idiopathic pruritis ani is due to a coffee-induced fall in anal sphincter pressure.

Several studies have shown abnormal anal sphincter function and/or anal leakage in patients with idiopathic pruritis ani, leading to the hypothesis that pruritis is secondary to irritation due to mild soilage in these patients. Examination of the fecal flora has failed to show a significant difference between the flora of pruritis patients and that of matched controls. While excision of non-specific hypertrophied anal papillae has been proposed as treatment for idiopathic pruritis ani, a randomized trial failed to show an improvement with this approach. Other causes of pruritis ani include pinworms, psoriasis, eczema, dermatitis, anal infections, and underlying anal pathology such as fissures or hemorrhoids.

Traditionally, it was felt that the majority of patients with pruritis ani had the primary or idiopathic form of the disease, but recent evidence suggests that underlying pathology may be present more often than previously thought. In a study of 109 patients with the chief complaint of perianal itching and/or burning, patients were examined thoroughly for the presence of underlying colon or anorectal disease. Only 26% of these patients were found to have idiopathic pruritis ani without an underlying pathology. For the remaining 75% of patients the associated pathologies were as follows: hemorrhoids (20%), anal fissures (12%), rectal cancer (11%), idiopathic proctitis (6%), squamous cell cancer of the anus (5%), ulcerative proctitis (5%), condyloma accuminata (5%), adenomatous polyps (4%), colon cancer (2%), fistulas and abscesses (2% each) and premalignant anal lesions (1%). While perianal skin conditions such as lichen sclerosis, Paget's disease, and Bowen's disease are always discussed as potential etiologies of pruritis ani, in the study above these conditions were rarely present.

The clinical presentation is usually characterized by a gradual onset of symptoms, including perianal itching and burning. As symptoms progress, the perianal skin may become tender, friable and blistered secondary to scratching. Regardless of the underlying cause, pruritis ani can progress to the point where the patient is incapacitated by his or her symptoms.

Pruritis ani is usually categorized as primary (idiopathic) or secondary. Grading schemes of the severity of the perianal irritation have been proposed. One classification divides the condition into three grades of severity

1. mild – perianal erythema only
2. moderate – erythema with abrasions and some exudate
3. severe – all of the above plus skin ulcerations and severe exudate.

Another scheme classifies the macroscopic skin appearance into four groups

1. no gross abnormality
2. reddened skin
3. ridged and edematous skin
4. coarse, white, ridged, and edematous skin.

The work-up of pruritis ani includes a thorough history, which will often give clues to the etiology. The physical examination includes inspection of the perianal skin, which may reveal erythema, abrasions, thickening, or ulcerations. Any suspicious areas should be biopsied. Digital rectal examination, anoscopy, and proctosigmoidoscopy should be performed to rule out coexisting anorectal pathology, especially anal or rectal cancer. Colonoscopy should be considered, especially in patients over 50 years of age, given the possible association of pruritis with colorectal cancer and polyps. Any abnormal skin or lesion should be biopsied.

Treatment of secondary pruritis is obviously directed at the underlying pathology. Symptomatic treatment of pruritis ani includes improving perianal hygiene, increasing dietary fiber, and the application of topical steroid creams and drying agents. Recommendations for hygienic care include gentle washing with water or baby wipes, then using gauze, cotton, or corn-starch powder to keep the area dry. Soaps and medicated or perfumed powders should be discontinued. Also, scratching and vigorous cleaning or scrubbing should be avoided, as trauma will usually exacerbate the problem. Most patients will experience symptomatic relief with these measures.

Fecal incontinence

Fecal incontinence is the debilitating condition in which a patient is unaware of the occurence of defecation or is unable to control defecation until a socially acceptable time. This condition is present in 2.2% of community-dwelling adults in the US, but it is thought to be under-diagnosed because of the reluctance of patients and families to discuss it. Of concern is the fact that many patients and physicians do not realize that medical and surgical treatments are available. Fecal incontinence is the second most common cause of institutionalization in the elderly, and may be present in up to 47% of nursing-home patients. While a number of treatment options exist, the ideal procedure or medication to correct fecal incontinence has yet to be described.

Etiology

Incontinence is commonly caused by damage to the anal sphincters during childbirth or anorectal surgical procedures. Because of the link with vaginal delivery, 60% to 75% of patients with fecal incontinence are women. The external anal sphincter is the most important muscle in continence, and its function is often disrupted in incontinent individuals. It is important to note that even procedures that involve no direct cutting of the external anal sphincter muscle may result in damage because of uncontrolled stretching during digital examination or retractor placement. Furthermore, pudendal nerve injury secondary to prolonged labor, chronic excessive straining because of constipation, or pelvic floor descent may lead to sphincter dysfunction and incontinence.

Because normal continence requires intact pelvic floor muscles and anorectal sensation, as well as intact sphincters, abnormalities of the S2–S3 nerve roots or the levator ani muscles may contribute to incontinence. In addition, the reservoir function of the rectum is important for continence, and rectal accomodation must be adequate for the volume of stool presented. Even normal patients may experience leakage when an excessive volume of stool enters the rectum, for example in severe diarrhea. Finally, cognition is a requisite for continence, and severe dementia or delerium may lead to incontinence.

Incontinence is associated with rectal prolapse in several conditions. First, direct sphincteric stretching may occur when the rectum prolapses through the sphincter muscles. Second, the pudendal nerves may be damaged bilaterally because of inordinate stretching during prolonged straining to defecate. Finally, intussuscepted bowel may over-stimulate the rectoanal inhibitory reflex, resulting in reflex relaxation of the internal sphincter and stool leakage.

Clinical presentation

Patients often present to a colorectal surgeon, gynecologist, or gastroenterologist with the chief complaint of leakage or uncontrolled passage of gas or stool. Sometimes the patient will only obliquely discuss the problem, and the physician must question them directly regarding incontinence.

Evaluation

The history and physical examination are helpful in evaluating this problem. Important components include the number, types, and difficulties of vaginal deliveries, past history of anorectal surgery, frequency of incontinence, and its impact on the patient's lifestyle. Information on the frequency of incontinent episodes, and whether gas, liquid stool, or solid stool is involved, helps the physician to assess the severity of the problem. In women, urinary incontinence may be present as a component of pelvic floor weakness. A urologic assessment may be warranted, as certain surgical procedures for fecal incontinence may exacerbate a urinary problem. Furthermore, a urologic procedure may be able to be performed concurrently with surgery for fecal incontinence.

The lithotomy or prone jackknife position may provide good visualization for the evaluation of incontinence. Perineal, vaginal, and rectal examinations are indicated to look for signs of injury, adequacy of sensation, and the integrity of the levator and anal sphincter muscles. Some authors recommend further evaluation after straining on the commode to detect hemorrhoidal or rectal prolapse.

Anorectal physiology testing, including transanal ultrasound, anorectal manometry, and pudendal nerve testing, has been prospectively evaluated and found to change medical and surgical management decisions significantly. Anorectal manometry documents resting and squeeze pressures of the anal sphincters, urge threshold, and pudendal nerve function. Testing pudendal nerve terminal motor latency is important to determine whether or not surgery will be of benefit. There is a greater failure rate for primary sphincter repair in patients with pudendal neuropathy when compared to individuals with normal nerve function.

The degree and location of internal and external anal sphincter defects should be quantitated by endoanal ultrasound. Cine-defecography is another important preoperative test, especially if associated lesions such as a rectocele are suspected. Importantly, these tests may identify problems such as pelvic floor dyssynergia, that respond better to biofeedback treatments than to surgery.

Colonoscopy should be performed in most patients to detect the presence of associated or causative lesions. Validated questionnaires should be included in the preoperative and postoperative assessment of patients with incontinence. Several incontinence severity scales have been developed, including the Wexner fecal incontinence score, the Pescatori scale, the American Medical Systems scale and the Rockwood et al. scale; these are valuable for assessing the severity of incontinence and response to treatment.

Treatment

Mild fecal incontinence and incontinence due to dyssynergia of the pelvic floor muscles may be treated successfully by non-surgical means. Dietary modifications, bulk-forming agents, and anti-diarrheal medications may be extremely helpful. Self-administration of enemas or suppositories in the morning may clear the rectum and allow patients to avoid defecation, and therefore incontinence, during daytime activities. Biofeedback exercises may be therapeutic in patients with impaired pudendal nerve function. Patients with incontinence in the setting of diarrhea may achieve continence with successful diagnosis and treatment of the diarrhea.

A number of surgical options exist for fecal incontinence, depending on the etiology. The most common operations are primary sphincter repair or muscle flap repairs, and these are most appropriate for patients with well-defined sphincter defects. Primary sphincter repair (sphincteroplasty) and the puborectalis transfer procedure have the advantages of using local muscle under voluntary control. Success rates of 50% to 80% have been reported with sphincteroplasty operations. Obviously, normal pudendal nerve function is required for muscular control with these repairs.

For patients with sphincter defects larger than 90 degrees or abnormal pudendal nerves, muscle flap procedures such as the gracilis or gluteal flap are indicated. In these procedures, a pedicled flap of muscle is mobilized, transferred, and wrapped around the anal sphincters. Patients learn to voluntarily control contraction of the muscle to control continence. Alternatively, the muscle flap may be stimulated artificially to improve contraction, as with the "dynamic graciloplasty". Success rates of approximately 60% have been achieved using the dynamic gracilloplasty, and 40% to 80% success rates have been reported for the flap repairs in general. Postoperative biofeedback treatments help with motor control of the transposed muscle.

Another surgical option is the total pelvic floor repair, which combines anterior external sphincter plication, levatorplasty, and postanal repair. This combined repair is recommended for women with neurogenic fecal incontinence and pelvic floor weakness.

Chronic sacral spinal nerve root stimulation with an implanted electrode has shown early promise in patients with neurogenic fecal incontinence, however, it is available only at specialized centers. Artificial or mechanical anal sphincters have been developed but have been associated with frequent infection, malfunction, and erosion, and are therefore used infrequently. A multi-center, prospective, controlled trial is ongoing to examine this approach. A novel non-surgical treatment is the Procon device, a balloon catheter with an electronic sensor inserted into the anus, to prevent soilage and allow rectal emptying at an appropriate time. The device is in experimental use. Finally, patients with incontinence and severe neurologic or cognitive disease are probably best treated with a permanent diverting sigmoid colostomy.

Rectovaginal fistulas

A rectovaginal fistula is an abnormal communication between the vagina and the rectum or anus, the latter is properly termed an anovaginal fistula. Because the distal 9 cm of the anterior rectum is separated from the posterior vagina only by the thin rectovaginal septum, this area is susceptible to the formation of such connections after injury.

Etiology

The common etiologies of this uncommon entity include obstetric injuries, penetrating and blunt perineal trauma, complications of gynecological or colorectal operations, inflammatory bowel disease, anorectal fistula disease, radiation injury, cancer of the anus, rectum, or vagina, infections such as lymphogranuloma venereum or tuberculosis, endometriosis, diverticulitis, lymphoproliferative malignancies, and congenital abnormalities. Only the acquired forms of the disease will be discussed.

Obstetric injuries are the most common etiology for rectovaginal fistulas, and approximately 1 in 1000 vaginal births is complicated by rectovaginal fistula formation. Complicated deliveries, including forceps deliveries, midline episiotomies, and prolonged second stage of labor with possible ischemia of the rectovaginal septum are associated with fistula formation. While most such injuries are recognized and successfully repaired, some injuries remain unrecognized, and some repairs are complicated by infection, breakdown of the repair, and fistula formation.

Up to 10% of women with Crohn's disease may develop rectovaginal fistulas. Amongst women with perianal disease complicating Crohn's disease, the presence of a rectovaginal fistula confers a worse prognosis, and such patients are more likely to require proctectomy or fecal diversion surgery. With Crohn's disease, the origin of an enterovaginal fistula may be elsewhere in the gastrointestinal tract. Patients with ulcerative colitis also may develop rectovaginal fistulas, although with lesser frequency.

Radiation treatment for endometrial and cervical cancer is complicated by rectovaginal fistulas more frequently than is radiation treatment for other diseases. The incidence of fistula formation is between 0.3% and 6%, is related to the radiation dose, and is more common in the setting of a previous hysterectomy. Most fistulas resulting from radiation therapy are high in the vagina and present within 2 years of treatment, although delayed presentations may occur. A fistula presenting very early – during treatment – is most likely to be due to tumor eroding through the rectovaginal septum. Some radiation-induced fistulas are associated with rectal strictures, and patients should be questioned and examined for the presence of a stricture. Many patients have a history of radiation proctitis with anterior anorectal ulceration developing into a fistula. It is important to rule out recurrent cancer as the etiology of the fistula, and biopsies should be taken.

Clinical presentation and evaluation

The symptoms of a rectovaginal fistula may vary from infrequent passage of flatus from the vagina to the passage of stool from the vagina. Vaginitis with a foul-smelling discharge may be present. Sometimes the fistula may be overlooked when associated with fecal incontinence due to obstetric trauma or other anorectal fistulas, as in Crohn's disease.

Examination of the patient with symptoms or signs of a rectovaginal fistula is performed in order to visualize the fistula and assess its size and location. Anoscopy and proctoscopy are the tools generally used. Small fistulas may be difficult to visualize, and may be better identified by using a lacrimal duct probe through the vaginal opening while viewing the distal rectum with an anoscope.

Examination under anesthesia may be required, and instillation of saline into the vagina and air into the rectum with the patient in the lithotomy position can be helpful. If the fistula is not identified directly, a tampon may be placed in the vagina, followed by the administration of a saline-retention enema colored with blue dye, such as methylene blue. After 15 minutes the tampon should be examined and the diagnosis of rectovaginal fistula must be questioned if there is no blue staining on the tampon. In these cases, a fistula originating from another portion of the gastrointestinal tract may be present. Examination should also assess the condition of the anal sphincters, and rule out associated anorectal diseases such as additional fistulas, strictures, or malignancy.

Diagnostic studies are occasionally needed in the evaluation of a rectovaginal fistula. Contrast gastrointestinal studies such as a barium enema, upper gastrointestinal series, vaginogram, or fistulogram may be helpful, especially in patients with Crohn's disease, in whom a colonoscopy is usually indicated as well. Some radiologists have reported good success rates using endoanal ultrasound or MRI to identify the site of rectovaginal fistulas.

Anal manometry, and possibly endoanal ultrasonography, should be used to quantify the degree of sphincter dysfunction in patients with any signs or symptoms of fecal incontinence. Some authors recommend endoanal ultrasonography and/or formal functional testing prior to rectovaginal fistula repair in all patients, given the high rate of associated sphincter injury and the need to alter the surgical approach if incontinence is contributing to the clinical picture. In patients with rectovaginal fistula secondary to obstetrical injury, the rate of associated incontinence is as high as 48%, and even this may be an underestimation, given the masking of incontinence symptoms by the symptoms of the fistula. Preoperative ancillary continence testing is mandatory in patients with symptoms of incontinence, sphincter disruption, or a history of prior failed repairs, especially if trauma is the etiology of the fistula.

Treatment

Some rectovaginal fistulas, such as small fistulas associated with obstetric trauma, are likely to heal spontaneously and watchful waiting for several months is reasonable. In the setting of active proctitis or active infection, for example with Crohn's disease, medical therapy is indicated and is required prior to surgery, as discussed below. However, definitive treatment for rectovaginal fistulas is primarily surgical.

In inflammatory conditions such as Crohn's disease, the disease must be aggressively treated medically prior to any attempt at surgical repair. Only with successful remission of associated proctitis is a repair likely to succeed. Some minor fistulas may close with aggressive medical therapy alone. Acute infection must also be resolved prior to attempting surgical repair. A waiting period of 3 to 6 months is suggested in such cases. Many authors recommend waiting a minimum of 10 weeks following surgical or other trauma prior to operative repair of a fistula.

Many procedures for repair of rectovaginal fistulae have been described, and the options have been reviewed in detail in several excellent surgical articles. The basic principles that guide all repairs include

1. excision of the fistula tract
2. interposition of healthy tissue
3. not attempting repair in the setting of active inflammation or infection
4. always repairing associated anal sphincter injuries.

For low rectovaginal fistulas, transvaginal, transanal, and perineal approaches have all been successfully used by gynecologists and colorectal surgeons. Probably the most commonly used approach by colorectal surgeons is the transanal advancement flap repair, in which a flap of rectal mucosa, submucosa, and circular muscle is mobilized and distally advanced to cover the rectal defect with healthy tissue.

High rectovaginal fistulas are usually repaired using a transabdominal approach. If the fistula is secondary to surgical or other trauma, mobilization of the rectovaginal septum with debridement and closure of the two defects plus interposition of omentum is usually successful. However, if the rectal and vaginal tissues are abnormal because of radiation, inflammatory bowel disease, or malignancy, bowel resection or other means of interposing normal colon will generally be required for successful healing.

Reported outcomes after rectovaginal fistula repairs vary widely in the literature, depending on the underlying etiologies and technical procedures used. While standard repairs have been reported to have cure rates in excess of 80% in some series, other authors have reported high rates of initial failure requiring multiple procedures. In addition, patients with healed fistulas may not be satisfied with their surgery because of persistent incontinence that was unrecognized preoperatively or not successfully treated by the procedure chosen. Patients suffering from recurrent rectovaginal fistulas – those that have failed previous attempts at repair – comprise a difficult group of patients who should seek treatment by a specialized surgeon.

The treatment of rectovaginal fistulas in inflammatory bowel disease deserves special attention. As discussed above, failure of any surgical approach is likely in the presence of active inflammation. Therefore, intensive medical therapy aimed at resolving the active proctitis is required prior to surgery. Patients who are relatively asymptomatic may be best treated by medical therapy alone. For symptomatic patients in whom the proctitis can be controlled medically, several retrospective series have shown eventual success in a majority of patients. For low rectovaginal fistulas, local procedures are ultimately successful in approximately 70% of patients, however, multiple surgeries and fecal diversion may be required. For high fistulas treatment is often unsuccessful and some authors recommend permanent colostomy for all such patients because of the poor results.

Patients with radiation-induced fistulas also present a difficult management scenario, and many surgeons recommend permanent diversion with colostomy or ileostomy. If surgical repair is chosen, incorporation or interposition of non-irradiated tissue is recommended, such as proctectomy with a pull-through coloanal anastamosis. In the setting of radiation, it is critical to rule-out recurrent malignancy as the etiology of the fistula, and to identify and treat associated strictures if present.

One novel approach, the fibrin glue technique, has been described recently. In this procedure the fistula tract is curretted to remove granulation tissue, then commercial or autologous fibrin glue is applied into the tract. While several series have shown promising results, several others have shown poor success with this technique and it has not gained wide popularity. Finally, for patients in poor medical condition or in whom a repair is extremely unlikely to be successful, permanent fecal diversion provides excellent palliation and is probably the best treatment option.

Rectal prolapse

Rectal prolapse is full-thickness intussusception of the rectal wall resulting in protrusion of the rectum through the anus (procidentia). This disease is more common in women, and it is a component of the category of diseases associated with weakness of the pelvic floor. Anatomic features in complete rectal prolapse include circumferential rectorectal intussuscption, lack of sacral fixation of the rectum, redundancy of the sigmoid colon, weakness or diastasis of the levator ani muscles, and a deep rectovaginal pouch.

Evaluation

Patients with rectal prolapse may present initially with the complaint of protrusion of the rectum through the anus. Alternatively, they may complain of constipation, difficulty with evacuation of the rectum and the need to digitally assist with defecation. Fecal incontinence may be a sequelum of chronic rectal prolapse, and mucus or bloody discharge is common. Between 80% and 90% of adult patients with rectal prolpse are women. Other patients at risk include elderly and infirm patients, patients with severe psychiatric illnesses, and those with sacral nerve or spinal cord injuries. In addition, a history of chronic constipation, obstetric trauma, or prior anorectal or gynecologic surgical procedures is often present.

Internal rectal intussusception (internal prolapse) may present as difficult or painful defecation or tenesmus, and may lead to full rectal prolapse in a few patients. While up to 50% of normal patients may demonstrate internal prolapse during straining, only a few of these patients will develop full rectal prolapse.

Certain positions and maneuvers, such as straining in the sitting position on the commode, may be required in order to demonstrate rectal prolapse in the office setting. The prolapsed rectum contains circumferential mucosal folds. Longitudinal folds suggest an isolated mucosal prolapse, not procidentia. A patulous anus or pelvic descent may be obvious. The perineal skin may show evidence of pruritis ani, mucus discharge, or decreased sensation because of perineal nerve damage. Digital rectal examination and proctosigmoidoscopy reveal the resting and squeeze strength of the anal sphincters, as well as focal colitis or a solitary rectal ulcer. A colorectal mass must be excluded by colonoscopy in any patient presenting with bloody discharge or obstructed defecation.

Diagnostic studies may help in selecting the optimal surgical approach. Defecography and a balloon expulsion test may demonstrate the internal or full intussusception and rule out associated disorders such as anismus, or anatomic abnormalities such as a rectocele. If there is a question of fecal incontinence or constipation, it is helpful to have anal manometry and/or colonic transit studies. These will help to determine whether a perineal or abdominal approach, with or without colon resection, can correct the prolapse without making other problems worse. Colonoscopy is often indicated to screen for associated tumors or lesions that would change the operative approach. A solitary rectal ulcer, due to injury and ischemia of the prolapsing mucosa, may be seen on lower endoscopy.

Treatment

Rectal prolapse requires operative treatment to prevent incarceration and possible strangulation of the bowel, and to prevent progressive sphincter and perineal nerve damage. An operation may be performed electively, unless the patient has incarceration of the prolapsed rectum, in which case the procedure must be urgently or emergently performed to prevent strangulation of the bowel.

For patients with complete rectal prolapse, the most effective operation is the suture rectopexy via an abdominal approach, with or without colon resection. Laparoscopic techniques have been advocated to lessen the perioperative morbidity. The operation is similar technically to a sigmoid colectomy, with similar recovery and potential complications. An alternative approach is through the perineum. With perineal procedures, the rectosigmoid is resected and reanastamosed transanally or the redundant rectal mucosa is stripped off the rectum transanally, while the muscularis of the rectum is "bunched up" distally. Thereby the laxity is removed from the rectum. These procedures are especially useful for cases of very symptomatic internal prolapse and for extremely elderly and bedridden patients.

It is important to consider the functional status of patients in selecting a surgical approach to the internal or complete prolapse. Patients suffering from preoperative fecal incontinence, diarrhea, or irritable bowel syndrome are good candidates for an abdominal rectopexy procedure without sigmoid resection, but may be worsened by sigmoid resection or by perineal approaches. Conversely, preoperative constipation may be worsened by abdominal fixation procedures, unless sigmoid colon resection is also performed. Patients with associated cystocele or bladder or uterine prolapse may be better treated transabdominally, because the associated disorders can be corrected simultaneously.

Potential complications of surgery vary with the operative approach. While abdominal operations for prolapse have low recurrence rates of 0% to 3%, they may result in greater physiologic stress and an increased risk of perioperative cardiopulmonary complications when compared to the perineal approach. Laparoscopic techniques have improved the morbidity of this approach for high-risk patients. Another concern with the abdominal approach is the potential for sexual dysfunction because of injury to the hypogastric and other sacral nerves. Finally, the abdominal rectopexy carries a significant risk of constipation, unless sigmoid resection is also performed.

Perineal approaches have the major disadvantages of increased recurrence and decreased improvement of incontinence. These concerns are countered by a lower operative morbidity and the possibility of using locoregional anesthesia. In some centers, very low recurrence rates of 5% to 10% are reported, however, rates of 16% to 27% are more typical with perineal approaches. The abdominal approach is therefore the preferred operation for patients who are candidates for general anesthesia.

Internal intussusception requires treatment only if it is severely symptomatic, particularly with obstructed defecation that does not respond to non-operative treatments such as dietary fiber. Multiple rubber-band ligations of the redundant rectal mucosa may be therapeutic, or a formal operation for prolapse may be required.

Anorectal stenosis

Anorectal stenosis is narrowing of the anal or rectal canal because of a functional disorder or scar tissue, in the latter case it is termed a "stricture".

Etiology

The most common cause of anal stenosis is surgical trauma, most frequently hemorrhoidectomy. In a series of 212 anal strictures, 87.7% were caused by hemorrhoidectomy. The proper technique of hemorrhoidectomy leaves bridges of normal anoderm intact between the resected segments and minimizes the risk of this rare complication. Rates of stricture formation from 0% to 1.5% have been reported after open hemorrhoidectomy. Other etiologies of anorectal stenosis include inflammatory bowel disease, radiation therapy, chronic diarrhea, chronic laxative abuse, anorectal abscess or fistula, sexually transmitted diseases, and previous reconstruction of a congenital abnormality.

Anal stenosis may be classified either by its severity or by the level of the abnormality. In "mild" stenosis, a well-lubricated index finger can be inserted through the stenosis. In "moderate" stenosis, forceful dilation is required for insertion of the index finger, and in "severe" stenosis the little finger cannot be inserted without forceful dilation. In terms of the location, "low" is at least 0.5 cm distal to the dentate line, "middle" is within 0.5 cm of the dentate line, and "high" is at least 0.5 cm proximal to the dentate line.

Clinical presentation

The most common presenting symptoms and signs are difficult stool evacuation, painful bowel movements, decreased caliber of the stool, and bleeding. The history will usually reveal a previous anorectal surgery or a disease associated with anorectal scarring. Patients will often have a long history of self-treatment with laxatives, enemas, and suppositories to maintain bowel movements. Examination with anoscopy or proctoscopy usually confirms the diagnosis; examination under anesthesia may be required. A functional stenosis will relax under anesthesia and may be accompanied by a fissure, while a stricture due to scarring will not relax. Obviously, examination should rule out a malignant, premalignant, or inflammatory lesion, especially if the stricture is secondary to surgery for polyp or mass removal. Biopsies of any suspicious tissue should be taken.

Treatment

Mild anal strictures may be treated initially by non-operative methods, including stool softening agents and bulk-forming agents. In the past, repeated dilation with a finger or dilator was recommended; this approach may be helpful in patients with Crohn's disease, or in those who have had previous radiation, in whom perineal surgery carries greater risk. However, operative or patient dilation must be prescribed with extreme caution because of the risk of incontinence or uncontrolled sphincter disruption if the scarring is made worse.

Cases of stenosis that fail to resolve with these measures usually require surgery. It is generally recommended that patients wait at least 3 to 6 months after the original procedure to allow postoperative inflammation to completely resolve. The type of procedure performed depends on the etiology and location of the stenosis. Most of the procedures can be performed as "outpatient" surgery.

For patients with functional stenosis low in the anal canal caused by a hypertonic anal sphincter, a sphincterotomy is the best option. For anal strictures due to scarring, simple stricture incision or "release" has been used, but should probably be avoided because of the possibility of rapid contraction of the resulting scar tissue, making the stricture worse.

Anoplasty procedures are designed to bring pliable tissue into a scarred, narrowed anal canal. Many variations on the anoplasty procedure have been designed, including advancement flaps, adjacent tissue transfer flaps, and rotational flaps. Complications are rare and include infection, failure to correct the stenosis, recurrent stenosis, ischemia and slough of the flap, suture line dehiscence, pruritis ani and minor incontinence, which is usually temporary.

When the etiology of the stricture is irradiation or inflammatory bowel disease, the outcome is less favorable, and patients should be notified of a higher risk of failure. Proctectomy or diversion is sometimes required in these cases if anoplasty procedures are unsuccessful. As with rectovaginal fistulas, any active infection or inflammation must be treated prior to an attempt at surgical stricture correction.

High rectal strictures

High rectal strictures are uncommon in the absence of previous surgery or cancer. Possible etiologies include inflammatory conditions such as inflammatory bowel disease or diverticulitis. Several case reports of actinomycosis as the etiology of rectal stricture have been published. These strictures should respond to treatment directed at the underlying cause. Ischemic rectal strictures have been reported following aortic surgery. These can often be treated with endoscopic dilation procedures, however, surgical resection, myotomy, or fecal diversion may also be required.

Anastomotic strictures

A special category of anorectal stenosis is that of anastomotic strictures, these strictures occur after rectal or anal anastomosis. A definition of an anorectal anastomotic stricture is a chronic narrowing or obstruction to the flow of intestinal contents resulting in clinical signs or symptoms of obstruction. Some authors consider anastomoses through which a 12 mm sigmoidoscope cannot pass to be strictures. The incidence of anorectal anastomotic strictures is between 5% and 80%.

Additional predisposing factors that contribute to this complication include postoperative anastomotic dehiscence, tissue ischemia at the anastomosis, excessive tension at the anastomosis, and the use of a 25 mm or smaller circular stapling device. Other possible factors are obesity, radiation therapy, incomplete "donuts" at the time of a stapled anastomosis, and postoperative pelvic sepsis. In one retrospective series of 27 patients with severe rectal anastomotic strictures, 21 (78%) had precedent anastomotic leaks. This is a key factor in the pathogenesis of strictures, especially those that cannot be treated by endoscopic dilation because of extensive scarring. Furthermore, because lower anastomoses have a higher risk of dehiscence and leak, they are at higher risk for stenosis. While any type of anastomosis may be complicated by stricture formation, a recent meta-analysis concluded that stapled colorectal anastomoses are more likely to form a stricture than hand-sewn anastomoses.

The diagnosis is established radiologically with a barium enema or by the inability to pass a 12 mm colonoscope through the anastomosis. A key step in the diagnostic evaluation of a patient with an anastomotic stricture is to exclude recurrent cancer.

Most anastomotic strictures are less than 1 cm in length, and are amenable to endoscopic treatment such as dilation with a bougie, finger, or hydrostatic balloon. While this is safe and effective in most patients with short strictures, perforation may be a rare complication. Occasionally laser or electrocautery incision is combined with dilation techniques. More recently, successful transanal use of a stapling device has been reported for treatment of short strictures. All of these techniques are suitable for short strictures less than 1 cm in length. Up to 28% of patients have a severe stenosis that cannot be treated effectively by endoscopic measures. In such patients, several operative techniques may be used, depending on the location of the anastomosis, the length of the stricture, and the condition of the pelvis at re-operation.

In situations where pelvic scarring is not prohibitive, particularly in the high rectum, the anastomotic stricture may be resected with the creation of a new anastomosis. When conditions are unfavorable, rectal resection is avoided by using the "Soave" technique for coloanal anastomosis. The rectal musculature is left *in situ*, and a coloanal "pull-through" anastomosis is performed. This avoids dissection in an extensively scarred pelvis, with potential for severe bleeding or injury to surrounding structures. In a recent series, 19 patients were successfully treated with this technique with relatively good functional results.

A permanent ostomy is the final common pathway for patients whose strictures cannot be treated by other means. The use of an expandable metal stent in the setting of rectal anastomotic stricture has been reported, similar to its palliative use in patients with malignant strictures who are not candidates for surgical resection. The stent was reportedly effective and tolerated for at least 1 year, and surgery was avoided. This approach should be limited to patients in whom other measures have failed and for whom surgery poses an unacceptable risk, given the unknown safety of long-term rectal stenting for benign disease.

Sexually transmitted diseases of the anus

Many patients with anorectal sexually transmitted diseases will present to the gastroenterologist or colorectal surgeon with anorectal pain, sepsis, or mass. Diagnoses include condyloma accuminata, herpes simplex, syphilis, gonorrhea, chlamydia, lymphogranuloma venereum, and AIDS. These problems are particularly prevalent in homosexual men and HIV-positive patients. Collaboration with a specialist in infectious diseases may be extremely helpful in these cases.

Anal condylomata

Human papillomavirus (HPV) infection may lead to condyloma accuminata of the anus or perianal skin. The HPV-6 and HPV-11 subtypes most commonly cause anal warts. Patients with HIV and patients who engage in anal intercourse are predisposed to the development of anal condylomata, although this is not universal. The lesions are grossly visible as typical warts, papules, and flat erythematous lesions that may be painful, pruritic, or friable. It is important to perform proctoscopic examination of patients with the presentation of anal warts to evaluate associated internal disease.

There is a risk of dysplasia and squamous cell carcinoma in patients with anal warts, especially in the setting of immunosuppression. In a series of 174 patients treated for anal condylomata, 20 high-grade dsyplasias and 1 invasive cancer developed during follow-up, with rates much higher in HIV-positive patients. Some authors recommend screening immunosuppressed patients with anal warts every 3 to 12 months with proctosigmoidoscopy and anorectal Papanicolaou smears, depending on the severity of the lesions.

Treatment options include topical solutions such as podofilox, imiquimod, bichloroacetic acid, trichloroacetic acid, and fluorouracil; local injections such as interferon; and surgical excision or destruction with electrocautery, cryotherapy, or laser. Surgical excision or destruction provides a more complete and durable elimination of warts compared with topical therapies. None the less, recurrence rates with surgical or topical therapies are extremely high in immunodeficient patients. Furthermore, surgical, laser, and electrocautery techniques place the health-care team at risk for HPV and HIV infection because of sharps exposures and aerosolized virus.

When treating anal condylomata, any indurated, ulcerated, or fixed lesion and lesions greater than 1 cm in size should be biopsied to exclude malignant or pre-malignant disease. Widespread or invasive disease such as the giant condyloma acuminatum, or "Buschke–Lowenstein tumor", may require wide excision with flap reconstruction, with or without fecal diversion.

Herpes simplex virus

Herpes simplex virus can cause a chronic, relapsing anorectal infection, similar to genital herpes. Symptoms include constipation, tenesmus, and severe anorectal pain or burning, exacerbated by a bowel movement. Pruritis may also be present, as well as inguinal lymphadenopathy. Unlike genital herpes, more severe neurologic dysfunction may occur such as urinary retention and sacral neuralgias. Painful vesicles or ulcerations may be present in the anal canal or on the anoderm during an acute episode. Viral cultures and/or microscopic examination of scrapings from ulcers are diagnostic, revealing multinucleated giant cells and intranuclear inclusions. Antiviral treatment with systemic or topical acyclovir may reduce duration and frequency of episodes, but is not curative. Chronic suppression with acyclovir may be used, particularly in AIDS patients.

Syphilis

The presentation of anorectal syphilis is similar to that of syphilis elsewhere, but with the presence of a chancre. However, unlike chancres in other locations, an anal chancre may be painful. Secondary syphilis may ensue if the infection is untreated, with systemic signs of illness, diffuse rash, and possibly condylomata lata at the anal area. Diagnosis is made by serologic testing or by scraping lesions and identifying spirochetes by darkfield microscopy.

Penicillin is the recommended treatment for both patients and contacts.

Gonorrhea

Gonococcal proctitis is a common condition in homosexual men, and women with genital gonorrhea may develop this condition from the adjacent spread of disease. Many patients are asymptomatic, however, symptoms can include constipation, pruritis, tenesmus, and a mucoid or bloody discharge. The anal canal is usually spared, with rectal proctitis predominating. A mucopurulent discharge in the rectum is the most common finding. Systemic disease can cause severe illness. The diagnosis is made by rectal culture swab with gram stain showing intracellular gram-positive diplococci. Rectal culture increases diagnostic sensitivity and should be performed. Antibiotic treatment according to local susceptibilities is recommended for the patient and their contacts.

Chlamydia

Chlamydia proctitis and lymphogranuloma venereum are caused by infection with *Chlamydia* spp., which are obligate intracellular pathogens. Proctitis and inguinal lymphadenopathy are the dominant features. Proctitis may be severe and may extend into the proximal sigmoid colon. Strictures and fistulas resembling Crohn's disease may develop if the disease is untreated. Unfortunately, the diagnosis may be difficult because of the intracellular location of the parasite.

Human immunodeficiency virus

Patients with AIDS, especially homosexual patients, have a high prevalence of gastrointestinal and anorectal diseases. This may be due in part to decreased mucosal resistance because of decreased CD4 T lymphocytes in the intestinal mucosa. In addition, anoreceptive intercourse may predispose an individual to anorectal problems. Patients with AIDS are susceptible to the infectious diseases described previously, as well as to a number of opportunistic infections and tumors.

Opportunistic anorectal infections that may be found in AIDS patients include *Mycobacterium avium-intercellulare*, candida, cryptosporidium, isospora, and cytomegalovirus. Perianal sepsis or ulceration may be the presenting symptom of *Mycobacterium avium-intercellulare* infection, or the symptoms may be diarrhea and abdominal pain due to proximal intestinal involvement. Biopsy with staining for acid-fast bacilli is diagnostic. Therapy is primarily medical, with surgery reserved for complications such as fistulas, abscesses, or intestinal obstruction. Other opportunistic infections are also medically treated.

Anal ulcers

Anal ulcers are common in patients with AIDS. These may be due to infectious or other benign diseases or malignant disease. Etiologies include fissures, syphilis, chancroid, chlamydia, cytomegalovirus, herpes simplex virus, cryptococcus, mycobacterial infection, AIDS-specific ulcers, lymphoma, squamous cell carcinoma, Kaposi's sarcoma, trauma, and idiopathic causes. Because of the wide variety of etiologies, clinical diagnosis is difficult. Biopsies and cultures are the best means of diagnosis. These should be performed in a controlled environment under anesthesia, where risks to the patient and health-care personnel are minimized. Biopsies, culture swabs, and ulcer scrapings should be sent for routine histology, acid-fast and gram stain, bacterial and viral culture, and darkfield microscopy. Treatment is directed toward the underlying etiology, although fecal diversion is sometimes required when pain is unremitting.

Anal neoplasms

Anal cancers account for only 1.5% of digestive tract cancers in the US. These neoplasms differ from the more common colorectal adenocarcinomas in histology, staging, biologic behavior, and treatment.

In recent years, our understanding of the etiology of anal cancer has changed significantly, as have the treatment algorithms. Epidemiologic studies have shown that the development of anal cancer is usually associated with HPV infection. Furthermore, the traditional treatment of anal canal cancer, namely abdominoperineal resection with permanent colostomy, has been replaced for most patients by organ-preserving chemotherapy and radiation therapy.

The American Joint Committee on Cancer and the Union Internationale Contre le Cancer use "anal canal" to refer to tumors from the anal verge to the anorectal ring and "anal margin" only for tumors outside the anal verge. However, several authors recommend classification of anal cancers according to their location above or below the dentate line, because of different lymphatic drainage. We use the former classification because the treatment of anal cancers follows this division. In clinical practice, however, it is important to specify the anatomic location of a tumor with respect to the anatomic landmarks of anal verge, dentate line, and anorectal ring, given the published inconsistency in the use of the terms "anal canal" and "anal margin".

Cancers of the anal canal

Epidermoid carcinoma

Squamous cell cancer and its variants are the most common anal cancers. Squamous cell, basaloid (cloacogenic), and mucoepidermoid carcinomas of the anal canal may be grouped together as epidermoid cancers. These cancers arise from the transitional or cloacogenic mucosa above the dentate line. Histologically they can be non-keratinizing or keratinizing. Cancers below the dentate line are usually well-differentiated squamous cell cancers with keratinization. "Basaloid" carcinoma is a variant of squamous cell cancer, with characteristic palisade nuclei in the periphery of clumps of tumor cells. Eosinophilic necrosis, nuclear atypia, and giant cells may also be found in these lesions.

Epidemiologically, anal cancers are rare tumors with a female preponderance. About 3400 new cases are diagnosed each year in the US. Inflammatory conditions were once thought to be risk factors for anal cancer, but subsequent studies have shown no definite link between anal cancer and inflammatory bowel disease, hemorrhoids, fissures, or fistulas. On the other hand, sexually transmitted diseases in general and HPV infection in particular have been strongly linked with anal cancer. The evidence for this association includes population-based and case-control studies surveying sexual behavior and history of sexually transmitted diseases in patients with anal cancer, as well as the finding of HPV DNA in 88% of anal cancer specimens by polymerase chain reaction analysis. Furthermore, women with cervical cancer, known to be caused by HPV, are at significantly increased risk of developing anal cancer. However, obvious anogenital warts are absent in the majority of patients.

Another risk factor for anal cancer is chronic immunosuppression, especially post-solid organ transplantation immunosuppression but probably also AIDS. Renal transplant recipients have a risk 100 times that of the general population. Long-term corticosteroid use and cigarette smoking may also be risk factors, but the evidence for these associations is less clear.

Some authors have advocated screening high-risk patients for anal canal cancer. Populations particularly at risk include homosexual men, immunosuppressed individuals, and women with a history of cervical cancer, especially when a history of HPV infection coexists. Possible screening tools include anal cytology smears and/or anoscopy with biopsy. However, unlike cervical cancer, anal cytology for high-grade dysplasia or cancer is relatively difficult to interpret. Furthermore, the presence of high-grade dysplasia is less predicitve of progression to cancer than in cervical cancer. In several small series, no patients followed for anal dysplasia progressed to invasive cancer over a 5-year period. In summary, screening for anal cancer is not currently performed because of the rarity of the disease and technical limitations.

Bleeding is the most common symptom of anal cancer and is present in 45% of patients, it leads to the misdiagnosis of hemorrhoids in many patients. Other symptoms include pain, the sensation of an anal mass, tenesmus, pruritis, and change in bowel habits. Physical examination in patients presenting with these complaints should include examination of the inguinal and femoral lymph nodes, examination of the perianal skin, anoscopy, and proctoscopy. Squamous cell cancers are often flat, firm, indurated, and/or ulcerated lesions. Incisional biopsy of any suspicious mass should be performed. Excisional biopsy should be performed only for very small and superficial lesions. Transanal ultrasound is helpful in defining the depth of invasion of the mass.

Staging work-up includes a history and physical examination, focusing on the findings and risk factors mentioned above. Blood tests include a complete blood count, electrolytes and liver function tests. A CT scan or MRI of the abdomen and pelvis can determine the local extent of disease and pelvic nodal and liver metastasis. Chest X-ray is indicated to evaluate for pulmonary metastasis.

The diagnosis of anal canal cancer is often delayed, and involvement of the underlying sphincter muscles and/or lymph node involvement are often present at the time of diagnosis. Anal cancer can spread by local extension, lymph node metastasis or hematogenous, dissemination. The size of the tumor is the most important prognostic factor.

Patients with tumors greater than or equal to 5 cm have a decreased survival compared to patients with smaller tumors. Nodal metastasis is also related to the size of the primary tumor, and is a major negative prognostic factor. The grade of the tumor also appears to affect the prognosis. Cancers above the dentate line metastasize to the superior rectal lymph nodes in approximately 40% of cases, and to the inguinal nodes in about 33% of cases, making it difficult to predict the draining lymph node basin. Cancers below the dentate line should drain more consistently to inguinal lymph nodes.

Staging of anal cancers is now done by a clinical system, reflecting the non-surgical treatment employed in the majority of patients. The prognostic value of tumor size and lymph node metastases is underscored by the staging, where any lymph node disease places the patient in stage III.

Traditionally, local excision or abdominoperineal resection was used to treat anal canal squamous cell cancers, however, local and regional recurrence rates were high (25% to 35% for abdominoperineal resection). This may reflect the rich lymphatic drainage of the anal canal and the propensity of this tumor for local invasion. In the 1980s neoadjuvant radiation therapy and chemotherapy were developed to address this problem and, unexpectedly, complete tumor eradication was found in many patients with this treatment, making surgery unnecessary. Radical surgery is now reserved for cases where primary radiation therapy and chemotherapy fail to eliminate the disease.

The original Nigro Protocol included 30 Gy of external irradiation to the primary tumor, pelvic lymph nodes, and inguinal lymph nodes. More recent studies have suggested better tumor response with higher radiation doses, although the side effects are more severe. The chemotherapy regimen includes 5-fluorouracil and mitomycin C, although cisplatin has shown early promise and may replace one of these agents. If the lesion disappears and the biopsies are negative, no further treatment is required. Complete response rates as high as 70% to 90% have been demonstrated. Frequent follow-up with history and physical examination approximately every 3 months is required for patients treated with combination therapy who initially have a complete response.

If residual tumor exists, abdominoperineal resection of the rectum and anus is performed 4 to 6 weeks after completion of the radiation therapy. Approximately 50% of patients failing to show a complete response with combination therapy can still be cured by abdominoperineal resection.

Prophylactic inguinal lymph node dissection is not indicated. However, gross disease in the groin, which may be present at the time of diagnosis or present as a recurrence, should be treated with lymph node dissection or radiation therapy. Distant metastasis is most frequently to the liver, and less frequently to lung or bone. Hematogenous metastasis eventually occurred in 10% to 17% of patients in combination therapy treatment trials. The benefits of additional chemotherapy in this setting are unknown, therefore patients should be encouraged to enter clinical trials.

Follow-up should be every 3 months for the first 3 years after treatment for cure, especially with primary chemoradiation as treatment. Recurrent disease can be cured by salvage therapy, and therefore should be identified as quickly as possible.

Overall 5-year survival for anal cancer is about 50% to 80% in various series. As mentioned above, size (T stage) of the tumor is the most important prognostic indicator. In a large series of patients from Minnesota who were treated primarily with chemoradiation, but a minority were treated with primary or salvage surgery, the overall survival was 57%. Survival by T stage was

- T1 – 63%
- T2 – 57%
- T3 – 33%
- T4 – 14%.

Improvement in these survival rates has probably been achieved with higher-dose radiation therapy, and further improvement is possible with the addition of platinum-based chemotherapy as mentioned above. Diagnosis of these tumors at an early stage is important to maximize survival. Clinicians must therefore maintain a high index of suspicion, especially when evaluating high-risk patients.

Adenocarcinoma

Adenocarcinomas of the anal canal are rare. They can arise from the spread of rectal adenocarcinomas or from the glandular tissue of the anal crypts. Their behavior and treatment are similar to that of rectal adenocarcinomas. Patients may present with complaints of pain, bleeding, or the presence of a mass. Local excision is used for small lesions less than 3 cm in size that are limited to the submucosa and have a well-differentiated histology. Otherwise, abdominoperineal resection is indicated. Adjuvant therapy is of unknown benefit.

Melanoma

Malignant melanoma accounts for 0.5% to 1% of anal canal cancers. These tumors present with rectal bleeding. Many patients have metastatic disease at the time of presentation, including lymphatic spread to the mesenteric lymph nodes and hematogenous spread to the liver and lungs. These tumors are resistant to chemotherapy, immunotherapy, and radiation therapy, therefore surgical therapy is usually recommended. However, survival is poor and 5-year survival rates are 15% to 17% following wide local excision or abdominoperineal resection. Abdominoperineal resection provides improved local control but may not improve survival over local excision.

Cancers of the anal margin

In general, cancers of the anal margin resemble skin cancers of the same histology elsewhere. Most patients present with symptoms of mild discomfort, itching, or bleeding. Most anal margin cancers are diagnosed late and misdiagnosis is common. Any questionable perianal lesion should be biopsied. Staging of anal margin cancers is the same as that for skin cancers elsewhere. The definitive treatment is usually wide local excision, as with skin cancers elsewhere.

Squamous cell cancer

The perianal skin may give rise to squamous cell carcinomas that resemble their counterparts in the skin elsewhere. Grossly, these tend to be slow-growing, ulcerated lesions with "rolled" edges. Histologically, these cancers are usually well differentiated with keratinization. Lymphatic spread, when present, is usually to the inguinal lymph node basin. Wide local excision with an approximate 1 cm margin can be curative if the lesion does not invade the underlying sphincter muscles. A 5-year survival rate of up to 88% has been achieved with selected patients treated with local excision alone, although local or inguinal lymph node recurrences occur relatively often, and are treated with re-excision or inguinal lymphadenectomy respectively.

If sphincter muscle invasion has occurred, abdominoperineal resection was traditionally the treatment of choice, because resection of the sphincter muscles will render the patient incontinent, and because metastasis along the superior and middle rectal nodes can occur. Currently, some authors advocate chemoradiation as primary treatment for sphincterinvasive anal margin cancers, and preliminary series of patients receiving such treatment are promising. For tumors greater than 5 cm in size, irradiation of the inguinal lymph nodes should also be performed.

Even with recurrent disease, prognosis of anal margin cancers appears to be much better than anal canal tumors, and local re-excision and inguinal lymphadenectomy should be performed when recurrences present, given the relative rarity of distant metastatic disease.

Basal cell cancer

Basal cell cancer of the anal margin is rare, and is more common in men than women. Central ulceration may occur as in squamous cell cancers. These lesions rarely metastasize, but inguinal lymphadenopathy may result from tumor-induced inflammation. Mild discomfort, itching or bleeding may occur, but misdiagnosis is common and delays treatment. Local excision with a margin of normal mucosa is the standard treatment. Local recurrence can occur in up to one third of patients and is treated with re-excision.

Perianal Bowen disease

Bowen disease of the perianal skin is a nonkeratinizing squamous cell carcinoma-in-situ. Like anal squamous cell cancer, perianal Bowen disease is associated with HPV infection. Epidemiologically, these lesions are most common in women in the fifth decade of life.

Perianal itching, burning, and bleeding are common presenting symptoms. On physical examination, an irregular plaque is seen that may have a scaly or moist surface. Invasive cancer rarely develops in these lesions, in only 2% to 6% of patients. Earlier studies suggested a high risk of associated skin or internal malignancies, as in Paget's disease. However, recent data suggest only a 5% incidence of other cancers in these patients, therefore a work-up for other malignancies is probably not indicated. Because these patients would be expected to be at higher risk for anal squamous cell cancer, vulvovaginal cancer, and cervical cancer because of the common viral etiology, examination of these areas should be performed. Examination is facilitated by the use of colposcopy and acetic acid "painting" to identify condylomata. It is worth noting that condyloma may contain high-grade dysplasia without a change in their gross appearance.

Treatment of perianal Bowen disease consists of wide local excision or destruction by other means. For excision, biopsies should be taken in four quadrants approximately 1 cm from the edge of the gross lesion to rule out microscopic extension of the disease. For larger lesions or lesions extending into the anal canal, wide excisions may be impossible to close without skin grafting or anal mucosal advancement flaps to prevent stricture formation. Given the lack of progression to invasive cancer, some clinicians have advocated other therapies for larger lesions that would require extensive surgery and flap closure, such as photodynamic therapy, laser ablation, topical 5-fluorouracil cream, or observation. Ablative techniques have the disadvantage of destroying the tissue so pathologic examination for invasive cancer is impossible. Also, large areas of ablation may be painful and slow to heal. Microscopic Bowen disease is not infrequently discovered incidentally on pathologic examination of specimens resected for other reasons such as hemorrhoidectomy. In these cases, many surgeons choose observation alone. Follow-up at 3- to 6-month intervals is recommended for all patients with Bowen disease, with ablation or resection of macroscopic recurrences.

Perianal Paget disease

Perianal Paget disease is a rare adenocarcinoma of the apocrine glands, which can present as an itchy, scaly plaque. Histologically, large, vacuolated cells are seen, called Paget cells, with eccentric nuclei and containing acid mucosubstances. If untreated, invasive adenocarcinoma will develop. Early lesions without invasion are treated with wide local excision; however, local recurrence is frequent and an adequate resection margin is essential. The margin may be difficult to identify, requiring multiple biopsies to determine adequate resection. Advanced lesions with underlying cancer may require an abdominoperineal resection. Clinically positive inguinal lymph nodes should be excised. About 25% of patients have metastatic disease at diagnosis, most commonly inguinal lymph nodes, pelvic lymph nodes, and liver, bone, lung, and brain. Between 52% and 73% of patients with Paget's disease harbor or will develop an underlying malignancy, therefore a work-up for other cancers is indicated.

Further reading

ANAL CANCER
Ryan DP, Compton CC, Mayer RJ. Medical progress: carconoma of the anal canal. *N Engl J Med* 2000; 342(11): 792–800.

ANAL FISSURE
Jonas M, Scholefield JH. Anal fissure. *Gastroenterol Clin N Am* 2001; 30(1): 167–181.

Richard CS, Gregoire R, Plewes EA, et al. Internal sphincterotomy is superior to topical nitroglycerin in the treatment of chronic anal fissure: results of a randomized, controlled trial by the Canadian Colorectal Surgical Trials Group. *Dis Colon Rectum* 2000; 43(8):1048–1057.

ANORECTAL ABSCESS AND FISTULA IN ANO
Schwartz DA, Pemberton JH, Sandborn WJ. Diagnosis and treatment of perianal fiistulas in crohn disease. *Ann Intern Med* 2001; 135: 906–918.

ANORECTAL SEXUALLY TRANSMITTED DISEASES
Beutner KR, Reitano MV, Richwald GA, et al. External genital warts: report of the American Medical Association Consensus Conference. *Clin Infect Dis* 1998; 27: 796–806.

ANORECTAL STRICTURES
Liberman H, Thorson AG. Anal Stenosis. *Am J Surgery* 2000; 179: 325–329.

FECAL INCONTINENCE
Rudolph W, Galandiuk S. A practical guide to the diagnosis and management of fecal incontinence. *Mayo Clin Proc* 2002; 77: 271–275.

Whitehead WE, Wald A, Norton NJ. Treatment options for fecal incontinence. *Dis Colon Rectum* 2001; 44(1): 131–142.

HEMORRHOIDS
Rowsell M, Bello M, Hemingway DM. Circumferential mucosectomy (stapled haemorrhoidectomy) versus conventional haemorrhoidectomy: randomised controlled trial. *Lancet* 2000; 355: 779–781.

HIDRADENITIS SUPPURATIVA
Endo Y, Tamura A, Ishikawa O, Miyachi Y. Perianal hidradenitis suppurativa: early surgical treatment gives good results in chronic or recurrent cases. *Brit J Dermatol* 1998; 139: 906–910.

PILONIDAL DISEASE
Akinci OF, Coskun A, Uzunkoy A. Simple and effective surgical treatment of pilonidal sinus. *Dis Colon Rectum* 2000; 43:701–707.

Da Silva JH. Pilonidal cyst: cause and treatment. *Dis Colon Rectum* 2000; 43: 1146–1156.

PRURITIS ANI
Daniel GL, Longo WE, Vernava AM. Pruritis ani: causes and concerns. *Dis Colon Rectum* 1994; 37: 670–674.

RECTAL PROLAPSE
Felt-Bersma RJF, Cuesta MA. Rectal prolapse, rectal intussusception, rectocele, and solitary rectal ulcer syndrome. *Gastroenterol Clinics N Am* 2001; 30(1): 199–222.

RECTOVAGINAL FISTULA
Tsang CBS, Rothenberger DA. Rectovaginal fistulas: therapeutic options. *Surg Clinics N Am* 1997; 77: 95–113.

Index

abdominal approaches to surgery
　rectal prolapse, 275–6
　rectovaginal fistulas, 274
abdominal examination, diarrhea (chronic), 39
abdominal pain
　colonic motility disorders, 207
　diverticular disease, 131
　ulcerative colitis, 58
abdominal wall defects, 12–14
abscesses
　anorectal, 264–6
　　anatomical aspects, 258, 264–5
　　clinical presentation and evaluation, 264–5
　　Crohn's disease, 107, 108, 267–8
　　etiology, 264
　　fistulas and, association, 266, 267–8
　　treatment, 265–6
　Crohn's disease, 106–7, 107, 108, 267–8
　in diverticulitis, intra-abdominal, 132
absorption see malabsorption and specific nutrients
abuse (physical and sexual) and irritable bowel syndrome, 247
acid steatocrit, 117
adenocarcinoma
　anal canal, 281
　anal margin, 283
　colorectal, histology, 178–9
　see also cancer
adenoma(s)/adenomatous polyps, 159
　in familial adenomatous polyposis, 137
　　chemoprevention, 139, 163
　　screening for/treatment, 139
　prior colorectal adenoma as risk factor for cancer, 173–4
　surveillance for cancer with, 188, 189
adenomatous polyposis, familial, 137–9, 167, 169

　cancer associated with, 137, 138, 139, 170
　　chemoprevention of, 139, 163
　clinical features, 136
　genetic testing, 138, 151, 153, 153–4, 172–3, 187–8
　genetics, 138, 167
　screening, 138–9, 187–8
　surveillance, 138–9, 188–9
　treatment, 139
adenomatous polyposis coli (APC) gene, 138, 167, 169
　common familial colorectal cancer and, 150
　function, 167
　testing for, 138, 151, 153, 154, 172–3, 182–3
　ulcerative colitis-associated cancer and, 73
adhesion molecule antagonists, Crohn's disease, 98
adjuvant therapy
　colon cancer, 190–1
　rectal cancer, 192–3
age-related occurrence
　colorectal cancer, 173
　diverticulitis, 129
　ulcerative colitis, 56
agenesis
　anal/anorectal, 17
　gastric, 6
AIDS see HIV disease
AJCC staging of colorectal cancer, 181
alosetron, irritable bowel syndrome, 248–9, 253
alpha-1-antitrypsin, fecal, 118
American Cancer Society, colorectal cancer
　screening guidelines, 184
　surveillance guidelines, 189
American College of Gastroenterology, colorectal cancer
　screening guidelines, 184
　surveillance for guidelines, 189
American Joint Committee on Cancer staging of colorectal cancer, 181

5-aminosalicylic acid see mesalamine
5-aminosalicylic acid-containing drugs
　Crohn's disease, 85–9, 104
　　efficacy, 87–8
　　in pregnancy and breastfeeding, 109
　　side-effects, 88, 88–9
　ulcerative colitis, 66–8
ampulla of Vater, familial adenomatous polyposis involving, 137
Amsterdam diagnostic criteria for hereditary non-polyposis colorectal cancer, 146, 147, 157, 170, 171
anal canal
　anatomy, 257–8
　cancers, 280–2
　development, 17
　see also anorectal region; anus
anal sphincters
　in anal fissure, hypertonicity and its management, 263–4
　anatomy, 206, 257, 258
　anorectal fistula in relationship to, 266
　　treatment of, 267
　EMG studies, 210–11
　fecal incontinence due to, 271
　　assessment, 271
　　treatment, 272
　function/physiology, 206, 259
　in manometry, 209, 210
　preservation in rectal cancer surgery, 192
　ultrasonography see ultrasonography, anal
anastomoses, intestinal
　in acute mesenteric ischemia surgery, 235
　stricturing, 277–8
　see also ileal pouch–anal anastomosis; ileal pouch–distal rectal anastomosis

285

Index

anemia
  Crohn's disease, 103
  in malabsorption, 120, 122
aneuploidy, 169
angiography
  diverticular hemorrhage, 133
  selective mesenteric, in mesenteric venous thrombosis, 239
  see also arteriography; magnetic resonance angiography
angioplasty, chronic mesenteric ischemia, 228
ankylosing spondylitis and Crohn's disease, 102
annular pancreas, 9
anoplasty, 277
anorectal function, assessment, 209–11
  manometry *see* manometry
anorectal region, 257–83
  acquired diseases, 259–83
    evaluation for, 259
  anatomy, 257–9
  developmental anomalies, 17
    see also anus
  physiology, 259
anorexia, laxative abuse, 47
anoscopy, 259
  hemorrhoids, 260
anovaginal fistulas, 272–4
Antegren®, Crohn's disease, 98
antibiotic(s)
  Crohn's disease, 91
    side-effects, 88–9
  diarrhea, 28, 29
    traveler's, 26, 28
  postoperative, in acute mesenteric ischemia, 235
antibiotic-associated *C. difficile see Clostridium difficile*
antibodies
  in Crohn's disease diagnosis, 83–4
  monoclonal *see* monoclonal antibodies
  in ulcerative colitis pathophysiology, 54, 54–5
anticoagulants, mesenteric venous thrombosis, 240
antidepressants, irritable bowel syndrome, 252
antidiarrheal agents, 27–8
antimotility agents, 28
antisense oligonucleotide, Crohn's disease, 98
a-1-antitrypsin, fecal, 118
antroduoden(ojejun)al manometry, 198–201

anus
  abscesses *see* abscesses
  anatomy, 257–9
  development, 17
  developmental anomalies, 17
  fissure, 262–4
  fistula between vagina and, 272–4
  physiology, 259
  pruritus, 269
  sexually-transmitted diseases *see* sexually-transmitted diseases
  stenosis *see* stenosis
  tumors, 279–83
  see also anal canal; anorectal function; anorectal region; perianal region; proctocolectomy with ileal pouch–anal anastomosis
aorta
  coarctation, mesenteric ischemia following repair, 236
  infrarenal (in mesenteric ischemia), bypass grafting from, 226, 227–8
  supraceliac (in mesenteric ischemia), bypass grafting from, 225, 226, 227, 228
APC see adenomatous polyposis coli gene
aphthous ulceration, Crohn's disease, 80
appendicitis, acute, vs Crohn's disease, 84
arterial supply, anorectum, 258
arterial thrombosis, mesenteric, 230
arteriography
  acute mesenteric ischemia, 231
  chronic mesenteric ischemia, 221–2
  nonocclusive mesenteric ischemia, 237
  see also angiography
arteriosclerosis/atherosclerosis, mesenteric arteries, 217, 220
arthropathy
  Crohn's disease, 101–2
  malabsorption, 122
  ulcerative colitis, 65–6
Asacol®
  Crohn's disease, 86, 87
  ulcerative colitis, 67
ascorbate (vitamin C) intake in colon cancer prevention, 165
Ashkenazi Jews
  common familial colorectal cancer in, 150
  ulcerative colitis in, 56
aspirin, colorectal cancer prevention, 163

Astler-Coller classification and modified system, 180–1
atherosclerosis/arteriosclerosis, mesenteric arteries, 217, 220
atresia
  biliary, 10
  duodenal, 7
  esophageal, 3–4
  gastric, 6
  intestinal, 14
  rectal, 17
autoantibodies
  Crohn's disease, 83
  ulcerative colitis, 54, 54–5
autonomic nervous system
  anorectum, 259
  dysfunction, in chronic intestinal pseudo-obstruction etiology, 203
azathioprine
  Crohn's disease, 92–4, 104, 105, 106
    in pregnancy, 109
  metabolism, 92
  side-effects, 89
  in ulcerative colitis, 68–9
    in pregnancy, 75

B cells, ulcerative colitis, 54
bacterial flora
  Crohn's disease pathogenesis, 79
  overgrowth in small intestine, 48, 205
    presentation, 121
    test for, 118, 121
bacterial infections, diarrhea, 22, 25
balloon distension in anal manometry, 210
balloon expulsion test, anorectal functional assessment, 211
balsalazide
  Crohn's disease, 86, 87
  structure, 86
  ulcerative colitis, 67–8
band ligation, hemorrhoids, 260–1
Bannayan–Ruvalcaba–Riley syndrome, 142
barium studies (incl. enemas)
  colorectal cancer screening, 185–6
    guidelines, 184
  Crohn's disease, 82–3
  malabsorption, 115
  small bowel transit, 196–7
  ulcerative colitis, 60–1
basal cell carcinoma, anal margin, 282
basal cell nevus syndrome, 143
BAX and Bax, 147, 169
behavioral treatment, irritable bowel syndrome, 254

Index

bentiromide test, 44, 119
Bethesda diagnostic criteria for hereditary non-polyposis colorectal cancer, 146, 147, 157, 170, 171
bile acids
  in colorectal cancer causation, 161, 176
  malabsorption by ileum, 36, 42, 44, 47–8, 119
    cholestyramine therapy, 119, 252
    tests for, 119
bile ducts
  congenital dilatation (=Caroli's disease), 11, 12
  development, 9
biliary tree/system
  in Crohn's disease, involvement, 101, 104
  development, 9
    anomalies, 10–12
  in ulcerative colitis, involvement, 66
biochemical tests, malabsorption, 122–3
biopsy, small bowel in malabsorption, 116
  see also histology
bismuth subsalicylate, 28
bleeding, rectal (and GI hemorrhage)
  diverticular disease, 131
    management, 133
  hemorrhoids, 260
  ulcerative colitis, 57
  see also blood, fecal
blood, fecal (rectal bleeding), occult, testing
  in chronic diarrhea, 41
  colorectal cancer screening, 184–5
    guidelines on, 184, 185
  see also bleeding, rectal
blood supply, anorectum, 258–9
bloody diarrhea see inflammatory diarrhea
BMPPR1A gene, 142
bone disease, metabolic, Crohn's disease and, 102
bone morphogenetic protein receptor 1A gene, 142
botulinum A toxin, anal fissure, 264
bowel movements in diarrheal illness, history-taking, 38
Bowen's disease, perianal, 282–3
brain and irritable bowel syndrome, 246, 248–9
breast cancer, Cowden syndrome, 142, 143
breast-feeding, Crohn's disease medications and, 109

breath tests
  bacterial overgrowth, 48
  carbohydrate malabsorption, 116, 117
  fat malabsorption, 117–18
  small-bowel transit studies, 197
brush border enzymes, 112
  deficiencies, 112
budesonide, Crohn's disease, 90
bulimia, laxative abuse, 47
bulking agents, 213
bypass grafting
  acute mesenteric ischemia, 233–4
  chronic mesenteric ischemia, 225–6, 227

C-reactive protein
  Crohn's disease, 123
  ulcerative colitis, 58, 59
calcium
  deficiency, signs and symptoms, 120
  intake, in colon cancer prevention, 162–3, 165, 166
  levels, measurement, 122–3
camptothecin analog, advanced colorectal cancer, 191
cancer (colorectal - predominantly carcinoma), 159–93
  chemoprevention, 139, 163–4
  common familial, 135–6, 149–50
    clinical features, 149
    genetics, 149–50
    screening/surveillance/treatment, 150
  diet as protective/preventive strategy, 73, 164–5, 166
  epidemiology, 160
  etiology/pathogenesis, 160–73
  hereditary, 135–7, 145–57, 169–71
    genetic discrimination, 152–3
    non-polyposis see non-polyposis colorectal cancer
    see also genetic testing; genetics
  in hereditary polyposis syndromes, 175
    familial adenomatous polyposis, 139, 174–5
    juvenile polyposis, 141–2, 175
  in inflammatory bowel disease see Crohn's disease; inflammatory bowel disease; ulcerative colitis
  natural history, 179–80
  pathology, 176–82, 182
  prior, as risk factor for second occurrence, 173–4
  process of progression to, 180
  prognostic factors, 178–9, 182
  risk factors, 173–6

  screening and surveillance for see screening; surveillance
  sites/distribution, 177
  staging, 180–2
  symptoms and signs, 182
  treatment, 190–3
    surgical see surgery
cancer (non-colorectal or in general)
  abdominopelvic (in general), Crohn's disease vs, 84
  anal, 279–83
    and HPV, 278, 280
  deaths in US (2002), 160
  in hereditary non-polyposis colorectal cancer, 145–6, 170
  in hereditary polyposis syndromes, 175
    Cowden syndrome, 142, 143
    familial adenomatous polyposis, 137, 138, 139, 170
    in Peutz–Jeghers syndrome, 140–1, 141, 175
  screening and surveillance for see screening; surveillance
carbohydrate(s)
  absorption, 111–12
  ingestion of poorly absorbed (and carbohydrate derivatives), 34
  malabsorption, 49, 112
    signs and symptoms, 120
    tests, 116–17
carbohydrate antigens, tumor-associated, prognostic value, 183
carcinoembryonic antigen, prognostic value, 183
carcinogenesis, colorectal, 180
carcinoid syndrome, diarrhea, 214
carcinoma
  anal canal, 280–1
  anal margin, 282, 283
  colorectal see cancer
  in Gorlin syndrome, 143
  see also specific histological types
carcinoma-in-situ, perianal, 282–3
Caroli's disease, 11, 12
ß-carotene intake in colon cancer prevention, 165
cataract, Crohn's disease, 103
ß-catenin, 169
  familial adenomatous polyposis and, 138, 167
CCK antagonist, irritable bowel syndrome, 249, 253
CD4+ (T helper) cells, Crohn's disease, 78
CDP571, Crohn's disease, 97
cecal disease, Crohn's disease vs other conditions, 84, 85

Index

celecoxib in prevention of cancer in familial adenomatous polyposis, 163
celiac axis, anatomy, 217, 218
celiac disease (celiac sprue; gluten enteropathy), 112
   diagnosis/investigations, 115–16, 123
   management, 124
   presentation, 121
cell-mediated immunity and ulcerative colitis, 54–5
central nervous system and irritable bowel syndrome, 246, 248–9
CHARGE syndrome, 3
chemoprevention, colorectal cancer, 139, 163–4
chemotherapy
   anal cancer, 281
   colon cancer
      adjuvant, 190–1
      advanced disease, 191–2
   rectal cancer, adjuvant, 192–3
childbirth *see* obstetric injuries
children
   abuse, irritable bowel syndrome in later life, 247
   celiac disease, presentation, 121
chlamydia, 279
cholangiopancreatography, endoscopic retrograde, chronic pancreatitis, 116
cholangitis, primary sclerosing
   in Crohn's disease, 104
   in ulcerative colitis, 66
      effect on colorectal cancer risk, 73
cholecystectomy, bowel cancer risk, 176
cholecystokinin receptor antagonist, irritable bowel syndrome, 249, 253
choledochal cysts, 10–11
choledochocele, 11
cholestyramine
   bile acid malabsorption, 119, 252
   irritable bowel syndrome with diarrhea, 252
chromosome instability, 168, 169
chymotrypsin, fecal, 119
cilansetron, irritable bowel syndrome, 249, 253
ciprofloxacin in Crohn's disease, 91
   side-effects, 88–9, 91
cisapride, chronic intestinal pseudo-obstruction, 204
cloaca, development of terminal portion, 15–17
Clostridium difficile, antibiotic-associated (and pseudomembranous colitis), 24–5, 63–4
   elderly, 26
   hospitalized patients, 26
   ulcerative colitis vs, 63–4
CMV infection, 63
coagulability, excessive *see* hypercoagulable states
cobalamin *see* vitamin B_{12}
cobblestoning, Crohn's disease, 81
colectomy (colonic resection)
   in colorectal cancer, 190
      surveillance following, 189
   diarrhea with, 45
   in diverticular hemorrhage, 133
   in familial adenomatous polyposis, 139
   in ulcerative colitis, with ileorectal anastomosis, 70, 71
   see also proctocolectomy
colipase, 113
colitis
   Crohn's, surgery, 101
   infectious *see* infections
   microscopic, 47
   pseudomembranous *see Clostridium difficile*
   ulcerative *see* ulcerative colitis
   see also pancolitis
colloid (mucinous) colorectal carcinomas, 178
colon
   adenomas, in familial adenomatous polyposis, 137
   cancer *see* cancer
   cell proliferation, abnormal, 165–6
   Crohn's disease vs other conditions affecting, 84, 85
   giant *see* megacolon
   motility *see* motility; motility disorders
   perforation *see* perforation
   resection *see* colectomy
   strictures in ulcerative colitis, 72
   transit *see* transit
colonoscopy
   Crohn's disease, 81, 82
   diarrhea
      acute, 25
      chronic, 41, 43
   hemorrhoids, 260
   screening and surveillance (for cancer), 186–7, 189
      in common familial colorectal cancer, 150
      in Cowden syndrome, 143
      in familial adenomatous polyposis, 139, 188–9
      guidelines for, 189
      in hereditary non-polyposis colorectal cancer, 148
      in juvenile polyposis, 142
      in Peutz–Jeghers syndrome, 141
      in ulcerative colitis, 74–5, 176
      virtual colonoscopy, 187
   ulcerative colitis, 60
      cancer surveillance, 74–5, 176
   see also sigmoidoscopy
colony stimulating factor therapy, Crohn's disease, 98
colorectal tumors
   benign, 159
   malignant *see* cancer
colostomy, diverticular disease, 132
computed tomography
   Crohn's disease, 83
   diverticulitis, 130
   malabsorption, 115
   mesenteric ischemia
      acute, 231
      chronic, 222–3
computed tomography colonography, colorectal cancer screening, 187
computerized tomography, in diarrhea (chronic), 41, 44
condylomata (warts), anal, 278
   dysplastic areas, 282
congenital malformations *see* developmental anomalies
consent for genetic testing (hereditary colorectal cancer predisposition), 152
constipation, 212–14
   causes, 206–7
   chronic functional, 212–14
   in irritable bowel syndrome, 214, 252
   treatment, 212–14, 252
continence, fecal, 259
   loss *see* incontinence
contractions, small bowel, 195–6
   assessment of contractile activity, 198–201
corticosteroids
   Crohn's disease, 89–91, 104, 105
      dependency, 85, 90
      newer preparations, 90
      steroid-sparing properties of infliximab, 96
   in diverticulitis etiology, 129
   side-effects, 88, 90–1
   ulcerative colitis, 68
cost, economic
   genetic testing for colorectal cancer predisposition, 153, 172
   irritable bowel syndrome, 246

Index

counselling, genetic, hereditary colorectal cancer, 152
Cowden syndrome, 142–3
COX-2 inhibitors in colorectal cancer prevention, 139, 163
CPT-11, advanced colorectal cancer, 191
Crohn's disease, 77–110
  activity assessment, 82
  clinical features, 79–82, 121
    extraintestinal, 101–4
    fistulas see subheading below
  colorectal cancer risk, 108, 175–6
  diagnosis, 82–4
  differential diagnosis, 84
  epidemiology, 55–6
  fistulas, 106–7, 267–8
    management, 85, 106–7, 107, 108, 267–8
    perianal, 107, 108, 267–8
    rectovaginal, 273
  laboratory tests see laboratory tests
  management, 84–101, 106–9, 125
    approaches, 104–6
    fistulas, 85, 106–7, 107, 108, 267–8
    of specific clinical problems and complications (other than fistulas), 106–9
  pathogenesis, 78–9
  pathology, 81–2
  in pregnancy, 108–9
  see also inflammatory bowel disease
Cronkhite–Canada syndrome, 144–5
crypts
  aberrant crypt foci, 164, 179–80
  in ulcerative colitis, 62
culture, in bacterial overgrowth, 48
cutaneous features see skin
cyclo-oxygenase-2 inhibitors in colorectal cancer prevention, 139, 163
cyclosporin A
  Crohn's disease, 94–5
  side-effects, 95
  ulcerative colitis, 69–70
cysts, choledochal, 10–11
cytokines
  in Crohn's disease
    in pathogenesis, 78
    therapeutic use, 09
  in ulcerative colitis
    in pathogenesis, 54
    therapeutic use, 70
cytolethal distending toxin *E. coli*, 27
cytomegalovirus infection, 63

DCC gene, 167
deaths/mortalities
  cancer (all sites), in US (2002), 160
  ulcerative colitis, 65
defecation, 206, 259
  anorectal manometry during, 210
defecography, 211
  rectal prolapse, 275
deleted in colon cancer gene (*DCC*), 167
dermatologic diseases see skin
desmoids in familial adenomatous polyposis, 137–8
development (normal), 1
  foregut, 2
    duodenum, 7
    esophagus, 2–3
    hepatobiliary, 9
    pancreas, 7–9
    stomach, 4–6
  hindgut, 15–17
  midgut, 12
developmental anomalies
  in Cowden syndrome, 142
  foregut
    duodenum, 7
    esophagus, 3–4
    hepatobiliary, 9–12
    pancreas, 9
    stomach, 6–7
  hindgut, 17–19
  midgut, 12–15
  pilonidal disease as, 268
dexoxyglutamide, irritable bowel syndrome, 249, 253
diarrhea, 21–51
  acute, 21–9
    chronic diarrhea vs, 32
    special situations, 26–7
  in AIDS, 123–4, 125
  chronic, 31–51
    classification, 33–4, 41
    difficult-to-diagnose, 44
    further evaluation, 41–4
    initial evaluation, 36–41
  definition, 21, 32
  epidemiology, 36–7
  functional (in motility disorders), 36, 50, 205, 214
  irritable bowel syndrome see subheading below
  iatrogenic, 45
  inflammatory (exudative/bloody) see inflammatory diarrhea
  irritable bowel syndrome with, 50, 205
    treatment, 248–9, 252
  management, 27–8, 214, 252
    algorithm, 23

osmotic see osmotic diarrhea
outbreak, 27, 50
pathophysiological mechanisms, 21–3, 32–3
secretory see secretory diarrhea
traveler's, 26, 28
in ulcerative colitis, 57–8
watery see watery diarrhea
diet
  in colorectal cancer
    as causative factor, 160–3
    as protective/preventive strategy, 73, 164–5, 166
  in diarrhea causation, 22, 34, 38
  in irritable bowel syndrome treatment, 251, 252
difluoromethylornithine, 164
digital rectal examination in fecal incontinence, 44–5, 214
digital subtraction arteriography, chronic mesenteric ischemia, 221–2
Dipentum® see olsalazine
diverticular disease/diverticulosis, 127–34
  epidemiology, 127–8
  etiology, 128–9
  pathology, 128
  surgical management, 131–3
  symptomatic, 129–31
diverticulitis
  acute, 129–30
  perforation, 132–3
  surgery, 131–2
diverticulum, Meckel's, 14–15
DNA
  colorectal cancer sample, content, prognostic value, 182–3
  fecal, mutation detection, 173, 187
DNA mismatch repair genes (in hereditary non-polyposis colorectal cancer), 146, 147, 169, 170, 175
  testing for, 151, 152, 153, 172, 173
DNA sequencing, mutation detection via, 151
doctor–patient relationship and irritable bowel syndrome, 251
Doppler studies, post-revascularization in acute mesenteric ischemia, 234
DPC4 (*SMAD4*), 142, 167–8, 175
drug-induced conditions (of GI tract)
  diarrhea, 46
    acute, 22
    chronic, 35, 45, 46
  diverticulitis, 129
  dysmotility in small bowel, 203
  mesenteric ischemia, 236

Index

drug therapy
  anal fissure, 263–4
  constipation, 212, 213
  Crohn's disease, 84–98, 267–8
    approaches, 104–6
    perianal fistulas, 267–8
    in pregnancy and breast-feeding, 109
  diarrhea, 27–8, 214
  irritable bowel syndrome, 206, 248–9, 251
  mesenteric ischemia (nonocclusive), 237
  pseudo-obstruction (chronic) in small bowel, 204
  ulcerative colitis, 66–70
    colorectal cancer risk and effects of, 73
    cutaneous side-effects, 65
    in pregnancy, 75
  see also chemoprevention *and specific (types of) drugs*
Dukes' classification, 180
  prognostic markers and, 183
"dumping syndrome", 205
duodenal cancer risk in familial adenomatous polyposis, 137
duodenal development, 7
  anomalies, 7
duodenal polyposis in familial adenomatous polyposis, 137
duodenoscopy, malabsorption, 115–16
duplex ultrasonography
  mesenteric ischemia
    acute, 231
    chronic, 223
  mesenteric venous thrombosis, 239
duplications
  gastric, 6
  intestinal, 15
dysplasia, anal, in condylomata, 282
dysplasia, colorectal
  aberrant crypt foci, 164, 179–80
  in inflammatory bowel disease, 74
  surveillance for, 189–90

economic cost *see* cost
elastase, fecal, 118
elastic-band ligation, hemorrhoids, 260–1
elderly
  acute diarrhea, 26
  malabsorption, 124
electrolytes
  mucosal transporter, congenital absence, 36
  stool, measurement in watery diarrhea, 40
electromyography, anal, 210–11

embolism, superior mesenteric artery, 230
  removal, 233
EMG, anal, 210–11
endocrine diarrhea, 33, 35, 36, 49–50
  diagnosis/differential diagnosis, 35, 41
  see also multiple endocrine neoplasia; neuroendocrine tumors
endoscopic retrograde cholangiopancreatography, chronic pancreatitis, 116
endoscopy
  Crohn's disease, 81, 82
  malabsorption, 115–16
  ulcerative colitis, 60
  see also anoscopy; colonoscopy; enteroscopy; laparoscopy; proctoscopy; proctosigmoidoscopy; sigmoidoscopy
endosonography, anal *see* ultrasonography, anal
enemas
  in constipation, 213
  in Crohn's disease, 5-ASA-containing drug, 87
  in ulcerative colitis, hydrocortisone, 68
  see also barium studies; enteroclysis
Entamoeba histolytica, 24
enteral nutrition
  chronic pseudo-obstruction (small bowel), 204
  Crohn's disease, 99–100, 125
enteroaggregative *E. coli*, 27
enteroclysis (small-bowel enema)
  Crohn's disease, 82–3
  malabsorption, 115
  transit studies, 196–7
enterocolitis in Hirschsprung's disease, 18
enterocutaneous fistulas, Crohn's disease, 107
enteroenteric fistulas, Crohn's disease, 107
enterohemorrhagic *E. coli*, 26
enteroinvasive *E. coli*, 27
enteropathogenic *E. coli*, 27
enteroscopy in chronic diarrhea, 41
Entocort®, Crohn's disease, 90
environmental risk factors
  Crohn's disease, 79
  ulcerative colitis, 56–7
epidermoid carcinoma, anal, 280–1
episcleritis, Crohn's disease, 103

erythema nodosum
  in Crohn's disease, 102–3
  in ulcerative colitis, 65
erythrocyte sedimentation rate
  Crohn's disease, 123
  ulcerative colitis, 58–9
Escherichia coli, 26–7
  enterohemorrhagic, 26
  non-hemorrhagic diarrheogenic, 27
  O157, 24
esophageal development, 2–3
  anomalies, 3–4
Etanercept, Crohn's disease, 97
Eudragit®, ulcerative colitis, 67
exomphalos (omphalocele), 12–13
extrasphincteric fistulas, 266, 267
exudative diarrhea *see* inflammatory diarrhea
eye involvement
  in Crohn's disease, 101, 103
  in familial adenomatous polyposis, 137
    examination for, 154
  in ulcerative colitis, 65

familial adenomatous polyposis *see* adenomatous polyposis, familial
familial colorectal cancer, common *see* cancer (colorectal)
familial primary intestinal pseudo-obstruction, 203
family history (of colorectal cancer), 188
  history-taking, 171
  incidence of colorectal cancer related to, 149
  risk of colorectal cancer based on, 149, 174, 188
fat (lipid)
  absorption, 113
  in colorectal cancer etiology, intake, 162
  fecal, estimation, 40–1, 117, 118, 123
  malabsorption, 113–14
    signs and symptoms, 120
    tests, 40–1, 117–18
fatty acids
  absorption, 113
  in colorectal cancer etiology, 161, 162
fatty diarrhea, chronic, 34, 36
  diagnosis and differential diagnosis, 34, 35, 36
  further evaluation, 44
feces *see* constipation; defecation; defecography; diarrhea; incontinence; stools

Index

fedotozine, irritable bowel syndrome, 253
fiber, dietary
  and colorectal cancer, 162, 164–5
  in constipation treatment, 213, 252
  and diverticular disease, 127–8, 128–9
  in irritable bowel syndrome treatment, 251, 252
fibrin glue, rectovaginal fistulas, 274
fissure in ano, 262–4
fistulas
  anorectal, 266–8
    clinical presentation and evaluation, 266
    etiology, 266
    treatment, 266–8
  anovaginal, 272–4
  Crohn's disease *see* Crohn's disease
  rectovaginal, 272–4
  tracheoesophageal, 3–4
fluid administration, diarrhea, 27
fluorouracil
  colon cancer
    adjuvant, 190–1
    advanced disease, 191–2
  rectal cancer, adjuvant, 193
folate/folic acid
  absorption, 115
  intake in colorectal cancer prevention, 73, 165
  malabsorption, 115
    signs and symptoms, 120
food-borne pathogens, 24
foregut development and anomalies *see* development; developmental anomalies

gadolinium-enhanced MR angiography, chronic mesenteric ischemia, 222, 223
gallbladder removal (cholecystectomy), bowel cancer risk, 176
Gardner's syndrome, colorectal cancer risk, 174–5
gastric cancer risk in familial adenomatous polyposis, 137
gastric development, 4–6
  anomalies, 6–7
gastric emptying, rapid, 205
gastric polyps/adenoma in familial adenomatous polyposis, 137
gastrinoma, 114
  see also Zollinger–Ellison syndrome
gastroschisis, 14
GDNF and Hirschsprung's disease, 18

genetic counselling, hereditary colorectal cancer, 152
genetic discrimination, hereditary colorectal cancer, 152–3
genetic testing (colorectal cancer predisposition), 136–7, 150–5, 171–3
  available tests, 150–1, 172–3
  common familial colorectal cancer, 149–50
  costs, 153, 172
  Cowden syndrome, 143
  familial adenomatous polyposis, 138, 151, 153, 153–4, 168, 172–3, 187–8
  hereditary non-polyposis colorectal cancer, 148, 151–2, 155, 156–7, 172, 173, 188
  indications and strategy, 153
  Peutz–Jeghers syndrome, 141
  see also mutation detection
genetics (genes and genetic factors)
  colorectal cancers, 166–73
    hereditary non-polyposis colorectal cancer, 146–7
    ulcerative colitis-associated, 73
  Crohn's disease, 78–9
  Hirschsprung's disease, 18, 211
  polyposis
    Cowden syndrome, 142–3
    familial adenomatous polyposis, 138
    Gorlin syndrome, 143
    juvenile polyposis, 142
    multiple endocrine neoplasia, 144
    neurofibromatosis type 1, 144
    Peutz–Jeghers syndrome, 141
  ulcerative colitis, 56
genitourinary manifestations, Crohn's disease, 101, 103–4
genomic instability, 168–9
  see also microsatellite instability
geographic distribution, inflammatory bowel disease, 55–6
glial cell line derived neurotrophic factor and Hirschsprung's disease, 18
gluten enteropathy *see* celiac disease
glyceryl trinitrate, anal fissure, 263–4
gonorrhea, 279
Gorlin syndrome, 143
graciloplasty, fecal incontinence, 272
grafts *see* transplantation
granulocyte colony stimulating factor therapy, Crohn's disease, 98

granulocyte–macrophage colony stimulating factor therapy, Crohn's disease, 98
granulomas, Crohn's disease, 81–2
growth hormone, Crohn's disease, 99

hamartomatous polyp syndromes, hereditary, 140–3, 175
harmonic scalpel®, hemorrhoids, 261
haustration, loss, 61
health insurance and hereditary colorectal cancer, 152–3
hematologic evaluation, mesenteric venous thrombosis, 240
hematologic manifestations
  Crohn's disease, 101, 103
  malabsorption, detection, 122
hemodialysis patients, nonocclusive mesenteric ischemia, 236
hemolytic *E. coli*, diarrhea-associated, 27
hemorrhage, GI *see* bleeding, rectal; blood, fecal
hemorrhoids, 259–62
  excision *see* surgery
  external, 262
  internal, 260–2
heparin
  mesenteric venous thrombosis, 240
  ulcerative colitis, 70
hepatic artery infusion of chemotherapy, liver metastases, 192
hepatic disease *see* liver
heredity *see* cancer; genetics; polyposis
hernia, umbilical, 14
herpes simplex virus infection, anorectal, 278
heterotopic tissue (mucosa)
  in esophagus, 4
  in stomach, 7
hidradenitis suppurativa, 269
Hinchey's grading system, diverticulitis, 132
hindgut development, 15–17
  anomalies, 17–19
Hirschsprung's disease (congenital megacolon), 17–19, 211
  genetic factors, 18, 211
histology
  colorectal cancer, 178–9
    prognostic value, 178–9, 182
  Crohn's disease, 81–2
  ulcerative colitis, 61–2
  see also biopsy
history-taking
  diarrhea (chronic), 36–8
  irritable bowel syndrome, 250

Index

HIV disease/AIDS
  anorectal disease, 279
  malabsorption, 123–4, 125
HLA (human leukocyte antigens)
  ankylosing spondylitis (and Crohn's disease) and, 102
  ulcerative colitis and, 56
HMG-CoA reductase inhibitors, colorectal cancer prevention, 164
homocholic acid taurine, Tc-99m-labelled selenium-75-, 119
homocystinemia, mesenteric arterial thrombosis, 230
hospital-acquired diarrhea, 26
HPV (human papilloma virus)
  anal cancer and, 278, 280, 282
  anal condylomata see condylomata
HSV (herpes simplex virus) infection, anorectal, 278
human immunodeficiency virus see HIV
human leukocyte antigens see HLA
human papilloma virus see HPV
hydrocortisone enemas, ulcerative colitis, 68
hydrogen breath test
  lactose, 116
  lactulose, small-bowel transit measurement, 197
hydrophilic agents, 213
7-a-hydroxy-4-cholesten-3-one measurement, 119
5-hydroxytryptamine see serotonergic agents; serotonin
hypercoagulable states
  mesenteric arterial thrombosis, 223
  mesenteric venous thrombosis, 238, 240
  tests for, 240
hyperhomocystinemia, mesenteric arterial thrombosis, 230
hyperosmolar agents, 213
hyperplastic polyposis, 144

iatrogenic diarrhea, 45
IBD genes, 79
ICAM–1 (intercellular adhesion molecule–1) inhibition, Crohn's disease, 98
ileal pouch–anal anastomosis
  anastomotic strictures, 277–8
  proctocolectomy with see proctocolectomy
ileal pouch–distal rectal anastomosis
  anastomotic strictures, 277–8
  colectomy with, in ulcerative colitis, 70, 71
ileococcygeus, 258

ileostomy diarrhea, 45
ileum
  bile acid malabsorption by see bile acids
  Crohn's disease vs other conditions affecting, 84, 85
ileus, acute, 204–5
iliac to superior mesenteric artery bypass, 225
imaging
  anorectal abscesses, 265
  anorectal fistulas, 266
  Crohn's disease, 80–1, 82–3
  diverticulitis, 130
  malabsorption, 115, 123
  mesenteric ischemia
    acute, 231
    chronic, 221–3
    nonocclusive, 237
  rectovaginal fistulas, 273
  small bowel motility/transit, 196–7, 197–8
  ulcerative colitis, 60–1
  see also specific modalities
immunocompromised patients, diarrhea (acute), 27
immunohistochemistry, hereditary non-polyposis colorectal cancer, 152
immunopathogenesis
  Crohn's disease, 78
  ulcerative colitis, 54–5
immunosuppression, chronic, anal cancer risk, 280
immunosuppressive drugs
  Crohn's disease, 91–6
  ulcerative colitis, 68–70
imperforate anus, 17
incontinence, fecal, 44–5, 214–15, 270–2
  clinical presentation, 271
  etiology, 271
  evaluation/diagnosis, 214, 271–2
    physical examination, 39, 44–5, 214, 271
  rectovaginal fistulas and, 273
  treatment, 214–15, 272
infarction, intestinal
  in acute mesenteric ischemia (due to venous thrombosis), 238
  in chronic mesenteric ischemia, 223–4
infections (GI tract - primarily bowel)
  Crohn's disease vs, 84
  diarrhea with, 22, 32–3
    in AIDS, 123–4, 125
    causative organisms, 22, 25
    chronic, 32–3
    diagnosis, 24–5

  exclusion, 41
  traveler's, 26, 28
  mesenteric venous thrombosis following, 238
  opportunistic, in AIDS, 123–4, 125, 279
  sexually-transmitted see sexually-transmitted diseases
  in ulcerative colitis etiology, 54
  ulcerative colitis vs, 63
inflammatory bowel disease
  anorectal strictures in, 274
  colorectal cancer in, 72–4, 175–6
    surveillance for, 189–90
  rectovaginal fistulas in, 274
  see also Crohn's disease; ulcerative colitis; ulcerative proctitis
inflammatory diarrhea (bloody/exudative diarrhea), 22, 36, 43–4
  acute, 22
  E. coli, 26
  chronic, 34, 36
    further evaluation, 43–4
  diagnosis and differential diagnosis, 34, 34–6, 36
inflammatory disorders (of bowel), diarrhea in, 33
inflammatory factors in irritable bowel syndrome, 247
inflammatory pseudopolyps/polyposis, 60, 145
inflammatory response, ulcerative colitis, 54
inflammatory veno-occlusive disease, mesenteric, 238
infliximab
  Crohn's disease, 96–7, 104, 106
    in pregnancy, 109
    side-effects, 89, 96–7
  ulcerative colitis, 70
informed consent for genetic testing (hereditary colorectal cancer predisposition), 152
inheritance see genetics
injection sclerotherapy, hemorrhoids, 261
injury see traumatic etiology
insurance (health) and hereditary colorectal cancer, 152–3
α-4-integrin inhibitor, Crohn's disease, 98
intercellular adhesion molecule-1 inhibition, Crohn's disease, 98
intersphincteric fistulas, 266, 267
intersphincteric space, 258
  abscesses, 264–5
  treatment, 266
intrinsic factor, 114
ion-transport defects, diarrhea, 33

Index

irinotecan, advanced colorectal cancer, 191
iron
  absorption, 114
  malabsorption and deficiency, 114–15
    laboratory findings, 120, 122
    signs and symptoms, 120
irritable bowel syndrome, 205, 243–55
  constipation, 214, 252
  definition, 243
  diagnosis, 249–50
    symptom-based criteria, 205, 243–5, 250
  diarrhea see diarrhea
  economic impact, 246
  epidemiology, 245–6
  pathophysiology, 246–9
    dysmotility, 205, 246
  prognosis, 254
  therapy, 251–4, 255
    drugs, 206, 248–9
    with mild symptoms, 251
    with moderate symptoms, 251
    with severe symptoms, 251
ischemia, intestinal see mesenteric ischemia
ischioanal space, 258
  abscesses, 264
  treatment, 265
ISIS-2302, Crohn's disease, 98
itching, perianal, 269

jejunostomy, venting, chronic intestinal pseudo-obstruction, 204
Jews
  common familial colorectal cancer in, 150
  ulcerative colitis in, 56
joint manifestations see arthropathy
juvenile polyposis, 141–2, 175

kappa opiate antagonist, irritable bowel syndrome, 253
kidney involvement, Crohn's disease, 103–4

laboratory tests/results
  Crohn's disease, 80, 83–4, 121, 123
    in activity assessment, 82
  diarrhea, 24–5, 25, 37, 39
  malabsorption, 120, 121, 122–3
  ulcerative colitis, 58–9
lactase, 112
  deficiency, 34, 49, 112
Lactobacillus GG therapy, Crohn's disease, 99

lactose intolerance, 34, 49, 112
  presentation, 121
  testing for, 116, 121
lactulose in hydrogen breath test, small-bowel transit measurement, 197
lamina propria in ulcerative colitis, 62
laparoscopy
  second-look, in acute mesenteric ischemia, 235
  therapeutic
    diverticulitis, 133
    mesenteric venous thrombosis, 240
    rectal prolapse, 275–6
laparotomy, second-look, revascularization for acute mesenteric ischemia, 234–5
large bowel
  motility see motility; motility disorders
  tumors see colorectal tumors
laxatives, 213
  abuse, 45–7
    diagnosing, 38, 42
lens cataract, Crohn's disease, 103
leukocytes in malabsorption, 122
levator ani, 258, 259
Lhermitte–Duclos syndrome, 142
linkage analysis, hereditary polyposis and colorectal cancer, 151
lipase, 113
lipid see fat
liver
  in Crohn's disease, involvement, 101, 104
  development, 9
    anomalies, 9–10
  metastases, treatment, 190, 191, 192
  methotrexate toxicity, 94
  in ulcerative colitis, involvement, 66
LKB1 (*STK11*), 141, 175
loperamide, irritable bowel syndrome with diarrhea, 252
lymph node involvement (metastases)
  anal cancer, 280–1
  colorectal cancer
    prognostic value, 182
    in TNM staging system, 181
lymphatic drainage, anorectum, 259
lymphatic vessels, small, involvement in colorectal cancer, prognostic value, 182
lymphogranuloma venereum, 279
lymphoma, intestinal, 145

lymphomatous polyposis, 145
Lynch syndrome see non-polyposis colorectal cancer, hereditary

M (distant metastases) in TNM staging system for colorectal cancer, 181
magnetic resonance angiography
  chronic mesenteric ischemia, 222
  mesenteric venous thrombosis, 239
magnetic resonance imaging
  Crohn's disease, 83
  malabsorption, 115
major histocompatibility antigens, human see HLA
malabsorption, 111–25
  definition and distinction from maldigestion, 111
  diarrhea due to, 35, 36
  management, 124–5
  mechanisms, 111–15
  patient evaluation for, 119–24
  presentation of common diseases causing, 121
  in special circumstances, 123–4
  tests for, 115–19
  see also specific malabsorbed substances
maldigestion, 111
  diarrhea due to, 35, 36
  distinction from malabsorption, 111
malignancy see cancer
malrotation, midgut, 14
Manning criteria, irritable bowel syndrome, 244
manometry
  anorectal, 45, 209–10
    in fecal incontinence, 45, 214, 271
  antroduoden(ojejun)al, 198–201
Meckel's diverticulum, 14–15
Mediterranean-type lymphoma, 145
medullary colorectal carcinomas, 178
megacolon
  acute, 211–12
  congenital see Hirschsprung's disease
  toxic, in ulcerative colitis, 71–2
melanoma, anal, 281
6-mercaptopurine
  Crohn's disease, 92–4, 104, 105, 106
    in pregnancy, 109
    side-effects, 89, 93
  in ulcerative colitis, 68–9
    in pregnancy, 75

293

Index

mesalamine (5-ASA)
  Crohn's disease, 85–6, 86, 87
  structure, 86
  ulcerative colitis, 66–7
    delayed-release, 67
mesenteric circulation, anatomy, 217, 218
mesenteric inflammatory veno-occlusive disease, 238
mesenteric ischemia, 217–37
  acute, 230–5
    diagnosis and imaging, 230–1
    pathophysiology, 230
    treatment, 231, 232–5
  chronic, 217
    causes/associated conditions, 217, 219
    imaging, 221–2
    pathophysiology, 217–19
    presentation and differential diagnosis, 220–1
    treatment, 223–8
  nonocclusive, 235–7
    diagnosis and imaging, 236–7
    outcome in, 237
    pathophysiology and presentation, 235–6
    treatment, 237
mesenteric venous thrombosis, 238–40
mesogastrium, dorsal and ventral, 4
mesorectal excision, rectal cancer, 192
metabolic bone disease and Crohn's disease, 102
metastases, distant
  anal cancer, treatment, 281
  colorectal cancer
    in TNM staging system for colorectal cancer, 181
    treatment, 190, 191, 191–2
metastases, lymph node *see* lymph node involvement
methotrexate
  Crohn's disease, 94, 106
  side-effects, 89, 94
  ulcerative colitis, 69
metronidazole
  Crohn's disease, 91
  side-effects, 88, 91
MHC, human *see* HLA
micelle formation, 113
  impaired, 114
microflora *see* bacterial flora
microsatellite instability, 168, 169
  in hereditary non-polyposis colorectal cancer, 147
    testing, 151–2, 155, 170, 171, 172, 173
microscopic colitis, 47

midgut development, 12
  anomalies, 12–15
Milligan–Morgan procedure, hemorrhoids, 261
mismatch repair genes *see* DNA mismatch repair genes
MLH1 mutations, 146, 147, 169, 170, 175
  testing for, 151, 152, 153, 172, 173
molecular markers for colorectal cancer, 182–3
monoclonal antibodies
  a-4-integrin, Crohn's disease, 98
  TNF *see* CDP571; infliximab
mortalities *see* deaths
motility (intestinal)
  anorectal, assessment, 45, 209–11
  drugs decreasing (and delaying transit), 201
    see also antimotility agents
  drugs increasing (and accelerating transit), 201
    see also prokinetic agents
  large bowel/colonic, 206
    diverticulosis and role of, 128
  serotonin and, 206, 248
  small intestine, 195, 195–6
    testing, 196–8
motility disorders, 195–215
  diarrhea in *see* diarrhea, functional
  in irritable bowel syndrome pathophysiology, 205, 246
  large bowel/colonic, 195, 211–15
    symptoms, 206–7
  small bowel, 195, 201–6
    evaluation, 203
    symptoms, 196
motor function
  colon, causes of dysfunction, 207
  small bowel, 195–6
    causes of dysfunction, 196
mouth *see* oral manifestations
MSH2 genes/mutations, 146, 147, 169, 170, 175
  testing, 151, 152, 155, 172, 173
MSH3 genes/mutations, 169
MSH6 genes/mutations, 169
mucin detection, colorectal cancer, 178
mucinous colorectal carcinomas, 178
mucosa
  anal canal, 258
  electrolyte transporter, congenital absence, 36
  heterotopic *see* heterotopic tissue
  surface area, diarrhea with reduction of, 33
  in ulcerative colitis, 60, 61, 62

Muir–Torre syndrome, 146, 175
Multidisciplinary Expert Panel, colorectal cancer
  screening guidelines, 184
  surveillance guidelines, 189
multiple endocrine neoplasia type 2, 144
  ret proto-oncogene and, 18, 144
Munchausen's syndrome, 47
Munchausen's syndrome by proxy, 47
muscle flap procedures, fecal incontinence, 272
musculoskeletal manifestations
  Crohn's disease, 101
  ulcerative colitis, 65–6
mutation detection methods (in hereditary polyposis and cancers), 151
  fecal DNA, 173, 187
  see also genetic testing; genetics *and specific genes*
mycophenolate mofetil
  Crohn's disease, 95
  side-effects, 95
myopathic causes of chronic intestinal pseudo-obstruction, 202–3

N (lymph node involvement) in TNM staging system for colorectal cancer, 181
near infrared reflectance analysis, fecal fat, 118
neoplasms *see* cancer; tumors
nerve supply, anorectum, 259
  in fecal incontinence etiology *see* neuropathic causes
  see also perineural invasion
neural polyposis syndromes, hereditary, 143–4
neuroendocrine tumors
  diarrhea due to, 33, 35, 36, 49–50
  fat malabsorption with, 114
neurofibromatosis type 1, 143–4
neurologic manifestations, malabsorption, 122
neuromuscular blockade, anal fissure, 264
neuropathic causes
  chronic intestinal pseudo-obstruction, 202–3
  fecal incontinence, 271
    testing for, 271
    treatment, 272
neutrophil cytoplasmic antibodies (pANCA)
  Crohn's disease, 83, 84
  ulcerative colitis, 55
NF1 gene, 144
nicotine, ulcerative colitis therapy, 70

nitrates, topical, anal fissure, 263–4
NOD2 gene and Crohn's disease, 79
non-polyposis colorectal cancer,
         hereditary (Lynch syndrome),
         145–9, 169–70, 175
    clinical features, 145–6
    diagnostic criteria, 146, 170
    genetics, 146–8, 169, 169–70
        genetic testing, 148, 151–2,
            155, 156–7, 172, 173, 188
    screening, 148, 188
    surveillance, 148
    treatment, 148–9
non-steroidal anti-inflammatory drugs
    in colorectal cancer and precancer
        prevention, 163–4, 166
    in familial adenomatous
        polyposis, 139, 163
    in diverticulitis etiology, 129
nosocomial (hospital-acquired)
    diarrhea, 26
nuclear factor kappa B and Crohn's
    disease, 79
nutritional therapy
    chronic pseudo-obstruction (small
        bowel), 204
    Crohn's disease, 99–100, 125
    ulcerative colitis, 66
    see also diet

obesity and diverticulitis, 129–30
obstetric injuries (incl. childbirth)
    fecal incontinence etiology, 271
    rectovaginal fistula etiology,
        271–2, 273
    see also pregnancy
obstruction
    bowel
        in colorectal cancer, prognostic
            value, 183
        Crohn's disease, 107
        mechanical obstruction in
            diverticular disease etiology,
            129
    duodenal, 7
    mesenteric vessels see embolism;
        mesenteric ischemia, acute;
        mesenteric ischemia, chronic;
        thrombosis
    urinary tract, Crohn's disease,
        103–4
    see also pseudo-obstruction;
        stenosis; strictures
octreotide
    chronic intestinal pseudo-
        obstruction, 204
    irritable bowel syndrome, 206
ocular manifestations see eye
    involvement
Ogilvie's syndrome, 211–12

oligonucleotide, antisense, Crohn's
    disease, 98
olsalazine (Dipentum®)
    Crohn's disease, 86, 87
    structure, 86
    ulcerative colitis, 67–8
omental bursa, formation, 5
omphalocele, 12–13
oncogenes see proto-oncogenes
ophthalmological manifestations see
    eye involvement
opiate antagonist, irritable bowel
    syndrome, 253
oral manifestations
    Crohn's disease, 102
    ulcerative colitis, 65
oral rehydration therapy, diarrhea, 27
organogenesis see development;
    developmental anomalies
osmotic diarrhea, 22, 34, 42
    acute, 22
    chronic, 34
        further evaluation, 42
    differential diagnosis, 34, 35
    secretory vs, 25, 34
osmotic gap, fecal, 40
osmotic laxatives, 213
osmotically active substances,
    ingestion of poorly absorbed,
    33, 34
osteomalacia
    Crohn's disease and, 102
    laboratory findings, 123
osteoporosis and Crohn's disease,
    102
oxaliplatin, advanced colorectal
    cancer, 192

p53 and colorectal cancer, 167, 168
Paget disease, perianal, 283–4
pain, abdominal (incl. colonic) see
    abdominal pain
pancolitis in ulcerative colitis, 64
pancreatic development, 7–9
    anomalies, 9
pancreatic duct development, 8
pancreatic exocrine insufficiency,
    44, 48–9, 112, 113
    tests for/diagnosis of, 44, 118–19,
        120, 123
pancreatic rests, 7
pancreatitis, chronic
    investigations, 123
        endoscopic retrograde
            cholangiopancreatography, 116
    management, 124–5
    presentation, 121
pancreolauryl test, 119
papaverine infusion, nonocclusive
    mesenteric ischemia, 237

parasite infections, diarrhea, 22, 25
parasympathetic nervous supply,
    anorectum, 259
parenchyma, liver, congenital
    abnormalities, 9–10
parenteral nutrition
    chronic pseudo-obstruction (small
        bowel), 204
    Crohn's disease, 100, 125
    ulcerative colitis, 66
pelvic floor muscles, anatomy and
    function, 258
Pentasa®
    Crohn's disease, 86, 87
    ulcerative colitis, 67
percutaneous revascularization
    acute mesenteric ischemia, 231
    chronic mesenteric ischemia, 228
perforation, colonic
    diverticulitis, 132–3
    iatrogenic (with colonoscope), 187
    in ulcerative colitis, 72
perianal region and anal margin
    cancer/precancer, 282–3
    Crohn's disease, 107–8, 268
        management, 85, 107–8, 268
    pruritus, 269–70
perianal space, 258
    abscesses, 264
        treatment, 265
perineal approaches, rectal prolapse
    surgery, 276
perineal Crohn's disease,
    management, 91
perineural invasion in colorectal
    cancer, prognostic value, 182
peritonitis with perforated
    diverticulum, 132
peroxisome proliferation-activated
    receptor (PPAR) agonist,
    Crohn's disease, 70
Peutz–Jeghers syndrome, 140–1, 175
pH, fecal, 40
physical abuse and irritable bowel
    syndrome, 247
physical examination
    anorectal complaints, 259
        fistulas (anorectal), 266
        fistulas (rectovaginal), 273
        hemorrhoids, 260
        prolapsed rectum, 275
    Crohn's disease, 80
    diarrhea
        acute, 24
        chronic, 37, 39
    diverticulitis, 130
    fecal incontinence, 39, 44–5, 214,
        271
    irritable bowel syndrome, 250
    malabsorption, 120–2

295

Index

physician–patient relationship and irritable bowel syndrome, 251
pilonidal disease, 268–9
plasmacytosis, lamina propria, 62
PMS1/PMS2 genes/mutations, 169, 170
Polle syndrome, 47
polyposis
  acquired, 144–5
    inflammatory polyposis (pseudopolyps), 60, 145
    hereditary, 136, 137–45, 175
      familial adenomatous polyposis *see* adenomatous polyposis; adenomatous polyposis coli
      hamartomatous polyposis, 140–3, 175
      juvenile polyposis, 141–2, 175
      neural polyposis, 143–4
  see also adenoma
portal vein infusion for adjuvant chemotherapy of liver metastases, 191
postanal space, 258
  abscesses, 264
  treatment, 266
PPAR agonist, Crohn's disease, 70
prednisone, ulcerative colitis, 68
pregnancy
  Crohn's disease, 108–9
  ulcerative colitis, 75
  see also obstetric injuries
pressure measurements *see* manometry
probiotics
  Crohn's disease, 99
  diarrhea, 28
procalopride, irritable bowel syndrome, 253
proctitis
  chlamydial, 279
  ulcerative, 57, 64
proctocolectomy with ileal pouch–anal anastomosis
  in familial adenomatous polyposis, 139
  in ulcerative colitis, 70–1
proctoscopy, hemorrhoids, 260
proctosigmoidoscopy, anorectal complaints, 259
prokinetic agents, 201
  chronic pseudo-obstruction (small bowel), 204
  constipation, 213
prolapse
  hemorrhoids, 260
  rectal *see* rectum
protein
  absorption, 112–13
  malabsorption, 113

signs and symptoms, 120
tests for, 118
protein immunohistochemistry, hereditary non-polyposis colorectal cancer, 152
protein-losing enteropathy, laboratory findings, 122
protein truncation test, 151
proto-oncogenes
  colorectal cancer and, 167
  Hirschsprung's disease and, 18
  multiple endocrine neoplasia type 2 and, 18, 144
pruritus ani, 269
pseudomembranous colitis *see Clostridium difficile*
pseudo-obstruction
  colonic, acute, 211–12
  small-bowel
    acute, 204–5
    chronic, 201–4
pseudopolyps, inflammatory, 60, 145
psychiatric comorbidity, irritable bowel syndrome, 247
psychological treatment, irritable bowel syndrome, 254
psychosocial factors in irritable bowel syndrome, 247
  diagnosis related to, 249
  treatment related to, 249, 254
PTC gene, 143
PTEN gene, 142–3, 175
pubococcygeus, 258
puborectalis, 257, 258
pudendal nerves, 259
  testing in fecal incontinence, 271
purine analogs
  Crohn's disease, 92–4, 104, 105, 106
  side-effects, 89, 93
  ulcerative colitis, 68–9
  in pregnancy, 75
pyloric stenosis, 6
pyoderma gangrenosum
  in Crohn's disease, 102–3
  in ulcerative colitis, 65

radiation-induced conditions
  anorectal strictures, 277
  diarrhea, 45
  rectovaginal fistulas, 273, 274
radiation treatment
  anal cancer, 281
  rectal cancer, adjuvant, 192–3
radiography
  Crohn's disease, 80–1, 82–3
  mesenteric venous thrombosis, 239
  ulcerative colitis, 60–1
  see also barium studies

radiology *see* imaging *and specific modalities*
radionuclide studies *see* scintigraphy
radiopaque markers, colonic transit studies, 208–9
radiotherapy *see* radiation treatment
ras and colorectal cancer, 167
rectopexy
  abscesses *see* abscesses
  circular stapler, hemorrhoids, 261–2
rectovaginal fistulas, 272–4
rectum
  anatomy, 257–9
  bleeding from *see* bleeding, rectal; blood, fecal
  cancer *see* cancer
  in Crohn's disease
    abscesses involving anus and, 107, 108, 267–8
    sparing, 80
  development, 17
  developmental anomalies, 17
  evacuation *see* defecation; defecography
  in fecal incontinence
    examination, 44–5, 214, 271
    prolapse in etiology, 271
  physiology, 259
  prolapse, 274–6
    evaluation, 275
    in fecal incontinence etiology, 271
    treatment, 275–6
  stenosis *see* stenosis
  see also anorectal function; anorectal region; ileal pouch–distal rectal anastomosis *and entries under* proct-
renal involvement, Crohn's disease, 103–4
RET (and ret)
  and Hirschsprung's disease, 18, 144
  and multiple endocrine neoplasia type 2, 144
retinal pigment epithelium, congenital hypertrophy, 137, 138
  examination for, 154
revascularization surgery
  acute mesenteric ischemia, 231, 233–4
  chronic mesenteric ischemia, 224–8
    outcome (patency rates), 229
    postoperative management and complications, 228–9
  vasospasm following, 236

Index

Rome criteria
  functional constipation, 212
  irritable bowel syndrome, 205, 244–5, 250
rosiglitazone, ulcerative colitis, 70
rubber-band ligation, hemorrhoids, 260–1

Saccharomyces cerevisiae antibodies (ASCA), Crohn's disease, 83, 84
sacral nerves and nerve roots (and the anorectum), 259
  in fecal incontinence, 271
    chronic stimulation, 272
sacroileitis, ulcerative colitis, 66
Schatzki ring, 4
Schilling test, 118
scintigraphy
  colonic transit, 209
  small-bowel transit, 197–8
sclerosing cholangiitis, primary *see* cholangitis
sclerotherapy, hemorrhoids, 261
screening (for anal cancer), 280
screening (for colorectal cancer), 183–8
  hereditary/familial conditions (high-risk groups), 183–4, 187–8
    common familial colorectal cancer, 150
    Cowden syndrome, 143
    familial adenomatous polyposis, 138–9, 187–8
    hereditary non-polyposis colorectal cancer, 148, 188
    juvenile polyposis, 142
    Peutz–Jeghers syndrome, 141
  techniques, 184–7
    new, 187
secretatogues causing diarrhea, 33
secretin test, 44, 119
secretory diarrhea, 22–3, 34–6, 41–2
  acute, 22–3
  chronic, 34, 34–6, 41–2
    further evaluation, 41–2
    idiopathic, 50
  differential diagnosis, 34–6
  osmotic vs, 25, 34
selenium, colorectal cancer prevention, 165
selenium-75-homocholic acid taurine, Tc-99m-labelled, 119
serologic tests
  Crohn's disease, 83–4
  malabsorption, 123
serotonergic agents, irritable bowel syndrome, 248–9, 252–3
serotonin (5-HT) in gut function, 248
  motility, 206, 248

sexual abuse and irritable bowel syndrome, 247
sexually-transmitted diseases of anus, 278–9
short bowel syndrome, 112, 125
short esophagus, congenital, 4
sigmoid diverticulosis, 128
sigmoidoscopy
  colorectal cancer screening, 185
    guidelines, 184, 185
  diarrhea
    acute, 25
    chronic, 41, 43
  fecal incontinence, 214
  ulcerative colitis, 59, 60
  see also proctosigmoidoscopy
signet-ring cell colorectal carcinoma, 178
  prognosis, 178–9, 182
sinus, pilonidal, 268–9
Sitzmark, colonic transit studies, 208–9
skin manifestations
  Crohn's disease, 101, 102–3
  malabsorption, 122
  ulcerative colitis, 65
  see also enterocutaneous fistulas; perianal region
"skip lesions", Crohn's disease, 81
SMAD4 (*DPC4*), 142, 167–8, 175
small bowel
  bacterial overgrowth *see* bacterial flora
  Crohn's disease
    diagnostic imaging, 82–3
    surgery, 100–1
  in malabsorption, investigations, 115–16
  motility *see* motility; motility disorders
  short (short bowel syndrome), 112, 125
  transit *see* transit
  transplantation in chronic intestinal pseudo-obstruction, 204
small-cell colorectal carcinomas, 178
  prognosis, 178–9, 182
smoking, ulcerative colitis reduced incidence, 56–7
Spiegelman classification, duodenal polyposis in familial adenomatous polyposis, 137
splenectomy, mesenteric venous thrombosis following, 238
spondylitis, ankylosing, Crohn's disease and, 102
squamous cell carcinoma
  anal canal, 280–1
  anal margin, 282

squamous cell carcinoma-in-situ, perianal, 282–3
staging
  anal cancer, 281
  colorectal cancer, 180–2
stapled hemorrhoidectomy, 261–2
statins (MG-CoA reductase inhibitors), colorectal cancer prevention, 164
steatocrit, acid, 117
steatorrhea
  diagnosis, 40, 117
  management, 124
stenosis
  anorectal
    acquired, 276–8
    congenital, 17
  esophageal, congenital, 4
  intestinal, 14
  pyloric, 6
  see also obstruction; strictures
stenting
  chronic mesenteric ischemia, 228
  ureteral, in diverticulitis, 133
steroids *see* corticosteroids
sterols in colorectal cancer causation, 161
stimulant laxatives, 213
STK11, 141, 175
stomach *see entries under* gastric
stools (feces)
  blood in *see* bleeding, rectal; blood
  in diarrhea
    examination/analysis, 24, 34, 39–41, 42
    weight defining diarrhea, 21
  DNA, mutation detection, 173, 187
  elastase measurement, 118
  in malabsorption, 123
    alpha–1-antitrypsin measurement, 118
    chymotrypsin measurement, 119
    fat measurement, 40–1, 117, 118, 123
  see also constipation; continence; defecation; defecography; diarrhea; incontinence
strictures
  anorectal, treatment, 276–8
  colonic
    in diverticular disease, 130, 133
    in ulcerative colitis, 72
  small bowel in Crohn's disease, 107
    management, 100–1, 107
  see also obstruction; stenosis
Sudan stain, 117

Index

sugar alcohols, excessive ingestion, 34
sulfasalazine (sulfapyridine and 5-ASA combination)
   Crohn's disease, 85–6, 87
   side-effects, 88, 88–9
   structure, 86
   ulcerative colitis, 66–7
sulindac in prevention of cancer in familial adenomatous polyposis, 163
suppositories
   constipation, 213
   Crohn's disease, 5-ASA-containing drug, 87
supralevator spaces, 258
   abscesses, 265
      treatment, 266
suprasphincteric fistulas, 266, 267
surgery
   anorectal, complications
      anorectal stenoses, 276
      fecal incontinence, 271
   anorectal complaints
      anal cancer, 281, 282, 283
      anal fissure, 263
      anorectal abscesses, 265–6
      fecal incontinence, 215, 272
      fistulas (anorectal), 266–7, 268
      fistulas (rectovaginal), 273–4
      hemorrhoids see subheading below
      pilonidal disease, 268–9
      rectal prolapse, 275–6
   colorectal cancer, 190
      advanced/metastatic disease, 190
      colon cancer, 190
      hereditary non-polyposis, 148–9
      rectal cancer, 192
      surveillance following, 189
   constipation (intractable), 213
   Crohn's disease, 100–1
      abscesses and fistulas, 106–7
   diarrhea due to, 45
   diverticular disease, 131–3
   familial adenomatous polyposis, 139
   hemorrhoids, 261–2, 262
      complications, 261, 262, 273
   mesenteric ischemia, acute, 231, 232–5
      postoperative care, 235
      re-operation, 234–5
   mesenteric ischemia, chronic, 224–8
      postoperative management and complications, 228–9
   mesenteric venous thrombosis, 240
   pseudo-obstruction (chronic intestinal), 204
   stenoses and stricture, 276–8

ulcerative colitis, 70–1
surveillance (for cancer), 188–90
   common familial colorectal cancer, 150
   Cowden syndrome, 143
   Crohn's disease, 176
   familial adenomatous polyposis, 138–9, 188–9
   hereditary non-polyposis colorectal cancer, 148
   juvenile polyposis, 142
   Peutz–Jeghers syndrome, 141
   ulcerative colitis, 74–5, 176
sympathetic nervous supply, anorectum, 259
syphilis, 278–9
systemic disorders
   chronic intestinal pseudo-obstruction in, 202–3
   in ulcerative colitis, 58

T cells
   Crohn's disease, 78
   ulcerative colitis, 54
tacrolismus
   Crohn's disease, 95–6
   side-effects, 96
   ulcerative colitis, 70
taurine analog ingestion, 119
technetium-99m-labelled selenium-75-homocholic acid taurine, 119
tegafur + uracil, advanced colorectal cancer, 191
tegaserod
   chronic intestinal pseudo-obstruction, 204
   irritable bowel syndrome, 249, 253
tenesmus, ulcerative colitis, 58
TGF-ß receptor type II gene and hereditary non-polyposis colorectal cancer, 147, 169
thalidomide, Crohn's disease, 97–8
thiopurine methyltransferase, 92
   gene polymorphisms, 93–4
thrombosis
   mesenteric artery, 230
   mesenteric venous, 238–40
TNF-a-blocking agents see tumor necrosis factor-a-blocking agents
TNM staging system, 181–2
a-tocopherol intake in colon cancer prevention, 165
topical agents
   5-ASA-containing compounds in Crohn's disease, 87
   nitrates in anal fissure, 263–4
Torre's (Muir–Torre) syndrome, 146, 175

toxic megacolon in ulcerative colitis, 71–2
tracheoesophageal fistula, 3–4
transforming growth factor-ß receptor type II gene and hereditary non-polyposis colorectal cancer, 147, 169
transit
   colonic, drugs reducing, 214
   colonic, evaluation, 207–9
   in chronic functional constipation, 212
   small bowel
      drugs accelerating, 201
      drugs delaying, 201
      measurement, 196–8
      rapid, 205–6
transplantation/grafting
   blood vessels see bypass grafting
   small-bowel, in chronic intestinal pseudo-obstruction, 204
transsphincteric fistulas, 266, 267
traumatic etiology
   fecal incontinence, 271
   rectovaginal fistula, 272–3, 273
traveler's diarrhea, 26, 28
tricyclic antidepressants, irritable bowel syndrome, 252
triolein breath tests, C–14, 117–18
Truelove and Witts classification of ulcerative colitis, 59
tumor(s)
   anal, 279–83
   Crohn's disease vs, 84
   malignant see cancer
   neuroendocrine see neuroendocrine tumors
tumor markers, prognostic value, 183
tumor necrosis factor-a-blocking agents
   Crohn's disease, 96–8
   ulcerative colitis, 70
tumor suppressor genes and colorectal cancer, 167–8
Turcot's syndrome, 146, 175

UFT (uracil + tegafur), advanced colorectal cancer, 191
ulceration
   anal, AIDS-related, 279
   in Crohn's disease, 80, 81
ulcerative colitis, 53–76
   clinical features/manifestations, 57–9
      extraintestinal, 65–6
   complications, 71–5
      colorectal cancer, 72–4, 175–6
   diagnosis, 59–62

differential diagnosis, 63–4
   Crohn's disease, 84
distribution and natural history, 64–5
epidemiology, 55–6
pathophysiology and etiology, 54–5
in pregnancy, 75
severity, assessment, 59
treatment, 66–71
   colorectal cancer risk and effects of, 73
   drug see drug therapy
   general approach, 66
see also inflammatory bowel disease
ulcerative proctitis, 57, 64
ultrasonography
   anal, 211
     in fecal incontinence, 214
   diverticulitis, 130
   see also Doppler studies; duplex ultrasonography
umbilical hernia, 14
uracil + tegafur, advanced colorectal cancer, 191
ureteral stenting, diverticulitis, 133
urogenital manifestations, Crohn's disease, 101, 103–4
US Preventative Services Task Force, colorectal cancer screening guidelines, 184
uveitis, Crohn's disease, 103

VACTERL syndrome, 3
vagina, fistula between anorectum and, 272–4
vascular disorders (bowel), 217–41
vascular supply, anorectum, 258–9
vasoactive drugs, mesenteric ischemia caused by, 236
vasoactive peptide hormone (VIP)-secreting tumor, 49
vasoconstriction, mesenteric, 235–6
vasospasm (mesenteric arteries)
   after revascularization, 236
   reversal, 237
VATER syndrome/complex, 3
Vater's ampulla, familial adenomatous polyposis involving, 137
venography, magnetic resonance, mesenteric venous thrombosis, 239
veno-occlusive disease, mesenteric inflammatory, 238
venous drainage, anorectum, 258–9
venous thrombosis, mesenteric, 238–40
viability, intestinal, assessment after revascularization in acute mesenteric ischemia, 234
Vienna classification, Crohn's disease, 80
VIPoma, 49
viral infections, diarrhea, 22, 25
virtual colonoscopy, colorectal cancer screening, 187
visceral hypersensitivity and irritable bowel syndrome, 246
vitamin(s), supplementation in ulcerative colitis and effects on colorectal cancer risk, 73

vitamin B_{12}
   absorption, 114
   malabsorption and deficiency, 114, 120
     diagnosing cause, 118
     laboratory findings, 120, 122
     signs and symptoms, 120
vitamin C intake in colon cancer prevention, 165
vitamin D
   intake in colon cancer prevention, 162–3
   malabsorption/deficiency, signs and symptoms, 120
vitamin E intake in colon cancer prevention, 165
vitamin K malabsorption/deficiency, signs and symptoms, 120
volume expansion, diarrhea, 27
volvulus, gastric, 6–7
von Recklinghausen's disease, 143–4

warts see condylomata
water transport, diarrhea and, 32
watery diarrhea, 34–6
   chronic, 34, 34–6
   differential diagnosis, 34–6
   E. coli, 27
Whipple's disease, presentation, 121
white cells in malabsorption, 122

X-ray radiography see radiography
D-xylose breath test, 117
D-xylose test, 116–17

Zollinger–Ellison syndrome, 114, 119–20
   presentation, 121